Intelligent Quality of Service Technologies and Network Management:
Models for Enhancing Communication

Pattarasinee Bhattarakosol
Chulalongkorn University, Thailand

INFORMATION SCIENCE REFERENCE
Hershey · New York

Director of Editorial Content:	Kristin Klinger
Director of Book Publications:	Julia Mosemann
Acquisitions Editor:	Lindsay Johnston
Development Editor:	Christine Bufton
Publishing Assistant:	Sean Woznicki
Typesetter:	Myla Harty
Production Editor:	Jamie Snavely
Cover Design:	Lisa Tosheff
Printed at:	Yurchak Printing Inc.

Published in the United States of America by
Information Science Reference (an imprint of IGI Global)
701 E. Chocolate Avenue
Hershey PA 17033
Tel: 717-533-8845
Fax: 717-533-8661
E-mail: cust@igi-global.com
Web site: http://www.igi-global.com/reference

Library of Congress Cataloging-in-Publication Data

Intelligent quality of service technologies and network management : models for enhancing communication / Pattarasinee Bhattarakosol, editor.
p. cm.

Includes bibliographical references and index.
Summary: "This book "quality of service" in organizations, offering fundamental knowledge on the subject, describing the significance of network management and the integration of knowledge to demonstrate how network management is related to QoS in real applications"--Provided by publisher.

ISBN 978-1-61520-791-6 (hbk.) -- ISBN 978-1-61520-792-3 (ebook) 1. Network performance (Telecommunication) 2. Computer networks--Quality control. I. Bhattarakosol, Pattarasinee.
TK5105.5956.I58 2010
004.6--dc22

2009040563

British Cataloguing in Publication Data
A Cataloguing in Publication record for this book is available from the British Library.

List of Reviewers

Chairat Phongphanphanee, *Chulalongkorn University, Thailand*
Pattarasinee Bhattarakosol, *Chulalongkorn University, Thailand*
Ohm Sornil, *National Institute of Development Administration, Thailand*
Pramote Kuacharoen, *National Institute of Development Administration, Thailand*
Luck Charoenwatana, *Ubon Ratchathani University, Thailand*
Morris Chang, *Iowa State University, USA*
Jennifer Rexford, *Princeton University, USA*
Sunyoung Han, *Konkuk University, Korea*
Jongwon Choe, *Sookmyung Women's University, Korea*
Yongtae Shin, *Soongsil University, Korea*
Hyunseung Choo, *Sungkyunkwan University, Korea*

Table of Contents

Section 3
Integrations of Quality of Service and Network Management Model

Detailed Table of Contents

The advent and rise of broadband technologies and new applications and services have led to a complex heterogeneous scenario in which providing Quality of Service (QoS) has become a compelling issue. Furthermore, the competitive condition of the telecommunications environment has caused user's perception of quality to become one of the most differential factors for service providers. Due to this fact, QoS must not only attend to specific technical metrics, but more important, QoS criteria should be defined to assure the level of quality to fulfill the users' requirements. In this new context, the definition of effective user-oriented QoS management models and frameworks has become a matter of contention. This chapter aims to provide readers a comprehensive analysis of the entire significance of a user-centered approach for quality of service management. For this purpose, a review of the most important issues related to the subject is provided.

During the last years Internet evolution demanded for new and richer applications. To fulfill the novel and more complex application requirements, new solutions in many domains were required. One of these domains is the network support, assuring, into some extend, a specific or predictable treatment to traffic; therefore, in this chapter, we present a broad view of the main efforts available on the literature in order to provide Quality of Service (QoS) in both wired networks and wireless sensor networks (WSNs). For this purpose, the authors present: (1) the more relevant QoS architectures and technologies along with some of its recent improvements; (2) the different perspectives that combine some of those architectures and technologies into more complex solutions, in order to achieve stronger QoS and/or performance; (3) the most relevant QoS issues in WSNs environments; and (4) through the comparison of the several solutions, the authors list the advantages and limitations and reveal some relations among the existing QoS solutions.

Currently the Internet offers a point-to-point delivery service, which is based on the "best effort" delivery model. In this model, data will be delivered to its destination as soon as possible, but with no commitment about bandwidth or latency. Using protocols such as the Transmission Control Protocol (TCP), the highest guarantee the network provides is reliable data delivery. This is adequate for traditional data applications like e-mail, web browsing, File Transfer Protocol (FTP) and Telnet, but inadequate for applications requiring timeliness. For example, multimedia conferencing or audio and video streaming applications, which require high bandwidth capacity and are sensitive to delay and delay variation. For these applications to perform adequately, Quality of Services (QoS) must be quantified and managed, and the Internet must be modified to support real-time QoS and controlled end-to-end delays. The efforts to enable end-to-end QoS over the Internet Protocol version 4 (IPv4) networks have led to the development of two different architectures, the Integrated services architecture (Intserv) and the Differentiated services architecture (Diffserv), which although different, support services that go beyond the best effort service. This chapter will present a detailed discussion on these IPv4 quality of services models. First, the Integrated services architecture with its related issues such as the reservation setup protocol will be demonstrated. Second, the Differentiated services architecture with a description of the services they provide will be described. Finally, a comparison between the Best-effort, the Integrated and Differentiated services will be done.

Wireless Sensor Networks (WSNs) have been envisioned as a new and effective means for creating and deploying previously unimaginable applications. These networks generally have the capabilities of observing the physical phenomena, communication, data processing and dissemination. Limited resources of sensor nodes like energy, bandwidth and processing abilities, make these networks excellent

Section 2
Network Management Model

The present day Internet traffic largely caters for the multimedia traffic throwing open new and unthinkable applications such as tele-surgery. The complexity of data transactions increases with a demand for in time and real time data transfers, demanding the limited resources of the network beyond their capabilities. It requires a prioritization of data transfers, controlled dumping of data over the network etc. To make the matter worse, the data from different origin combine together imparting long lasting detrimental features such as self similarity and long range dependency in to the traffic. The multimedia data fortunately is associated with redundancies that may be removed through efficient compression techniques. There exists a provision to control the compression or bitrates based on the availability of resources in the network. The traffic controller or shaper has to optimize the quality of the transferred multimedia data depending up on the state of the network. In this chapter, a novel traffic shaper is introduced considering the adverse properties of the network and counteract with the same.

This chapter presents a multiple constraint optimization algorithm called routing decision system (RDS) that uses the concept of preference functions to address the problem of selecting paths in core networks that satisfy traffic-oriented QoS requirements while simultaneously satisfying network resource-oriented performance goals. The original contribution lies in the use of strong scales employed for constructing a multiple criteria preference function in an affine space. The use of preference functions makes it possible for paths that match both traffic-oriented and resource-oriented goals to be selected by the algorithm. The RDS algorithm is used in conjunction with a heuristic path finding algorithm called Constraint Path Heuristic (CP-H) algorithm which is a novel approach to finding a set of constraint paths between source and destination nodes in a network. The CP-H algorithm finds multiple paths for each metric and then passes all the paths to the RDS algorithm. Simulation results showed that the CP-H/RDS algorithm has a success rate of between 93 and 96% when used in Waxman graph topologies, and is shown to be significantly better than other heuristic based algorithms under strict constraints. In addition, it is shown that the associated execution time of the CP-H/RDS algorithm is slightly higher than other heuristic based algorithms but good enough for use in an online traffic engineering (TE) application. Simulations to assess the performance of CP-H/RDS algorithm in a TE environment show that the algorithms has lower call block rates than other TE algorithms. It is also shown that the CP-H/RDS has a 96% probability of providing at least two distinct feasible backup paths in addition to the main QoS path. A framework for implementing the CP-H/RDS as a routing server is proposed. The routing decision system server (RDSS) framework is novel in that the complexity introduced by QoS awareness remains outside the network.

The Internet relies on the cooperation of competitive network operators that typically administrate their networks unilaterally and autonomously to interconnect people and companies in different locations. Recent work calls for extending this organizational model with augmented interactions between network operators, to provide a higher level of endtoend quality of service and to ease certain aspects of traffic management in backbone networks. This chapter presents the emerging collaborative network management models as well as related technologies. In particular, it describes recent techniques for interdomain traffic engineering and for qualityofservice aware routing. The detailed methods are of great interest for network operators and permit the development of new types of commercial relationships between them, ranging from simple interconnection agreements to collaborative traffic management and automated provisioning.

In this chapter, the authors examine two important network traffic issues: estimation of effective bandwidth and data loss probability in communication networks. They focus on estimation approaches based on network traffic modeling. Initially, the authors review some concepts related to network traffic modeling such as monofractal and multifractal properties. Further, the authors address the issue of estimating the effective bandwidth for network traffic flows. Besides effective bandwidth, the knowledge of the loss probability explicitly allows us to guarantee some QoS parameters required by the traffic flows, for example, by discarding flows with intolerable byte loss rate. In this sense, they present an overview of loss probability estimation methods including an approach that considers multifractal characteristics of network traffic. That is, given the model parameters, the data loss probability for network traffic can be directly computed. The authors conclude that both the multifractal based effective bandwidth and loss probability estimation methods can be powerful tools for really providing QoS to network flows.

activities including perception of dynamic conditions in the environment, reasoning for interpretation of the perceptions, solve problems, draw inferences and determine actions.

The Internet is an interconnection of multiple networks called domains. Inter-domain routing is ensured by BGP which preserves each domain's independence and announces routes arbitrarily chosen by domains. BGP messages carry no information concerning quality parameters of announced routes. Our goal is to provide domains with information regarding the congestion state of other domains without any changes in BGP. A domain, which is aware of heavily congested domains, can choose a bypass instead of a route exhibiting possible problems with QoS satisfaction. The authors propose a mechanism which sends alert messages in order to notify domains about the congestion state of other domains. The major difficulty consists in avoiding flooding the Internet with signaling messages. Their solution limits the number of alerts by taking advantage of the hierarchical structure of the Internet set by P2C and P2P relationships. Their algorithm is distributed and heuristic because it is a solution to an NP-complete and inapproximable problem. They prove these properties by reducing the Steiner problem in directed acyclic graphs to our problem of alert diffusion. The simulations show that our mechanism significantly diminishes the number of unavailable domains and routes compared to those obtained with BGP routing and with a theoretical centralized mechanism.

Network multimedia applications constitute a large part of Internet traffic and guaranteed delivery of such traffic is a challenge because of their sensitivity to delay, packet loss and higher bandwidth requirement. The need for guaranteed traffic delivery is exacerbated by the increasing delay experienced by traffic propagating through more than one QoS domain. Hence, there is a need for a flexible and a scalable QoS manager that handles and manages the needs of traffic flows throughout multiple IPv6 domains. The IPv6 QoS manager, presented in this paper, uses a combination of the packets' flow ID and the source address (Domain Global Identifier (DGI)), to process and reserve resources inside an IPv6 domain. To ensure inter-domain QoS management, the QoS domain manager should also communicate with other QoS domains' managers to ensure that traffic flows are guaranteed delivery. In this scheme, the IPv6 QoS manager handles QoS requests by either processing them locally if the intended destination is located locally or forwards the request to the neighboring domain's QoS manager. End-to-end QoS is achieved with an integrated admission and management unit. The feasibility of the proposed QoS management scheme is illustrated for both intra- and inter-domain QoS management. The scalability of the QoS management scheme for inter-domain scenarios is illustrated with simulations for traffic flows propagating through two and three domains. Excellent average end-to-end delay results have been achieved when traffic flow propagates through more than one domain. Simulations show that packets belonging to non-conformant flows experience increased delay, and such packets are degraded to lower priority if they exceed their negotiated traffic flow rates. Many pricing schemes have been proposed for QoS-enabled networks. However, integrated pricing and admission control has not been studied in detail. A dynamic pricing model is integrated with the IPv6 QoS manager to study the effects of increasing traffic flows rates on the increased cost of delivering high priority traffic flows. The pricing agent assigns prices dynamically for each traffic flow accepted by the domain manager. Combining the pricing strategy with the QoS manager allows only higher priority traffic packets that are willing to pay more to be processed during congestion. This approach is flexible and scalable as end-to-end pricing is decoupled from packet forwarding and resource reservation decisions. Simulations show that additional revenue is generated as prices change dynamically according to the network congestion status.

In this chapter, the authors present some of the latest developments related to the provisioning of Quality of Service (QoS) in today's networks and the associated network management structures that are or will be deployed to support them. They first give a brief overview of the most important Quality of Service proposals in the areas of Layer 2 (L2) and Layer 3 (L3) QoS provisioning in backbone networks, and we discuss the network management structures and brokers that have been proposed in order to implement these services. As a case study, they describe the pan-european research and academic network, which is supported centrally by GEANT and which encompasses multiple independent NRENs (National Research and Education Networks). In the last few years, GEANT has developed and deployed a number of production and pilot services meant for the delivery of quality network services to the end users across Europe.

Every community in the world expects to have a high value of life. Therefore, budgets are pooling to the local healthcare unit to increase healthcare and medical services to their citizen. One common implementation in the healthcare system is a healthcare network, where all necessary information are transferred to safe patients' lives. Various developments in medical equipments integrate communication circuit to enhance ability to transmit data direct from patients to medical staffs so that their lives can be safe in time. Since the implementation of wireless network is widely spread, this paper proposes

Foreword

This book edited by Prof. Pattarasinee Bhattarakosol, "Intelligent Quality of Service Technologies and Network Management: Models for Enhancing Communication", is an excellent reference for QoS administrators, developers, graduate students, research workers, or anyone who needs to understand QoS technology and network management. This book is comprehensive in its coverage of QoS technologies and network management, providing enough theories, models and practical examples in each chapter.

Each chapter in this book is independent of each other. Nevertheless, there is a common theme through all chapters. QoS and network management are the link that holds all chapters. Also, this book deals with various QoS subjects very thoroughly and considers many aspects even though it discusses QoS technologies and network management at large.

This book covers a diversity of QoS research fields, environment and systems. Especially, as a case study, research and academic networks, which are supported by GEANT and which encompasses multiple independent NRENs(National Research and Education Networks) and other international and national R&D networks, are a distinguished example.

The effective bandwidth management and data loss probability allow us to guarantee the QoS parameters required by the traffic flows. This book includes estimation concepts and approaches based on network traffic modeling.

The network of today requires a flexible and a scalable QoS management mechanism in order to handle traffic flows throughout multiple domains, like IPv6 domain, mobile domain and private domain. The manager in charge of QoS management communicates with other domains managers to ensure that traffic flows are guaranteed. This book introduces the mechanism of QoS manager to process and reserve QoS inside a domain.

The optimization of network carrier and traffic flow using routing decision system presented in this book enables dynamic admission control to admit user flows into the network. Also, it creates a management environment in which it is easy to deploy network policies that benefit both network carrier and user traffic flows.

In addition, this book involves principal QoS issues with relation to heterogeneous networks, pricing scheme, various routing methods, traffic modeling, QoS case studies, intra/inter domain management, and so forth. Also, although a reader is not a well-informed person, they can get the point because this book describes primary issues clearly and concisely.

To sum up, "Intelligent Quality of Service Technologies and Network Management: Models for Enhancing Communication" will put the reader inside QoS technologies and network management using diverse ideas and approaches in each high quality chapter. Experts who have interests in QoS and Network Management will find this book very helpful.

Sunyoung Han
June 2009
Seoul, Korea

Sunyoung Han *is the Dean and Professor at College of Information & Telecommunications, Konkuk University, Hwayangdong Kwangjinku, Seoul, Korea. He is a specialist in the area of computer network and has many publications related to Internet, Mobile IP, Multicasting, Wireless/Mobile Networks, Future Internet, Distributed Systems, including Web Services.*

Preface

WHY NETWORK IS IMPORTANT?

People use data in various reasons; some use data to evaluate their performance, while some use data to create value of human's lives. Although there are various objectives of using data, the most important problem is "how people gain access to the right data in the right time?" because data are distributed in different form and places.

The above problem leads to the invention and installation of data communication and networking system in the previous age. These systems are installed to support data exchange process and remote access to serve human's activities. Moreover, in order to serve people with the requested data in the suitable time interval, the communication system classifies applications over the network in two different categories: real time applications, and non-real time applications. These classifications help manipulating the condition of time to deliver the data packets. The real time applications refer to applications that the delay from data transfer situation can damage the waiting process; the non-real time applications refer to the application that the delay from data transfer situation has no affect to the waiting process. The example of the real time applications is the money-transfer application that allows a bank customer to transfer his money between banking accounts; this case cannot allow having delay because the financial situation of the customer will be unsecured. The example of the non-real time application is the e-mail application; this case the delay of the message will not have any affect to any process of the receiver.

PROBLEMS OVER NETWORK TECHNOLOGY

The results from the implementing network technologies lead to the growth rate of data communication among organizations, and accommodations. However, there are some errors, or defects during the communication process, such as data packet lost, high delay, high error rate, etc. These errors or defects can cause critical damages to organization or human's lives. For example, if there are missing packets of security warning system while an intrusion occurs, then the system inspector will not receive any warning signals and the system will not be protected. In some situation, a long delay of packets also initiates severe lost such as life. For example, the message from a fire alarm system tc a fire station must not have a long delay because the lost from the fire can be lives or valuable assets.

Why & What Quality of Service (QoS)?

According to problems mentions above, all services over network must be fixed and guaranteed in order to prevent all lost and damages. Therefore, it is the obligation of network providers to provide reliable and available networks for their customers. So, the network providers must find mechanisms to protect and detect all defects and errors that might occur during their services in order to maintain their quality of services (QoS) or services capabilities.

When considering about the quality of services of a network, it usually related to the users' appreciation rather than the measurement metrics. However, the quality of services usually refers to the ability to manage all kinds of packets over the network based on the payload of those packets. Moreover, these abilities include the efficiency to which packets are classified by network providers towards their customers and service level agreements (SLAs). Thus, each customer and their applications and devices will be differentiated according to their requirements.

Factors and Indicators of QoS

Currently, QoS is a significant issue for all network providers. The fundamental concept about QoS measurement is based on the traffic over the network. Nevertheless, this traffic condition is relied on various factors, such as network's queuing mechanism, network's load balancing mechanism, process time at destination, etc. Consequently, different indicators are used to determine the level of QoS.

Generally, QoS metric is measured in a certain period of time. These measurement values will be stored in the management information based, or log file of each network. Network administrator is responsible to analyze these values to indicate the QoS of the network over the measurement time, including making a plan for further growth of the network. Thus, it is the truth that the successes or failures of QoS are the main responsibility of the network administrator. Consequently, the network administrators are responsible for a qualified network management policy.

Network Management & QoS

The network management means a control mechanism to maintain the network so that it can continuously grant services to customers as needed with trust, available and reliable. Even though network management is important as described in their definition, it is usually applied to a large scale network with high complexity, and a large number of connecting nodes over the network.

When a network is in a proper managed, all traffics flow and reach to destinations as requested in time; otherwise, the data packets flood over the network and may be cascaded during the transmission time because of a long delay. Without a good management policy, the transmission condition over a network cannot be guaranteed the arrival time of the delivered packets; some might be lost and some might have a long delay time. Unfortunately, these lost and long delay times can bring damages to the organization. Thus, a consequence of a good network management is a reliable and available network with high performance, high throughput, and low delay. These results indicate the quality of services of the network as defined above.

Based on the organizational profiles, different organizations implement different network model under diverse network requirement. So, the quality of services and their levels over networks based on network requirements are dissimilar. Furthermore, the diversity of QoS maps to miscellaneous network management policies.

THEMES OF THE BOOK

The book consists of three main sections, starting from giving fundamental knowledge on the subject of QoS. Then, the second section describes significant of network management before the last section is the integration of knowledge to show how the network management is related to QoS in real applications.

Section 1: Quality of Services

The objective of this section is to give a clear picture of the word "Quality of Service". Thus, this section will start with the chapter of *Eva et al.* who have elaborated all contexts relevant to QoS in network and telecommunication. This chapter includes the evaluation and measurement metrics that are usually applied to maintain QoS over the communication system. Then, in the second chapter written by *Marques et al.* describes the broad concept of improving QoS over wired and wireless sensor network (WSN). This article presents from the fundamental mechanism up to the complicate mechanisms that are obtained from combining of several architectures and technologies. After reading this chapter, readers will have various solutions for supporting end-to-end QoS on heterogeneous networks. Afterwards, the dept literature reviews of the IP QoS model and the comparisons among the best-effort services, the Integrated and Differentiated services are stated in the chapter of *El-Kader.* Furthermore, the characteristics of QoS for WSN on different network layers are illustrated by *Shah et al* in following chapter. Therefore, readers will understand QoS mechanisms that are implemented on different layers of network to support and provide optimize performance for various types of applications. The last chapter of this section is written by *Marwaha et al.* who have pointed out the factors of achieving QoS of MANET. Moreover, the various QoS models of MANET have been clearly elaborated with mechanisms to support these models.

Section 2: Network Management Model

The intention of this section is to state network management models that are implemented to maintain the QoS of a network. The first chapter of this section focuses on the method to control multimedia transfer mechanism over a network where a significant loss of multimedia data over a wireless network occurs. The implementation of round trip time control was proposed by *Ramachandra and Jain* with the experimental results, evaluation and analysis.

Another network management mechanism is related to the traffic engineering, especially the routing algorithm, or path finding. Presently, various protocols and algorithms have been introduced and implemented. However, there are some defects remained. Therefore, in the second chapter, a new routing algorithm is implemented in conjunction with a heuristic path finding algorithm was proposed by *Goodridge, et al.* to find the best routing path for network traffic flow. So, the QoS for data transmitting can be obtained because the call back rate is lower than normal routing mechanism. Moreover, this proposed mechanism enables dynamic admission control and manageable environment. Besides, the emerging collaborative network management models is proposed by *Bertrand et al.* in order to gain the traffic management in backbone networks in the following chapter. Finally, *Vieira and Bozinis* proposed the use of network traffic models. This application is considered to increase the QoS because it leads to the correct estimation of bandwidth. Therefore, the loss probability can be guaranteed.

Section 3: Integrations of Quality of Service and Network Management Model

After readers have a clear understanding of QoS and roles of network management models, the integration of QoS and network management models will be displayed in this section. The first chapter of this section begins with the evolution of voice network technology where the transitions from circuit-switched public telephone network to IP packet-switched network are described by *Bross et al.* The paper has indicated requirements and QoS evaluation metrics of these indicators. Therefore, the QoS of each technology is clarified. Then the traffic and performance of mobile monitoring system have been elaborated by *Papantoni-Kazakos and Burrell* in the following chapter. This chapter described design, analysis, and evaluation of distributed and dynamic techniques that are used to manage the traffic and performance of sub-network. The readers will see the traffic model, including the network management context. Furthermore, the future research related to this area is also recommended. For the next chapter, *Ramachandra and Jain* had proposed a model based QoS constrained communication using multiple agents. These agents are used to exchange multimedia data over a network. The exchanged data performs via agents, including the integration of information from all agents. Moreover, the transmission rate is calculated using the result from neural networks.

In the forth chapter of this section, the authors, *Weisser and Tomasik,* provides an alternative solution for obtaining a QoS network management by introducing an inter-domain hierarchy. Therefore, the congestion problem of the entire domain can be avoided using the other domain congestion information. Then the inter-domain and intra-domain using IPv6 for QoS management will be demonstrated by *Fgee et al.* in the following chapter. This chapter provides useful information of IPv6 related to the network management area. Moreover, various pricing schemes are also elaborated.

For the chapter written by *Bouras et al.,* it gives an example of implementing a QoS network for the pan-european research and academic network project, GÉANT2. In this article, the QoS on each network layer is put in details. In addition, the network management structures and brokers of GÉANT2 system are described in details. After that a case study of a healthcare network in Thailand has been investigated by *Bhattarakosol and Tanchotsrinon.* This chapter demonstrates that applying a good network management policy can obtain a high quality of services without high investment cost. Then, the QoS of MANET focussing in the security issue will be discussed in the last chapter of this book by *Sornil.*

PRELIMINARY CONCLUSION

The contributions of this book are as follows.

1. Meaning and important of quality of services over networks has been clarified.
2. Various network management models and mechanisms that are applied for quality of services have been described.
3. Linkages between quality of services and network management methodologies are clearly presented with examples.

After reading these chapters, readers will realize that a high quality of services over various types of networks has many alternative solutions to be applied, with or without increasing the investment cost.

Pattarasinee Bhattarakosol
Editor

Section 1
Quality of Services

Chapter 1
Introduction to Quality of Service

Eva Ibarrola
University of the Basque Country, Spain

Fidel Liberal
University of the Basque Country, Spain

Armando Ferro
University of the Basque Country, Spain

ABSTRACT

The advent and rise of broadband technologies and new applications and services have led to a complex heterogeneous scenario in which providing Quality of Service (QoS) has become a compelling issue. Furthermore, the competitive condition of the telecommunications environment has caused user's perception of quality to become one of the most differential factors for service providers. Due to this fact, QoS must not only attend to specific technical metrics, but more important, QoS criteria should be defined to assure the level of quality to fulfil the users' requirements. In this new context, the definition of effective user-oriented QoS management models and frameworks has become a matter of contention. This chapter aims to provide readers a comprehensive analysis of the entire significance of a user-centered approach for quality of service management. For this purpose, a review of the most important issues related to the subject is provided.

INTRODUCTION

A deep comprehension of Quality of Service (QoS) is essential before attempting to understand any QoS management model. Quality of service may be thought, at first sight, a simple and obvious notion. Nonetheless, an inspection in related literature emerges the complexity of the subject. This chapter analyzes the full significance of quality of service concept. First, a review of the most relevant standards and definitions of QoS is provided. Then, this analysis will be expanded to consider its implications in telecom environments. In summary, this chapter offers an overview about the terms, standards and issues that may be of interest when managing QoS in communications.

DOI: 10.4018/978-1-61520-791-6.ch001

BACKGROUND

Quality of service (QoS) can be defined in many different ways. If we break the term down into its component parts, the word "service" can be understood as the provision of value in some domain. Therefore, the connotation of the term "service" will be tightly linked to the considered area: business, engineering, manufacturing, computer science. The meaning of "quality" has changed over time. Quality has been defined as the degree of excellence of a product (Abbott, 1955), bundle of characteristics desired by consumers (Lancaster, 1966), the degree to which a service conforms with specific requirements (Crosby, 1979; Juran, 1999) or the degree of user's satisfaction with the service (Ishikawa, 1985; Kano, 1984; Parasuraman, Zeithaml, & Berry, 1996). The most progressive views of quality include most of the issues that have been referred in the above definitions: products, services, characteristics, user's requirements and user's satisfaction. One example is how the International Standard Organization (ISO) defines quality in ISO 8402 (1986, p.3.1): *"The totality of features and characteristics of an entity (product or service) that bear on its ability to satisfy stated or implied needs"*. Considering this extension, several quality general frameworks and models like ISO 9000 (ISO, 2005), TQM/EFQM (Dale & Cooper, 1994) and Six-Sigma (Harry & Schroeder, 2000) have been widely adopted and deployed in business and other general environments but, still, none of them has been found to be fully satisfactory for telecommunication environment.

Despite the fact the term "Quality of Service" has been traditionally linked to one specific domain (communications), QoS definition has also evolved over the time. ITU-T Recommendation E.800 (ITU-T, 1994, p.3) defines quality of service as *"the collective effect of service performance which determines the degree of satisfaction of a user of the service"*. Some authors (TMF, 2005b) find this definition excessively narrow and ITU-T seem to agree with a later revision of this Recommendation (ITU-T, 2008, p.4) which changes the QoS definition to one derived from the ISO 8402: *"Totality of characteristics of a telecommunications service that bear on its ability to satisfy stated and implied needs of the user of the service"*. The amended Recommendation adds importance to the user's perception by remarking:

Of particular interest is QoS experienced by the user (expressed by QoSE or QoSP - QoS perceived). QoSE is influenced by the delivered QoS and the psychological factors influencing the perception of the user. Understanding of the QoSE is of primary importance to help to optimize revenue and resources of the service provider. (ITU-T, 2008, p.3)

This adjustment perfectly reflects the global transition of organizations and standardization bodies from the initial conception of the telecommunications quality of service, which was very much focused on network performance, to a more user-oriented approach. In addition, the increase of Internet use in all ranges of ages and domains has made QoS to become one of the most important differential factor between service providers. End-users are not passive users anymore since they have the opportunity to choose their own provider. Still, users may not know much about the technical aspects of the service and, therefore, they evaluate the level of QoS based on their own perception. This new context together with the current heterogeneous network environment makes it necessary to adopt practical QoS management models that may accomplish the difficult task of relating users' perception of QoS (QoP) to both network performance and non-network performance parameters.

The following sections summarize the main topics that need to be considered in order to define a QoS model adequate to be adopted in any heterogeneous network and for any kind of service.

QUALITY OF SERVICE IN TELECOMMUNICATIONS

In spite of the amount of research in the area of QoS in the telecommunication, the definition of QoS management models and frameworks is still a hot issue. Some authors have analyzed the reasons why so many QoS management models have failed to be widely adopted. A good approach can be found in *"QoS Downfall: At the bottom, or not at all!"* (Crowcroft, Hand, Mortier, Roscoe, & Warfield, 2003) where the reason of this failure is declared to be the timeliness of QoS mechanisms (they rarely arrive when they are needed), and the inherent contradiction of layering QoS mechanisms over a best-effort network. The authors of this article also state that, since networks are inherently dynamic and the ratio of resources available at the access and the core network changes over the time, the QoS research must be forward-looking and the proposed QoS models should be timely and inherent in the network.

Another important topic to consider in this analysis is that QoS can be studied from many different points of view: service provider, network operator, regulator or final user of the service. However, the key to make all these different points of view converge is reaching the user's satisfaction with the service. So, an effective QoS management model must achieve the level of quality to fulfil all the user's requirements. The customer's satisfaction is based on the user's QoS experienced (QoE) and many factors may shape the user's perception. Therefore, an effective QoS management model should consider an extensive collection of objective and subjective features than may influence on the QoS as perceived by the user. Capturing the user's requirements may be of interest in order to prioritize the QoS criteria most relevant for users.

Another issue that a QoS model should consider and clearly establish is how the set of criteria can be transformed into measurable parameters so evaluation of the achieved QoS can be performed. Some of the defined parameters will be metrics of network performance but others can be subjective indicators.

In order to avoid confusion and compose a consistent set of terms and definitions to specify all the technical and non-technical aspects in the context of QoS, ITU-T developed Recommendation E.800 (ITU-T, 2008) which clarifies the appropriate use, definition and application of the different terms. For a comprehensive understanding of QoS, next section analyze the implications of the most important QoS definitions as referred in this Recommendation.

Quality of Service and Network Performance

Network performance (NP) is defined in ITU-T Recommendation E.800 (ITU-T, 2008, p.6) as *"the ability of a network or network portion to provide the functions related to communications between users"*. Therefore, network performance must be evaluated in terms of metrics and technical parameters to cover all the technical aspects of the network. These technical parameters may influence the quality of the service but this influence is not necessary meaningful in the quality experienced by users. Many other factors may also contribute to the final user's QoS perception, i.e., user's previous experiences, user's expectations, customer care. Hence, an improvement in network performance not always leads to a better perception of the service. For example, improving delay conditions only sometimes may have consequences in user's perception, depending on the service and the user's tolerance.

Many studies (Bouch, Kuchinsky, & Bhatti, 2000; Varga, Kún, Sey, Moldován, & Gelencsér, 2006) have been carried out to analyze the relation between network performance and quality of service, and most of them conclude that the evaluation of QoS cannot be assessed based only on network performance measures. A more extended QoS framework was needed in order to consider

Figure 1. The four points of view of QoS and network performance

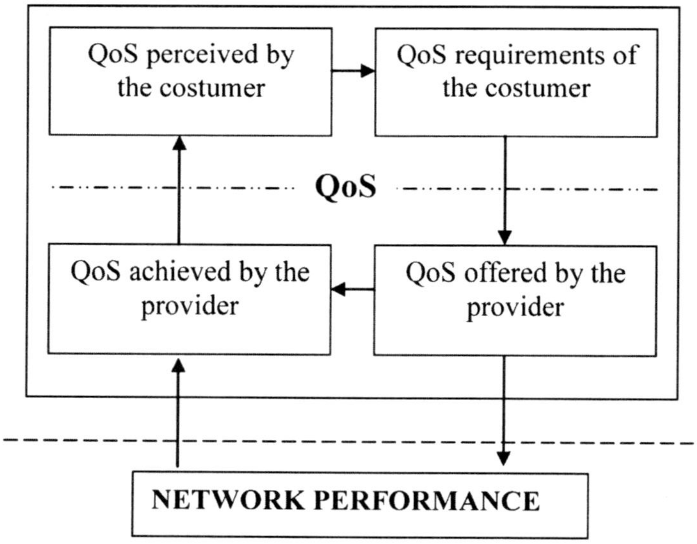

all the global aspects that may influence on final QoS users' perception.

To fill this gap, ETSI (1994) and ITU-T (2001a) have defined together a QoS framework approach that may be meaningful for all users, vendors, service providers and network operators. Figure 1 illustrates the key connections in this framework.

As figure 1 shows, this approach is a QoS user/costumer oriented framework but, in addition, network performance and QoS offered/achieved by provider are also considered. Furthermore, in order to cover all this different points of view and to assure successful mapping between them, four different QoS points of view have been defined: customer's QoS requirements, QoS offered by provider, QoS achieved by provider and QoS perceived by customers. The "customer's QoS requirements" define the level of quality required for a particular service quality and it can be expressed in technical or nontechnical language but anyway in a language understandable to both the customer and the service provider. An example of the requirements definition can be found in (ITU-T, 2001b). The "QoS offered by provider" establishes the level of quality expected to be offered to the customer by the service provider and is expressed by values assigned to parameters understandable to the customer and fixed within the Service Level Agreements (SLA) (ITU-T, 2002). Therefore, the offered QoS may be affected by the considerations of a service provider's strategy, benchmarking, service deployment cost, and other factors. The "QoS achieved by the service provider" asserts the level of quality delivered. It should be expressed in the same terms and with the same parameters as the offered QoS so they can be compared to evaluate if the offered service is achieved within the SLA terms. Finally, the most relevant data when assessing quality of service is the "QoS perceived by the customer". It represents the level of quality that users have experienced and is usually expressed in terms of satisfaction.

ITU-T Recommendation G.1000 (ITU-T, 2001a, p.4) states that *"for any framework of QoS to be truly useful and practical enough to be used across the industry, it must be meaningful from these four viewpoints"*. This statement implies that QoS assessment will necessary involve an assortment of objective and subjective parameters' measures which, if properly linked, may be used as a barometer of user's QoS perception.

Figure 2. The general QoS model, and ITU/ETSI and IETF approaches

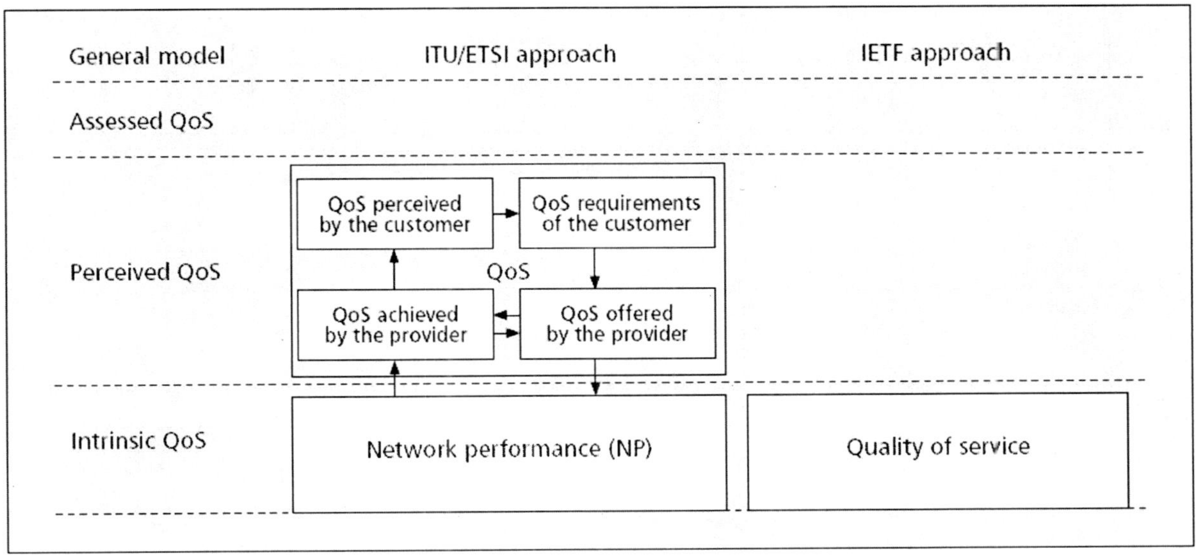

William C. Hardy in his book QoS: "Measurement and Evaluation of Telecommunications Quality of Service" (Hardy, 2001) develops a QoS framework very similar to the ITU-T's four points of view. This author identifies three different and interrelated notions: the intrinsic QoS, the perceived QoS, and the assessed QoS. The intrinsic QoS is related to network performance, the perceived QoS to customer's experience (QoE) and the assessed QoS refers to customer satisfaction and intention to repurchase the service. Some authors (Gozdecki, Jajszczyk, & Stankiewicz, 2003) have combined both Hardy's and ITU-T/ETSI's frameworks and, referring to IP Networks, compares them with the IETF approach, which is primarily network oriented. Figure 2 graphically describes the relationships between the three approaches. The Telemanagement Forum (TMF, 2005a) also describes this relationship in a very similar way but separating the service provider's and the network provider's viewpoints.

In the current competitive telecommunications scenario, it is evident that service provider pursue the satisfaction of the customer or, in other words, the customer intention to repurchase the service. Besides, it is widely accepted that customer satisfaction is determined as a function of user's perceptions together with the user's expectations/requirements (Anderson & Sullivan, 1993). Therefore, a general QoS framework should consider all the intrinsic QoS (NP), the perceived QoS (QoE) and the assessed QoS (user's satisfaction). The big challenge is to find the linkage between them for QoS reliable evaluation and, if necessary, for QoS improvement. In the next sections these relationships will be delved into.

QUALITY OF SERVICE EVALUATION AND MEASUREMENT

Quality of service evaluation is not an easy issue. As mentioned above, many factors may shape the user's perception and, therefore, the evaluation of quality of service should involve an extensive collection of objective and subjective data measures. This section introduces a review of the most extended QoS models and methodologies for the identification of the QoS criteria relevant to users and their conversion to measurable parameters. A discussion of the literature and standards for user's perceived evaluation will also be provided.

Figure 3. Matrix for identification of QoS criteria

		Service quality criteria						
		Speed 1	Accuracy 2	Availability 3	Reliability 4	Security 5	Simplicity 6	Flexibility 7
Service function								
Service manage-ment	Sales & pre-contract activities 1							
	Provision 2							
	Alteration 3							
	Service support 4							
	Repair 5							
	Cessation 6							
Connection quality	Connection establishment 7							
	Information transfer 8							
	Connection release 9							
Billing 10								
Network/service management by customer 11								

QoS Criteria Identification

Quality of service perceived by the user may be affected by network performance and many others contextual factors. For any management model to be practical and effective, it must be able to identify the set of QoS criteria that are relevant for users and establish how the set of criteria can be transformed into measurable parameters. In this way the evaluation of the achieved QoS can be performed. Some of the defined parameters will be metrics of network performance but others can be subjective indicators.

Some scientific contributions and standards can be found concerning the QoS criteria identification and related measurable indicators. One of the most widely used is the one defined by Richters (Richters & Dvorak, 1988). This model's approach focuses on the customer perspective and it is based on identifying the quality criteria of interest for users and the functional components of these criteria to infer the evaluable parameters or indicators. This model has been adopted by many authors (Seitz, Wolf, Voran, & Bloomfield, 1994), standardization bodies (ETSI, 1994; ITU-T, 2001a) and organizations (TMF, 2005b). ITU-T refers to it as "the performance model".

The principle of the model is a matrix (see figure 3) of rows and columns. Each row of the matrix represents service functions related to the performance of the service. Columns designate a set of quality criteria that can be perceived by users. Both the service functions and the quality criteria are meant to cover all the QoS criteria that may be related with user's requirements. Each cell of the matrix must be checked in order to identify quality parameters or indicators for later measures.

Even though ETSI (2003) used this model to determine the user's most relevant QoS criteria in the internet access, most of the authors agree that this model is mainly applicable in PSTN services and legacy networks. Due to this fact, the guide ETSI EG-202 009 (ETSI, 2007a) enhanced the model to allow a better understanding and to update it to a more current range of networks and services. In comparison with previous matrix, the service functions have been more detailed to cover all the aspects of the service life. Moreover, the simplicity criteria is encompass to usability criteria and security and capability criteria have been added. This ETSI guide thoroughly describes each cell of the matrix to evince how this new matrix can consider and capture all the user's QoS requirements of any specific service. The second part of this guide (ETSI, 2007b) together with the third part (ETSI, 2007b) fully undertakes the QoS assessment process (to be described later).

ITU-T has also updated the QoS framework and in Recommendation E.802 (ITU-T, 2007a) suggests three different models for QoS identification. One of them is the first version of the performance model mentioned above, but they also argue that it is suitable for legacy networks services. The second proposed model is the universal model. This model is very similar to the performance model, with a matrix structure where rows represent functions and columns the QoS criteria. The difference with the performance model is that QoS criteria are gathered under four categories: performance, aesthetic, presentational and ethical criteria. The third recommended model in Rec. E.802, especially suitable for multimedia services, is the four market model whose basic components are: customer's equipment, service transport, service provision and content creation. Besides, the E.802 Recommendation suggests some basic aspects that must be considered when identifying the criteria and determining the scope and measurement methods of parameters:

- QoS criteria and parameters are to be considered on a service-by-service basis.
- QoS criteria are to be specified on an end-to-end basis.
- QoS criteria and parameters are to be specified in terms understandable to the customers.
- Different segments of the customer population may require different orders of priorities.
- The preferred levels of performance for diverse segments of the population may be different for various user population segments.
- The QoS profile of a customer segment may vary with time and it is essential for the service provider to ascertain the customer's changing requirements. (ITU-T, 2007a, p.6-7)

Some authors have also proposed QoS models for the identification of user's requirements. For example, Oodan (2003) proposes the ACF model to analyze user's perspective of quality in the Internet-based-applications. In this model the evaluation of user's perception is based on the accessibility, continuity and fulfillment functions. Besides, various R&D projects have also made efforts to define user-centered QoS models. For instance, QUASIMODO (P906, 2000), TEQUILA (TEQUILA, 2002), SEQUIN (SEQUIN, 2002) or ENTHRONE (Ahmed et al., 2006).

QoS criteria (user's QoS requirements) can be identified from one or more of the above models and then their conversion into measurable parameters or indicators must be carried out. Still, when defining the suitable parameters, it is necessary to determine which of them will mainly contribute most decisively to user's perception. The ETSI EG 202 009 guide part II (ETSI, 2007b) is a perfect example of this exercise. In this guide a thorough analysis of a vast number of indicators and parameters is carried out. Still, the ETSI EG 202 009 contends that *"Measurements of every interesting parameter all the time might be very expensive and can even jeopardize the network performances"* (ETSI, 2007a, p.4). Therefore a deep analysis is necessary in order to designate appropriate parameters with the required granularity of quality evaluation. A lot of literature and standards deal with this issue. For example, for identification of parameters related with network performance the ETSI guide EG 202 057 (ETSI, 2005) can be a useful approach and for general parameters the TeleManagementForum (TMG) SLA Management book (TMF, 2005a) is also a helpful resource. Finally, together with the identification of the QoS parameters a measurement method for each of them must be defined.

End to End Performance Measurement

Usually both objective and subjective parameters may be involved in the evaluation of the user's perception. The objective parameters are generally related to network performance metrics. Regarding the subjective parameters usually survey methods will be required. Therefore, an extended collection of measures, of different nature, will be used when evaluating QoS as perceived by user.

The measurement methods to evaluate the objective or technical parameters have been largely studied since it was the first notion of QoS developed in the telecommunication environment. In this case the type of network and the nature of the service will have a profound influence in the measurements. For example, a lot of research and standards have been developed for IP networks over the last decade. For internet measurements the IETF has some pioneering work and a set of RFC's concerning metrics (IETF-IPPM, 1998a) has defined precisely the measurement methodology required for this network. IETF has also defined some QoS architectures as Intserv (IETF-IPPM, 1994), Diffserv (IETF-IPPM, 1998b) or MPLS (IETF-IPPM, 2001) widely extended over Internet community for QoS management from the network point of view.

ITU-T has also issued different standards about technical metrics measurements for general services (ITU-T, 2007c,, 2007d), for specific services (ITU-T, 2008b,, 2008c), and for the end-to-end measurement approach (ITU-T, 2001b,, 2005,, 2006). Hence, the measurement of network performance parameters is fairly well specified, not only over the internet services but also for legacy and new emerging networks Next Generation Networks (NGN). The network performance measurements will help network operators and service providers to define the offered QoS and the achieved QoS. Subjective parameters are more difficult to measure. They are not much related to network but, in many cases, they should be translatable into specific network parameters. An example of methods for subjective parameters measurement is provided in (ITU-T, 1996). There are also scientific contributions (Bouch, Kuchinsky, & Bhatti, 2000) and standards (ITU-T, 1996,, 2007) that may help to assess the desired measurement. Most of them use subjective tests, results of survey opinion, customer panels or opinion polls. The problem, once more, is to gather all this data measurements collection in order to evaluate user's perception.

User's Perceived QoS Evaluation

One of the biggest challenges in the QoS assessment process is gathering qualitative information about how different QoS levels are perceived by the user. As mentioned before, an extended number of objective and subjective parameters may have an incidence on QoS perceived and this influence may vary among different users. In addition, the "nature" of the evaluation of the subjective parameters (tests, opinion polls) may also pass out some important details.

In this context, a significant amount of research has been carried out in the study of user's perception. One of the most extensive is Bouch and Sasse's work. They analyze the influence of many network and other contextual factors like experience (Bouch, Kuchinsky, & Bhatti, 2000), pricing (A. Bouch & M. A. Sasse, 1999), user's circumstances (A. Bouch & M.A. Sasse, 1999), purpose of the service (Bouch, Sasse, & DeMeer, 2000).

Nowadays a lot of scientific research work is also being done on Quality of Experience (QoE). The increasing use of the multimedia services has caused an increase in the study of quality of experience since, in these services people become part of the service. The revision of the literature referring to this subject led to Jain's contributions. Jain aims for the necessity to develop systems to capture the nature of user's quality of experience (Jain, 2004). In this way, Siller in (Siller & Woods, 2003) proposes a QoE framework based on the hypothesis that a better QoE can be achieved when the QoS interactions of the network and application layers are considered holistically as whole rather than single entities. Similarly, in (J. Xiao & Boutaba, 2007) the perceived utility of the service is evaluated in terms of service utility based on network performance and availability, together with other non-network related factors like customer care.

QUALITY OF SERVICE ASSESMENT FRAMEWORKS

A considerable amount of research has been conducted over the past several years in the context of QoS assessment frameworks. Nevertheless, few of them cover all the QoS aspects that have been introduced in this chapter: the intrinsic QoS (network performance), the QoS perceived by user (quality of experience) and the user's satisfaction.

General Concepts

Before starting the review of the most relevant QoS assessment frameworks we will first resume the general stages that an effective QoS process should undertake. First of all, the analysis of the user's requirements must be accomplished. The study should be carried out on a service-by-service and on end-to-end (user's terminal) basis. Of course, the user's requirements may be different for different population's segments. The identified QoS criteria relevant to users will be converted into measurable indicators that will help to set the quality of service objectives. Then, the analysis of the quality of service that should be offered to fulfil with user's requirements must be carried out. A process to collect measurements of the decided parameters, on end-to-end and service-by-service basis, will be also accomplished. The resulting data measures will be useful to define the QoS delivered by provider. Still, these data measures must be adequately treated to obtain the QoS perceived by user. Finally, a deep analysis and comparison between QoS delivered, QoS perceived and the stated objectives will draw how far is the QoS assessment, or in others word, the grade of user's satisfaction.

Frameworks for QoS Management

The definition of a QoS management framework that will get along with all the analysis, the measurement process, and the improvement design required for the QoS process, is a very difficult burden. Besides, once the QoS enhancement methods have been found, powerful network management system will be required to deploy them. Therefore it will be necessary the integration of efficient QoS models with effective network management architectures and systems.

The ITU-T (ITU-T, 2007a) suggests some guidelines on the QoS process that must be considered. Figure 4 illustrates graphically the description of the process that is linked to the next QoS process steps:

1. **Quality objectives:** The service provider (or a regulatory body) first defines the target values to be applied to the telecommunication service. The respective parameters have already been created and the quality

Figure 4. Process of managing quality policy

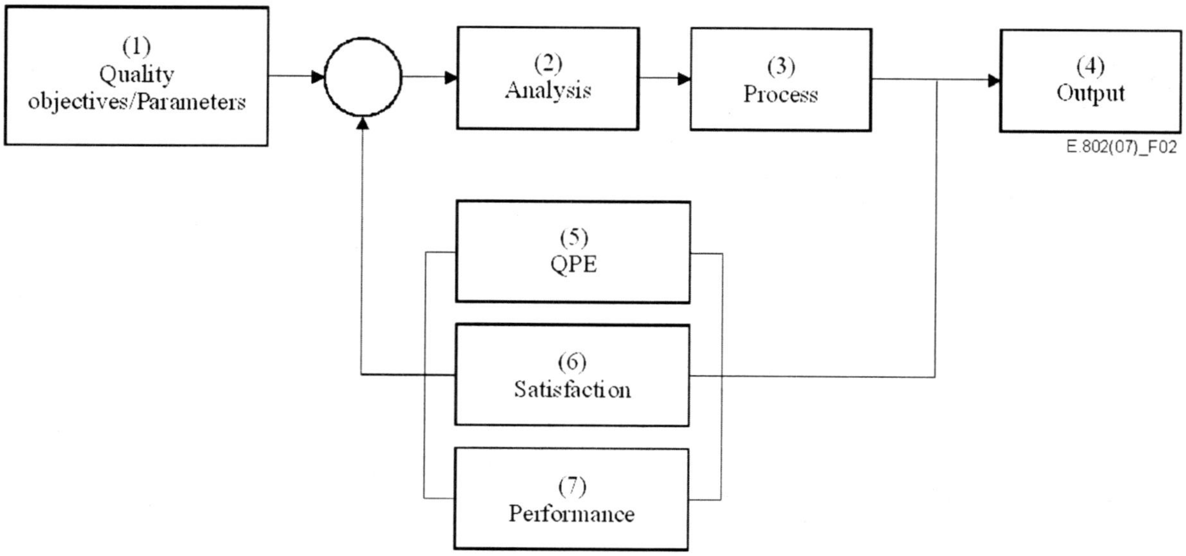

objectives were established within a close observation of the customer's requirements, historical evolution, benchmarking, etc.

2. **Analysis:** Initially, the action represented by this block is not applied. This block represents the action where studies, reflections, weights and comparisons are done taking into consideration the quality objectives established and the information provided by the feedback channels.
3. **Process:** This block represents the process developed by the service provider in order to deliver a service with a level of quality as specified by the quality objectives.
4. **Output:** It is the quality effectively delivered to the customer by the service provider as the result of the quality process.
5. **QPE (Quality Perception):** This feedback channel provides information on the perception of quality delivered by the service provider to the customers.
6. **Satisfaction:** This feedback channel provides information on the customer's level of satisfaction with the provided service.
7. **Performance:** This feedback channel provides information on the quality parameters as a result of the process of each service provider (the values reached, evolution in the period observed, difficulty to measure, etc.). (ITU-T, 2007a, p.20)

In addition, ITU-T provides specific recommendations to undertake the QoS process. For example, ITU-T Recommendation G.1030 (ITU-T, 2005) proposes different alternatives in the process of estimating the end-to-end performance of applications in IP networks. Figure 5 illustrates the alternatives approach. One of the alternatives is also applied in (Siller, 2003) where the same construction of network and application metrics interaction is used to improve quality of experience in multimedia services.

Another general and interesting approach to the QoS management process is eTOM (enhanced Telecom Operations Map). eTOM framework (TMF, 1999), was developed by the Telemanagement Forum and is part of the NGOSS program (New Generation Operation Systems and Software). eTOM is a business

Figure 5. Framework for developing end-to-end IP performance estimate

Inputs (beyond application of interest)	Network performance assessment	Application performance assessment	Perceptual performance assessment	
Access to live network for testing ►	Measurements • Ping • Unbiased sample • Application stream • Bulk transfer tool	Model for long-lived TCP flows (see Appendix I) Direct assessment with application tool	Model for web browsing (see Annex A)	► End-to-end performance estimate
Network design (detailed) ►	Modelling tools • Commercial products • Research tools	Embedded in network modelling tool	Future model for video teleconferencing	
Network design (limited info) ►	Simplified estimation (see Appendix I)	ITU-T Rec. G.1040 (Note)	Other models	

process framework defined to guide the key management process within the telecommunications service provider. Some authors (Huang, 2005) compares the eTOM framework with the ITIL (IT infrastructure Library) that is considered one of the best practice of Information Technology (IT) service management and it is also extended in QoS management processes (Ishibashi, 2007).

Some scientist contributions have also shed light to the QoS assessment process. One of them is the EQoS framework (Jensen, Grgic, & Espvik, 1999), a generic framework suitable for multi-provider environment, which captures many of the QoS-aspects of the QoS process. Another contribution is CyberPlanner (Jin Xiao, Boutaba, & Aib, 2008), an interesting management system that may help in assisting many key provider operations. A knowledge-based system and architecture for the formalization of quality of service (QoS) in telematic services is provided in (Sánchez-Macián, López de Vergara, Pastor, & Bellido, 2008) and a more user-centered approach is presented in (Patrick et al., 2004) to describe an architecture that takes into account the users' goals and needs.

Many other approaches could be mentioned but most of them only deal with some aspects of the QoS assessment process. A really effective QoS management framework must commit with the whole QoS process as described at the beginning of this section.

CONCLUSION

In this chapter the most important topics behind the QoS concept has been outlined. A revision of the most extended standards and contributions has led to user's oriented QoS frameworks in which QoS is specified in terms of different QoS points of views. QoS models have been described in order to establish the required linkage between the different viewpoints of quality of service. The complex process for QoS assessment has been defined in order to establish all the different tasks that must be accomplished when trying to achieve QoS. This process will require of intelligent QoS models and techniques together with powerful network management tools to manage the total aspects of QoS. Integration of the QoS models and the network managements system is essential to cover all the technical and subjective facets of quality of service. This book contents a deep analysis of the subject.

REFERENCES

P906. E. P. I. P. (2000). Project P906: QUASIMODO - *Quality of Service MethODOlogies and solutions within the service framework: measuring, managing and charging QoS.*

Abbott, L. (1955). *Quality and Competition: An Essay in Economie Theory*. New York: Columbia University Press.

Ahmed, T., Asgari, A., Mehaoua, A., Borcoci, E., Berti-Equille, L., & Georgios, K. (2006). End-to-end quality of service provisioning through an integrated management system for multimedia content delivery. *Computer Communications, 30*(3), 638–651. doi:10.1016/j.comcom.2006.10.009

Anderson, E. W., & Sullivan, M. W. (1993). The Antecedents and Consequences of Customer Satisfaction for Firms. *Marketing Science, 12*(2), 125–143. doi:10.1287/mksc.12.2.125

Bouch, A., Kuchinsky, A., & Bhatti, N. (2000). *Quality is in the eye of the beholder: meeting users' requirements for Internet quality*. Paper presented at the Proceedings of the SIGCHI conference on Human factors in computing systems The Hague, The Netherlands

Bouch, A., & Sasse, M. A. (1999). *It ain't what you charge, it's the way that you do it: a user perspective of network QoS and pricing*. Proceedings of the Sixth IFIP/IEEE International Symposium on Distributed Management for the Networked Millennium, Boston.

Bouch, A., & Sasse, M. A. (1999). *Network Quality of Service – An Integrated Perspective.* Paper presented at the 4th International distributed conference (IDC'99), Madrid, Spain.

Bouch, A., Sasse, M. A., & DeMeer, H. (2000). *Of packets and people: a user-centered approach to quality of service*. Paper presented at the Eight International Workshop on Quality of Service, Pittsburgh, PA, USA.

Crosby, P. B. (1979). *Quality is Free: The Art of Making Quality Certain.* New York: New American Library.

Crowcroft, J., Hand, S., Mortier, R., Roscoe, T., & Warfield, A. (2003). *QoS's downfall: at the bottom, or not at all!* Paper presented at the Conference ACM SIGCOMM workshop on Revisiting IP QoS: What have we learned, why do we care? Karlsruhe, Germany.

Dale, B. G., & Cooper, C. L. (1994). Introducing TQM. *Management Decision, 32*(1), 20–26. doi:10.1108/00251749410050660

ETSI. (1994). ETR 003: Network Aspects (NA); General aspects of Quality of Service (QoS) and Network Performance (NP).

ETSI. (2003). TR 102 276: User's Quality of Service Criteria for Internet Access in Europe.

ETSI. (2005). EG 202 057: Speech Processing, Transmission and Quality Aspects (STQ); User related QoS parameter definitions and measurements.

ETSI. (2007a). EG 202 009-1: Quality of telecom services; Part1: Methodology for identification of parameters relevant to the users.

ETSI. (2007b). EG 202 009-2: Quality of telecom services; Part 2: User related parameters on a service specific basis.

Gozdecki, J., Jajszczyk, A., & Stankiewicz, R. (2003). Quality of service terminology in IP networks. *IEEE Communications Magazine, 41*(3), 153–159. doi:10.1109/MCOM.2003.1186560

Hardy, W. C. (2001). *QoS: Measurement and Evaluation of Telecommunications Quality of Service*. Chichester, UK: John Wiley & Sons, Inc.

Harry, M. J., & Schroeder, R. R. (2000). *Six Sigma: The Breakthrough Management Strategy Revolutionizing the World's Top Corporations*. New York: Doubleday.

Huang, J. (2005). eTOM and ITIL: Should you be Bi-lingual as an IT Outsourcing Service Provider? *BPTrends*.

IETF-IPPM. (1994). *RFC 1633: Integrated Services in the Internet Architecture: an Overview*.

IETF-IPPM. (1998a). *RFC 2330: Framework for IP Performance Metrics*.

IETF-IPPM. (1998b). *RFC 2475: An Architecture for Differentiated Services*.

IETF-IPPM. (2001). *RFC 3031: Multiprotocol Label Switching Architecture*.

Ishibashi, K. (2007). Maintaining Quality of Service Based on ITIL-Based IT Service Management. *Fujitsu Scientific and Technical Journal*, *43*(3), 334–344.

Ishikawa, K. (1985). *What is total quality control? The japanese way*. Englewood Cliffs, NJ: Prentice Hall.

ISO 2005. (2005). *ISO 9000:2005. Quality management systems - Fundamentals and vocabulary*.

ISO 8402. (1986). *ISO 8402:1996. Quality management and quality assurance - Vocabulary*.

ISO/IEC 13236. (1998). *ISO/IEC 13236: Information technology -- Quality of service: Framework*.

ITU-T. (1994). [Terms and definitions related to quality of service and network performance including dependability.]. *E (Norwalk, Conn.)*, 800.

ITU-T. (1996). P.800: Methods for subjective determination of transmission quality.

ITU-T. (2001a). *G.1000: Communications quality of service: A framework and definitions*.

ITU-T. (2001b). *G.1010: End-user multimedia QoS categories*.

ITU-T. (2002). [*Framework of a service level agreement*.]. *E (Norwalk, Conn.)*, 860.

ITU-T. (2005). G.1030: Estimating end-to-end performance in IP networks for data applications.

ITU-T. (2006). [Framework for achieving end-to-end IP performance objectives.]. *Y (Dayton, Ohio)*, 1542.

ITU-T. (2007a). [Framework and methodologies for the determination and application of QoS parameters.]. *E (Norwalk, Conn.)*, 802.

ITU-T. (2007b). *G.1070: Opinion model for video-telephony applications: ITU-T*.

ITU-T. (2007c). [Internet protocol data communication service – IP packet transfer and availability performance parameters: ITU-T.]. *Y (Dayton, Ohio)*, 1540.

ITU-T. (2007d). [Measurements in IP networks for inter-domain performance assessment.]. *Y (Dayton, Ohio)*, 1543.

ITU-T. (2008a). [Definitions of terms related to Quality of Service.]. *E (Norwalk, Conn.)*, 800.

ITU-T. (2008b). *G.1081: Performance monitoring points for IPTV: ITU-T*.

ITU-T. (2008c). J.247: Objective perceptual multimedia video quality measurement in the presence of a full reference: ITU-T.

Jain, R. (2004). Quality of experience. *Multimedia, IEEE*, *11*(1), 96–95. doi:10.1109/MMUL.2004.1261114

Jensen, T., Grgic, I., & Espvik, O. (1999). *Managing Quality of Service in Multi-Provider Environment*. Paper presented at the TELECOM 99.

Juran, J. M. (1999). *Juran's Quality Handbook*. New York: McGraw-Hill.

Kano, N. (1984). Attractive quality and must-be quality. *The Journal of the Japanese Society for Quality Control*, *14*(2), 39–48.

Lancaster, K. J. (1966). A New Approach to Consumer Theory. *The Journal of Political Economy*, *74*(2), 132. doi:10.1086/259131

Oodan, A. P. Ward, K.E., Savolaine, C.G., Daneshmand, M. & Hoath, P. (2003). Telecommunications Quality of Service Management: from legacy to emerging services. Stevenage, UK: Institution of Engineering and Technology.

Parasuraman, A., Zeithaml, V. A., & Berry, L. L. (1996). The Behavioral Consequences of Service Quality. *Journal of Marketing*, *60*(2), 31–46. doi:10.2307/1251929

Patrick, A. S., Singer, J., Corrie, B., Noel, S., El Khatib, K., Emond, B., et al. (2004). *A QoE sensitive architecture for advanced collaborative environments*. Paper presented at the Quality of Service in Heterogeneous Wired/Wireless Networks, Dallas, TX.

Richters, J. S., & Dvorak, C. A. (1988). A framework for defining the quality of communications services. *IEEE Communications Magazine*, *26*(10), 17–23. doi:10.1109/35.7663

Sánchez-Macián, A., López de Vergara, J. E., Pastor, E., & Bellido, L. (2008). A system for monitoring, assessing and certifying Quality of Service in telematic services. *Knowledge-Based Systems*, *21*(2), 101–109. doi:10.1016/j.knosys.2007.02.003

Seitz, N. B., Wolf, S., Voran, S., & Bloomfield, R. (1994). User-oriented measures of telecommunication quality. *IEEE Communications Magazine*, *32*(1), 56–66. doi:10.1109/35.249792

SEQUIN. (2002). *SEQUIN (IST-1999-20841)*

Siller, M. (2003). *Improving Quality of Experience for Multimedia Services by QoS Arbitration on a QoE Framework*. Paper presented at the 13th Packed Video Workshop Nantes.

Siller, M., & Woods, J. C. (2003). *QoS arbitration for improving the QoE in multimedia transmission*. Paper presented at the Visual Information Engineering.

TEQUILA. (2002). *TEQUILA: Traffic Engineering for Quality of Service in the Internet at Large Scale* (IST-1999-11253).

TMF. Telemanagement Forum. (1999). *enhanced Telecom Operations Map (eTOM)*. Retrieved February 1st, 2009 from http://www.tmforum.org/BusinessProcessFramework/1647/home.html

TMF. (2005a). *Telemanagement Forum* (*Vol. 2*, p. 0). SLA Handbook Solution Suite.

TMF, Telemanagement Forum (2005b). SLA Management Book - Volume 2- Concepts and Principles (Vol. 2).

Varga, P., Kún, G., Sey, G., Moldován, I., & Gelencsér, P. (2006). Experimenting with QoE. In *Autonomic Principles of IP Operations and Management* (pp. 218–221). Correlating User Perception and Measurable Network Properties. doi:10.1007/11908852_19

Xiao, J., & Boutaba, R. (2007). Assessing Network Service Profitability: Modeling From Market Science Perspective. *IEEE/ACM Transactions on Networking, 15*(6), 1307-1320.

Xiao, J., Boutaba, R., & Aib, I. (2008). *Cyber-Planner: A comprehensive toolkit for network service providers*. Paper presented at the Network Operations and Management Symposium, 2008. NOMS 2008 Salvador, Bahia.

Chapter 2
An Analysis of Quality of Service Architectures:
Principles, Requirements, and Future Trends

Eduardo M. D. Marques
University of Madeira, Portugal

Lina M. P. L. de Brito
University of Madeira, Portugal

Paulo N. M. Sampaio
University of Madeira, Portugal

Laura M. Rodríguez Peralta
University of Madeira, Portugal

ABSTRACT

During the last years Internet evolution demanded for new and richer applications. To fulfill the novel and more complex application requirements, new solutions in many domains were required. One of these domains is the network support, assuring, into some extend, a specific or predictable treatment to traffic; therefore, in this chapter, we present a broad view of the main efforts available on the literature in order to provide Quality of Service (QoS) in both wired networks and wireless sensor networks (WSNs). For this purpose, the authors present: (1) the more relevant QoS architectures and technologies along with some of its recent improvements; (2) the different perspectives that combine some of those architectures and technologies into more complex solutions, in order to achieve stronger QoS and/or performance; (3) the most relevant QoS issues in WSNs environments; and (4) through the comparison of the several solutions, they list the advantages and limitations and reveal some relations among the existing QoS solutions.

INTRODUCTION

Traditional Internet offers to its users a simple service in terms of quality, called best-effort. This means that data will be transmitted as quickly as possible within the available resources, with some reliability, however without any other kind of guarantees. These network architecture mechanisms were mainly conceived to make a network

DOI: 10.4018/978-1-61520-791-6.ch002

very resilient and to handle all traffic similarly. The broader use of new applications, including real-time audio and video, imply new constraints to the Internet infrastructure in a way to provide control over end-to-end packet delay.

Different solutions have been proposed to overcome common network problems, such as providing extra bandwidth, ad-hoc prioritization of traffic for some applications and the development of adaptive applications (Teitelbaum & Shalunov, 2002). Nevertheless, they are not enough for sensitive applications in a congested network, thus, demanding the utilization of different service classes (Xiao & Ni, 1999). Therefore, the expected delivery of specific data traffic can only be assured if the network can support some kind of preferential treatment to the packets of this traffic.

Two principles emerge when handling special streams: reservation and provisioning. In the first one the nodes allocate enough resources to assure the expected requirements of the sender (or application) and try to give absolute guarantees to the flow of packets from that node. With provisioning, the intermediate node statistically assures an average treatment to the packets of a certain flow, but not guaranteeing that some particular packets will not be discarded or randomly delayed, in case of congestion. Each one of the QoS architectures presented in this chapter follows one of these principles.

Wireless Sensor Networks (WSNs) are a particular case of the general Wireless Networks. Differently to Wired Networks, Wireless Networks have a set of constraints related to the highly variable and unpredictable nature of the wireless link (in terms of dependence on time and location). Besides bringing some constrains WSNs still add some more challenges to the basic support of communication by the introduction of richer and more variable traffic in WSNs which lead to the need of more complete QoS solutions.

This chapter aims at providing a broad view of different existing QoS architectures for wired networks, and to provide a reflection on how these solutions can inspire the proposal of viable QoS implementations for WSNs.

This chapter is organized as follows: Section 2 describes some important QoS architectures for wired networks; Section 3 presents some hybrid architectures based on the previous architectures introduced; Section 4 introduces Wireless Sensor Networks and discusses how QoS can be achieved on these networks along with some solutions; Finally, this chapter is concluded with a comparison among the traditional and WSN QoS solutions and other relevant issues within both domains.

QUALITY OF SERVICE ARCHITECTURES

In the last two decades some architectures and technologies emerged as solutions to new applications and networks requirements. The proposed architectures had a strong and distinct principle guiding its creation and tried to solve some of the existing problems or limitations of the traditional networks. In some cases, these problems are still present in the current networks.

The architectures that will be presented in this section approach the issue of the traffic differentiation from different perspectives in wired IP networks, having as main goal, in some cases, the support of rich applications and, in other cases, the improvement of the network utilization.

Multiprotocol Label Switch (MPLS) and Traffic Engineering (TE) are also introduced in this section. The main goals and principles of each one of these technologies is not to provide native support to QoS, but instead to propose mechanisms to provide special treatment to flows crossing an MPLS or TE enabled network.

Integrated Services

The Integrated Services (IntServ) (Braden et *al.*, 1994) architecture represented an important

Figure 1. Integrated services example domain

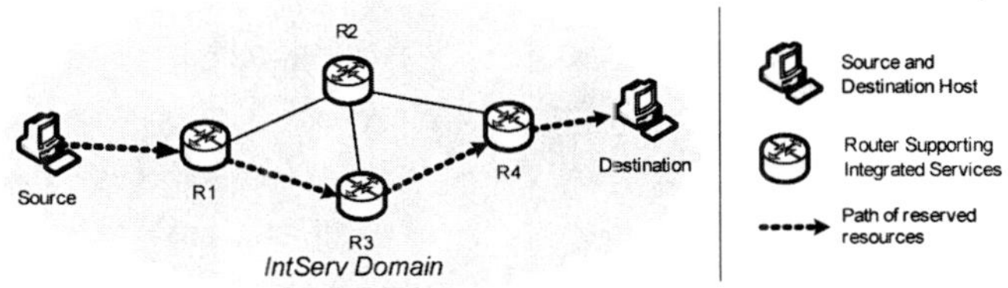

modification in the traditional Internet paradigm. With IntServ, the responsibility to maintain flow state information is distributed to all nodes along the network. This is a major shift in the Internet model; however, IntServ was defined as an extension and does not affect all the existing network components, which can continue to operate normally with the existence of IntServ in one or several network domains.

The IntServ philosophy determines that the needed resources must be reserved before a data flow could cross the network. All the network nodes along the path between two end hosts will have to support this resource reservation. The network represented in Figure 1 is a simple example of a domain that supports IntServ and, in this case, the nodes R1, R3 and R4 will forward, with some guarantees, the traffic between Source and Destination. This support is carried out reserving enough local resources to forward the packets of a flow within the expected delay and bandwidth requirements. If a node in the network cannot meet the flow requirements, the reservation in all nodes cannot be established and the flow will get across the network with a best-effort service.

Besides the best-effort service, IntServ offers two types of services for traffic requiring different treatments by the network. In the case of sensitive traffic which needs low latency, such as Voice over IP (VoIP), the Guaranteed Service (Shenker et *al.*, 1997) is the most appropriate. The traffic that needs a slightly better treatment than that offered by the best-effort service, will apply the Controlled Load Service (Wroclawski, 1997).

A signaling protocol is used to inform all nodes in one path between a sender and a receiver about the traffic characteristics and the network requirements. If all nodes confirm the resource availability then the reservation is set up and the data will start to be transmitted through the network assuring the reserved treatment. The most used signaling protocol is the Resource Reservation Protocol (RSVP) (Braden, 1997) and it is responsible to receive, establish and maintain QoS requests.

Advantages and Disadvantages

IntServ brings an important advantage to the Internet: guarantee. Therefore, it allows applications, if a reservation is set up, to expect from the network a predictable treatment. Still, this architecture presents some other advantages:

- Due to its flexibility, IntServ can meet the requirements of different applications based on its per-flow reservation;
- Network operators can apply IntServ guarantees to ensure some special treatment to a user or application, incrementing revenues, and;
- It supports the end-to-end model, allowing the network resources needed by an application to be selected.

The main weakness of IntServ is the scalability, a consequence of the per-flow reservation. This is caused by many factors:

- All nodes of a domain must be IntServ aware. If one node fails along the data path it is not possible to conclude the reservation. In an heterogeneous environment such as the Internet it is hard to overcome this limitation, and;
- Routers have to maintain state information of all the flows. In a small network this is not complex, however in the Internet core the predicted large number of flows will impose huge memory and processing overhead.

Currently, IntServ is not used in the Internet environment, but it is still considered an important mechanism available as an option to private networks' managers. IntServ is useful where a limited number of data flows, that need special treatment, exists.

The IntServ principles are relevant and they are applied in some recent contributions in the literature. In (Reid & Katchabaw, 2006) a simple architecture called SCalable Aggregate Reservations (SCAR) is proposed maintaining the basic IntServ principles to provide guarantees to a flow. It also partially overcomes the main IntServ limitation, the scalability. Other goals are simplicity, robustness and flexibility, and they are all achieved aggregating individual flows into classes, reducing the state information in the nodes only to the active classes.

Signaling is also an active on-going research area where much work has been done. Postigo-Boix et *al.* (2007) proposed a resource reservation managing mechanism which applies reservation only when congestion is detected. This detection is done by the analysis of a memory buffer in the end system application and requesting a reservation to assure network support in case of a predictable congestion.

Indeed, the reservation of network resources is a relevant innovation in IP networks, since network support to data was only assured on a best-effort basis. Thus, with IntServ it is possible to provide guarantees to the flows crossing a network. The main advantages of IntServ are flexibility, supported by its per-flow reservation capabilities, and guarantee, based on the reservation established prior to the process of sending data.

The scalability is IntServ major challenge, since it is not easy to control it in an Internet environment. Also, the reservation time can lead to some problems because (1) it imposes an extra delay to the applications that must wait until the reservation setup is concluded, which is unacceptable to some real-time applications, and (2) the use for short-lived sessions where the setup time could be longer than the data-time transfer (El-Gendy & Shin, 2003). Other disadvantages are related to the change in the traffic from the application which requires resetting the reservation and also IntServ lack of support to IP Security Protocol.

The next architecture presents how the Internet traffic can also be treated with some level of QoS, but under a different perspective. Moreover, it tries to overcome some of the IntServ limitations.

Differentiated Services

Differentiated Services (DiffServ) is a QoS architecture where traffic is classified according to a small number of classes. Each one of these classes is assigned with a different treatment following (1) a quantitative or statistical criteria based on the main QoS parameters or (2) the use of some relative priority sent across a network domain. DiffServ aims at allowing specific treatments to different applications having differentiated pricing for each network services (Blake et *al.*, 1998). Other important characteristics are: the applications on end hosts do not need to be modified; the need of a signaling protocol is discarded, and it can operate with non-DiffServ-compliant nodes or networks.

An important DiffServ principle is to have simple forwarding/routing in core nodes of a domain, keeping the heavy tasks in the boundary nodes. The treatment of each traffic aggregate in a

Figure 2. Differentiated services in a core domain example

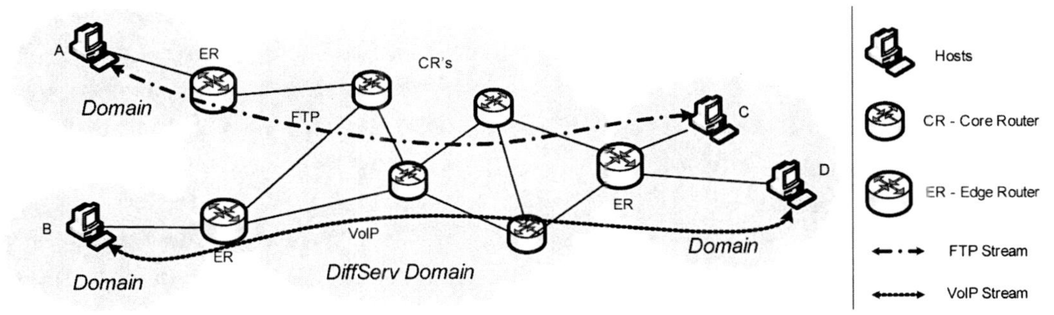

node is designated as the per-hop behavior (PHB). With the use of PHBs it is not necessary to maintain flows states in each node. The identification of each flow aggregate is done using a 6 bit code placed in the Type of Service field of the IP header designated DiffServ Code Point (DSCP).

The DiffServ domain architecture has two types of nodes in a domain: boundary and core nodes. Figure 2 contains several networks, represented only with one or two hosts, connected through a core DiffServ domain. In this example there are two different traffic streams: VoIP and FTP. In case of congestion, VoIP will expect a special treatment from the core network contrarily to FTP; VoIP is sensible to traffic delay or jitter, whereas for FTP best-effort is satisfactory.

The boundary nodes (Edge Routers in Figure 2) will perform the classification and, if needed, the conditioning of the traffic. This classification refers to the assignment of a behavior aggregate (BA) identified by the DSCP to the traffic. The conditioning includes some functions such as metering, shaping, policing and/or marking. The boundary nodes of a DiffServ domain also establish the connection to other domains (DiffServ or non-DiffServ compliant), based on Service Level Agreements (SLAs).

After the traffic classification, the core nodes (Core Routers in Figure 2) will forward the traffic packets based on the DSCP and on the associated PHB inside the domain. A PHB defines the node resources that are reserved to a behavior aggregate, and DiffServ are built over this hop-by-hop resource allocation mechanism. A PHB may be specified in terms of priority relative to other PHB's (e.g., buffer and bandwidth), or in terms of observable traffic characteristics (e.g., delay and loss). Its implementation is carried out through buffer management and packet scheduling mechanisms.

The number of PHB's possible to be defined is large, and two classes of services were normalized, within the range allowed: the Assured Forwarding (AF) and the Expedited Forwarding (EF). The AF class is indicated to traffic that needs special treatment, but can tolerate some delay and/or loss. The EF PHB is a specific PHB to accommodate less tolerant traffic in terms of loss, latency, jitter and bandwidth.

The PHB's configuration in a domain can be done statically. The provision of a network with predictable traffic patterns allows the definition of the initial PHB's needed. However, that is not a regular situation in current networks. The DiffServ already predicts the dynamically update of the PHB's to better respond to a specific network utilization. One example of it is the use of a central administration entity, normally called a Bandwidth Broker (BB) (Nichols et *al.*, 1999), which has the responsibility of making dynamic control and management of QoS provisioning. BB's are also able to manage inter-domains resources (DiffServ or non-DiffServ).

Advantages and Disadvantages

The DiffServ architecture is based on the provisioning of the nodes with the needed PHB to support the predictable traffic of a network. This principle presents the following advantages:

- Scalability, since there is no need to keep state information for each flow, but only for each class of traffic, making it more adequate to the Internet reality;
- Network optimization, using the traffic aggregation it is possible to accommodate more flows and achieve a better usage of the network resources, and;
- No setup time before sending data, on the fly admission control done by the traffic conditioner and the possibility to encrypt the data using IP Security protocol.

However, there are also some disadvantages when using DiffServ on a network domain, such as:

- No strict guarantees, only statistically guarantees are assured, making difficult to assure a minimum delay or maximum lost under heavy congestion;
- Low flexibility, since it can differentiate traffic only up to a certain number of classes;
- Lack of end-to-end support, making it not very adequate to some applications that need this characteristic from a network.

The different efforts carried out recently to improve DiffServ try to overcome some of its limitations and also to bring some new capabilities to the architecture. Chen et *al.* (2007) applied improved resource management to provide some reservation capabilities in a DiffServ Domain. Admission control is also a very important mechanism in DiffServ domains and is implemented in (Lima et *al.*, 2004), (Chen et *al.*, 2007) and (Marsan et *al.*, 2007). Another important requirement for QoS in DiffServ architecture is the end-to-end support which is also considered in (Lima et *al.*, 2004). At last, in (Yaghmaee et *al.*, 2005) some conventional modules are replaced with new ones using fuzzy logic aiming at improving performance.

When compared to IntServ, the DiffServ architecture brought, to some extent, important improvements, since it is much more scalable and allows the optimization of the network. This architecture is more oriented to core domains and gives to network administrators a good set of tools to manage their networks.

The next two topics will present some important mechanisms to optimize the use of the networks and, with that, the possibility to improve QoS.

Multiprotocol Label Switching and Traffic Engineering

Multiprotocol Label Switch (MPLS) is an architecture which allows to quickly forward packets in a network. Internet Traffic Engineering (TE) is a set of principles to control and optimize the use of a network. Although the different nature of both concepts, they tend to be applied together because of their complementary nature. In this section we first present MPLS and then we introduce some TE principles and characteristics. At last, the advantages and disadvantages of the usage of both approaches are discussed.

Multiprotocol Label Switching

MPLS (Rosen et *al.*, 2001) represents a convergence between an Internet Protocol (IP) connectionless environment and the ATM, or Frame Relay (FR), with its virtual circuit principles (Wang, 2001). MPLS brings to IP networks a simpler forwarding paradigm, reducing the time that each packet takes in a network node and also brings a mechanism to define an explicit path, creating conditions to the support of more complex services such as QoS and Traffic Engineering.

Figure 3. MPLS label description

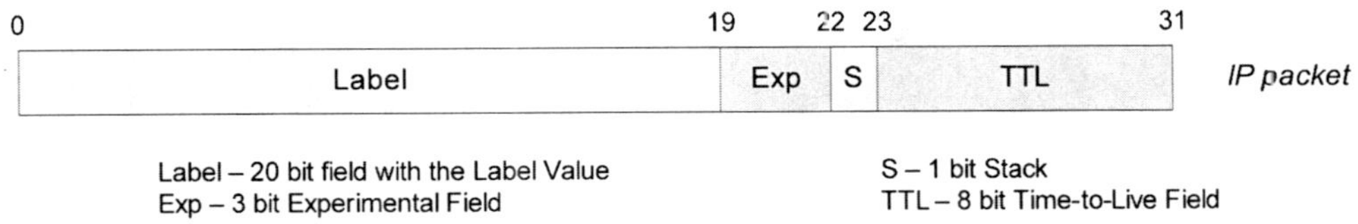

The packets entering an MPLS network are tagged by an ingress Label Edge Router (LER) with a fixed size label. By the analysis of this label, a Label Switch Router (LSR), located in the core of the network, is able to determine the next hop of each packet. In this process the packet label is updated by the LSR with a new value. When exiting the MPLS network the egress LER removes the label from the packet. In Figure 3 we can see the structure of an MPLS label. The field names are enough to explain themselves, but there is still the *Stack* field that is used to indicate the stacking of labels in a packet, used in nested MPLS domains.

All the packets tagged with the same label follow a predefined path, referred to as Label Switched Path (LSP), in the network and are in the same Forwarding Equivalent Class (FEC).

The creation of the LSPs is achieved by distributing through the LSRs of a network the labels that define each FEC. An LSP could be established with different objectives: to guarantee a certain level of performance, to route around network congestion, or to create IP tunnels for virtual private networks (Raj & Oliver, 2007).

An LSP configuration can be carried out manually by the network administrator or by the use of a signaling protocol. One of the first signaling protocols is the Label Distribution Protocol (LDP) (Andersson et *al.*, 2001), which used the information obtained from the IP routes and did not support QoS. A second group of signaling protocols allowed to create explicitly routed LSPs supporting QoS and Traffic Engineering (TE): the Constrained-based Routing LDP (CR-LDP) (Jamoussi et *al.*, 2002) and the Resource Reservation Protocol - TE (RSVP-TE) (Awduche et *al.*, 2001).

MPLS is an advanced forwarding scheme (El-Ghendy & Shin, 2003) which provides the packets in a node with a faster classification and forwarding. MPLS is also an efficient tunneling mechanism, where MPLS Virtual Private Networks (VPNs) are more flexible and simpler to manage than ATM/FR or IP-based VPNs (Kang & Lee, 2005). Another important advantage is the MPLS scalability (Wang, 2001) achieved through the use of switching technology. MPLS can work with many layer 2 protocols, such as ATM, Ethernet and Frame Relay, promoting interoperability. At last, an important characteristic of MPLS is that it enhances the traffic shaping and engineering capabilities, providing the efficient use of network resources.

The main disadvantage of this technology is the overhead for creating, maintaining and terminating the LSPs. Nevertheless, this disadvantage is largely compensated by the quick forwarding of the data packets. Another important advantage of MPLS is its efficient failure recovering schemes. Jorge & Gomes (2006) present some mechanisms to quickly recover from a node or link failure based on the use of a backup path, and compare them with other recovery schemes.

Traffic Engineering

The TE main concerns are the network evaluation and the network resources optimization. In (Awduche et *al.*, 2002) TE is defined as

Figure 4. Traffic flowing through different label switch paths

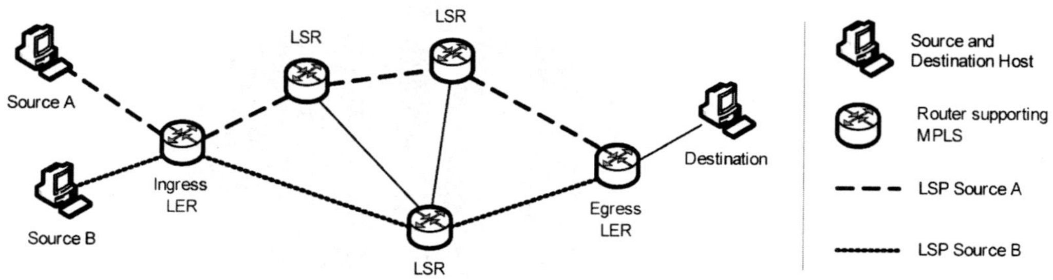

"... it encompasses the application of technology and scientific principles to the measurement, characterization, modeling, and control of Internet traffic".

The routing of the traffic associated with data flowing from a source node to a destination node is one of the most important functions of the Internet. The traditional routing algorithms, even in over provisioned networks, do not avoid network bottlenecks in inter-domain links between Autonomous Systems (AS). In (Hu et *al.*, 2004) measurements are made showing that the bottlenecks not only appear in inter-domain links, but also inside individual domains. Therefore, other mechanisms able to control and optimize the routing function are needed to improve network utilization and minimize network congestion.

The final purpose is to steer traffic trough the network the most effective way. Although network resources optimization is the main focus of TE, in some networks the operation objectives also depend on other aspects, such as: business model, network capabilities, and local constraints (Awduche et *al.*, 2002).

A common and simple scenario of the use of traffic engineering techniques is to balance the traffic between different network links, as demonstrated in Figure 4, having the purpose of, for example, avoiding bottlenecks and the degradation of the service provided to the network users.

Multiprotocol Label Switch and Traffic Engineering

Most of the MPLS/TE issues were already referred to in the individual sections of MPLS and TE. The use of CR-LDP and RSVP-TE signaling protocols are examples of having TE as a complement to MPLS to achieve QoS. The main advantage of this joint utilization is to provide network administrators with tools to optimize the management of their networks. With MPLS/TE it is possible to reduce congestion by means of a more effective load balancing and also MPLS offers mechanisms to recover from failures with better results than IP routing recovery. Although a better managed network provides better services to users, this solution does not support end-to-end.

The solutions presented in this section are individual QoS architectures based on simple principles. In the next section we present some efforts that combine to some extent the characteristics of the presented architectures in order to propose a more complete and richer solution to provide support to users and network administrators.

MULTI-ARCHITECTURE APPROACHES

The IntServ, DiffServ and MPSL/TE architectures provided some interesting background to traditional Internet, however they are not the ultimate

Figure 5. Combination of intServ and diffServ architectures

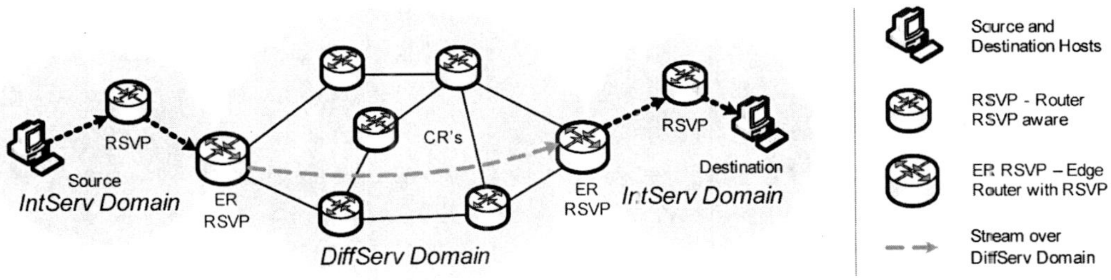

solutions because of the heterogeneity of traffic, networks and devices communication in current networks. A promising approach is to combine two or more architectures and technologies to try to: overcome individual architectures limitations, provide a good support to end-users applications and to make available to network administrators a richer set of tools to manage their networks. The solutions presented in the next sub-sections are the more relevant available in the literature and they are a good demonstration of the benefits of associating the assets of each architecture.

Integrated Services over Differentiated Services

A combination of IntServ and DiffServ architectures is presented in (Bernet et *al.*, 2000) and is based on the strengths of both approaches, guarantees and scalability, respectively for IntServ and DiffServ. This work proposes the existence of DiffServ regions in an IntServ network. The IntServ, for instance, could be used in boundary domains where the number of flows is small, not having scalability problems. The DiffServ could be used in the core, where only a fixed number of classes will exist, to be used by aggregated traffic, having a per-hop treatment and not presenting any scalability issues.

From the IntServ perspective, the DiffServ regions are virtual links connecting IntServ enabled nodes. To the DiffServ regions the management of traffic with IntServ characteristics brings some benefits, such as: resource admission control, policy based admission control, assistance in traffic identification/classification and traffic pre-conditioning.

Figure 5 illustrates the utilization of both architectures. The hosts are the entities exchanging messages where the signaling process starts. The IntServ domains are regions where signaling is fully supported. The DiffServ regions may or may not have all nodes supporting signaling, but are required to carry signaling messages.

The routers between two domains, designated as edge routers, are important elements. They support IntServ and DiffServ and are responsible for admission control, policing and mapping between both domains. Besides the individual issues of IntServ and DiffServ, there are also some problems related to this aggregated architecture. The first issue is how to carry signaling, using for instance RSVP, in DiffServ regions. Other problem is how to map IntServ flows to DiffServ classes. At last, how to make resource management in this context in DiffServ.

The carrying of IntServ signaling messages over the DiffServ domain depends on this one being RSVP aware or unaware. In the first case the messages are carried out and admission control and reservation will also be supported inside the DiffServ regions. In the second case, at least, the RSVP messages will pass the DiffServ domain unhindered.

In the case of service mapping the DiffServ domains are analogous to an IntServ capable node, and the IntServ services must be mapped into one or several DiffServ classes. The mapping must be agreed between the administration entities of neighbor regions and could be done statically, where the DiffServ region PHBs provisioning is negotiated (used when the domain is RSVP unaware). Other option is to have dynamic provisioning using some mechanisms such as aggregated RSVP, per-flow RSVP or a bandwidth broker.

The resource management in DiffServ regions, as referred before, can be static (based on a Service Level Specification - SLS agreed between domains administrators) or dynamic (done, for example, with RSVP or by a centralized oracle).

Advantages and Disadvantages

The advantages of having both architectures are: the ability to make resource reservations in a large heterogeneous domain or domains, with end-to-end capability being flexible enough to allow different applications and requirements.

The disadvantages result from the association of both architectures, posing new challenges: (1) how to map IntServ services into DiffServ classes, (2) how to transport IntServ signaling inside a DiffServ domain, and (3) how to make resource management in DiffServ in order to maintain IntServ guarantees. Also, another important issue is how to define billing rates between domains, owned by different entities. Some efforts and solutions to these limitations are presented further on.

Pereira & Monteiro (2006) propose two new modules, *mapper* and *meter*, to handle the admission control. The mapping problem is also referred on this work where dynamic mechanisms and statically provisioned solutions to map between IntServ and DiffServ are presented.

One option to carry signaling messages in DiffServ is implemented with the Common Open Policy Service (COPS) (Durham et *al.*, 2000), which is used essentially to carry policy information in DiffServ domains, but can also be used to carry RSVP messages. In (Chen, 2006) COPS is modified to reduce setup time in signaling, by simplifying the messages involved. A new protocol, SRRP, to be used transparently in IntServ and DiffServ domains is proposed by (Zhang & Mouftah, 2001).

A proposal to the inter-domain billing can be found in (El-Haddadeh et *al.*, 2006) and is based on relating the costumer's fares to the level of network congestion, driving customers to moderate the network use in case of congestion.

Multiprotocol Label Switching and Differentiated Services

DiffServ is a QoS architecture where, by means of several existing classes, it is possible to differentiate traffic flows into Behavior Aggregates (BA). It is a scalable QoS architecture; however, it does not offer mechanisms to improve the network efficiency.

The MPLS architecture basically allows explicit routing which is not possible in traditional IP networks. It is a fast method to forward traffic and, with TE, can balance the load of a network. Although it can manipulate traffic paths, MPLS is not a QoS architecture and it lacks of mechanisms to handle traffic in case of network congestion.

The DiffServ and MPLS architectures can be applied over the same domain because they are in different network layers. The DiffServ mechanisms are applied at the layer 3 and the MPLS label attached to the packet stands between layers 2 and 3. Also, in terms of network functions, they can complement each other. DiffServ provides queuing, scheduling and policing, while MPLS enhances the forwarding of the packets and the possibility to use Traffic Engineering. Another similar aspect in both architectures is the processing of intensive functions being executed on the edges of the domain. DiffServ executes the classification and conditioning while MPLS does the FEC classification.

In (Le Faucher et *al.*, 2002) a solution is presented to support DiffServ over MPLS networks.

The most important issue is how to map the DiffServ BA to MPLS LSPs. The two methods to convey this information are: EXP-Inferred PHB Scheduling Class LSPs (E-LSP) and Label-Only-Inferred PHB Scheduling Class LSPs (L-LSP). In the case of a limited number of BA (up to eight) the use of the EXP field from the MPLS Shim Header is enough to contain the indication of the packet PHB, being the designated E-LSP paths. In the case of the L-LSP, only a PHB Scheduling Class (PSC) is carried in each L-LSP and it is identified by the label value. A PSC could represent one or more PHBs and the EXP field is used to differentiate the treatment in terms of drop precedence among several PHBs.

Advantages and Disadvantages

The major advantage of using DiffServ and MPLS is to join a QoS-oriented architecture with a network load balancing mechanism. The resulting advantages are:

- The optimization of the network, achieved essentially by the use of the MPLS mechanisms;
- A better support to applications, gained with the traffic differentiation provided by DiffServ, the flexible control of flows provided by MPLS and, also from MPLS, the LSP strong protection schemes, and;
- It is a scalable solution, since the resulting architecture still maintains the complexity in the edges, having quick forward in the core.

The major disadvantage of this solution is the additional complexity to configure both architectures.

The solution discussed in the next section, besides MPLS and DiffServ, will incorporate TE mechanisms to improve performance.

Differentiated Services Aware MPLS/TE

The technologies presented so far are in most of the cases intended to be deployed in networks with enough resources and with predictable patterns of traffic. The mechanisms are implemented to prevent and recover from several problems such as periods of congestion or network failures, for instance. However, there are networks with very limited resources and heavy usage, where the bandwidth is scarce, the amount of delay-sensitive traffic is high and the volume of traffic across classes is very unbalanced. For this reason, a very flexible solution with a high-level of managing capabilities is needed.

The combination of the DiffServ traffic differentiation and the MPLS/TE mechanisms can provide the set of tools to perform traffic engineering at a per-class level, obtaining a fine-grained optimization of the transmission resources. The requirements for a DiffServ aware MPLS/TE architecture (DS-TE) are described in (Faucheur, 2003).

Two important requirements were considered for DS-TE: it must not cause a conflict with already deployed TE mechanisms and it could be implemented to a certain level of granularity and scope, in terms of classes and network topology, respectively. The concept of Class-Type (CT) is introduced to relate a class or type of traffic to a set of bandwidth constraints. It is used for the allocation of link bandwidth, constrained routing and admission control.

Two models of bandwidth constraints are discussed and evaluated in (Lai, 2005): Maximum Allocation Model (MAM) and Russian Dolls Model (RDM). In the first, the bandwidth defined for each class is for its exclusive use and cannot be shared among classes. In RDM each class gets an amount of bandwidth and can use higher priority class bandwidth if available. Basically, the differences between MAM and RDM concern the sharing policies of the CT resources and the type of preemption priorities necessary to provide some guarantees to a specific CT.

The complexity of this solution is its major disadvantage. It is applied mainly in situations where it is very difficult or very expensive to add more resources (e.g., transatlantic connections). In the last years this solution raised a lot of interest and some authors tried to confirm the advantages of deploying this kind of solution. In (Zhang & Mouftah, 2001) the authors evaluated the QoS performance of the services Voice-over IP (VoIP) and video in a DS-TE network, and concluded that in VoIP it is possible to achieve some guarantees; however, the bandwidth calculation in the video service is more complex and the probability of loss is very variable, because of the variable-bit-rate property of video. In (Barakovic et *al.*, 2007) the authors compare the behavior of the traffic under different architectures in a defined network. Partly, some conclusions confirmed the advantages of using DS-TE over just DiffServ or over only traditional routing mechanisms and also showed to E-LSP and L-LSP some favorable network environments. Secondly, some other conclusions verified the constrained-based routing mechanism of MPLS/TE in case of link or node error, having results showing improvements in all network traffics.

A limitation in the DS-TE architecture is its lack of usage, the small number of evaluation studies and tools to carry out these studies. In some recent works, such as in (Hu et *al.*, 2004) and (Adami et *al.*, 2005) the authors proposed new modules and platforms to speed-up the design, development and deployment of DS-TE.

The solutions presented so far are applied essentially in wired networks. The differences in the communication framework of wired and wireless networks are essentially in the two lower layers (data link and physical), and, as a consequence, we could conclude that the QoS architectures can be applied straightforward in both domains. In fact, this is not correct and the next section will characterize some of the constraints present in wireless environments, in particular in wireless sensor networks, which makes the use of traditional QoS architectures difficult or in some cases impossible to be applied in these networks.

QOS IN WIRELESS SENSOR NETWORKS

Wireless Networks can be classified in two main groups: infrastructure-based wireless networks and wireless ad hoc networks. Wireless Local Area Networks (WLANs), or IEEE 802.11 networks, are infrastructure-based wireless networks and can be seen as an extension of wired networks to mobile users. All mobile hosts under the communication range of an access point can reach it in one hop. QoS challenges usually arise from the shared bandwidth (that can become scarce, depending on the number of mobile hosts) and from the added complexity caused by user mobility. Therefore, it is possible to integrate the QoS architectures used in wired networks in the wireless MAC protocols. The QoS schemes explored by the IEEE 802.11 protocol mainly cover (Zhu et *al.*, 2004): service differentiation at the MAC layer, admission control and bandwidth reservation at the MAC and higher layers, and link adaptation at the physical layer.

Wireless ad hoc networks are autonomous systems typically deployed in highly dynamic environments; therefore, they are bandwidth constrained and have a highly dynamic network topology. Consequently, mechanisms used to support QoS in wired networks cannot be applied to ad hoc networks. Most QoS provisioning methods in wireless ad hoc networks are based on end-to-end path discovery, resource reservation along the path, and path recovery in case of topology changes (Wang et *al.*, 2006). However, these approaches are not suitable to Wireless Sensor Networks (WSNs), a special case of wireless ad hoc networks, because these networks impose many specific requirements.

Figure 6. Wireless sensor network

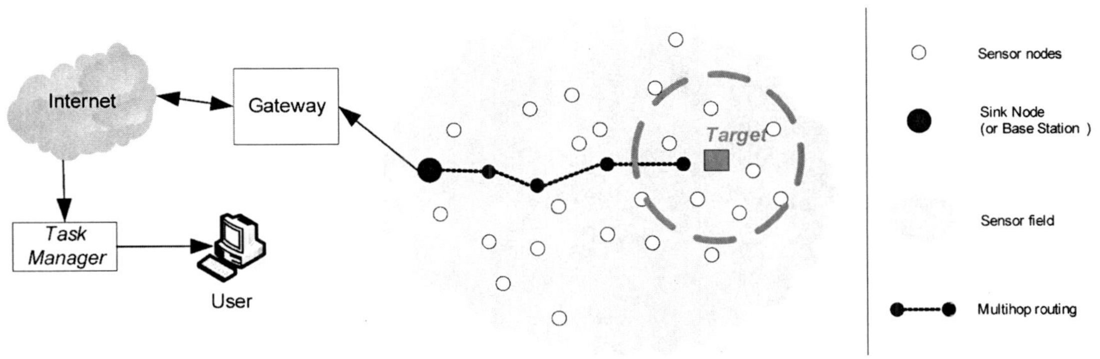

In general, a WSN consists of a large number of tiny wireless sensor nodes (often referred to as nodes) that are, typically, densely deployed. Nodes measure ambient conditions in the environment surrounding them. Then, data collected by sensor nodes is routed to a special node, the sink node (or Base Station), in a multi-hop basis, as shown in Figure 6. In the case of remote monitoring, the sink node sends data to the user via Internet or satellite, through a gateway.

WSNs represent a significant improvement over traditional sensor networks concerning: cost, size, flexibility, distributed intelligence, etc. However, the main advantage of WSNs is the possibility of being deployed anywhere, in irregular or inaccessible terrains or even in hostile environments, where cable installation is not a viable solution. Combining the advantages of wireless communications with some computational capabilities, the application areas of WSNs are quite numerous: environmental monitoring, health, surveillance, traffic monitoring, military, home, disaster monitoring, industry, agriculture, structures monitoring, etc.

However, these networks require unattended operation. Consequently, protocols and algorithms for sensor networks must possess self-organizing capabilities. The failure of sensor nodes due to lack of power, environmental interferences or physical damage, should not affect the overall task of sensor nodes. Moreover, due to their reduced size, sensor nodes face severe resource limitations (restricted energy, reduced memory and processing capabilities, and limited transmission range). Besides, when comparing the WSNs to other traditional networks, there are some strict constraints for sensor nodes that need to be considered (Akyildiz, et *al.*, 2002; Chen & Varshney, 2004; Karl & Willig, 2005; Martínez et *al.*, 2007; Rentala et *al.*, 2002; Wang et *al.*, 2006; Xia, 2008): 1) they have to consume extremely low power (energy); 2) scale (they have to operate in high volumetric densities); 3) simplicity; 4) scalability; 5) low cost; 6) auto-configuration (be autonomous, operate unattended, be adaptive to changes in the environment and to the network dynamics); 7) ambient interaction; 8) application specific; 9) data centric; 10) data redundancy; 11) unbalanced traffic (traffic mainly flows towards a small subset of sink nodes); 12) multiple traffic types (due to the inclusion of heterogeneous sets of sensors, and to the mixture of periodic and non-periodic traffic types); and 13) multiple sinks (there may exist multiple sink nodes, which may impose different requirements on the network).

All these challenges have to be considered when supporting QoS in WSNs.

QoS Metrics

Due to the WSNs' specific characteristics, some of the QoS metrics differ from the ones used in other networks. Usually, the packet delivery ratio is not a significant QoS metric in WSNs; the amount and quality of information that can be extracted about the observed phenomenon are considered more relevant metrics. Also, it is crucial to consider the amount of energy spent in the process of obtaining these metrics. Besides, it is critical to find a balance between accuracy, latency and energy costs. Depending on the application, the network should adapt to different accuracy and latency requirements, with minimal energy expenses. Hence, in WSNs the QoS requirements are strongly application-dependent.

Therefore, the QoS metrics can comprise (Chen & Varshney, 2004; Martínez et *al.*, 2007; Pereira et *al.*, 2003; Rentala et *al.*, 2002):

- **Energy efficiency and system lifetime:** As sensor nodes are equipped with batteries, protocols should be energy-efficient in order to extend the system lifetime;
- **Latency and accuracy:** A user is interested in some specific phenomenon, during a certain time period (latency). Besides, the main goal of the user is to obtain accurate information. The intended latency and accuracy levels depend on the application scenario;
- **Fault tolerance and easy recovery:** Sensor nodes can fail due to adverse physical conditions or due to lack of battery. It can be very difficult or even impossible to substitute these nodes, so the network has to be fault tolerant and recover from these failures as quickly as possible;
- **Scalability:** In order to assure the system's scalability, which is very important in large-scale WSNs, the interaction between the hierarchy of nodes and data aggregation are critical factors;
- **Sensors exposition:** One major concern of WSNs is the ability to detect objects. The term exposition can be defined as: "the network ability to sense an object, moving in an arbitrary path, during a certain time period" (Pereira et *al.*, 2003);
- **Coverage and optimum number of active sensors:** The area and/or event to be monitored should be covered by enough active sensor nodes;
- **Reliability:** Multipath routing can ensure reliability in case of failure of nodes or paths;
- **Bandwidth:** Usually, bandwidth is not a concern for a single sensor node; however, it may be a concern for a group of sensor nodes for certain time periods, due to the bursty nature of traffic, and;
- **Packet losses:** It can be tolerated to a certain limit, since there is usually much redundancy in the data.

Chen & Varshney (2004) even proposed some new collective QoS parameters (collective latency, collective packet loss, collective bandwidth and information throughput), which are associated with the data related to monitoring a certain phenomenon or event, instead of being associated with the data generated from an individual sensor node.

QoS Solutions

In WSNs, the great majority of contributions in the literature concerning QoS mainly focus on routing protocols (network layer) and on protocols and mechanisms at the MAC layer.

- **Routing protocols:** Directed Diffusion (Intanagonwiwat et *al.*, 2000), Sensor Protocols for Information via Negotiation (SPIN) (Kulik et *al.*, 2002) and dual-path energy-aware routing protocol (Mahapatra et *al.* 2006) do not implement any QoS mechanism; they essentially eliminate redundant data, which allows for: energy saving (the number of transmissions decreases), reducing the routing delay, and increasing bandwidth in the links near to the sink node; this increases efficiency, robustness, scalability and, thus, the network lifetime. TEEN and Adaptive TEEN (APTEEN), proposed by Manjeshwar & Agarwal (2001) and Manjeshwar & Agarwal (2002), Real-time Power-Aware Routing (RPAR), proposed by Chipara et *al.* (2006), and SPEED, proposed by He et *al.* (2003) have been designed for time-critical applications, providing some real-time guarantees, since they focus on guaranteeing minimum delay. Sequential Assignment Routing (SAR) (Akyildiz et *al.*, 2002) makes routing decisions based on QoS metrics, namely: energy resources, QoS planned for each path, and the type of traffic to which each packet belongs to; it also ensures fault tolerance and easy recovery using a multi-path approach. Multi-path and Multi-SPEED Routing Protocol (MMSPEED) (Felemban et *al.* 2006) provides QoS differentiation based on two domains: timeliness, by guaranteeing the packet delivery speed, and reliability, through multi-path routing. MultiConstrained MultiPath (MCMP) (Huang & Fang, 2008) utilizes multiple paths to provide QoS under multiple constraints (e.g., delay and reliability). Energy-aware QoS Routing (Akkaya & Younis, 2003) divides traffic in two classes: best effort and real-time; nodes maintain two queues, one for each traffic type.

- MAC layer protocols and mechanisms: From the MAC layer perspective, the concerns regarding the QoS provision cover essentially: avoiding collisions, ensuring efficiency in channel occupation, guaranteeing tolerance to changeable environments, and ensuring scalability. B-MAC (Polastre et *al.*, 2004) is designed to avoid collisions, to ensure efficiency in the channel occupation either at low or high data rates, to guarantee tolerance to changeable environments (topology changes, etc.), and to ensure scalability. Zebra MAC (Z-MAC) (Rhee et *al.*, 2005) is a hybrid scheme; under low contention it has a CSMA behaviour, and under high contention it has a TDMA behaviour, which is important for applications with delay and/or reliability requirements. Implicit GTS Allocation Mechanism (i-GAME) (Koubâa et *al.*, 2008) is the MAC protocol for the IEEE 802.15.4 standard; it consists in sharing the same guaranteed time slot (GTS) between multiple nodes, instead of being exclusively dedicated to a single node; this allows for more efficiency and smaller delays. Mahapatra et *al.* (2006) propose an adaptive prioritized MAC protocol that provides a differentiated service model for real-time packets (reducing the delay). PEDAMACS (Ergen & Varaiya, 2006) implements a TDMA-based scheduling algorithm to determine when a node should transmit and receive data; this eliminates network congestion and guarantees delay.

The routing and MAC protocols alone cannot provide all the QoS requirements described above; therefore, depending on the QoS requirements of the application, other protocols and mechanisms may have to be implemented to enhance the QoS provision, such as:

- Sleeping mechanisms to save energy - Most of the times it is a bit contradictory to guarantee QoS and, yet to reduce energy consumption, since the provision of a better QoS is usually associated with bigger energy expenses. Zhao et *al.* (2006) propose a periodic sleeping mechanism (not all sleeping nodes wake up every second) that reduces the whole energy consumption without affecting the QoS;

- Data processing strategies – Data aggregation can improve energy efficiency, and decrease delay and the system overhead (Li et *al.*, 2007);
- Cross-layer solutions - An example is the architecture (AMoQoSA) proposed by Troubleyn et *al.* (2008). It is an adaptive architecture that uses several QoS techniques that can be activated according to the nodes' remaining capabilities. This allows the network to dynamically adapt to the current network conditions and to continuously deliver QoS in heterogeneous sensor networks. Other solutions (Li et *al.*, 2007) include RAP (cross-layer communication architecture that includes a transport-layer protocol, a geographic routing protocol, a scheduling mechanism and a contention-based MAC protocol) and MERLIN (integrates routing and MAC protocols to support energy efficiency and low latency), and;
- Topology control schemes – Liu et *al.* (2008) propose a topology control algorithm that improves QoS performance, by reducing packet loss rate and latency and considering energy reduction.

CONCLUSION

In order to better identify and compare the QoS technologies in the wired networks as discussed in this chapter, Table 1 presents some important characteristics of each one of these solutions. These characteristics summarize the main advantages, disadvantages and differences among the several architectures. The *Main Goals* column provides us with a perspective of the existing problems and which concerns guided the design of the several solutions. The *Traffic Granularity* and the *Core vs. End-to-End* columns identified the approach to the traffic and the possible domains of implementation. The *Network Optimization* and the *Overall Complexity* lead us to understand the balance between having a better solution and the difficulty to achieve it.

The analysis of Table 1 allows us to obtain some conclusions. The first one is that the direct support to application is hard to obtain. Only IntServ allows the design of applications that could specify their needs to the network. All the other solutions join the traffic in classes or in an aggregation of flows, not providing much flexibility to the end user applications. This is an important issue because of the heterogeneity of the networks, devices and applications. We can find in the literature some contributions that try to improve the flexibility of the architectures with low or without end-to-end support. In (Lima et *al.*, 2004) the authors proposed a Distributed Admission Control component to the DiffServ architecture to provide more control over the guarantees offered to applications, enabling the support of a predictable end-to-end treatment. In (Chiu et *al.*, 2003) the authors optimize the LSP selection with the objective of minimizing the LSP preemption (overlapped by higher priority LSPs). The algorithm proposed is based on the LSP preemption probability and reducing the LSP preemption increases the guarantees of a better end-to-end support.

Another conclusion from the analysis of Table 1 shows us that each one of the architecture was created considering a set of particular requirements and constraints. Those aspects are important during the characterization of a network in order to guide the application of an appropriate QoS solution or architecture for this network. For instance, if we consider DS-TE which is the more complete solution, in general it is not the best one for all networks due to its complexity.

There are several approaches that generally explore the interoperability between IEEE 802.11 and DiffServ or IntServ in wireless networks, at the Access Point. Since MAC layer protocols are

Table 1. Comparison of QoS architectures and technologies

Architecture	Main Goals	Traffic Granularity	Core vs. End-To-End	Network Optimization	Overall Complexity	Main Advantages	Main Disadvantages
IntServ	Strong Support to Applications	Individual Flows	End-to-End	Very Low	Low	Guarantees	Scalability
DiffServ	Traffic Differentiation	Traffic Classes	Core	Low	Low	Scalable	Low flexibility
MPLS with TE	Traffic Forwarding Control	Aggregated Flows	Core	Good	High	Network Efficiency and Resilience	Not a QoS Architecture
IntServ and DiffServ	End-to-End in Heterogeneous Networks	Individual Flows over Traffic Classes	End-To-End over Core	Low	Average	End-To-End Support	Low Network Efficiency
DiffServ over MPLS	Traffic Differentiation over some Network Optimization	Traffic Classes within Explicit Paths	Core	Medium	High	Network Optimization with Traffic Differentiation	Complex
DS aware MPLS/TE	High Network Optimization and Strong QoS Protection	Traffic Classes within Explicit Paths	Could be Both	Very Good	Very High	Fine Tuning of Network Usage	Very Complex

prevalent in IEEE 802.11 WLANs cross-layer interaction is necessary (Zhu et *al.*, 2004). WSNs have several particular constraints that impose unprecedented challenges. Consequently, the traditional QoS approaches are not feasible since they are too complex to be applied to WSNs. However, some efforts are being developed towards the implementation of the IP protocol in WSNs. The work of the IETF 6LoWPAN group, which has specified the use of IPv6 over low-power wireless networks, aims especially at ensuring interoperability between networks of different manufacturers. Indeed, this integration can be considered as one possible future direction for QoS assurance and control at the routing layer. Besides, as WSNs evolve to support more complex applications, research should focus more on the problem of differentiating QoS provision for traffic with different QoS requirements.

REFERENCES

Adami, D., Callegari, C., Giordano, S., Mustacchio, F., Pagano, M., & Vitucci, F. (2005). Signalling protocols in diffserv-aware MPLS networks: design and implementation of RSVP-TE network simulator. *IEEE Global Telecommunications Conference (GLOBECOM '05)*, 792-796.

Akkaya, K., & Younis, M. (2003). An energy-aware QoS routing protocol for wireless sensor networks. In *Proceedings of the 23rd International Conference on Distributed Computing Systems Workshops*, (pp. 710–715).

Akyildiz, I., Su, W., Sankarasubramaniam, Y., & Cayirci, E. (2002). A Survey on Sensor Networks. *Computer Networks*, *38*(4), 393–422. doi:10.1016/S1389-1286(01)00302-4

Andersson, L., Doolan, P., Feldman, N., Fredette, A., & Thomas, B. (2001). *LDP Specification, RFC 3036.*

Awduche, D., Berger, L., Gan, D., Li, T., Srinivasan, V., & Swallow, G.. (2001). *RSVP-TE: Extensions to RSVP for LSP Tunnels, RFC 3209, updated by RFCs 3936, 4420.*

Awduche, D.O., Chiu, A., Elwalid, A., Widjaja, I:, & Xiao,X (2002). *Overview and Principles of Internet Traffic Engineering, RFC 3272.*

Barakovic, J., Bajric, H., & Husic, A. (2007). QoS Design Issues and Traffic Engineering in Next Generation IP/MPLS Network. In *proceedings of the 9th International Conference on Telecommunications (ConTel 2007)*, (pp. 203-210).

Bernet, Y., Ford, P., Yavatkar, R., Baker, F., Zhang, L., Speer, M., Braden, R., Davie, B., Wroclawski, J., & Felstaine, E., (2000). *A Framework for Integrated Services Operation over Diffserv Networks, RFC 2998.*

Blake, S., Black, D., Carlson, M., Davies, E., Wang, Z., & Weiss, W. (1998). *An Architecture for Differentiated Services, RFC 2475.*

Braden, R., Clark, D., & Shenker, S. (1994). *Integrated Services in the Internet Architecture: an Overview, RFC 1633.*

Braden, R., Zhang, L., Berson, S., Herzog, S., & Jamin, S. (1997). *Resource ReSerVation Protocol (RSVP), RFC 2205.*

Chen, C.-L. (2006). *The signaling protocol for intserv operation over diffserv model.* Tech Rep. No. 2002 ICS, Feng Chia University, Taiwan.

Chen, D., & Varshney, P. (2004). QoS Support in Wireless Sensor Networks: A Survey. In *Proceedings of the International Conference on Wireless Networks (ICWN 2004)*, Las Vegas, NV, (pp. 227-233).

Chen, J.-L., Chen, M.-C., & Chian, Y.-R. (2007). QoS management in heterogeneous home networks. *Computer Networks*, *51*(12), 3368–3379. doi:10.1016/j.comnet.2007.01.032

Chipara, O., He, Z., Xing, G., Chen, Q., Wang, X., Lu, C., et al. (2006). Real-time Power-Aware Routing in Sensor Networks. In *Proc. 14th IEEE International Workshop on Quality of Service (IWQoS 2006)*, (pp. 83-92).

Chiu, J.-F., Huang, Z.-P., Lo, C.-W., Hwang, W.-S., & Shieh, C.-K. (2003). Supporting end-to-end QoS in DiffServ/MPLS networks. In *10th International Conference on Telecommunications (ICT 2003), 1*, (pp. 261-266).

Durham, D., Boyle, J., Cohen, R., Herzog, S., Rajan, R., & Sastry, A. (2000). *The COPS (Common Open Policy Service) Protocol, RFC 2748.*

El-Gendy, M. A., & Shin, K. G. (2003). Evolution of the Internet QoS and Support for Soft Real-time Applications. *Proceedings of the IEEE*, *91*(7). doi:10.1109/JPROC.2003.814615

El-Haddadeh, R., Watts, S. J., & Taylor, G. A. (2006). Charging QoS Inter-Domain Networks: IntServ over DiffServ. In *IEEE Global Telecommunications Conference, (GLOBECOM '06)*, (pp. 1-5).

Ergen, S. C., & Varaiya, P. (2006). PEDAMACS: Power Efficient and Delay Aware Medium Access Protocol for Sensor Networks. *IEEE Transactions on Mobile Computing*, *5*(7), 920–930. doi:10.1109/TMC.2006.100

Felemban, E., Lee, C.-G., & Ekici, E. (2006). MMSPEED: Multipath Multi-SPEED protocol for QoS guarantee of reliability and timeliness in wireless sensor networks. *IEEE Transactions on Mobile Computing*, *5*(6), 738–754. doi:10.1109/TMC.2006.79

He, T., Stankovic, J., Lu, C., & Abdelzaher, T. (2003). SPEED: A stateless protocol for real-time communication in sensor networks. In *Proceedings of 23rd International Conference on Distributed Computing Systems*, (pp. 46–55).

Hu, N., Li, L., Mao, Z. M., Steenkiste, P., & Wang, J. (2004). Locating Internet bottlenecks: algorithms, measurements, and implications. In *Proceedings of the 2004 Conference on Applications, Technologies, Architectures, and Protocols for Computer Communications*, Portland, OR, (pp. 41-54).

Huang, X., & Fang, Y. (2008). Multiconstrained QoS Multipath Routing in Wireless Sensor Networks. *Wireless Networks*, *14*(4), 465–478. doi:10.1007/s11276-006-0731-9

Intanagonwiwat, C., Govindan, R., & Estrin, D. (2000). Directed diffusion: A scalable and robust communication paradigm for sensor networks. In *Proceedings of the 6th Annual ACM/IEEE International Conference on Mobile Computing and Networking (MobiCom'00)*, Boston, (pp. 56-67).

Jamoussi, B., Andersson, L., Callon, R., Dantu, R., Wu, L., & Doolan, P., et al. (2002). *Constraint-based LSP Setup Using LDP, RFC 3212.*

Jorge, L., & Gomes, T. (2006). Survey of Recovery Schemes in MPLS Networks. *International Conference on Dependability of Computer Systems (DepCos-RELCOMEX '06)*, (pp. 110-118).

Kang, Y.-H., & Lee, J.-H. (2005). The implementation of the premium services for MPLS IP VPNs. In *The 7th International Conference on Advanced Communication Technology (ICACT 2005)*, (pp. 1107-1110).

Karl, H., & Willig, A. (2005). *Protocols and Architectures for Wireless Sensor Networks*. Chichester, UK: John Wiley & Sons. doi:10.1002/0470095121

Koubâa, A., Alves, M., Tovar, E., & Cunha, A. (2008). An Implicit GTS Allocation Mechanism in IEEE 802.15.4 for Time-sensitive Wireless Sensor Networks: Theory and Practice. *ACM Real-Time Systems*, *39*(1-3), 169–204. doi:10.1007/s11241-007-9038-x

Kulik, J., Heinzelman, W. R., & Balakrishnan, H. (2002). Negotiation-based protocols for disseminating information in wireless sensor networks. *Wireless Networks*, *8*(2/3), 169–185. doi:10.1023/A:1013715909417

Lai, W. (2005). *Bandwidth Constraints Models for Differentiated Services (Diffserv)-aware MPLS Traffic Engineering: Performance Evaluation, RFC 4128.*

Le Faucheur, F. (2003). *Requirements for support of Differentiated Services-aware MPLS Traffic Engineering, RFC 3564.*

Le Faucheur, F., Wu, L., Davie, B., Davari, S., Vaananen, P., Krishnan, R., Cheval, P., & Heinanen, J., (2002). *Multi-Protocol Label Switching (MPLS) Support of Differentiated Services, RFC 3270.*

Li, Y., Chen, C. S., Song, Y.-Q., & Wang, Z. (2007). Real-time QoS support in wireless sensor networks: a survey. In *7th IFAC International Conference on Fieldbuses & Networks in Industrial & Embedded Systems (FeT'2007)*, Toulouse, France.

Lima, S. R., Carvalho, P., & Freitas, V. (2004). Distributed Admission Control for QoS and SLS Management. *Journal of Network and Systems Management. Special Issue on Distributed Management*, *12*(3), 397–426.

Mahapatra, A., Anand, K., & Agrawal, D. P. (2006). QoS and Energy Aware Routing for Real-time Traffic in Wireless Sensor Networks. *Computer Communications*, *29*(4), 437–445. doi:10.1016/j.comcom.2004.12.028

Manjeshwar, A., & Agarwal, D. P. (2001). TEEN: a routing protocol for enhanced efficiency in wireless sensor networks. In *Proceeding of 15th International Parallel and Distributed Processing Symposium (IPDPS 2001)*, (pp. 2009-2015).

Manjeshwar, A., & Agarwal, D. P. (2002). APTEEN: A hybrid protocol for efficient routing and comprehensive information retrieval in wireless sensor networks. In *Proceeding of 16th Proceedings International Parallel and Distributed Processing Symposium (IPDPS 2002)*, (pp. 195-202).

Marsan, M., Casetti, A. C., Mardente, G., & Mellia, M. (2007). A framework for admission control and path allocation in DiffServ networks. *Computer Networks*, *51*(10), 2738–2752. doi:10.1016/j.comnet.2006.11.022

Martínez, J. F., García, A. B., Corredor, I., López, L., Hernández, V., & Dasilva, A. (2007). QoS in wireless sensor networks: survey and approach. In *Proceedings of the 2007 Euro American conference on Telematics and Information Systems (EATIS '07)*.

Nichols, K., Jacobson, V., & Zhang L. (1999). *A two-bit differentiated services architecture for the Internet, RFC 2638*.

Pereira, A., & Monteiro, E. (2006). Admission Control in IntServ to DiffServ mapping. *International conference on Networking and Services (ICNS '06)*, (pp. 83).

Pereira, M., Amorim, C., & Castro, M. (2003). Tutorial sobre Redes de Sensores. Universidade do Estado do Rio de Janeiro, Cadernos do IME. *Série Informática*, *14*, 39–53.

Polastre, J., Hill, J., & Culler, D. (2004). Versatile low power media access for wireless sensor networks. In *Proceedings of the 2nd International Conference on Embedded Networked Sensor Systems (SenSys '04)*, 95--107, New York.

Postigo-Boix, M., Garcia-Haro, J., & Melus-Moreno, J. L. (2007). A cost-efficient method for streaming stored content in a guaranteed QoS Internet. *Computer Networks*, *51*(1), 309–335. doi:10.1016/j.comnet.2006.05.002

Raj, A., & Oliver, C. I. (2007). A survey of IP and multiprotocol label switching fast reroute schemes. *Computer Networks*, *51*(8), 1882–1907. doi:10.1016/j.comnet.2006.09.010

Reid, D. & Katchabaw, M. (2006). Achieving Quality of Service through SCalable Aggregate Reservations. *INFOCOMP - Journal of Computer Science*, *5*(4), 9-18.

Rentala, P., Musunuri, R., Gandham, S., & Saxena, U. (2002). *Survey on Sensor Networks*. Technical Report No.UTDCS-33-02, University of Texas, Dallas, TX.

Rhee, I., Warrier, A., Aia, M., & Min, J. (2005). Z-MAC: a Hybrid MAC for Wireless Sensor Networks. In *Proceedings of the 3rd International Conference on Embedded Networked Sensor Systems (SenSys '05)*, (pp. 90 – 101), San Diego, CA.

Rosen, E., Viswanathan, A. & Callon, R. (2001). *Multiprotocol Label Switching Architecture, RFC 3031*.

Shenker, S., Partridge, C., & Guerin, R. (1997). *Specification of Guaranteed Quality of Service, RFC 2212*.

Teitelbaum, B., & Shalunov, S. (2002). *Why Premium IP Service Has Not Deployed*. Retrieved 01/12/2009 from http://qbone.internet2.edu/papers/non-architectural-problems.txt

Troubleyn, E., Poorter, E., Moerman, I., & Demeester, P. (2008). AMoQoSA: Adaptive Modular QoS Architecture for Wireless Sensor Networks. In *2nd IEEE International Conference on Sensor Technologies and Applications (SENSORCOMM 2008)*, (pp. 172 – 178), Cap Esterel, France.

Wang, Y., Liu, X., & Yin, J. (2006). Requirements of Quality of Service in Wireless Sensor Networks. In *Proceedings of the International Conference on Networking, International Conference on Systems an International Conference on Mobile Communications and Learning Technologies (ICNICONSMCL'06)*.

Wang, Z. (2001). *Internet QoS: Architectures and Mechanisms for Quality of Service*. San Mateo, CA: Morgan Kaufmann Publishers.

Wroclawski, J. (1997). *Specification of the Controlled-Load Network Element, RFC 2211*.

Xia, F. (2008). QoS Challenges and Opportunities in Wireless Sensor/Actuator Networks. *Sensors*, *8*(2), 1099–1110. doi:10.3390/s8021099

Xiao, X., & Ni, L. M. (1999). Internet QoS: a big picture. *IEEE Network*, *13*(2), 8–18. doi:10.1109/65.768484

Yaghmaee, M. H., Menhaj, M. B., & Amintoosi, H. (2005). Design and performance evaluation of a fuzzy based traffic conditioner for differentiated services. *Journal on Computer Networks, Elsevier*, *47*(6), 847–869. doi:10.1016/j.comnet.2004.09.003

Zhang, G., & Mouftah, H. T. (2001). End-to-end QoS guarantees over Diffserv networks. In *Proceedings of the Sixth IEEE Symposium on Computers and Communications*, (pp. 302-309).

Zhao, L., Xu, C., Xu, Y., & Li, X. (2006). Energy-Aware QoS Control for Wireless Sensor Network. In *1st IEEE Conference on Industrial Electronics and Applications (ICIEA 2006)*, 1–6.

Zhu, H., Li, M., Chlamtac, I., & Prabhakaran, B. (2004). A Survey of Quality of Service in IEEE 802.11 Networks. *IEEE Wireless Communications*, *11*(4), 6–14. doi:10.1109/MWC.2004.1325887

Chapter 3
IP Quality of Service Models

Sherine M. Abd El-Kader
Electronics Research Institute, Egypt

ABSTRACT

Currently the Internet offers a point-to-point delivery service, which is based on the "best effort" delivery model. In this model, data will be delivered to its destination as soon as possible, but with no commitment about bandwidth or latency. Using protocols such as the Transmission Control Protocol (TCP), the highest guarantee the network provides is reliable data delivery. This is adequate for traditional data applications like e-mail, web browsing, File Transfer Protocol (FTP) and Telnet, but inadequate for applications requiring timeliness. For example, multimedia conferencing or audio and video streaming applications, which require high bandwidth capacity and are sensitive to delay and delay variation. For these applications to perform adequately, Quality of Services (QoS) must be quantified and managed, and the Internet must be modified to support real-time QoS and controlled end-to-end delays. The efforts to enable end-to-end QoS over the Internet Protocol version 4 (IPv4) networks have led to the development of two different architectures, the Integrated services architecture (Intserv) and the Differentiated services architecture (Diffserv), which although different, support services that go beyond the best effort service. This chapter will present a detailed discussion on these IPv4 quality of services models. First, the Integrated services architecture with its related issues such as the reservation setup protocol will be demonstrated. Second, the Differentiated services architecture with a description of the services they provide will be described. Finally, a comparison between the Best-effort, the Integrated and Differentiated services will be done.

INTRODUCTION

The current Internet consists of multitude of networks built from various link-layer technologies and relies on the Internet protocol to interwork between them. IPv4 makes no assumptions about the underlying protocol stacks and offers an unreliable, connectionless network-layer service that is subject to packet loss, reordering, packet duplication, and

DOI: 10.4018/978-1-61520-791-6.ch003

queuing delay in router buffers, all of these will increase with the network load. Because of the lack of any firm guarantees, the traditional IP delivery model is often referred to as Best-Effort (BE), so additional higher-layer end-to-end protocol such as TCP required to provide end-to-end reliability. TCP does this through the use of such mechanisms as packet retransmission, which further adds to the overall information transfer delay.

For traditional non-real-time Internet traffic such as FTP data, the best-effort delivery model of IPv4 has not been a problem. However, as we move further into the age of multimedia communications, many real-time applications are being developed that are delay-sensitive to the point where the best-effort delivery model of IP can be inadequate (Kamel, Elzarki, Eissa, & Abd El-kader, 2002). So there is still a firm need to provide many applications with additional service classes offering enhanced QoS with regard to bandwidth, packet queuing delay, and loss (Huston, 2000). These additional enhanced QoS delivery classes would supplement the BE delivery service in what could be described as an Integrated services Internet (Braden, Clark, & Shenker, 1994) and Differentiated services Internet (Blake, Black, Carlson, Davies, Wang, & Weiss, 1998).

The Integrated Services architecture provides QoS guarantees, but due to per flow management of traffic introduces severe scalability in the core network element, i.e. router where the number of flows reaches up to millions. It has proven to be easily deployable only in access networks where the number of flows is rather moderate in terms of scalability issues. Learning from the first experiences with Intserv, researchers developed a new architecture, i.e. Diffserv, which is intended to avoid the scalability problems and complexity of Intserv Architecture. Diffserv provides quality differentiation on aggregates without strict guarantees on individual flows, where QoS is attained by marking packets at the boundaries. Even though it seems that the Diffserv architecture has lots of obvious advantages towards Intserv as being relatively simple and more scalable, Intserv has also advantages applicable to specific network environments. Intserv provides end-to-end per-flow guarantees on the applications requirements and consequently achieves high utilization of the network resources, while Diffserv is not intended to provide end-to-end per application guarantees, rather it provides service differentiation on aggregates. These Intserv characteristics are especially desirable in an environment where the network resources are scarce, the available bandwidth is difficult to predict and where the guaranteed service for flows and high utilization is essential for the overall operation.

INTEGRATED SERVICE

The Internet Integrated services framework provides the ability for applications to choose among multiple, controlled levels of delivery service for their data packets. To support this capability, two things are required; first, individual network elements (subnets and IP routers) along the path followed by an application's data packets must support mechanisms to control the quality of service delivered to those packets. Second, a way to communicate the application's requirements to network elements along the path and to convey QoS management information between network elements and the application must be provided.

In the integrated services framework the first function is provided by QoS control services such as Controlled-Load service (Wroclawski, 1997) and Guaranteed service (Shenker, Partridge, & Guerin, 1997). The second function may be provided in a number of ways, but it is frequently implemented by a Resource Reservation Setup Protocol such as RSVP (Black, Brim, Carpenter, & Le Faucheur, 2001).

Reference Implementation Framework

A reference implementation framework is proposed to realize the Intserv mode. This framework includes four components: the packet scheduler, the classifier, the admission control routine, and the reservation setup protocol.

Traffic Control

For Intserv, a router must implement an appropriate QoS for each flow, in accordance with the service model. The router function that creates different qualities of service is called traffic control. Traffic control in turn is implemented by three components: the packet scheduler, the classifier, and admission control.

- **Packet Scheduler:** The packet scheduler manages the forwarding of different packet streams using a set of queues. The packet scheduler must be implemented at the point where packets are queued. The basic function of packet scheduling is to reorder the output queue. There are many possible ways to manage the output queue, and the resulting behavior. Perhaps the simplest approach is a priority scheme, in which packets are ordered by priority, and highest priority packets always leave first. An alternative scheduling scheme is round –robin, which gives different classes of packets access to a share of the link. A variant called Weighted Fair Queuing (WFQ), has been demonstrated to allocate the total bandwidth of a link into specified shares (Chandrasekaran, 2001). There are more complex schemes for queue management, most of which involve observing the service objectives of individual packets, such as delivery deadline, and ordering packets based on these criteria.
- **Classifier:** For the purpose of traffic control, each incoming packet must be mapped into a class; all packets in the same class get the same treatment from the packet scheduler. This mapping is performed by the classifier. Choice of a class may be based upon the contents of the existing packet header(s) and/or some additional classification number added to each packet.
- **Admission Control:** Admission control implements the decision algorithm that a router or host uses to determine whether a new flow can be granted the requested QoS without impacting earlier guarantees. Admission control is invoked at each node to make a local accept/reject decision, at the time a host requests a real-time service along some path through the Internet.

Reservation Setup Protocol

The RSVP protocol is used by a host to request specific qualities of service from the network for particular application data streams or flows. RSVP is also used by routers to deliver QoS requests to all nodes along the path(s) of the flows and to establish and maintain state to provide the requested service. RSVP requests will generally result in resources being reserved in each node along the data path (Braden, Zhang, Berson, Herzog, 1997).

RSVP operates on top of IPv4 or IPv6, occupying the place of a transport protocol in the protocol stack. However, RSVP does not transport application data but is rather an Internet control protocol, like ICMP, IGMP. RSVP is not also a routing protocol; RSVP is designed to operate with current and future unicast and multicast routing protocols. An RSVP process consults the local routing database(s) to obtain routes. In the multicast case, for example, a host sends IGMP messages to join a multicast group and then sends RSVP messages to reserve resources along the delivery path(s) of that group. Routing protocols determine where packets get forwarded; RSVP is only concerned with the QoS of those packets that are forwarded in accordance with routing. The two principle characteristics of RSVP are; first, the RSVP provides reservations for bandwidth in multicast trees (unicast is handled as special case).

Figure 1. The direction of the RSVP messages

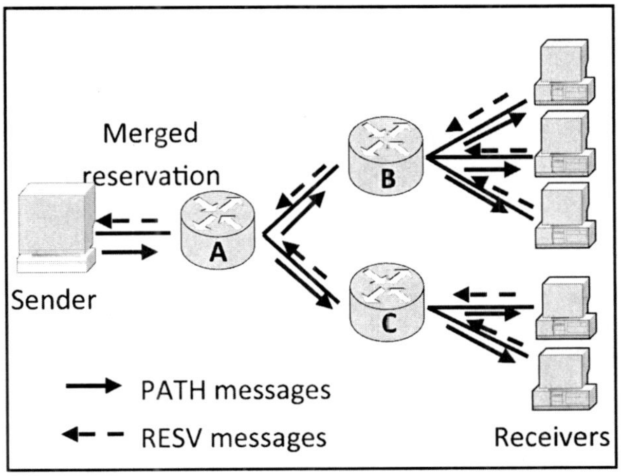

Second, It is receiver-oriented, i.e., the receiver of a data flow initiates and maintains the resource reservation used for that flow.

In order to efficiently accommodate large groups, dynamic group membership, and heterogeneous receiver requirements, RSVP makes receivers responsible for requesting a specific QoS. A QoS request from a receiver host application is passed to the local RSVP process. The RSVP protocol then carries the request to all the nodes (routers and hosts) along the reverse data path(s) to the data source(s), but only as far as the router where the receiver's data path joins the multicast distribution tree. As a result, RSVP's reservation overhead is in general logarithmic rather than linear in the number of receivers (Postigo-Boix, Melu´s-Moreno, 2007).

RSVP Messages

The primary messages used by RSVP are the Path message, which originates from the traffic sender, and the Resv message, which originates from the traffic receivers. Figure (1) shows an example of RSVP for a multicast session.

The primary roles of the Path message are first to let the routers know on which links they should forward the reservation messages. Specifically, a path message sent within the multicast tree from a Router A to a Router B contains Router A's unicast IP address. Router B puts this address in a path-state table, and when it receives a reservation message from a downstream node it accesses the table and learns that it should send a reservation message up the multicast tree to Router A. And second to provide receivers with information about the characteristics of the sender traffic and end-to-end path so that they can make appropriate reservation requests. Each Path message includes the following information:

- *Previous HOP (PHOP)*, the address of the last RSVP-capable node to forward this Path message. This address is updated at every RSVP-capable router along the path.
- *The Sender Template*, a filter specification identifying the sender. It contains the IP address of the sender and optionally the sender port.
- *The Sender Tspec* defining the sender traffic characteristics.
- *An optional Adspec* containing One Pass With Advertising (OPWA) information which is updated at every RSVP-capable router along the path to attain end-to-end significance before being presented to

receivers to enable them to calculate the level of resources that must be reserved to obtain a given end-to-end QoS.

The primary role of the Resv message is to carry reservation requests to the routers along the distribution tree between receivers and senders.

Reservation Styles

RSVP offers several different reservation styles, which determine the manner in which the resource requirements of multiple receivers are aggregated in the routers. These styles allow the reserved resources to more efficiently meet application requirements. There are currently three reservation styles defined: wildcard-filter style; fixed-filter style; and shared-explicit style.

- *Wildcard-Filter Style*: When a receiver uses the wildcard-filter style in its reservation message, it is telling the network that it wants to receive all flows from all upstream senders in the session and that its bandwidth reservation is to be shared among the senders.
- *Fixed-Filter Style:* When a receiver uses the fixed-filter style in its reservation message, it specifies a list of senders from which it wants to receive a data flow along with a bandwidth reservation for each of these senders. These reservations are distinct, i.e., they are not to be shared.
- *Shared-Explicit Style:* When a receiver uses the shared-explicit style in its reservation message, it specifies a list of senders from which it wants to receive a data flow along with a single bandwidth reservation. This reservation is to be shared among all the senders in the list.

Shared reservations, created by the wildcard filter and the shared-explicit styles, are appropriate for a multicast session whose sources are unlikely to transmit simultaneously. Packetized audio is an example of an application suitable for shared reservations; because a limited number of people talk at once, each receiver might issue a wildcard-filter or a shared-explicit reservation request for twice the bandwidth required for one sender to allow for over speaking. On the other hand, the fixed-filter reservation, which creates distinct reservations for the flows from different senders, is appropriate for video teleconferencing.

Integrated Services Classes

Once an appropriate reservation has been installed in each router along the path, the data flow can expect to receive an end-to-end QoS commitment provided no path changes or router failures occur during the lifetime of the flow, and provided the data flow conforms to the traffic envelope supplied in the request. Service-specific policing and traffic reshaping actions will be employed within the network to ensure that nonconforming data flows do not affect the QoS commitments for behaving data flows. The IETF has considered two QoS classes, Guaranteed Service and Controlled-Load Service.

Guaranteed Service

Guaranteed Service provides an assured level of bandwidth, a firm end-to-end delay bound, and no queuing loss for conforming packets of a data flow. It is intended for applications with stringent real-time delivery requirements, such as certain audio and video applications that use "playback" buffers and are intolerant of any datagram arriving after their playback time (Shenker, Partridge, & Guerin, 1997).

Each router characterizes the guaranteed service for a specific flow by allocating a bandwidth, *R*, and buffer space, *B*, that the flow may consume. This is done by approximating the "fluid model" of service (Tang, & Charles, 1999) so that the flow effectively sees a dedicated wire of bandwidth R between source and receiver. In a perfect fluid model, a flow conforming to a token bucket of rate r and depth b will have its delay bound by b/R provided $R \geq r$. To allow for deviations from this perfect fluid model in the router's approximation, two error terms, C and D, are introduced; consequently, the delay bound now becomes $b/R + C/R + D$. Where C is the rate-dependent error term, which represents the delay a datagram in the flow might experience due to the rate parameters of the flow. And D is the rate-independent error term which represents the worst case non-rate-based transit time variation through the service element, it is generally determined or set at boot or configuration time. However, with guaranteed service a limit is imposed on the peak rate p of the flow, which results in a reduction of the delay bound. In addition, the packetization effect of the flow needs to be taken into account by considering the maximum packet size M. These additional factors result in a more precise bound on the end-to-end queuing delay as follows:

$$Q_{\text{end-to-end delay}} = \frac{(b-M)(p-R)}{R(p-r)} + \frac{(M+C_{tot})}{R} + D_{tot} \; (\text{case } p > R \geq r) \quad (2.1)$$

$$Q_{\text{end-to-end delay}} = \frac{(M+C_{tot})}{R} + D_{tot} \; (\text{case } R \geq p \geq r) \quad (2.2)$$

Where C_{tot} and D_{tot} represent the summation of the C and D error terms, respectively, for each router along the end-to-end data path. In order for a router to invoke guaranteed service for a specific data flow, it needs to be informed of the traffic characteristics, *Tspec*, of the flow along with the reservation characteristics, *Rspec*. Furthermore, C_{tot} and D_{tot} are required to enable the router to calculate sufficient local resources to guarantee a lossless service.

Tspec parameters:

- p = peak rate of flow (bytes/s),
- b = bucket depth, can range from 1 byte to 250 gigabytes,
- r = token bucket rate, can range from 1 bytes/s to maximum 40 terabytes/s,
- m = minimum policed unit (Any IP datagram < m will be of size m, bytes),
- M = maximum datagram size (bytes).

Rspec parameters:

- R = bandwidth, i.e., service rate (bytes/s),
- S = slack term (ms).

Where S represents the amount by which the end-to-end delay bound will be below the end-to-end delay required by the application.

Guaranteed service traffic must be policed at the network access points to ensure conformance to the *Tspec*. The usual enforcement policy is to forward nonconforming packets as BE datagrams; if and when a marking facility becomes available, these nonconforming datagrams should be marked to ensure that they are treated as BE datagrams at all subsequent routers. In addition to policing of data flows at the edge of the network, guaranteed service also requires reshaping of traffic to the token bucket of the reserved *Tspec* at certain points on the distribution tree. Any packets failing the reshaping are treated as BE and marked accordingly if such a facility is available. Reshaping must be applied at any points where it is possible for a data flow to exceed the reserved *Tspec* even when all senders associated with the data flow conform to their individual *Tspecs*.

Controlled-Load Service

Unlike guaranteed service, controlled-load service (Wroclawski, 1997) provides no firm quantitative guarantees. A *Tspec* for the flow desiring controlled-load service must be submitted to the router as for the case of guaranteed service, although it is not necessary to include the peak rate parameter. If the flow is accepted for controlled-load service, the router makes a commitment to offer the flow a service equivalent to that seen by a BE flow on a lightly loaded network. The important difference is that the controlled-load flow does not noticeably deteriorate as the network load increases. This will be true regardless of the level of load increase. By contrast, a BE flow would experience progressively worse service (higher delay and loss) as the network load increased. Controlled-load service is intended for those classes of applications that can tolerate a certain amount of loss and delay provided it is kept to a reasonable level. Examples of applications in this category include adaptive real-time applications.

Routers implementing the controlled-load service must check for conformance of controlled-load data flows to their appropriate reserved *Tspecs*. Any nonconforming controlled-load data flows must not be allowed to affect the QoS offered to conforming controlled-load data flows or to unfairly affect the handling of BE traffic. Within these constraints the router should attempt to forward as many of the packets of the nonconforming controlled-load data flow as possible. This might be done by dividing the packets into conforming and nonconforming groups and forwarding the nonconforming group on a BE basis. Alternatively, the router may choose to degrade the QoS of all packets of a nonconforming controlled-load data flow equally.

DIFFERENTIATED SERVICES

As work on Intserv has proceeded, researchers involved with these efforts have begun to uncover some of the difficulties associated with the Intserv model and per-flow reservation of resources, which is listed below:

- *Scalability:* Per-flow resource reservation implies the need for a router to process resource reservations and to maintain per-flow state for each flow passing though the router. So per-flow reservation processing represents a considerable overhead in large networks.
- *Flexible Service Models:* The Intserv framework provides for a small number of pre-specified service classes. This particular set of service classes does not allow for more qualitative or relative definitions of service distinctions (e.g., "Service class A will received preferred treatment over service class B").
- *Better-than-best-effort service to applications without the need for host RSVP signaling:* Few hosts in today's Internet are able to generate RSVP signaling or express their traffic characteristics or performance requirements in the detail needed by the Intserv mode. As noted above, many applications and users may only want to specify a more qualitative notion of the service they require e.g., "Better service than class B receives".

These considerations have led to the Differentiated Services. The diffserv working group is developing an architecture for providing scalable and flexible service differentiation, i.e., the ability to handle different classes of traffic in different ways within the Internet. The need for scalability arises from the fact that hundreds of thousands simultaneous source-destination traffic flows may be present at a core router. This need is met by placing only simple functionality within the network core, with more complex control operations being implemented towards the edge of the network. The need for flexibility arises from the fact that new service classes may arise and old service classes may become obsolete. The Diffserv architecture is flexible in the sense that it does not define specific services or service classes as in the case of Intserv. Instead, the Diffserv architecture provides the functional components, i.e., the "pieces" of a network architecture, with which such services can be built.

Differentiated Services Architectural Model

The Differentiated Services (DS) architecture consists of two sets of functional elements implemented in network nodes (Blake, Black, Carlson, Davies, Wang, & Weiss, 1998):

- *Edge functions* (packet classification and traffic conditioning): At the incoming edge of the network, i.e., at either a DS -capable host that generates traffic and/or at the first DS -capable router that the traffic passes through, arriving packets are marked by setting the DS field of the packet header to some value. The mark that a packet receives identifies the class of traffic to which it belongs. Different classes of traffic will then receive different service within the core network. Conditioning functions including metering, marking, shaping and policing.
- *Core function* (forwarding): When a DS-marked packet arrives at a DS-capable router, the packet is forwarded onto its next hop according to the so-called per-hop behavior associated with that packet's class. The per-hop behavior will influence the sharing a router's buffers and link bandwidth among the competing classes of traffic. A crucial tenet of the DS architecture is that a router's forwarding behavior will be based only on packet markings, i.e., the behavior aggregate (the class of traffic) to which a packet belongs.

Differentiated Services Domain

A DS domain is a contiguous set of DS nodes which operate with a common service provisioning policy and set of Per-Hop Behavior (PHB) groups implemented on each node (Nichols, Blake, Baker, & Black, 1998). A DS domain normally consists of one or more networks under the same administration; for example, an organization's Intranet or an Internet Service Provider (ISP). The administration of the domain is responsible for ensuring that adequate resources are provisioned and/or reserved to support the Service Level Agreement (SLA) offered by the domain.

A DS domain consists of DS boundary nodes and DS interior nodes. DS boundary nodes interconnect the DS domain to other DS or non-DS-capable domains, while DS interior nodes only connect to other DS interior or boundary nodes within the same DS domain. Both DS boundary nodes and interior nodes must be able to apply the appropriate PHB to packets based on the DS codepoint (Nichols, Blake, Baker, & Black, 1998); otherwise unpredictable behavior may result. In addition, DS boundary nodes may be required to perform traffic conditioning functions as defined by a Traffic Conditioning Agreement (TCA) between their DS domain and the peering domain which they connect to. Interior nodes may be able to perform limited traffic conditioning functions such as DS codepoint re-marking. Interior nodes which implement more complex classification and traffic conditioning functions are analogous to DS boundary nodes.

A host in a network containing a DS domain may act as a DS boundary node for traffic from applications running on that host; we therefore say that the host is within the DS domain. If a host does not act as a boundary node, then the DS node topologically closest to that host acts as the DS boundary node for that host's traffic (Abd El-kader, 2003).

Traffic Classification and Conditioning

The packet classification policy identifies the subset of traffic which may receive a differentiated service by being conditioned and/ or mapped to one or more behavior aggregates (by DS codepoint re-marking) within the DS domain. Traffic conditioning performs metering, shaping, policing and/ or re- marking to ensure that the traffic entering the DS domain conforms to the rules specified in the TCA, in accordance with the domain's service provisioning policy.

1. Classifiers Packet classifiers select packets in a traffic stream based on the content of some portion of the packet header. There are two types of classifiers, the Behavior Aggregate (BA) Classifier which classifies packets based on the DS codepoint only and the MF (Multi-Field) classifier that selects packets based on the value of a combination of one or more header fields, such as source address, destination address, DS field, protocol ID, source port and destination port numbers, and other information such as incoming interface. Classifiers are used to "steer" packets matching some specified rule to an element of a traffic conditioner for further processing. Classifiers must be configured by some management procedure in accordance with the appropriate TCA.
2. Traffic Profiles A traffic profile specifies the temporal properties of a traffic stream selected by a classifier. It provides rules for determining whether a particular packet is in-profile or out-of-profile. For example, a profile based on a token bucket (Tang, & Charles, 1999) may look like:

Codepoint = X, use token-bucket r, b

The above profile indicates that all packets marked with DS codepoint X should be measured against a token bucket meter with rate r and burst size b. In this example out-of-profile packets are those packets in the traffic stream which arrive when insufficient tokens are available in the bucket. The concept of in- and out-of-profile can be extended to more than two levels, e.g., multiple levels of conformance with a profile may be defined and enforced. Different conditioning actions may be applied to the in-profile packets and out-of-profile packets. In-profile packets may be allowed to enter the DS domain without further conditioning. Out-of- profile packets may be queued until they are in-profile (shaped), discarded (policed), marked with a new codepoint (re-marked), or forwarded unchanged while triggering some accounting procedure. Out-of-profile packets may be mapped to one or more behavior aggregates that are "inferior" in some dimension of forwarding performance to the BA into which in-profile packets are mapped (Abd El-kader, Eissa, & Baraka, 2001).

TRAFFIC CONDITIONERS

A traffic conditioner may contain the following elements: meter, marker, shaper, and dropper. A traffic stream is selected by a classifier, which steers the packets to a logical instance of a traffic conditioner. A meter is used to measure the traffic stream against a traffic profile. The state of the meter with respect to a particular packet (whether it is in- or out- of-profile) may be used to affect a marking, dropping, or shaping action. When packets exit the traffic conditioner of a DS boundary node the DS codepoint of each packet must be set to an appropriate value. Figure (2) shows the block diagram of a classifier and traffic conditioner. Note that a traffic conditioner may not necessarily contain all four elements. For example, in the case where no traffic profile is in effect, packets may only pass through a

Figure 2. Logical view of a packet classifier and traffic conditioner

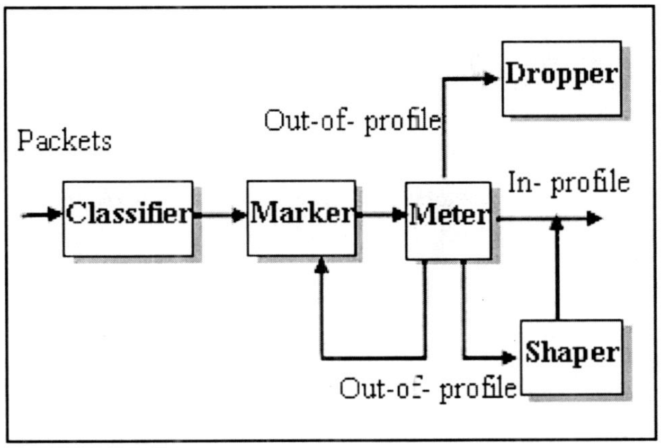

classifier and a marker (Abd El-kader, Eissa, & Baraka, 2002).

- *Markers:* Packet markers set the DS field of a packet to a particular codepoint, adding the marked packet to a particular DS behavior aggregate. The marker may be configured to mark all packets which are steered to it to a single codepoint, or may be configured to mark a packet to one of a set of codepoints used to select a PHB in a PHB group, according to the state of a meter. When the marker changes the codepoint in a packet it is said to have "re-marked" the packet.
- *Meters*: Traffic meters measure the temporal properties of the stream of packets selected by a classifier against a traffic profile specified in a TCA. A meter passes state information to other conditioning functions to trigger a particular action for each packet which is either in- or out-of-profile.
- *Shapers:* Shapers delay some or all of the packets in a traffic stream in order to bring the stream into compliance with a traffic profile. A shaper usually has a finite-size buffer, and packets may be discarded if there is not sufficient buffer space to hold the delayed packets.
- *Droppers:* Droppers discard some or all of the packets in a traffic stream in order to bring the stream into compliance with a traffic profile. This process is known as "policing" the stream. Note that a dropper can be implemented as a special case of a shaper by setting the shaper buffer size to zero (or a few) packets.

Location of Traffic Conditioners and MF Classifiers

Traffic conditioners are usually located within DS ingress and egress boundary nodes, but may also be located in nodes within the interior of a DS domain, or within a non-DS-capable domain.

- *Within the Source Domain:* The source domain is defined as the domain containing the node(s) which originate the traffic receiving a particular service. Traffic sources and intermediate nodes within a source domain may perform traffic classification and conditioning functions. The traffic originating from the source domain across a boundary may be marked by the traffic sources directly or by intermediate nodes before leaving the source domain. This is referred to as initial marking or "pre- marking". There are some advantages to marking packets close to the traffic source. First, a traffic source can more easily take an application's preferences into account when deciding which packets should receive better forwarding treatment. Also, classification of packets is much simpler before the traffic has been aggregated with packets from other sources, since the number of classification rules which need to be applied within a single node is reduced.

- *At the Boundary of a DS Domain*: Traffic streams may be classified, marked, and otherwise conditioned on either end of a boundary link (the DS egress node of the upstream domain or the DS ingress node of the downstream domain). The SLA between the domains should specify which domain has responsibility for mapping traffic streams to DS behavior aggregates and conditioning those aggregates in conformance with the appropriate TCA. However, a DS ingress node must assume that the incoming traffic may not conform to the TCA and must be prepared to enforce the TCA in accordance with local policy. When packets are pre-marked and conditioned in the upstream domain, potentially fewer classification and traffic conditioning rules need to be supported in the downstream DS domain. In this circumstance the downstream DS domain may only need to re-mark or police the incoming behavior aggregates to enforce the TCA. However, more sophisticated services which are path- or source-dependent may require MF classification in the downstream DS domain's ingress nodes.
- *In non-DS-Capable Domains*: Traffic sources or intermediate nodes in a non-DS-capable domain may employ traffic conditioners to pre-mark traffic before it reaches the ingress of a downstream DS domain. In this way the local policies for classification and marking may be concealed.
- *In Interior DS Nodes:* Although the basic architecture assumes that complex classification and traffic conditioning functions are located only in a network's ingress and egress boundary nodes, deployment of these functions in the interior of the network is not precluded. For example, more restrictive access policies may be enforced on a transoceanic link, requiring MF classification and traffic conditioning functionality in the upstream node on the link. This approach may have scaling limits, due to the potentially large number of classification and conditioning rules that might need to be maintained.

Per-Hop Behaviors

The first key component of the DS architecture as mentioned early is the edge functions and the second key component involves the packet forwarding function performed by DS-capable routers (Nichols, & Carpenter, 2001). The Per-Hop Behavior (PHB) is defined as "a description of the externally observable forwarding behavior of a DS node applied to a particular DS behavior aggregate." Currently, two PHB's are under active discussion within the Diffserv working group; an Expedited Forwarding (EF) PHB (Jacobson, Nichols, & Poduri, 1999) and an Assured Forwarding (AF) PHB (Heinanen, Baker, Weiss, & Wroclawski, 1999):

Premium Service

Premium Service provides low-delay and low-jitter service for applications that generate fixed peak bit-rate traffic (Jacobson, Nichols, & Poduri, 1999). Each application will have a SLA with its ISP. The SLA specifies a desired peak bit-rate for a specific flow or an aggregation of flows. The application is responsible for not exceeding the peak rate. Otherwise, excess traffic will be dropped. The ISP guarantees that the contracted bandwidth will be available when traffic is sent. Premium Service is suitable for Internet Telephony, Video Conferencing, or for creating *virtual lease lines* for *Virtual Private Networks* (VPNs).

Because Premium Service is more expensive than Assured Service, it is desirable for ISPs to support both static SLAs and dynamic SLAs. Dynamic SLAs allow applications to request for Premium Service on demand without subscribing to it. Admission control is needed for dynamic SLAs. Premium Service can be implemented as follows. At the applications side, some entity will decide which application flow can use Premium Service. The leaf routers directly connected to the senders will do MF classifications and shape the traffic. The exit routers of the application domain may need to reshape the traffic to make sure that the traffic does not exceed the peak rate specified by the SLA. At the provider side, the ingress routers will police the traffic. Excess traffic is dropped. All packets that demand Premium Service enter a *Premium Queue* (PQ), packets in the PQ will be sent before packets in the *Assured Queue* (AQ).

Assured Service

Assured Service is intended for applications that need reliable services from their service providers, even in time of network congestion (Heinanen, Baker, Weiss, & Wroclawski, 1999). Applications will have SLAs with their ISPs. The SLAs will specify the amount of bandwidth allocated for the applications. Senders are responsible for deciding how their applications share that amount of bandwidth. SLAs for Assured Service are usually static, meaning that the senders can start data transmission whenever they want without signaling their ISPs.

The Assured Forwarding PHB is more complex. AF divides traffic into four classes, where each AF class is guaranteed to be provided with some minimum amount of bandwidth and buffering. Within each class, packets are further partitioned into one of three "drop preference" categories. When congestion occurs within an AF class, a router can then discard (drop) packets based on their drop preference values. Assured Service can be implemented as follows. First, classification and policing are done at the ingress routers of the ISP networks. If the Assured Service traffic does not exceed the bit-rate specified by the SLA, they are considered as *in* profile. Otherwise, the excess packets are considered as *out* of profile. Second, all packets, *in* and *out*, are put into an AQ to avoid out of order delivery. Third, the queue is managed by a queue management scheme called *RED with In and Out*, or *RIO* .

Random Early Detection *(RED)* is a queue management scheme that drops packets randomly. This will trigger the TCP flow control mechanisms at different end hosts to reduce send rates at different time. By doing so, RED can prevent the queue at the routers from overflowing, and therefore avoid the tail-drop behavior (dropping all subsequent packets when a queue overflows). Tail-drop triggers multiple TCP flows to decrease and later increase their rates simultaneously. It causes network utilization to oscillate and can hurt performance significantly. RED has been proved to be useful and has been widely deployed.

RIO is a more advanced RED scheme. It basically maintains two RED algorithms, one for *in* packets and one for *out* packets. There are two thresholds for each queue. When the queue size is below the first threshold, no packets are dropped. When the queue size is between the two thresholds, only *out* packets are randomly dropped. When the queue size exceeds the second threshold, indicating possible network congestion, both *in* and *out* packets are randomly dropped, but *out* packets are dropped more aggressively. In addition to breaking the TCP flow-control synchronization, RIO prevents, to some extent, greedy flows from hurting the performance of other flows by dropping the *out* packets more aggressively. Because *in* packets have low loss rate even in the cases of congestion, the applications will perceive a predictable service from the network if they keep traffic conformant. When there is no congestion, *out* packets will also be delivered. The networks are thus better utilized.

QBone Architecture

The goal of the Quality of service backBone model (*QBone*) is to provide an interdomain testbed for Diffserv, where the engineering, behavior, and policy consequences of new IP services can be explored (Teitelbaum, 1999). The *QBone* will be the first wide-area test of the evolving Diffserv architecture and the first experimental deployment of interdomain Diffserv. It is obviously that the *QBone* will grow incrementally as new QoS services. By establishing a highly instrumented test bed that is open and accessible to researchers and advanced development efforts, the *QBone* initiative seeks to advance the state of Diffserv technology.

A high-level architectural requirement of the *QBone* is contiguity. Unlike IPv6 and MBone technology, quality of service cannot be implemented as an overlay network service based on address aggregation only. The *QBone* is necessarily a contiguous set of DS domains. Within the *QBone*, each participating network is a DS Domain that interoperates with other *QBone* networks to provide the end-to-end *QBone* services.

QBone Premium Service (QPS)

A QPS reservation makes a simplex, peak-limited bandwidth assurance through multiple DS domains. The extent of a QPS reservation may be entirely within a *QBone* domain, from one edge of a *QBone* domain to another edge of the same domain, or through multiple *QBone* domains and is defined by a service source and service destination, each of which is, in general, defined by a network prefix.

The *QBone* architecture seeks to remain consistent with the Diffserv standards, so each network participating in the *QBone* will be considered a "DS domain" and the union of these networks - the *QBone* itself - a "DS region". *QBone* participants must cooperate to provide one or more interdomain services besides the default, traditional best effort IP service model. The first such service to be implemented is the Virtual Leased Line ("Premium") Service. Every *QBone* DS domain must support the Expedited Forwarding Per-Hop Behavior and configure its traffic classifiers and conditioners (meters, markers, shapers, and droppers) to provide a VLL service to EF aggregates.

Initiators of QPS reservations request and contract for a peak rate *peakRate* of EF traffic, at a specified maximum transmission unit *MTU* for transmission with a specified jitter bound *jitter*. Each QPS reservation is also parameterized by a DS-domain-to-DS-domain route *route* and a specified time interval {*startTime*, *endTime*}. In summary, a QPS reservation {*source, dest, route, startTime, endTime, peakRate, MTU, jitter*} is an agreement to provide the transmission assurances of the QBone Premium Service starting at *startTime* and ending at *endTime* across the chain of DS-domains *route* between source *source* and destination *dest* for EF traffic ingressing at *source* and conforming to a "CBR-like" traffic profile parameterized by a token bucket profiler with a token rate equal to *peakRate* bytes per second and bucket depth equal to *MTU* bytes.

The transmission assurance offered by the *QBone* Premium Service is as follows:

- *Low loss:* This should be very close to zero, but will not be quantified in this service definition.
- *Low latency:* The queuing delay within a QPS reservation will be minimal; however, no assumptions regarding minimal latency routing are made.
- *Low jitter:* The instantaneous packet delay variation within a QPS reservation should

be minimal; for each QPS reservation, an explicit jitter bound (jitter) is provided that captures the worst case variation in delay for traffic conforming to its QPS reservation profile; the bound jitter explicitly does not apply in the presence of IPv4 routing changes.

The transmission assurances of a QPS reservation remain valid only if the EF traffic ingressing at the source of the reservation extent conforms to the agreed upon token bucket profile *{peakRate, MTU}*. This can be achieved either by discarding non-conformant packets or by reshaping them until they are conformant. Because of synchronization effects, conformant EF behavior aggregates may be merged within a *QBone* domain to form an EF behavior aggregate that does not conform to a downstream QPS traffic profile. Consequently, each egressing EF behavior aggregate should be shaped to conform to the QPS traffic profile of the downstream *QBone* domain. Depending on the capabilities of the border router equipment, a QBone domain may shape on behalf of an upstream domain. If two adjacent *QBone* domains offer different transmission MTUs, then reshaping must occur at the boundary going from a larger to a smaller value.

Qbone Service Level Specifications (SLS)

Consistent with the Diffserv architectural model, all SLSs are determined bilaterally between adjacent *QBone* networks. However, to implement QPS, certain minimum requirements for any *QBone* SLS must be met. The following is a list of recommendations and requirements that needed for any *QBone* SLS supporting QPS. The list assumes a bilateral SLS between an upstream QBone DS domain U and a downstream *QBone* DS domain D.

1. Within the *QBone*, the DS Byte Codepoint 101110 should be used for the EF PHB.
2. D must respond to reservation requests from U. The protocol by which a reservation is established specifies how D must respond to admissions requests.
3. A necessary part of any SLS is a TCA that specifies how traffic is conditioned and policed on ingress. The TCA is a dynamic component of the SLS, which may need to be adjusted with the creation or teardown of every reservation across the boundary. To implement QPS, a TCA must specify:
   - *Traffic conditioning:* First, traffic must be conditioned into EF and non-EF traffic. Then EF traffic may be conditioned into either a single EF behavior aggregate or a set of EF BAs, each of which could be defined by destination prefix or by the egress link in domain D.
   - *Traffic profiles:* A traffic profile must be specified for each behavior aggregate. Given a peak rate *peak Rate* and MTU " *MTU*", the traffic profile is defined by a token bucket with:
   - A token rate equal to *peakRate* bytes per second;
   - A bucket depth equal to *MTU* bytes.
   - *Disposition of excess traffic:* Traffic within a BA that exceeds the aggregate's profile should be discarded.
   - *Shaping:* Shaping of individual traffic flows or aggregates may be supported by ingress/egress *QBone* boundary nodes as an option.
4. EF traffic conforming to the traffic profiles of the TCA will be given EF treatment across DS domain U toward its destination. The EF PHB requires the same low-loss, low-latency, low-jitter packet-delivery assurances discussed for the QPS above.
5. EF packets should be routed identically to packets with the default PHB (best-effort).

Every SLS must specify the jitter assurance made to conforming EF traffic.

COMPARISON BETWEEN BE, INTSERV, AND DIFFSERV

The BE is a single service model in which an application sends data whenever it must, in any quantity, and without requesting permission or first informing the network. For BE service, the network delivers data if it cans, without any assurance of reliability, delay bounds, or throughput, i.e., it doesn't make any promises about the QoS an application will receive. An application will receive whatever level of performance that the network is able to provide at that moment. Also it doesn't allow delay-sensitive multimedia application to request any special treatment. All packets are typically treated equally at the routers, including delay- sensitive audio and video packets.

The Integrated Service is a multiple service model that can accommodate multiple QoS requirements. The level of QoS provided by these enhanced QoS classes is programmable on a per-flow basis according to the end application requests. In this model the application requests a specific kind of service from the network before it sends data. The request is made by explicit signaling using a reservation protocol such as RSVP; the application informs the network of its traffic profile and requests a particular kind of service that can encompass its bandwidth and delay requirements. The application is expected to send data only after it gets a confirmation from the network. It is also expected to send data that lies within its described traffic profile. The network performs admission control, based on information from the application and available network resources. It also commits to meeting the QoS requirements of the application as long as the traffic remains within the profile specifications. The network fulfills its commitment by maintaining Per-flow State and then performing packet classification, policing, and intelligent queuing based on that state.

Nearly a decade of research has gone into this approach and the protocols have nearly become an Internet standard. It is a ready to use technology. However the breakthrough hasn't come yet. The reasons could be:

1. The amount of state information increases proportionally with the number of flows. This places a huge storage and processing overhead on the routers. Therefore, this architecture doesn't scale well in the Internet core,
2. The requirement on the routers is high. All routers must implement RSVP, admission control, MF classification and packet scheduling,
3. The IS service framework provides for a small number of pre-specified service classes. This particular set of services classes doesn't allow for more qualitative services,
4. Many applications need Better-than-best-effort service without the need for host RSVP signaling, because only few hosts in today's Internet are able to generate RSVP signaling or express their traffic characteristics or performance requirements in the detail needed by the Integrated Services model,
5. High complexity,
6. And insufficient application support.

Integrated Services can be useful in multicast environments (receiver-initiated reservation, request merging) and mission critical environment (hard real time applications like robot/machine control). Flow and Traffic Specifications can define fine-grained bandwidth and delay requirements.

Because of the difficulty in implementing and deploying Intserv and RSVP, Differentiated Ser-

Table 1. Comparison between BE, IS and DS

	BE	IS	DS
Setup	No	Dynamic per session	Static for long term
Model Functionality	Delivers data if it cans	Classification, scheduling, admission control and RSVP	Classification, marking, shaping, and PHB
QoS Guarantees	No	Yes	Yes
Services Classes	one	Guaranteed &control load service classes	One EF, four AF service classes
Complexity	Simple	complex	Simpler than IS
Scalability	Yes	No	Yes
Cost	Low	High	High

vices is introduced. Diffserv is a multiple service model that can satisfy differing QoS requirements. However, unlike the integrated service model, an application using Diffserv does not explicitly signal the router before sending data. The network of Diffserv tries to deliver a particular kind of service based on the QoS specified by each packet. This specification can occur in different ways, for example, using the IPv4 Precedence bit settings in IP packets or source and destination addresses. The network uses the QoS specification to classify, mark, shape, and police traffic, and to perform intelligent queuing.

Diffserv is significantly different from Intserv in:

1. The amount of state information is proportional to the number of classes rather than the number of flows. So Differentiated Service is more scalable,
2. Sophisticated classification, marking, policing and shaping are only needed at boundary of the networks. Core routers need only to implement behavior aggregate classification. Therefore, it is easier to implement and deploy Diffserv,
3. The Diffserv architecture is flexible in the sense that it does not define specific services or service classes as in the case of Intserv. Instead, the Diffserv architecture provides the functional components, i.e., the "pieces" of a network architecture, with which such services can be built,
4. Much simpler approach.

The differentiated service model is used for several mission-critical applications. Typically, this service model is appropriate for aggregate flows because it performs a relatively coarse level of traffic classification.

However Differentiated Services are in the stage of an Internet Draft, and there are still big changes in the architecture. Service models and the semantic of the TOS byte needs to be defined. Signaling could provide dynamic reservations and extensions toward receiver initiated reservation are thinkable. This makes the Differentiated Services approach even more attractive. However the changes in the TOS byte can become a big obstacle for Differentiated Services since it involves a major change in one of the fundamentals of the Internet: the IPv4 Header definition.Table (1) summarizes the above discussion about the differences between best effort, integrated services, and differentiated services.

REFERENCES

Abd El-kader, S., Eissa, H. & Baraka, H. (2001). A New Proposed No-Loss\No-Delay Effective Network Resources Consumer Meter. The Egyptian Computer Journal. Institute of Statistical Studies and Research, 29(1), 34–44.

Abd El-kader. S., Eissa, H. & Baraka, H. (2002). Real-time Voice Quality Guarantee on the IP Based Networks. In The 8th IEEE International Conference On Communication Systems, (pp. 510-514).

Abd El-kader. S. (2003). A New Scalable Quality Guaranteed Model For The Real-Time Multimedia Communications Across the Internet. Ph.D thesis, Faculty of Engineering, Cairo University, Cairo, Egypt.

Black, D., Brim, S., Carpenter, B., & Le Faucheur, F. (2001). Per Hop Behavior Identification Codes. RFC 3140.

Blake, S., Black, D., Carlson, M., Davies, E., Wang, Z. & Weiss, W. (1998). An Architecture for Differentiated Services. RFC 2475.

Braden, R., Clark, D., & Shenker, S. (1994). Integrated Services in the Internet Architecture: an Overview. RFC 1633.

Braden, R., Zhang, L., Berson, S., & Herzog, S. (1997). Resource Reservation Protocol (RSVP) - Version 1 Functional Specification. RFC 2205.

Chandrasekaran, G. (2001). Performance Evaluation of Scheduling Mechanisms for Broadband Networks. Chennai, India: Master of Science, Anna University.

Heinanen, J., Baker, F., Weiss, W. & Wroclawski, J. (1999). Assured Forwarding PHB Group. RFC 2597.

Huston, G. (2000). Next Steps for the IP QoS Architecture. RFC 2990.

Jacobson, V., Nichols, K. & Poduri, K. (1999). An Expedited Forwarding PHB. RFC 2598.

Kamel, T., Elzarki, M., Eissa, H. & Abd El-kader, S., (2002). Bandwidth and Capacity Study for Multimedia Applications over IP Backbone Networks. US-Egypt Science & Technology Joint Fund, ID Code: OTH3-009-001.

Nichols, K., Blake, S. Baker, F. & Black, D. (1998). Definition of the Differentiated Services Field (DS Field) in the IPv4 and IPv6 Headers. RFC 2474.

Nichols, K. & Carpenter, B. (2001). Definition of Differentiated Services Per Domain Behaviors and Rules for their Specification. RFC 3086.

Postigo-Boix, M., Melu's-Moreno, J. (2007). Performance evaluation of RSVP extensions for a guaranteed delivery scenario. Computer Communications. ScienceDirect., 30, 2113–2121.

Shenker, S., Partridge, C. & Guerin, R. (1997). Specification of Guaranteed Quality of Service. RFC 2212.

Tang, P., & Charles, T. (1999). Network Traffic Characterization Using Token Bucket Model. In Proceedings of the Conference on Computer Communications (IEEE Infocom).

Teitelbaum, B. (1999). QBone Architecture (v1.0).

Wroclawski, J. (1997). Specification of the Controlled Load Quality of Service. RFC 2211.

Chapter 4
QoS in Wireless Sensor Networks

Ghalib A. Shah
National University of Sciences and Technology (NUST), Pakistan

Shaleeza Sohail
National University of Sciences and Technology (NUST), Pakistan

Faisal B. Hussain
National University of Sciences and Technology (NUST), Pakistan

ABSTRACT

Wireless Sensor Networks (WSNs) have been envisioned as a new and effective means for creating and deploying previously unimaginable applications. These networks generally have the capabilities of observing the physical phenomena, communication, data processing and dissemination. Limited resources of sensor nodes like energy, bandwidth and processing abilities, make these networks excellent candidates for incorporating QoS framework. The possible applications of WSNs are numerous while being diverse in nature which makes analyzing and designing QoS support for each application a non-trivial task. At the same time, these applications require different type of QoS support from the network for optimum performance. A single layer cannot address all these issues, hence, numerous researchers have proposed protocols and architectures for QoS support at different network layers. In this chapter, the authors identify the generic QoS parameters which are usually supported at different layers of WSNs protocol stack and investigate their importance in different application models. A brief overview of significant research contribution at every network layer is provided. It is worthwhile to mention that same QoS parameter may be supported at multiple layers, hence, adequate selection of suitable mechanism would be application's choice. On the other hand, it is quite possible that a single QoS parameter, such as energy conservation or real-time delivery, can be efficiently supported through interaction of multiple layers. It is difficult, if not impossible to optimize multi layer QoS architecture. Hence, a number of researchers have also proposed the idea of cross layer architecture for providing QoS support for a number of sensor applications, which is also discussed in this chapter. At the end, the authors highlight the open research issues that might be the focus of future research in this area.

DOI: 10.4018/978-1-61520-791-6.ch004

INTRODUCTION

Wireless Sensor Networks (WSNs) are emerging as one of the most effective mechanism to sense, collect, process and disseminate physically dispersed information. Small sensing devices provide flexibility and ease of deployment as well as self configuring wireless networks for communication. Advances in sensor hardware resulted in a huge number of different type of sensors like: thermometers, barometers, moisture gauges, motion and glass break detectors, RFID access control badges and so many more (Conner et al., 2004). Most importantly, the economy of this type of solution is responsible for development of a huge number of applications in this area. Following are few of the interesting applications of WSNs:

- Habitat monitoring requires access to the remote area which may not be safe and/or feasible to be accessed regularly for data collection. WSNs provide a robust and safe alternative and hence, a large number of such applications have developed in last few years (Szewczyk et al., 2004; Polastre et al., 2004).
- Environmental observation and forecasting systems have benefited a lot with the emergence of WSNs as the means to sense, monitor, model and forecast the physical processes like rain fall, flooding, temperature changes, pollution etc.
- Disaster management is the area that has emerged as the perfect candidate for applying WSN technology. Monitoring, assistance and management provided by a WSN based disaster management system provides critical information without risking human lives.
- Surveillance and security in buildings and secure areas can be provided by WSNs. Motion tracking sensors are perfect to detect intruders as provide required services round the clock.
- Military applications like battlefield assistance, troop management and enemy tracking are one of the driving forces behind the success of WSNs.

In addition to the above mentioned possibilities, the applications in the area of WSN are unlimited and are emerging everyday. Before going into further details, a brief and simple introduction of WSN is provided here. WSNs are essentially composed of a large number of small sensing devices, deployed in an ad-hoc manner to collectively sense a physical phenomenon (Tilak et al., 2002). The sensor nodes disseminate the collected data after limited processing to the sink node using wireless technology. The sink node can have the ability to query sensor nodes for any information. The exterior networks are connected to the sink node which enables these networks to collect data from WSN.

The following sets of distinguishing features of WSNs are responsible for a tremendous amount of research in this area (Wang et al., 2006):

- The topology of the sensor networks is application dependent while being self configuring and ad-hoc in nature (Conner et al., 2004). Generally, a star-tree type topology is resulted due to the presence of a single sink node at the root of the tree. Multi-hop flat or hierarchical networks may form depending upon the number of sensor nodes and the requirements of the applications.
- The applications of the WSNs are very diverse in nature, as previously discussed. Due to this diversity the QoS requirements of different applications can vary a lot. A generic QoS framework for WSN needs to address all these requirements if to be deployed at a large scale.
- The traffic of WSN has a particular pattern. Generally, upstream traffic exists due to the messages send by sensors to the sink. However, sink can query and/

or reconfigure sensor nodes which results in downstream traffic from sink to sensor nodes. The handling and QoS requirements of both upstream and downstream traffic are different (discussed in detail in Section 5).

- Resources in WSN are constrained and must be used optimally. Computation capability, battery life, wireless communication ability and memory size of the sensor nodes are limited. For any application to be realistically deployed and effectively used, it is a mandatory requirement to make best of the available resources in an optimized manner.
- The messages exchanged among the nodes in the sensor networks are small in size. Limited amount of data can generally be sent in a single message which puts the restriction on the amount of data that can be transferred.

The above mentioned characteristics of WNSs mold the research directions in this field. The following sections discuss the proposed QoS provisions in WSNs at different network layers after briefly describing the concept and implications of QoS in these networks.

QOS IN WSNS

The notion of QoS is very different in WSN as compared to traditional wire-line and wireless networks. The QoS requirements in commonly used networks include end-to-end reliability, jitter control, delay bounds and dedicated bandwidth allocation. In such networks generally, the aspects of reliability are handled by the transport layer protocol like TCP. IETF has proposed a number of architectures that can provide QoS guarantees in the Internet like DiffServ (Blake et al., 1998), IntServ (Braden et al., 1994) etc. Various QoS models for mobile ad hoc networks have been also proposed, which might be thought as potential possible solutions for WSNs. Service Differentiation in Stateless Wireless Ad hoc networks (SWAN) (Ahn G. et al., 2002) offers a stateless QoS model for MANETs in which intermediate nodes do not maintain per-flow reservation states. INSIGNIA (Lee B., et al, 2000) is another signaling protocol which is specially designed for MANETs. It supports algorithms like fast flow reservation, restoration and adaptation; which are designed to deliver adaptive real-time service. These QoS models are not possible to implement in WSN due to differences between MANET and WSN. The major difference is the resource limitation in WSN. Therefore, in WSN it is difficult to determine available resources along end-to-end path and reserve them. Yet more important is the higher density of nodes, which raises the question on the performance of these candidate protocols in WSNs.

However, when we turn our attention to WSNs then the above mentioned features of these networks make the QoS provision more challenging and have resulted in numerous research proposals at different network layers. Before going into the details of such protocols and architectures, it is imperative to classify the large number of WSN applications into categories, as discussing each application independently is impractical while being infeasible. Due to the obvious importance of data delivery mechanism, we are using the classes which are based on common characteristics in data delivery requirements of each application (Tilak et al., 2002):

- **Event-Driven:** The events that are to be detected by sensors are very important for event-based applications. On the occurrence of the event a number of sensors send messages to sink, hence, the data is correlated and highly redundant. The nature of traffic is usually bursty as a set of sensors start transmitting on the occurrence of an event. Message of a single sensor is

Table 1. QoS parameters in wireless sensor networks

QoS Parameter	Event-driven	Query-driven	Continuous
Energy consumption	Low	Low	Low
Delay tolerance	Low	Medium	Medium
Bandwidth utilization	Low	Medium	High
Loss tolerance	Low	Low	Medium
Throughput	Medium	Low	High
Coverage	High	High	High
Fairness delivery	High	Medium	Medium
End-to-end reliability	High	High	Low

usually small and a number of messages are required to detect particular event properly. These applications require interactive, delay intolerant (real-time), mission-critical and non end-to-end services. The example of such application would be surveillance services in which the geographically dispersed sensors detect intruder entry and relay messages to the sink.

- **Query-Driven:** The data is pulled by sink on demand generally, which is the only difference among these types of applications and event driven ones. Sink has control over the flow of traffic and can be programmed to avoid congestion and provide reliability in the network. These applications have the same characteristics as event driven applications except the delay tolerance that is query-specific. Few environmental sensing applications which focus on observing temperature and humidity like parameters fall in this category.
- **Continuous:** These applications require a continuous flow of data to the sink at pre-configured intervals. The sensed information needs to be delivered in continuation in order to study the phenomenon under consideration. This class of applications demands real-time services for voice, image, or video data with bandwidth provisions but packet losses can be tolerated to a certain extent. However, non real-time traffic is also possible that is delay and packet loss tolerant. Habitat monitoring applications require continuous stream of data from the sensors sensing different parameters related to the living species at the target area.
- **Hybrid:** The data delivery models of the above mentioned three types of applications can also coexist. In such applications, the QoS constraints are to be fulfilled according to the application's requirement. Battlefield surveillance applications can lie in this class as they can provide continuous information about own troops and event driven information about the intrusion of enemy troops.

Defining the number and type of parameters for providing QoS to the above mentioned application classes is a difficult task. However, on the basis of relative importance, we have established criteria for a number of commonly used QoS parameters for each class, which is provided in Table 1. Keeping these parameters as guidelines, we will be categorizing different research efforts, discussed in this chapter.

QOS AT MEDIUM ACCESS CONTROL LAYER

Medium access control (MAC) is an essential function of all the shared medium networks, which employs a coordination mechanism to provide a transmission opportunity to a node among the contenders of that medium. MAC protocol for WSNs needs to be much more sophisticated than in any of its counterparts in wired or wireless due to the inherent limitations of sensor nodes. Therefore, supporting QoS on the MAC layer of WSNs is quite a challenging task, particularly, when the QoS parameters are diverse in nature. For instance, real-time delivery and energy efficiency are two contradictory requirements, which are fundamental in event-driven applications. The important question that arises here is that what type of support can be provided by the MAC layer, particularly if that is also possible at some higher layer.

The important difference between MAC and higher layer is the level of QoS. MAC ensures QoS by controlling medium access or provisioning resources among nodes. While network or higher layer provision resources by differentiating applications or flows on a single node. Hence, QoS cannot be achieved without the assistance of MAC protocol, since the transmission of packets relies on the operations of MAC. In the following section, we identify different QoS parameters that can be supported on the MAC layer and the techniques through which they can be achieved are investigated.

Energy Efficiency

Energy efficiency is the most demanding requirement of the applications that must be provided in order to prolong the life of nodes and in turn the life of wireless sensor network. MAC can play an important role in controlling energy consumption. Although other layers also incorporate some measures to minimize energy consumption or utilize it efficiently, but major factors of energy consumption are driven by MAC layer. In WSN energy efficiency has become an important objective of MAC as medium access is generally driven by the energy consuming factor. If we look at the sources of energy consumption then it is observed that the energy is uselessly consumed for most of the time, which can be minimized through a proper design of a MAC protocol.

The major sources of energy consumption are collision, retransmission, idle listening, overhearing and over-emitting (Demirkol et al., 2006). Collision occurs when the MAC protocol is unable to resolve medium contention among nodes that results in unsuccessful transmission wasting the transmission power and bandwidth. Such a scheme is classified as contention-based MAC and the probability of frames collision increases with the offered load, which degrades channel utilization and further reduces battery life. This motivates the need for collision-free protocol that establishes transmission schedules statically or dynamically to allow nodes to receive data packets without collisions and thus avoids wasteful transmissions.

In contention free protocols, transmission opportunity is granted to nodes in some predefined order, which may be based either on round robin fashion or traffic priority. This requires some central node that negotiates with the contenders and forms a transmission schedule. IEEE 802.11 (WLAN Standard, 1997) defines point coordination function (PCF) to provide collision free transmission in wireless LAN. However, such a centralized technique is not possible in WSN and particularly when the topology is highly dynamic due to the failure of nodes, addition of new nodes, mobility of nodes and hostile deployment field. A distributed hybrid MAC protocol (Rajendran et al., 2003) and (Busch et al., 2004) might solve the frame collision problem more efficiently. In such a technique, medium access is divided into super-frames which are composed of two parts; contention period and contention-free period. This

Figure 1. Contention-free access technique in which nodes first reserve slots in short contention period and later transmit data in their reserved slots during contention-free period

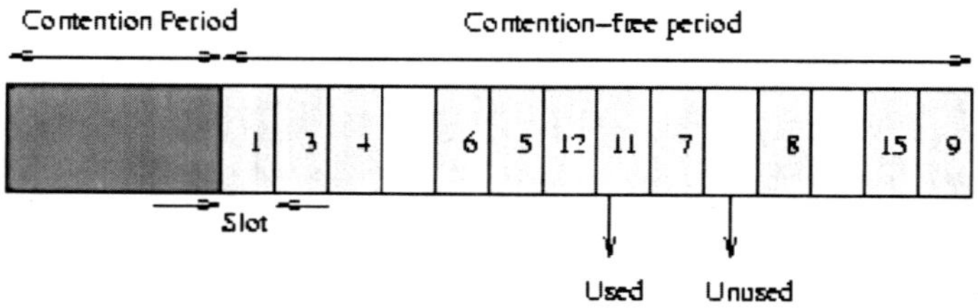

idea is similar to coexistence of nodes operating in PCF and DCF modes of IEEE 802.11. In contention phase, nodes transmit short transmission desire frames using any contention-based MAC protocol to reserve the channel in contention-free period. At the end of contention period, they transmit data frames in their respective time slots of contention-free period as shown in Fig. 1. Hence, collision-free transmission is achieved in a distributed environment, which is even more scalable compared to centralized contention-free mechanism.

Besides collision, the hostile propagation conditions may damage the frame that may trigger retransmission if reliability is desired. The noisy conditions can be overcome by using some adaptive forward error correction (FEC) technique (Ahn et al., 2005) that changes the redundancy in frames according to link conditions. That is, lower redundancy is introduced when the error rate is lower, higher redundancy otherwise. Thus a hybrid MAC protocol with adaptive FEC algorithm would solve the collision and retransmission issues quite nicely which will eventually save energy and bandwidth. Idle listening and overhearing are the other major sources of energy consumption during which the transceiver remains *on* unnecessarily. This is generally dealt by switching a node to sleep/off mode when there is no frame waiting for transmission or it is expecting any frame reception.

In a very simple technique, nodes define their static duty cycle in which they switch between wake-up and sleep mode periodically. Thus frames are queued during sleep mode and transmitted as soon as the node switches back to wake up mode. Obviously, such an energy conserving mechanism would pay the price in terms of higher frames delay. Lower duty cycle conserves more energy at cost of higher delay and vice versa (Bacco et al., 2004). There is a tradeoff between energy conservation and frame delay. However, this simple technique can be made adaptive to the traffic in such a way that duty cycles are adjusted dynamically according to current traffic conditions. This will make the approach little more complex. By integrating such an adaptive duty cycling scheme with hybrid MAC, a concrete energy efficient solution is achieved. In this case, all the nodes are switched to wakeup state during contention period to establish transmission schedule. During contention-free period, only a pair of transmitter and receiver at any given time slot will remain in wake up mode according to the schedule and rest of nodes will switch to sleep mode.

Real-Time Delivery

Real-time applications are very common in wireless sensor networks these days ranging from industrial process automation to military surveillance. Routing protocols generally claim to provide real-time assurance to applications by sending packets through delay constrained paths. However such a guarantee cannot be provided if appropriate duty cycle is not chosen at any given time or under heavy traffic load and higher network density. In former case, if the duty cycle of MAC

Figure 2. Transmission of frames in different energy saving MAC protocols

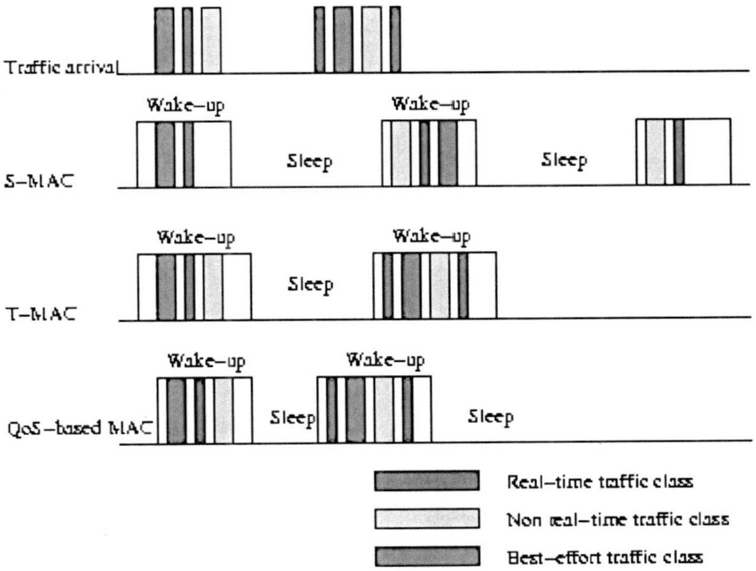

is low and non-adaptive SMAC (Ye et al., 2004) then higher delay is expected. Contrarily, making it adaptive to traffic (Dam & Langendoen, 2003), delay can be significantly minimized. These solutions are further optimized (Saxena et al., 2008; Fu et al., 2006) in which nodes are immediately switched to active mode if a higher priority packet with lesser delay tolerance is fed to MAC as shown in Fig 2. Yet energy-latency tradeoffs for data gathering are explored in DB-MAC (Bacco et al., 2004), whose objective is to find optimal data delivery trees subject to minimum latency and minimum energy.

So far, our discussion for real-time delivery mainly focused on turning transceiver of nodes in to wake up mode as soon as the frame is available for transmission or reception. Another aspect of real-time delivery is to refrain the transmission of nodes contending for low priority (non real-time) traffic in favor of higher priority (real-time) traffic. In a centralized fashion, central node polls the nodes according to the traffic priority or delay constraint. In distributed environment, an approach similar to enhanced distributed coordination function (EDCF), as specified in IEEE 802.11e, can be implemented in which medium access is controlled by contention window size, arbitrary inter-frame spacing and persistence factor. QoS based MAC (Saxena et al., 2008) addresses this by taking longer wake up period for real-time traffic and lower for best-effort traffic. This allows nodes of higher priority traffic to capture medium for longer time than nodes contending to transfer low priority traffic. Hence, in-time data delivery can be guaranteed through traffic adaptive duty cycling and nodes coordination.

Reliability

An event can be reliably detected, if the minimum information required for successful detection of an event is delivered by the nodes to the sink. CCMAC protocol (Vuran M. C., 2006) provides event-based reliability solution, which form virtual clusters and cluster-heads. The heads control the number of active nodes to maintain the required reporting rate of nodes. This eliminates the need of hop-by-hop frame acknowledgment. This fact is applicable in periodic or continuous monitoring applications. However, in query-driven or event-driven scenarios, application may need reliability on packet basis which is possible by using backward error correction (BEC) or forward error correction (FEC) technique at MAC layer. CSMA based MAC protocols (Ye et al., 2004; Dam & Langendoen, 2003) provide such reliability features, while contention-free MAC protocols (Busch et al., 2004) support implicit reliability assuming that nodes only transmit in their dedicated slots during contention-free period.

Fairness

Fairness is also an important aspect of QoS which ensures that all the nodes get due bandwidth share. It is a common practice that real-time traffic always get preference over best-effort traffic in QoS-aware MAC protocols. If there is a continuous flow of real-time traffic then it may capture medium for indefinite time period resulting in unfair channel utilization. This situation may arise in hybrid model of applications that contain mixed traffic. In a simple energy-efficient MAC protocol, all the nodes get equal transmission opportunity which implicitly implements fairness. Thus fairness is also an important QoS parameter that needs to be accounted while designing real-time delivery mechanism. The problem can be addressed by dividing medium access time into real-time and best-effort transmission periods. Real-time transmission period may be kept longer or adjusted dynamically according to the volume of both classes of traffic.

Bandwidth guarantees can be provided by MAC layer for reserving medium access time corresponding to the required bandwidth. This is possible with distributed contention-free MAC protocol in which nodes can reserve slots which will be unanimously utilized during contention-free period.

QOS AT NETWORK LAYER

Network layer is responsible to deliver data packets from source to destination node. This functionality generally requires knowledge of network state that includes available resources such as buffer space, bandwidth etc. as well as connectivity or possible routes towards destination. Network layer is assumed to be the most effective choice of implementing QoS since it has control over the carrier network. This role becomes even more prominent if QoS needs to be supported over resource constrained wireless sensor networks.

One of the key issues in providing QoS guarantees is how to determine paths that satisfy QoS constraints. Solving this problem is known as QoS routing or constraint-based routing. Despite its difficulty, QoS routing is invaluable in a network architecture that needs to satisfy traffic and service requirements. There can be a debate that a QoS mechanism can be implemented as an independent layer or middleware that will run on top of network layer like DiffServ, IntServ/RSVP. We argue that such resource reservation approaches are not possible in WSN because the sensor nodes are the sources as well as the routing nodes in these networks, have limited resources. Moreover, traffic can not be predicted unlike the general purpose nodes/routers with abundant resources implementing these techniques in traditional network.

In WSNs, routing protocols are highly influenced by the data delivery model. For instance, it has been concluded in (Heinzelman, 2000) that for a habitat monitoring application where data is continuously transmitted to the sink, a hierarchical routing protocol is the most efficient choice. This is due to the fact that such an application generates significant redundant data that can be aggregated on route to the sink, thus reducing traffic and saving energy. Contrarily, a hierarchical routing protocol implementing aggregation is unable to provide service to the event-driven applications since the real-time delivery is affected due to aggregation. Moreover, there always exists a single path from source to sink in hierarchical routing that can not ensure reliability. Eventually routing protocols are proposed based on different data delivery models. According to our discussion in Section I, we identify the QoS parameters listed in Table I, which can be potentially supported at network layer unlike sticking to a data model based QoS support. We define the following QoS requirements for the network layer: real-time delivery, reliability, energy efficiency, routing robustness and scalability.

Real-Time Delivery

Delay can be minimized collectively by both MAC and routing layers. MAC controls hop latency at forwarding nodes, whereas routing protocol selects the forwarding nodes such that end-to-end (E2E) delay is minimized. Generally, the level of QoS at routing layer is classified as *predictive or soft QoS* that relies on local link state information and *deterministic or hard QoS* that requires complete E2E path information. The traditional methods supporting hard-QoS are based on the end-to-end path discovery, resources reservation along the discovered path, and path recovery in case of topological changes. They are not suitable for WSN for several reasons. Firstly, path discovery time is not acceptable for event-driven applications. Secondly, it is not convenient to reserve resources for the unpredictable non-periodic packets. Even for periodic continuous flows, these methods are not practical in dynamic WSN since service disruption during the path recovery increases the data delivery delay which is not acceptable in mission critical application. Finally, the end-to-end path based approaches are not scalable due to huge overhead of path discovery and recovery in large scale sensor networks. The alternative approach is to include an end-to-end QoS provisioning based on local decisions at each intermediate node without path discovery and maintenance that can only support soft QoS.

The most commonly used technique is greedy routing in which nodes are presumably location-aware. Nodes select next hop based on its closeness to destination, i.e., each node chooses a forwarding node among its neighbors which has the shortest distance to destination node. This exhibits the characteristics similar to the shortest path routing. The important difference is that greedy routing is a stateless technique that only needs to know the location of its neighbors unlike the shortest path routing that needs to collect complete network state. However, it is not able to provide hard QoS support which is possible in shortest path routing. The simple greedy routing is modified to provide real-time routing by including timing constraint in addition to geographical location of nodes in its forwarding node selection criteria. The SPEED (He et al., 2003) and MMSPEED (Felemban et al., 2006) are geographical routing protocols which assume that end-to-end deadlines are proportional to the distance from the source to the destination, thus provide soft real-time guarantees by maintaining a uniform delivery speed in the network using feedback control.

A class-based QoS routing protocol (Akkaya & Yonus, 2003) is also proposed that aims to distribute the bandwidth fairly among real-time and best effort traffic by employing a class-based queuing model and supports bandwidth provision as required by the application. However, this approach may not be efficient in WSN (Ali & Faisal, 2008), where the topology is highly dynamic and link failure rate is high. In multi-constrained routing (Huang & Fang, 2007), energy constraint is also included in the forwarding criteria to achieve energy efficiency besides real-time delivery, which is based on local link state information and provides predictive or soft-QoS support.

Figure 3. Example topology of sensor nodes in which source S sends data to sink Z through different alternative routes ABD, CD and EFG

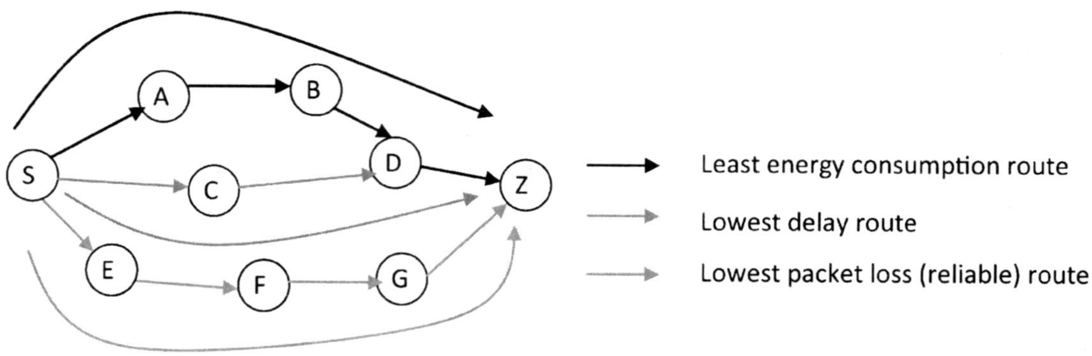

Reliability

Reliability can be defined in terms of packet delivery ratio (Huang & Fang, 2007). OMR (Du et al., 2007) provides reliability through hop to hop acknowledgment and nodes keep the packets in their cache for some time in case of negative acknowledgment transmitted by the sink. Nodes can also keep track of different alternative routes and a path with lowest packet loss ratio can be assumed as a reliable to transfer data as shown in Fig. 3.

Fault Tolerance

Fault tolerance is measured by the likelihood that alternate paths exist between a source and a destination in case the primary path fails. Source nodes maintain multiple paths (Vidhypria & Vanathi, 2007; Wang et al., 2006) with destination nodes associated with some cost metric. The lowest cost path is considered as a primary path and is preferred for routing, while the alternative paths are known as secondary or backup paths and are selected on failure of primary path only. These alternate paths are kept alive by sending periodic messages. Hence, network reliability can be increased at the expense of increased overhead of maintaining the alternate paths. Thus multipath solves the fault tolerance issue effectively when the network is highly dynamic and unreliable. However, when delay and reliability requirements are to be met collectively then redundancy can be made on multiple disjoint paths (Dulman et al., 2003) to achieve the high probability of reception in first attempt of transmission that will also minimize the delay.

Energy Efficiency

Routing protocol contributes in achieving energy efficiency by considering cost metric, i.e., energy consumption in route selection. The cost metric can be incorporated in one of the following ways (Akyildiz et al., 2002) to make energy efficient route:

- *Maximum Power Available (PA) route:* The route that has maximum total available power is preferred. The total PA is calculated by summing the PAs of each node along the route.
- *Minimum Energy (ME) route:* The route that consumes ME to transmit the data packets between the sink and the sensor node is the ME route.

Figure 4. (a) Direction of sensor-to-sink/event information flow (b) direction of sink to nodes information flow

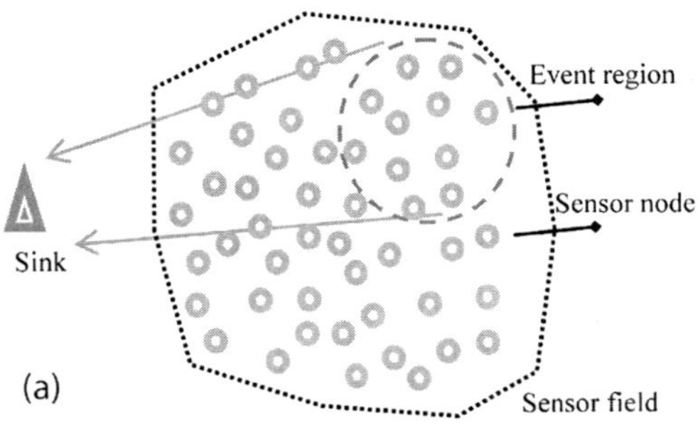

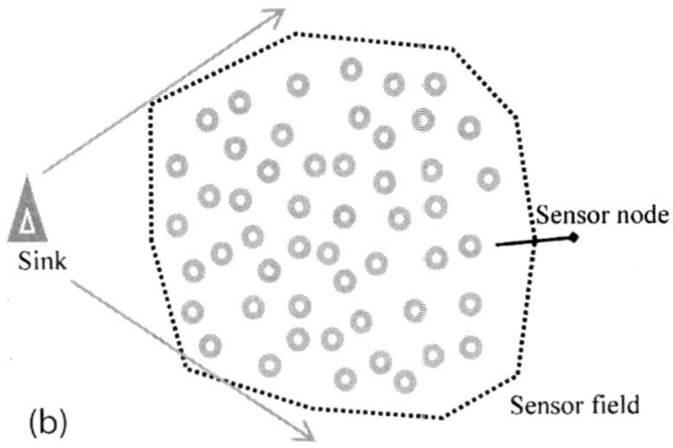

- *Maximum of Minimum PA node route:* The route along which the minimum PA is larger than the minimum PAs of the other routes is preferred.

All of these approaches require end-to-end route discovery and updated information which incurs overhead and can not be potential routing techniques in WSN. In order to avoid such network-wide state information, clustering techniques (Younis & Fahmy, 2004; Shah et al., 2006) has been proposed in which a subset of nodes called cluster-heads involve in routing decision which is more scalable and has lesser overhead to determine end-to-end path. In a stateless routing technique such as greedy routing, power metric is included in forwarding criteria such that a neighbor node is selected for routing having maximum residual energy. This condition is checked for every packet by all the nodes in path independently. Hence, packets from same source might follow different paths and result in balanced energy consumption.

Aggregation is also incorporated at network layer to reduce the volume of traffic that in turn conserves the energy of nodes (Hu et al., 2006; He et. al, 2007). In cluster-based configuration approach, data can be aggregated by cluster-heads that collect data from their members, apply aggregation function and forward to the clusters on the path towards sink (Yoon & Shahabi, 2004). Unlike clustering, nodes are configured to form an aggregation tree in which sink is the root of tree. Data is aggregated from leaf nodes towards root node hierarchically. The drawback of this technique to maintain aggregation trees which is a nontrivial task.

QOS AT TRANSPORT LAYER

Reliable transport protocols and congestion control mechanisms for WSNs have got late recognition from the researchers. Since energy conservation is the basic issue, the introduction of a transport solution increases the energy consumption by making extra reliability related transmissions. However, the shifting of sensor networks from research labs to industry and the increase in the application areas of WSNs, demands for different quality of service metrics along with reliability at the transport layer.

In normal wired and wireless networks reliability is defined as the complete transport of information from a source to the destination. However, in WSNs the definition of reliability is application dependent and is associated with the direction of information flow. There are two basic information flows in WSNs ash shown in Figure 4 a & b: sensors-to-sink and sink-to-sensors. The sensors-to-sink flow is also named as event flow, upstream flow, many-to-one flow and sensors to destination flow. While the sink-to-sensors flow is also named as downstream flow, one-to-many and destination to sensors flow.

The sensors-to-sink information flow is triggered on event occurrence and due to dense nature of these networks, a number of nodes detecting the event transmit information to destination. Redundant data travelling through multiple flows is forwarded to a sink and occasional loss of information is not deemed to affect the overall information delivery to the sink. Hence, instead of end-to-end reliability the concept of event-to-sink reliability (Akan & Akyildiz, 2005) is more useful in these networks. Another issue related to sensors-to-sink transport in WSNs is that of congestion. In case of event occurrence, the sudden flow of information from event nodes to a single destination results in congestion. The degree of congestion increases with the increase in the number of nodes sending the event information, resulting into high degree of packet and energy loss.

The large scale and random deployment of sensor networks demands for reliable information transport from sink-to-sensor nodes. The basic reason for this information transport includes updating of event definitions on sensor nodes or for changing the binary codes of sensor nodes. In these cases, the definition of reliability is 100% transport of all the information from the sink to the sensor nodes. Since sensor nodes are generally powered by standard batteries, providing reliability with minimum energy consumption is the basic issue at the transport layer. Apart from this, congestion control mechanisms and different QoS issues like per node fair bandwidth allocation, prioritized bandwidth allocation and real-time information transport have also been studied in existing literature.

Energy Efficiency

Energy conservation is the key issue in transport and congestion control protocols. Energy can be conserved by limiting the reliability related transmissions and decreasing the packet drops due to congestion. A number of studies (Hu, et. al., 2005; Rangwala et al., 2006; Shigang Na, 2006; Wang, et. al., 2007) had proposed different techniques for solving the issue of congestion in sensor networks with minimum overhead. These techniques have used different metrics like buffer size, packet inter-arrival time, packet service time, channel sampling and traffic load assessment to detect congestion. One protocol that has redefined the concept of reliability in order to conserve energy is Event to Sink Reliable Transport (ESRT) (Akan & Akyildiz, 2005). ESRT is based on the idea that on event occurrence correlated information from an event region is sent to the sink. Therefore, instead of transporting individual sensor based information to the sink, general event region information is sufficient for reliable detection of an event. This decreases the overhead of end-to-end transport from individual sensor nodes to the sink. As a result, ESRT measures reliability in terms of number of packets received at the destination in certain amount of time.

Fidelity of Knowledge

Packets from different sources may have different contribution to improve sink's information on the phenomenon of interest. Communication costs between sources and the sink may be different and may change dynamically. Therefore, reliability can not be simply measured by the total incoming packet rate at the sink. Price-Oriented Reliable Transport (PORT) (Yangfan et al., 2005) defines sensor to sink data transport to be reliable when the transport mechanism can assure that the sink can obtain enough fidelity of the knowledge on the phenomenon of interest.

Fairness

In some applications, where general event region information might not be sufficient to predict the event nature, it is required to have precise per node information at the sink. Therefore, fairness demands that the system bandwidth should be allocated to event reporting nodes in a way that all nodes have same throughput at the sink. Interference-aware fair rate control in wireless sensor networks, (IFRC) (Rangwala et al., 2006) monitors average queue size to detect incipient congestion and uses Additive Increase Multiplicative Decrease (AIMD) scheme to adjust the reporting rate of nodes. IFRC does not imply strict fairness and allows flows passing through less restrictive contention domains to have higher rates than the ones passing through higher contention domains.

Credit based fairness control in wireless sensor networks (CFRC) (Shanshan et al., 2007) proposes a mechanism to ensure that all data sources have equal or weighted access to end-to-end network bandwidth. CFRC allocates bandwidth to nodes based on credit; the effective amount of sensed information, which is dependent on node density and their distribution instead of uniformity. Congestion Control and Fairness for many-to-one routing in sensor networks (CCF) (Tien & Bajcsy, 2004) proposes an algorithm that ensure fairness by assuming that all the nodes are transmitting and routing data at the same time. CCF uses buffer size to detect for congestion. CCF implements a tree based technique in which each node calculates its sub-tree size. Reporting rate is allocated to nodes depending on their sub-tree sizes.

Prioritized Throughput

More than one event can occur within the sensor field at the same time or some nodes within the event region can have more importance than the other nodes. As a result, prioritized event reporting with respect to a certain event, region or node can be required in sensor networks. Priority-based congestion control in wireless sensor networks (PCCP) (Wang et al., 2007) uses packet inter-arrival time and packet service time to detect congestion level at a node and employs weighted fairness to allow nodes to receive priority-dependent throughput. PCCP suggests that sensor nodes might have different priority due to their function or location. Therefore, nodes with higher priority-index gets more share of the bandwidth in order to ensure priority dependent throughput. The priority based rate adjustment scheme of PCCP uses congestion degree and priority index of a node to adjust its reporting rate.

Real-Time Transport

Another QoS metric regarding transport layer is real-time transport of time-critical event information from the nodes to the sink, for instance, the location information of a mobile intruder from an intrusion detection system. Delay-aware reliable transport (DART) in wireless sensor networks (Gungor & Akan, 2007) provides time-bound and reliable event transport from the sensor field. DART defines transport to be reliable and delay-aware if the packets are received within application defined time bound and at application defined reporting rate. DART uses time critical event packet scheduling policy to forward packets according to their deadlines.\

Cross-Layer QOS Support

The general emphasis of the communication protocols in WSNs has been to improve the energy efficiency by exploiting the collaborative nature and correlation characteristics present in these networks.

The traditional layered protocol architecture when used in sensor networks, simplifies design, eases of implementation and provides the possibility of alternative layer implementations. Each layer makes use of the services provided by the

Figure 5. Cross-layer QoS architecture for WSN

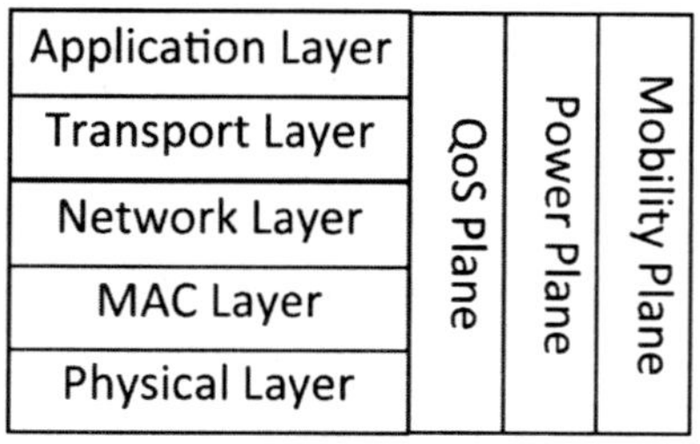

layer directly below it, and also provides service to the layer directly above it. However, the disadvantage of using simple layered approach is that communication is limited between adjacent layers with a minimum set of primitives.

Layered approach may achieve very high performance in terms of the metrics related to each of these individual layers. But they are not jointly optimized to maximize the overall network performance while minimizing the energy expenditure. Because of the direct coupling between the physical layer and the upper layers, the traditional protocol stack is not sufficient for wireless networks. In a wireless network, physical layer, MAC layer and routing layer together contend for the network resource. The physical layer affects MAC and routing decisions by its transmission power and rate. The MAC layer is responsible for scheduling and allocating the wireless channel, which finally determines the available bandwidth of the transmitter and the packet delay. This bandwidth and packet delay also can affect the decision at the routing layer to select the link. The routing layer chooses the wireless links to relay the packets to the destination. The routing decision changes the contention level at the MAC layer, and accordingly the physical layer parameters. Also, considering the scarce energy and processing resources of WSNs, joint optimization and design of networking layers, i.e., cross-layer design stands as the most promising alternative to inefficient traditional layered protocol architectures. Adding a QoS plane in the protocol stack would be helpful to optimize QoS as shown in Fig. 5.

The cross-layer approach depending on the existing work can be categorized as cross-layer interaction and cross-layer melting. In the former, the traditional layered structure is preserved, while each layer is informed about the conditions of other layers. While in the later, multiple traditional layers are melted into a functional module. In the remaining of this section, we present different cross-layer designs in which physical, MAC, routing and transport layers either interact with each other or are melted to form a single layer for more optimized performance.

MAC + Routing

MAC and routing layers can interact with each other to provide resilient routing with minimum energy consumption. In sensor networks, MAC layer protocols minimize energy consumption by using sleep and wake cycle. In this case, packets can suffer higher delay due to short wake up periods. Such issues can be addressed more effectively through a cross-layer solution. Hence, most of the cross-layer designs (Sichitiu, 2004; Galluccio et al., 2007; Fang & McDonald, 2004) have concentrated on MAC and routing layer interactions. For providing real-time routing with efficient energy consumption, all the nodes along the path can be informed to determine their wakeup and sleep schedule as they must be in wake up state when the packet arrives for forwarding. This idea has been presented in (R-MAC) (Yassad et al., 2007).

A joint scheduling and routing scheme is proposed in (Sichitiu, 2004) for periodic traffic in WSNs. In this scheme, the nodes form distributed on-off schedules for each flow in the network while the routes are established such that the nodes are only awake when necessary. Since the traffic is periodic, the schedules are then maintained to favor maximum efficiency. Similarly in (Galluccio et al., 2007), the routing decision is performed as a result of successive competitions at the medium access level. More specifically, the next hop is selected based on a weighted progress factor and the transmit power is increased successively until the most efficient node is found. Moreover, on-off schedules are used. The performance evaluations of all these propositions present the advantages of cross-layer approach at the routing and MAC layers.

Routing + PHY

The throughput optimization problem in multi-hop sensor networks can be solved by the coordinated effort of routing and physical layers. In (Fang & McDonald, 2004), the throughput optimization problem is split into two sub-problems, i.e., multi-hop flow routing at the network layer and power allocation at the physical layer. The throughput is tied to the per-link data flow rates, which in turn depend on the link capacities and hence, the per-node radio power level. On the other hand, the power allocation problem is tied to interference as well as the link rate. Based on this solution, a CDMA/OFDM based solution is provided such that the power control and the routing are performed in a distributed manner.

Transport + MAC

The interdependency between local contention and congestion calls for an adaptive cross-layer mechanism for efficient data delivery in WSNs (Vuran et al., 2005). A cross-layer design approach between the transport and MAC layer can easily decrease the degree of congestion by indicating the MAC layer of congested nodes to decrease their wait time at the MAC layer (in case of CSMA-based MAC protocols). This allows congested nodes to get more share of the medium than the surrounding nodes. As a result, the congested node can send more packets to the next hop nodes.

Application + MAC

The spatial correlation present in the observed physical phenomenon can be exploited for medium access control. A cross-layer solution among MAC layer, physical phenomenon, and the application layer for WSNs is proposed in (Vuran & Akyildiz, 2006). Since, a sensor node can act as a representative node for several other sensor nodes. Therefore, a collaborative medium access control (CC-MAC) is used to exploit the distributed spatial correlation available in the physical phenomenon. Such a cross-layer design can decrease latency and packet drop ratio while increasing the life time of the network. Another issue related to cross-layer design is that we might not require all the conventional layers in the protocol stack of all the applications. Considering the OSI model where end-to-end and link-to-link packet drops are detected by transport and data link layers respectively. In sensor networks few packet drops can be ignored without the enforcement of state-of-art protocols for data link and transport layers. On the other hand, an application may use either data link or transport protocol. Moreover, light weight reliability can be achieved at the routing layer by routing through less congested nodes.

QOS AT APPLICATION LAYER

In the last few sections, we have discussed the provisions of QoS in sensor networks at different layers in detail. It seems natural that there are certain aspects in the paradigm of QoS that can best handled at only the application layer. Keeping in mind the extra ordinary number of applications in this area it is almost impossible to discuss every application specific QoS issue here. Hence, we are only providing brief description of few relatively important aspects in this area.

Coverage and Deployment

For proper execution and efficient use of certain applications, it is a requirement that the area under consideration must be properly covered by sensor nodes. This means that the phenomena under study must be observed by a minimum number of sensor nodes in every part of the concerned area. Coverage can be a very important QoS requirement in two cases: firstly, if no sensor is placed at some part of the WSN area then the event in that area is not sensed. Secondly, imprecise measurements of some sensors require a set of minimum number of values to get required information.

The problem of coverage has been studied on its own and by combining it with connectivity and energy efficiency issues. Recently, more focus has been on designing algorithms that enable application developers to provide minimum coverage and required connectivity in the sensor area.

(Huang & Tseng, 2005) discusses the general problem of coverage and its solution as determining that the area under consideration is covered by at least k sensors. k is the parameter that application can define according to its requirements and i can vary widely as some applications may require higher value of k for fault tolerance or location monitoring purpose. The algorithm works in two modes; one assumes that all sensors have same sensing range and other without this explicit assumption. The complexity of the proposed algorithm is O(nd log d), where d is the number of sensors in the largest sensing neighbor set and n, which is the total number of sensors.

The coverage solutions for sensors having irregular sensing and communication ranges and mobile sensors have not been explicitly addressed (Thai et al., 2008). Application specific coverage details are still an open issue especially for the applications requiring high fault tolerance.

Data Management

The aim of any WSN application is to collect data effectively and efficiently from the network. The whole network can be considered as a database. Hence, collection, analysis and aggregation of appropriate data to get required information are non trivial tasks keeping in mind the energy constraints of these networks. One of the methods to simplify data aggregation is to group sensor nodes into clusters and to make a hierarchal structure of those clusters to minimize communication cost (Younis & Fahmy, 2004). Use of cluster hierarchy can reduce this data redundancy to minimize communication and hence, energy wastage. Keeping in view the resource constraints of these networks, some applications can sacrifice data accuracy and precision for other requirements like network lifetime.

Yates et al. (Yates et al., 2008) have discussed several caching policies to be used at the data server in the field of WSN. The relative importance of two application specific factors: accuracy and end to end delay for query driven applications, proposed the use of caching and different lookup policies depending upon applications' QoS requirements. Intanaganwiwot et al. (Intanaganwiwot et al., 2000) have proposed an application aware data dissemination paradigm, where, data represented as named attributes is sensed as interests by the sensors and disseminated to the sink. Data progation is in two rates, low and high, high rate is only used with very few selected neighbors to collect additional information. The important feature of the proposed approach is its flexibility. Depending upon the data importance, tuning of data sensing rate/value and data dissemination frequency efficient energy consumption can be application specific.

Security

Particular applications may require a level of security of data and network due to the inherent nature of some applications like battlefield surveillance and disaster management. Depending upon the application and its purpose, physical and data security measures can be emphasized. Among a huge set of research in this are we are briefly discussing few efforts here. Anand et al. (Anand et al., 2006) have discussed following security challenges specific to WSNs as compared to traditional networks:

- Probabilistic guarantees of data as compared to "all or nothing" security guarantees in traditional networks.
- Secure hiding of timing of sensor messages to minimize the possibility of inferring critical information from the frequency and instances of these messages.
- Special cryptographic approach for aggregated data, as data aggregation is one of the commonly used approach to reduce energy wastage due to communication of each individual message.
- Hiding topology information to protect critical and important nodes, like sink and nodes closer to the sink.
- Proper light weight key management for large number of sensor nodes.
- Privacy and anonymity of the aggregated data.

Robustness and Fault Management

Robustness is the quality that may be the primary requirement of certain set of applications in order to minimize the effect of failure scenarios. The failure incidences of the sensor nodes are a common occurrence and a robust application requires handling of these incidences effectively. Additionally, applications may require sensor nodes to be placed under harsh environmental conditions like sun, rain etc which increases the possibility of failure. Some important applications may be prone to malicious activities as well (as discussed in previous section) which can result in faults in the networks. Hence, WSN applications requiring QoS in terms of robustness and fault tolerance, management framework different than the traditional applications is required.

The existing research work in fault management is surveyed in terms of three phases of management: detection, diagnosis and recovery (Yu et al., 2007). The first and probably the most important factor of fault management is fault discovery, a number of central and distributed mechanisms have been proposed. Centralized approach requires a nominated sink/ central node/ manager to perform the energy intensive fault discovery tasks. Network flooding, querying sensor nodes and message piggybacking methods have been proposed to collect nodal information by the central manager (Staddon et al., 2002; Ramanathan et al., 2005; Perrig et al., 2001).

Query Management

Query based WSN applications send queries to particular sensor or set of sensors to collect required data. Depending upon the applications requirement, the query rate and/or query target may be changed depending upon previous query answer or any other factor. Hu et al. (Hu et al., 2007) have proposed the use of Virtual Grid Clustering protocol for query driven applications which establishes on demand cluster head in the interest region instead of using generic clustering technique. On the basis of the query, the interest region is selected and cluster heads are established. Model driven query management is proposed in (Deshpande et al., 2004) to answer queries optimally. Statistical calculations and modeling of the sensor data is used to find the required information for users' query. Hence, the numbers of actual queries send to the sensor nodes are minimized.

CONCLUSION

WSNs are essentially composed of a large number of small sensing devices, deployed in an ad-hoc manner to collectively sense a physical phenomenon. The notion of QoS is very different in energy-constrained WSN as compared to traditional wire-line and wireless networks. QoS metrics like energy consumption, delay, bandwidth utilization, reliability, throughput, coverage and fairness have been focus of research in WSNs. However, new applications in the field of WSN are coming up everyday and additional QoS requirements of these applications may evolve with time as well. Hence, each application may have to be designed individually for optimal management and QoS provisions. A better option would be to formalize a generic and standardized framework, probably with cross layer functionality, which can cater for every QoS requirement. Different applications requiring different QoS may turn on required features using that framework for efficient deployment.

REFERENCES

Ahn, G., Campbell, A., Veres, A., & Sun, L. (2002). Supporting Service Differentiation for Real-Time and Best Effort Traffic in Stateless Wireless Ad Hoc Networks (SWAN). *IEEE Transactions on Mobile Computing, 1*(3), 197–207.

Ahn, J. S., Hong, S. W., & Heidemann, J. (2005). An Adaptive FEC Code Control Algorithm for Mobile Wireless Sensor Networks. *Journal of Communication and Networks, 7*(4), 1–10.

Akan, O.B., & Akyildiz, I.F. (2005). Event-to-sink reliable transport in wireless sensor networks. *IEEE/ACM Transactions on Networking, 13*(5), 1003-1016.

Akkaya, K., & Younis, M. (2003). An energy-aware QoS routing protocol for wireless sensor network", *In Proc. of 23rd International Conference on Distributed Computing Systems, pp. 710-715.*

Akyildiz, I. F., Su, W., Sankarasubramaniam, Y., & Cayirci, E. (2002). Wireless Sensor Networks: A Survey. *Elsevier Computer Networks, 38*(4), 393–422. doi:10.1016/S1389-1286(01)00302-4

Ali, A. A., & Fisal, N. (2008). A real-time routing protocol with load distribution in wireless sensor networks. *Computer Communications, 31*(14), 3190–3203. doi:10.1016/j.comcom.2008.04.030

Anand, M., Cronin, E., Sherr, M., Blaze, M., Ives, Z., & Lee, I. (2006). Sensor Network Security: More Interesting Than You Think. In *Proc. of 1st USENIX Workshop on Hot Topics in Security.*

Bacco, G. D., Melodia, T., & Cuomo, F. (2004). A MAC protocol for Delay-Bounded applications in Wireless Sensor Networks. In *Proc of Third Annual Mediterranean Ad Hoc Networking Workshop (Med-Hoc-Net 2004),* (pp. 208-220).

Blake S., Black D., Carlson M., Davies E., Wang Z. & Weiss W. (1998). An Architecture for Differentiated Services. *RFC 2475, IETF, December 1998.*

Braden, R., Zhang, L., Berson, S., Herzog, S., & Jamin, S. (1997). *Resource reSerVation Protocol (RSVP) version 1, Functional Specification. RFC 2205.* IETF.

Busch, C., Ismail, M. M., Sivrikaya, F., & Yener, B. (2004). Contention-Free MAC Protocols for Wireless Sensor Networks", *In Proc. Of 18th International Conference on Distributed Computing, DISC'04, Amsterdam,* (pp. 245-259).

Conner, W., Heidemann, J., Krishnamurthy, L., Wang, X., & Yarvis, M. (2004). Workplace applications of sensor networks. In Bulusu, N., & Jha, S. (Eds.), *Wireless Sensor Networks: A Systems Perspective*. Boston: Artech House.

Dam, T. V., & Langendoen, K. (2003). An Adaptive Energy-Efficient MAC Protocol for Wireless Sensor Networks. In *Proc. of ACM Conference on Embedded Networked Sensor System, Los Angeles, CA*.

Demirkol, I., Ersoy, C. & Alagoz, F. (2006). MAC Protocols for Wireless Sensor Networks: A Survey. *IEEE Comm. Magzine,* 115-121.

Deshpande, A., Guestrin, C., Madden, S., Hellerstein, J., & Hong, W. (2004). Model-Driven Data Acquisition in Sensor Networks. In *Proc. of the 13th international conference on Very large data bases,* Canada.

Du, J., Liu, H., & Chen, P. (2007). OMR: An Opportunistic Multi-Path Reliable Routing Protocol in Wireless Sensor Networks. In *Proc. of International Conference on Parallel Processing Workshops*.

Dulman, S., Nieberg, T., Wu, J., & Havinga, P. (2003). Trade-off between Traffic Overhead and Reliability in Multipath Routing for Wireless Sensor Networks. In *Proc. of WCNC Workshop,* New Orleans, LA.

Fang, Y., & McDonald, B. (2004). Dynamic codeword routing (DCR): a cross-layer approach for performance enhancement of general multi-hop wireless routing. In *Proc. of IEEE SECON'04,* (pp. 255-263).

Felemban, E., Lee, C., & Ekici, E. (2006). MMSPEED: multipath Multi-SPEED protocol for QoS guarantee of reliability and Timeliness in wireless sensor networks. *IEEE Transactions on Mobile Computing*, *5*(6), 738–754. doi:10.1109/TMC.2006.79

Fu, Z., Yang, Y., Lee, T. S., & Park, M. S. (2006). Adapted Listening in Wireless Sensor Network MAC Protocol. In *Proc. of 3rd International Conference, UIC 2006, Wuhan, China*, (pp. 546-555).

Galluccio, L., Leonardi, A., Morabito, G., & Palazzo, S. (2007). A MAC/Routing cross-layer approach to geographic forwarding in wireless sensor networks. *Ad Hoc Networks*, *5*(6), 872–884. doi:10.1016/j.adhoc.2007.02.004

Gungor, V. C., & Akan, O. B. (2007). Delay aware reliable transport in wireless sensor networks. *International Journal of Communication Systems*, *20*(10), 1155–1177. doi:10.1002/dac.869

He, T., Stankovic, J., Chenyang, L., & Abdelzaher, T. (2003). SPEED: A stateless protocol for real-time communication in sensor networks. *In Proc. of 23rd International Conference on Distributed Computing Systems*, (pp. 46-55).

He, W., Liu, X., Nguyen, H., Nahrstedt, K., & Abdelzaher, T. (2007). PDA: Privacy-preserving Data Aggregation in Wireless Sensor Networks. In *Proc. of IEEE INFOCOM'07*.

Heinzelman, W. (2000). *Application specific protocol architectures for wireless networks*. PhD Thesis, MIT, Cambridge, MA.

Hu, Y., Hu, N., & Jia, X. (2006). Energy Efficient Real-Time Data Aggregation in Wireless Sensor Networks. In *Proc. of ACM IWCMC'06*.

Hu, Y., Xue, Y., Li, B., Xie, J., & Yang, H. (2005). A congestion control protocol for wireless sensor networks. *Journal of Information and Computational Science*, *2*(1), 41–50.

Hu, Y., Yu, F., & Deng, P. (2007). A Novel Data Query Method for Wireless Sensor Networks. In *Proc. of International Conference on Wireless Communications, Networking and Mobile Computing*.

Huang, C., & Tseng, Y. (2005). The Coverage Problem in a Wireless Sensor Network. [MONET]. *ACM Mobile Networks and Applications*, *10*(4), 519–528. doi:10.1007/s11036-005-1564-y

Huang C., Tseng Y. & Wu, H. (2008). Distributed Protocols for Ensuring Both Coverage and Connectivity of a Wireless Sensor Network. *ACM Transactions on Sensor Networks, 3*(1).

Huang, X., & Fang, Y. (2007). Multiconstrained QoS multipath routing in wireless sensor networks. *Springer Wireless Networks*, *14*(14), 465–478.

Intanagonwiwat, C., Govindan, R., & Estrin, D. (2000). Directed diffusion: A scalable and robust communication paradigm for sensor networks. In *Proc. of 6th Annual International Conference on Mobile Computing and Networking, USA*.

Lee, S.-B., Ahn, G. S., Zhang, X., & Campbell, A. T. (2000). INSIGNIA: an IPbased quality of service framework for mobile ad hoc networks. *Journal of Parallel and Distributed Computing*, *60*(4), 374–406. doi:10.1006/jpdc.1999.1613

Perrig, A., Szewczyk, R., Wen, V., Culler, D., & Tygar, J. (2001). SPINS: Security protocols for sensor networks. In *Proc. of ACM MobiCom'01, Italy*.

Polastre, J., Szewczyk, R., Mainwaring, A., & Culler, D. (2004). Analysis of Wireless Sensor Networks for Habitat Monitoring. In Raghavendra, C. S., Sivalingam, K. M., & Znati, T. (Eds.), *The book Wireless Sensor Networks*. Amsterdam: Kluwer Academic Publishers.

Rajendran, V., Obraczka, K., & Garcia-Luna-Aceves, J. J. (2003). Energy-Efficient, Collision-Free Medium Access Control for Wireless Sensor Networks. In *Proc. ACMSenSys '03, Los Angeles, CA,* (pp. 181-92).

Ramanathan, N., Chang, K., Kapur, R., Girod, L., Kohler, E., & Estrin, D. (2005). Sympathy for the Sensor Network Debugger. In *Proc. of 3rd Embedded networked sensor systems*.

Rangwala, S., Gummadi, R., Govindan, R., & Psounis, K. (2006). Interference-aware fair rate control in wireless sensor networks. *ACM SIGCOMM. Computer Communication Review*, *36*(4), 63–74. doi:10.1145/1151659.1159922

Saxena, N., Roy, A., & Shin, J. (2008). A QoS-Based Energy-Aware MAC Protocol for Wireless Multimedia Sensor Networks. In *Proc. of IEEE VTC'08*, (pp. 183-187).

Shah, G. A., Akan, O. B., & Bozyigit, M. (2006). (MEAC) Protocol for Heterogeneous Wireless Sensor Networks. In *Proc. of Mediterranean Ad Hoc Networking Workshop (MedHoc-Net'06)*. Multi-Event Adaptive Clustering.

Shanshan, L., Xiangke, L., Shaoliang, P., Peidong, P., & Jie, J. (2007). Credit based fairness control in wireless sensor network. In *Proc. of 8th ACIS, International Conference on SNPD, Qingdao, China, (*pp. 817-822).

Shigang, C., & Na, Y. (2006). Congestion avoidance based on light-weight buffer management in sensor networks. *IEEE Transactions on Parallel and Distributed Systems*, *17*(9), 934–946. doi:10.1109/TPDS.2006.115

Sichitiu, M. L. (2004). Cross-layer scheduling for power efficiency in wireless sensor networks. In *Proc. of IEEE INFOCOM'04*.

Staddon, J. Balfanz, D. & Durfee, G. (2002). Efficient Tracing of Failed Nodes in Sensor Networks. In *Proc. of 1st ACM International Workshop on Wireless Sensor Networks and Applications, USA*.

Szewczyk, R., Mainwaring, A., Polastre, J., & Culler, D. (2004). An Analysis of a Large Scale Habitat Monitoring Application. *ACM Conference on Embedded Networked Sensor Systems*.

Thai, M. T., Wang, F., Du, H., & Jia, X. (2008). Coverage Problems in Wireless Sensor Networks: Designs and Analysis. *International Journal of Sensor Networks*, *3*(3), 191–200. doi:10.1504/IJSNET.2008.018482

The Working Group for WLAN Standards. (1997). *Ieee 802.11tm Wireless Local Area Networks*. Retrieved from http://www.ieee802.org/11/

Tien, C., & Bajcsy, R. (2004). Congestion control and fairness for many-to-one routing in sensor networks. In *Proc. of 2nd International Conference on Embedded Networked Sensor Systems (SenSys), Baltimore, MD,* (pp. 148-161).

Tilak, S., Abu-Ghazaleh, N., & Heinzelman, W. (2002). A taxonomy of wireless microsensor network communication models. In ACM Mobile Computing and Communication Review(MC2R).

Vidhyapriya R. & Vanathi, P. T. (2007). Energy Efficient Adaptive Multipath Routing for Wireless Sensor Networks. *International Journal of Computer Science*.

Vuran, M. C. & Akyildiz, I. F. (2006). Spatial Correlation-based Collaborative Medium Access Control in Wireless Sensor Networks. *IEEE/ACM Transactions on Networking, 14*(2), 316-329.

Vuran, M. C., Gungor, V. B., & Akan, O. B. (2005). On the interdependency of congestion and contention in wireless sensor networks. In *Proc. of SENMETRICS'05*.

Wang, C., Daneshmand, M., Li, B. & Sohraby, K., (2006). A survey of transport protocols for wireless sensor networks. *IEEE Journal of Network*.

Wang, C., Li, B., Sohraby, K., Daneshmand, M., & Hu, Y. (2007). Upstream congestion control in wireless sensor networks through cross-layer optimization. *IEEE Journal on Selected Areas in Communications*, *25*(4), 786–795. doi:10.1109/JSAC.2007.070514

Wang, Y., Tsai, C., & Mao, H. (2006). HMRP: Hierarchy-Based Multipath Routing Protocol for Wireless Sensor Networks. *Journal of Science and Engineering*, *9*(3), 255–264.

Yangfan, Z., Micheal, R. L., Jiangchuan, L., & Hui, W. (2005). PORT: A price-oriented reliable transport protocol for wireless sensor networks. In *Proc. of 16th IEEE International Symposium on Software Reliability Engineering (ISSRE),* (pp. 117-126).

Yates, D. J., Nahum, E. M., Kurose, J. F., & Shenoy, P. (2008). Data quality and query cost in pervasive sensing systems. *Pervasive and Mobile Computing*, *4*(6), 851–870. doi:10.1016/j.pmcj.2008.09.003

Ye W., Heidemann, J. & Estrin, D. (2004). Medium Access Control with Coordinated Adaptive Sleeping for Wireless Sensor Networks. *IEEE/ACM Transaction on Network, 12*(3), 493-506.

Yessad, S., Abdesselam, F. N., Taleb, T., & Bensaou, B. (2007). R-MAC: Reservation Medium Access Control Protocol for Wireless Sensor Networks. In *Proc. of 32nd IEEE Conference on Local Computer Networks,* (pp. 719-724.)

Yoon, S., & Shahabi, C. (2005). Exploiting Spatial Correlation Towards an Energy Efficient Clustered AGgregation Technique (CAG). In *Proc. of ICC'05*.

Younis, S., & Fahmy, O. (2004). HEED: A Hybrid, Energy-Efficient, Distributed Clustering Approach for Ad Hoc Sensor Networks. *IEEE Transactions on Mobile Computing*, *3*(4). doi:10.1109/TMC.2004.41

Yu, M., Mokhtar, H., & Merabti, M. (2007). A Survey on Fault Management in Wireless Sensor Networks. In *Proc. of 8th Annual Postgraduate Symposium*.

Zhu, H., Li, M., Chlamtac, I., & Prabhakaran, B. (2004). *A Survey of Quality of Service in IEEE 802.11 Networks*. IEEE Wireless Communications.

Zorzi, M., & Rao, R. (2003). Geographic random forwarding (GeRaF) for ad hoc and sensor networks: multihop performance. *IEEE Transactions on Mobile Computing*, *2*(4), 337–348. doi:10.1109/TMC.2003.1255648

Chapter 5
Quality of Service Provisioning in Wireless Mobile Ad Hoc Networks:
Current State of the Art

Shivanajay Marwaha
The University of Queensland, Australia

Jadwiga Indulska
The University of Queensland, Australia

Marius Portmann
The University of Queensland, Australia

ABSTRACT

Wireless networks such as Bluetooth, WLAN and WiMax have transformed the way we access information and communicate seamlessly whether we are at home, in the office, or on the move on a train, bus or even aircraft. As mobile and embedded computing devices become more omnipresent, it will become increasingly difficult to interconnect them via wires and single-hop wireless links limited by radio transmission range. This has given rise to mobile ad hoc networks (MANET) where far away nodes communicate by requesting intermediate nodes to relay their information in order to reach the destination. MANETs self-organize, self-configure and self-heal themselves. MANETs are being used in many applications ranging from emergency response situations to wireless vehicular ad hoc networks. Many applications of MANETs such as Emergency Response and First Responders have strict Quality of Service (QoS) requirements for their communications systems, making MANET QoS provisioning mechanisms very crucial for supporting multimedia communications such as real-time audio and video. However, QoS provisioning in MANETs is quite tough in comparison to QoS provisioning in wireline IP networks. This is due to numerous reasons such as the dynamic network topology, unpredictable communication medium and limited battery power of mobile devices forming the network. This chapter describes the challenges and the current state of the art of QoS protocols and mechanisms in MANETs.

DOI: 10.4018/978-1-61520-791-6.ch005

Figure 1. Example of an ad hoc network

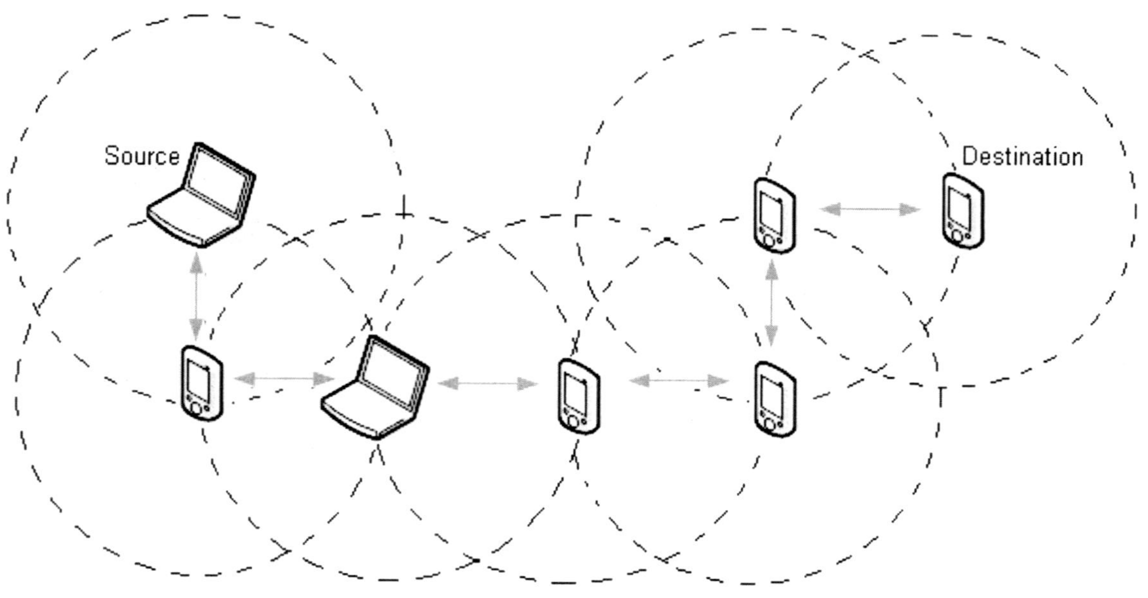

INTRODUCTION

Only "best effort" communication services existed in the Internet in its early design, treating every kind of data traffic as equal and not having any provision for Quality of Service (QoS) support. In recent years, many real-time multimedia communication applications such as Voice over Internet Protocol (VoIP) and Video on Demand (VoD) have gained popularity. Such applications require stringent QoS requirements in terms of delay, jitter and throughput. Many QoS models have been developed to support the required communication QoS over the Internet. In order to satisfy the QoS requirements, the communication network has to meet certain QoS bounds such as delay, jitter, throughput and packet loss for a data flow (Crawley, 1998).

Wireless Networks have grown to be ever more popular in the recent years, creating the requirement for supporting real-time multimedia communication applications on highly mobile network environments. Within the wireless networks domain, Mobile Ad hoc networks (MANET) have received a lot of interest and numerous deployments. MANETs (Perkins, 2001) are formed by a collection of mobile nodes, such as PDAs and laptops; using wireless connections amongst the nodes in the network, without using any pre-existing wired or wireless network infrastructure, such as WLAN access points. Computing devices in MANET communicate with each other using wireless medium and route of data in a multi-hop fashion, if the wireless nodes are not within direct wireless transmission range of each other as shown in Figure 1.

There are many applications of mobile ad hoc networking technology such as Satellite multi-hop networks (Vladimirova, 2008; Shen, 2004) as shown in Figure 2, public safety applications (Miller, 2005), planetary surface exploration (Alena, 2005), inter-planetary networks (Sekhar, 2004), intelligent transportation systems (Toh, 2007), metropolitan ad hoc networks (Conti, 2003), building automation (Reinisch, 2007)

Figure 2 Multi-hop routing in satellite networks

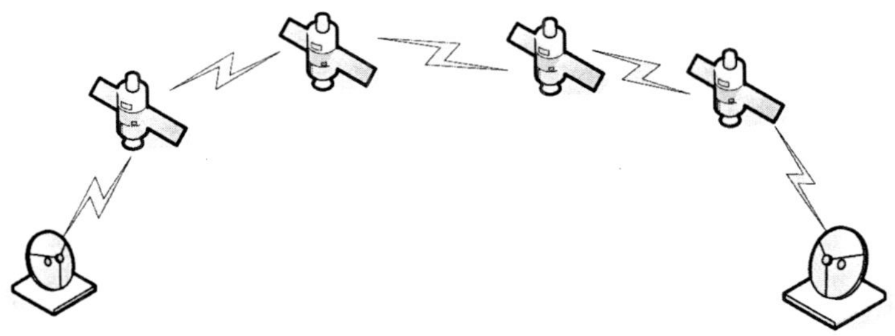

as well as providing connectivity to remote and inaccessible places (Wolff, 2005).

MANETs have many advantages; they can be set-up very fast, they do not require any pre-existing network infrastructure such as wiring or base stations etc. MANETs can also configure and organize themselves without requiring any manual intervention, for example when new nodes join or leave the network or when two MANETs merge together. Furthermore, due to the mesh topology of MANETs, if a path breaks due to node mobility or battery exhaustion, alternate redundant paths can be discovered quickly. Having shorter wire-less transmissions also increases the opportunity for frequency re-use.

In spite of the numerous advantages offered by MANET, there are still many challenges when it comes to supporting Quality of Service (QoS) on MANETs in comparison to supporting QoS in static wired networks due to many reasons as described in Section 3. Although initially most of the research on MANETs was focussed primarily on routing (Perkins, 1994; Perkins, 1999) and medium access control (Karn, 1990; Fullmer, 1995; Deng, 1998; & Tzamaloukas, 2001), in the past couple of years there has been an increased interest in QoS provisioning for MANETs with the aim to support real-time communication services such as voice and video (Ahn, 2002; Badis, 2006; Calafate, 2006; Reddy, 2007; Marwaha, 2008).

Figure3. MANET QoS mechanisms

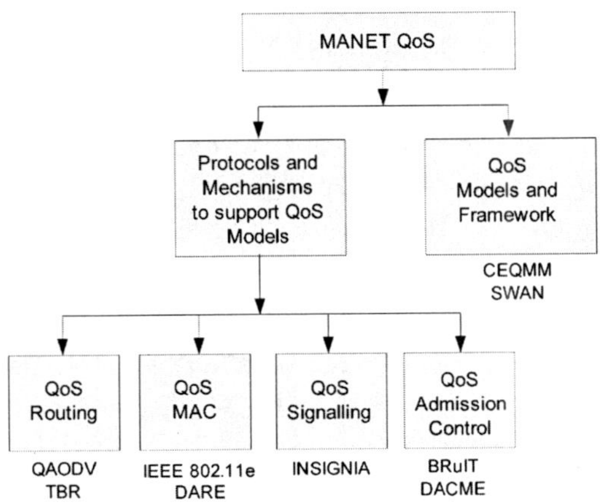

Many QoS protocols have been developed for MANETs and newer mechanisms are constantly being proposed. This chapter presents some of the important mechanisms and protocols for supporting QoS in MANETs. These range from QoS provisioning models to MANET QoS routing, signalling, admission control and MAC, as shown in Figure 3.

The structure of the chapter is as follows. Section 2 provides a brief background on basic QoS provisioning Models in IP Networks and basic routing schemes in MANETs as well as the Medium Access Control protocols used in MANET. Section 3 presents the challenges in QoS provisioning for MANETs. Section 4 presents the QoS provisioning models developed for MANETs, followed by Section 5 which presents the MANET QoS routing, signalling, Admission Control and Medium Access Control (MAC) schemes. Section 6 presents cross-layer frame-

Figure 4. RSVP resource reservation

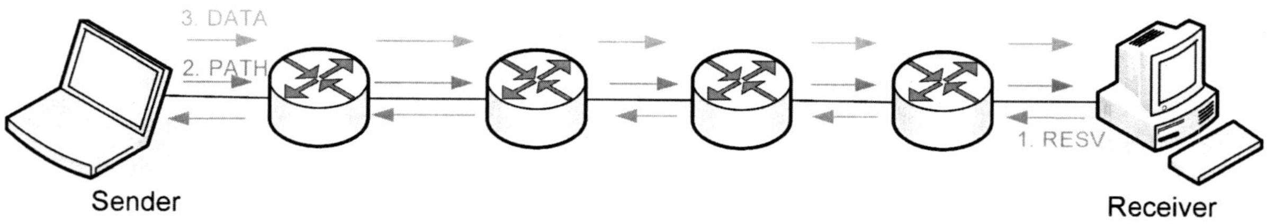

work for MANET QoS and Section 7 presents the concluding remarks.

BACKGROUND

This Section presents the brief background on IP Quality of Service (QoS) models, as well as the Mobile Ad hoc Networks (MANET) routing and IEEE 802.11 (IEEE Standard 802.11, 1999) Medium Access Control (MAC).

Background on IP QoS Models

QoS Models provide a framework for ensuring that the QoS requirements are met. There are three main QoS provisioning model in the Internet: (i) Integrated Services (IntServ) (Braden, 1994), (ii) Differentiated Services (DiffServ) (Blake, 1998) and (iii) Multi-Protocol Label Switching (Rosen, 2001).

Integrated Services

Integrated Services (IntServ) (Braden, 1994) model requires applications to inform the network about their QoS requirements. Resource ReSerVation Protocol (RSVP) (Braden, 1997) is used for signalling QoS requirements on a path to reserve and release a router's resources.

To set up resource reservation in the routers along the path between the sender and the receiver, the receiver sends RSVP Resource Reservation (RESV) messages (Braden, 1997) towards the source on the upstream path creating reservation state on the routers along the path as shown in Figure 4. When the RESV message reaches the Source, it sends a PATH message downstream towards the Receiver, setting the path reservation state on every node lying on the route.

Advantages and Disadvantages

IntServ provides guarantees on how a particular traffic flow will be handled inside the network in terms of the delay, throughput etc that it experiences. However, due to the need for per-flow reservation in routers, IntServ has scalability issues as it has high storage and processing overhead of reserved flow states on the QoS path nodes. Moreover, each reservation needs to be first set up, then refreshed regularly and lastly torn-down leading to high signalling overhead. This problem becomes even more severe in wireless networks where the bandwidth is scarce.

Differentiated Services

Differentiated Services (DiffServ) (Blake, 1998) is a model for QoS provisioning on a per-class basis, with requirement for storing and processing huge amounts of per-flow reservation state information at the routers ("stateless"). A class of traffic is an aggregate of multiple flows with similar traffic characteristics and performance requirements. In DiffServ, certain types of traffic classes get more QoS resources (CPU, buffer etc) compared to others.

Figure 5. DiffServ router

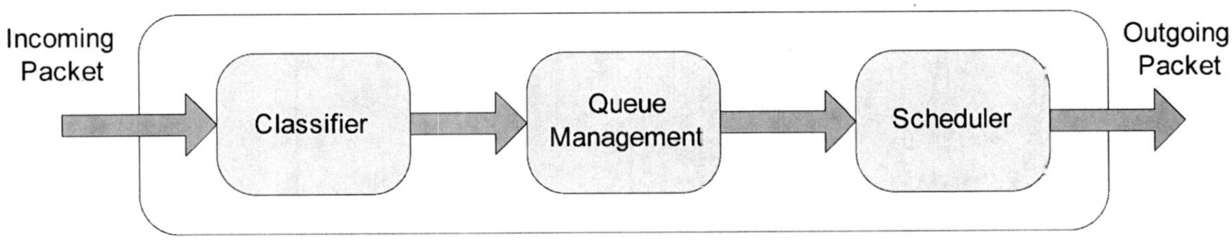

Figure 5 shows the basic block diagram of a DiffServ router, which consists of (i) a Classifier; (ii) a Queue Management module and; (iii) a Scheduler. The Classifier classifies the incoming packets and puts the packets in one of the various queues in the queue management module. The Queue management module is responsible for dropping packets if the queue overflows and marking packets if congestion is experienced at that node. The scheduler is responsible for providing priority to various classes of traffic over others.

The QoS class information is carried in-band in the header of each IP packet. The Type of Service byte is used for this purpose, wherein, the first 3 bits describe the precedence, the next 4 describe the Type of Service and the last bit is not used and Must Be Zero (MBZ) as shown in Figure 6.

Advantages and Disadvantages

DiffServ does not maintain per-flow state and therefore, does not suffer from the same scalability problems associated with IntServ. On the other hand, as the design and management of DiffServ routers is not necessarily controlled by a single entity, traffic flow may experience different levels of QoS as it traverses across networks.

Multi-Protocol Label Switching

MPLS provides fast packet forwarding and support for traffic engineering. MPLS can create virtual links between nodes far away in the network. Packets that enter an MPLS domain are labelled by Label Edge Routers (LERs). These labels are then processed very fast by Label Switched Routers (LSR) in the MPLS core as indicated in Figure 7.

Figure 6. IPv4 type of service field

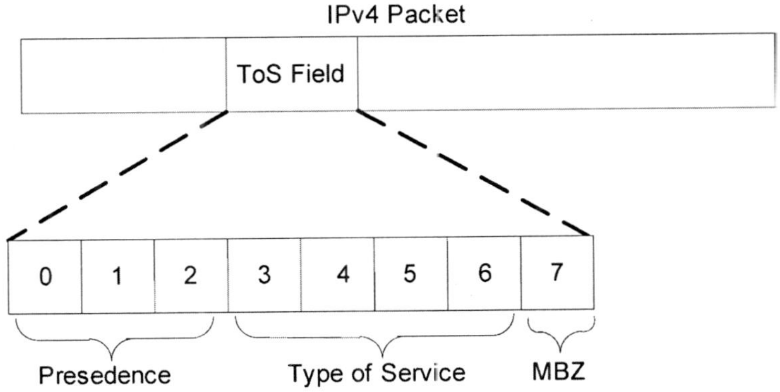

Figure 7. Example of an MPLS network

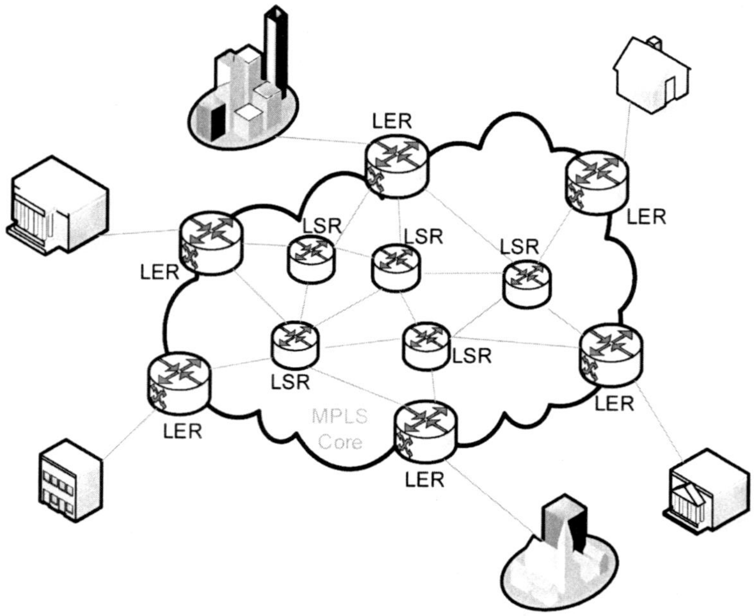

Advantages and Disadvantages

MPLS has many advantages. It has fast switching and it can support multiple protocols, traffic engineering as well as QoS. However, MPLS adds another layer in the protocol stack and the network equipment should be able to support it. It is also difficult to support MPLS in networks with the dynamic network topology which will require frequent re-establishment of Label Switched Paths, resulting in high control overhead and route establishment delay.

Background on Routing Schemes in MANETs

The two main routing schemes for MANETs are: (i) Proactive routing (Perkins, 1994) and (ii) Reactive or On-Demand routing (Perkins, 1999).

Proactive routing schemes continuously update the routing tables of mobile nodes and lead to the consumption of a huge amount of wireless bandwidth to update the frequent changes in routing tables, potentially leaving very little bandwidth for actual data communication.

Reactive routing protocols initiate an on-demand path discovery towards the destination from the source node, whenever a route is needed to be set up.

Destination-Sequenced Distance-Vector (DSDV) Routing Protocol

The Destination-Sequenced Distance-Vector (DSDV) (Perkins, 1994) Routing Algorithm is a Proactive routing protocol for MANET. DSDV is one of the earliest MANET routing protocols. Nodes using DSDV maintain a routing table and exchange it frequently with their neighbours. The routing table consists of entries of next hop nodes to reach the destinations in the network, including the sequence numbers assigned by those destination nodes. If a node receives multiple routes to a destination with the same sequence number, the one with the smallest number of hops is adopted.

Ad Hoc On-Demand Distance-Vector Routing

Ad hoc On-demand Distance-vector (AODV) (Perkins, 1999) routing protocol is a reactive routing scheme. AODV finds routes only when they are required, and saves the wireless bandwidth and battery power of mobile nodes, as it does not have to exchange routing tables frequently, as is the case in proactive routing schemes. The protocol operation is as follows. If a node using AODV does not have a route to the destination it needs to communicate with, that node broadcasts a Route Request (RREQ) message to its neighbours which in turn re-broadcast the message to their neighbours until the destination is found as shown in Figure 8 (a). When the Destination node receives the RREQ message it sends back a Route Reply (RREP) message back to the source as shown in Figure 8 (b). Also, if an intermediate node has a fresh enough route to the destination it replies with an RREP message in response to the RREQ message that it had received. Furthermore, if multiple copies of the same RREQ from different routes are received at an intermediate node, which discards the RREQs arriving later.

Local connectivity is maintained using regular HELLO messages which are exchanged between neighbouring nodes. If an active route fails, the node upstream to the point of failure sends a Route Error (RERR) message back to the source, which can then begin the discovery of a new route.

Medium Access Control in MANET

IEEE 802.11 MAC (IEEE Standard 802.11, 1999) protocol which uses Carrier Sense Medium Access with Collision Avoidance (CSMA/CA) is most commonly used in MANETs. As shown in Figure 9, every source node first listens to the wireless channel for carrier sensing to ensure no that one else is transmitting, before it can access the medium for transmitting a message. If no one is transmitting, the node first sends a Request-To-Send (RTS) message to the receiver node. The RTS message has the information of the receiver node's MAC address and the duration of transmission. Nodes in the vicinity which receive the RTS message then do not transmit during that duration. The receiver node after getting the RTS message transmits a Clear-To-Send (CTS) message back to the source node. The source node transmits the DATA packet to the receiver, after receiving the CTS message. If the receiver correctly receives the data packet, it replies by sending an Acknowledgement (ACK) message back to the source node.

CHALLENGES IN QOS PROVISIONING FOR MANET

In comparison to wired networks, QoS provisioning in MANETs is very hard because of numerous challenges and constraints as discussed below:

Resource constraints – The most important problem in QoS provisioning for MANETs is the limitation on various resources. The wireless bandwidth is scarce, the battery capacity of the mobile nodes is also limited as well as the range of the wireless communication which is limited by the transmission power of the mobile node. The Battery power resource must be utilised efficiently so as to prolong network lifetime and prevent the network from getting partitioned by battery exhaustion of certain key nodes with high connectivity. The wireless bandwidth has to be used efficiently by reducing the number of control messages.

QoS Routing – QoS routing protocol is an algorithm which finds paths that satisfies QoS constraints while transporting the data and multimedia traffic from the source to destination. QoS routing with multiple constrains is very challenging and becomes even more difficult in MANETs since the paths keep breaking due to the dynamic network topology. Obtaining the

Figure 8. Route discovery in AODV

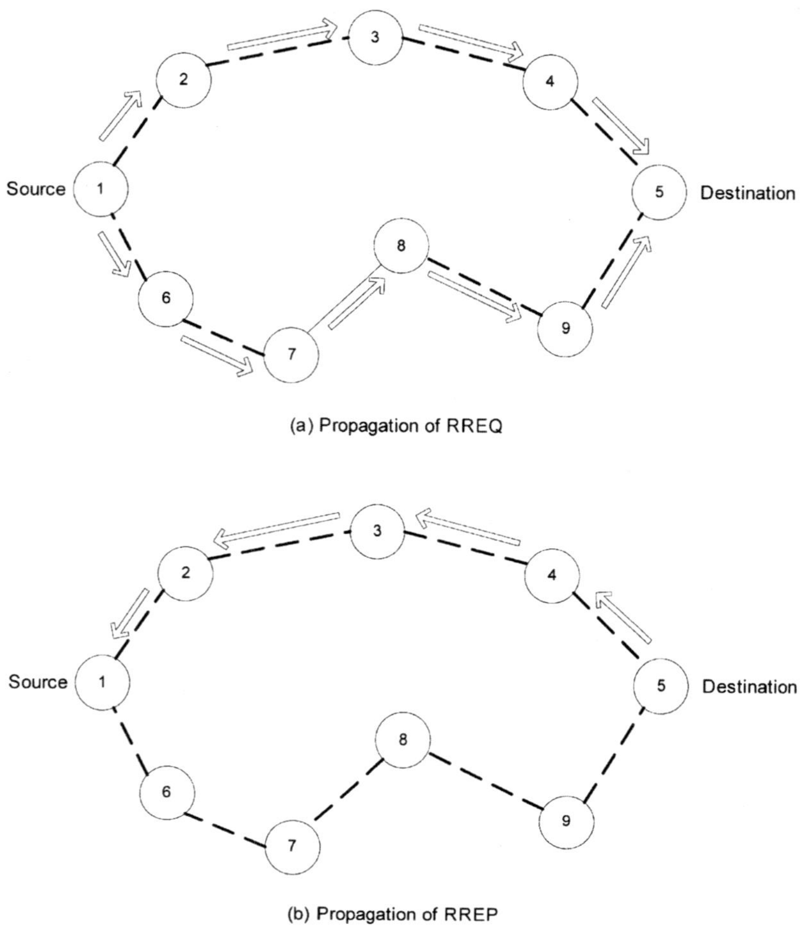

knowledge of QoS availability on each link in a dynamic network topology is quite hard.

Unpredictability of the Wireless Channel – The wireless medium is prone to many errors such as interference and fading etc. The wireless channel is shared among various nodes and is used in a decentralised manner. This makes the channel access delay unpredictable for different data packets belonging to the same stream of data. Bandwidth estimation of a shared channel is also difficult, as users are mobile and can come in and go out of the wireless interference and contention range of each other over time without any fixed pattern.

Heterogeneous nodes and applications – MANETs have different sizes, different types of nodes within them with varying capabilities in terms of battery power, number of interfaces etc and also different applications such as satellite networks, building automation and vehicular networks etc as mentioned in Section 1. Therefore, it is be difficult to develop one set of QoS requirements and protocols which suit all applications and types of MANETs.

Stateless QoS Model Related Problems – In QoS Models which do not maintain state information of the traffic flow reservations at intermediate nodes and rely on probing messages to gather instantaneous bandwidth, there can be a potential problem that multiple sources send probe messages to test the available bandwidth on the same path

Figure 9. Message exchange sequence in IEEE 802.11

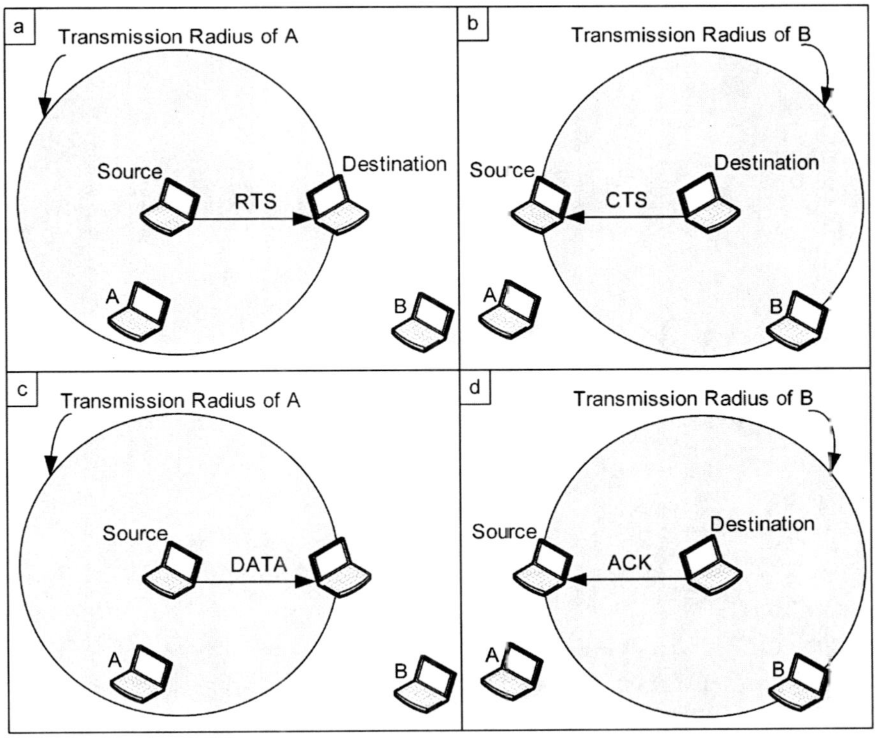

at the same time. In such a scenario the source nodes think that QoS resources are available when in fact they are not (Ahn, 2002).

This is explained as follows. Consider the network shown in Figure 10, where Source 1 and Source 2, send Probe messages Probe1 and Probe2 simultaneously towards Destination 1 and Destination 2 respectively for 10Mbps end-to-end bandwidth requirement for their traffic flows. When the two probe messages arrive at nodes 3 and 4, they both will read the instantaneous available bandwidth of say 12Mbps. However, when Source 1 and Source 2 start transmission of packets, nodes 3 and 4 will receive 10Mbs traffic from both the sources together. This will lead to congestion and queue overflows at the intermediate nodes.

QOS MODELS IN MANETS

This Section presents various QoS models proposed for MANET. Some of the MANET QoS models (Badis, 2006) use a combination of the IntServ and DiffServ frameworks, while some other QoS models (Ahn, 2002) make use of rate-control mechanisms like Explicit Congestion Notification (ECN) (Ramakrishnan, 2001).

Complete and Efficient QoS Model for MANETs

Complete and Efficient QoS Model for MANETs (CEQMM) (Badis, 2006) is a QoS model combining IntServ and DiffServ models. CEQMM makes use of QoS Optimized Link State Routing (QOLSR) (Badis, 2004) and nodes maintain a routing table for every traffic class using the neighbourhood and topology databases. Per-flow

Figure 10. Failure of probe messages in stateless QoS model

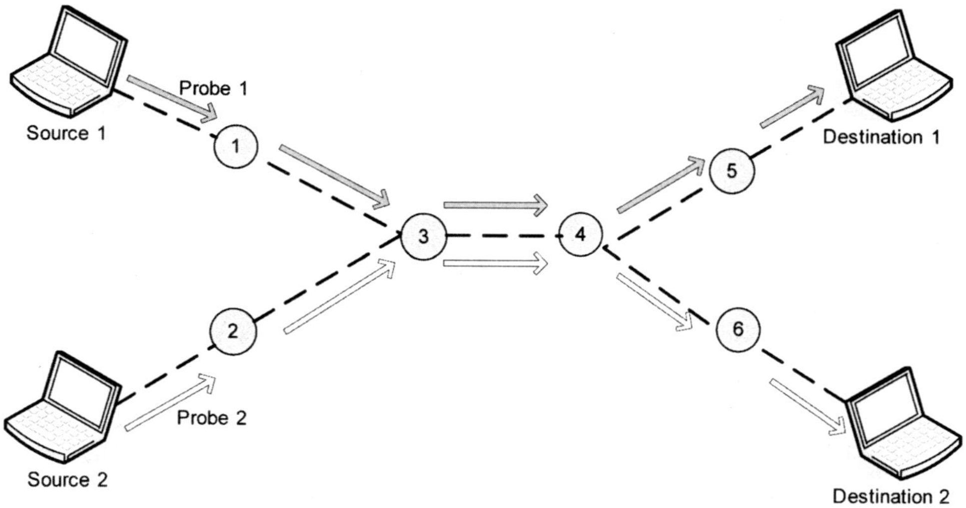

reservations are made for traffic flow with highest priority, and per-class QoS provisioning for other traffic flows. Admission Control is performed by sending a Check Request (CREQ) message on the path from the source to the destination node. The CREQ is forwarded by intermediate nodes, if they are able to support the QoS requirements. Reservations are maintained by using periodic CREQ messages. Queuing is separated for control traffic, QoS traffic and best-effort traffic, wherein the control traffic has the highest priority and the priority for the best-effort traffic being the least. It also uses an active queue management technique based on Random Early Detection (RED).

Advantages and Disadvantages

CEQMM uses a combination of both IntServ and DiffServ and therefore, can avoid the scalability problems seen with the IntServ model. Refreshing of soft-state increase the signalling overhead.

Stateless QoS Model for MANETs (SWAN)

Service Differentiation in Stateless Wireless Ad hoc networks (SWAN) (Ahn, 2002) does not require storing any state information for reserved traffic flows. However, SWAN differentiates between real-time and non-real-time packets. It uses a rate-control technique for the best-effort UDP and TCP traffic. For real-time traffic it uses sender based admission control. Early Congestion Notification is also used in SWAN for regulating UDP real-time traffic flows.

Before sending real-time data on a path, a source node sends a probing request message to gather information about the end-to-end bandwidth availability on that path. Intermediate nodes update the bottleneck bandwidth field if the available bandwidth at that node is less than the current value stored in that field. A probe response message is then sent by the destination node to the source with the information about the bottleneck bandwidth in it copied from the probing request.

The probe message reads the instantaneous value of the bandwidth availability. However, this may lead to a problem of "false admission" (Ahn, 2002), when multiple traffic sources send probe messages at the same time wherein, the source nodes will infer the result of the probe message as QoS resources being available on the path, when in reality they might not be. To solve this, a Congestion Experienced (CE) flag (Ahn, 2002) is used by the intermediate node experiencing congestion. The destination upon noticing the CE flag informs the source node to discover another path.

Advantages and Disadvantages

SWAN is stateless and therefore, it does not require storing and maintaining flow reservation states on the path, reducing the overhead involved in supporting QoS. However, the re-discovery of QoS paths when "false admission" happens may introduce jitter experienced by real-time flows as well as increases signalling overhead associated with multiple probe messages.

Dynamic RSVP for MANET

Dynamic RSVP (DRSVP) (Mirhakkak, 2000) solves the problem of crisp reservation requirements of RSVP, wherein a binary decision has to be made by the network whether or not the requested amount of resources can be reserved or not. Normally in RSVP, the reservation carries the following five QoS values specified by the application: average rate, token bucket depth, peak rate, minimum policed unit and maximum packet size. The reservation is accepted if the network is able to support these QoS reservation parameters. However, in the case of MANETs, the network capacity is dynamic and therefore, there is a need for more flexible QoS parameters. In DRSVP, average rate (r) is replaced by a range of minimum rate (rmin) and maximum rate (rmax).

Advantages and Disadvantages

DRSVP uses a range of QoS values for reserving QoS resources instead of using crisp values. This is a good way of accommodating more flows in resource constraint wireless networks such as MANETs. However, this could lead to higher complexity as compared to RSVP.

PROTOCOLS AND MECHANISMS TO SUPPORT QOS MODELS IN MANETS

To support the various MANET QoS Models, various protocols have been proposed such as: (i) QoS routing protocols to search for paths that can support the required QoS, (ii) signalling protocols for carrying the reservation information, (iii) admission control to limit the number of flows entering the network in order to maintain the QoS of existing flows and; (iv) Medium Access Control protocols to support QoS by giving high priority to certain traffic types at the time of transmission. This Section presents some of the key protocols and mechanisms which support QoS in MANETs.

MANET QoS Signalling

IntServ type QoS resource reservation models require a signalling protocol. The signalling protocol is responsible for carrying the QoS resource reservation and tears down messages as well as establishing appropriate QoS reservations on the intermediate nodes on a path.

The main QoS signalling protocol for MANETs is The INSIGNIA Signalling System (Lee, 2000; Ahn, 1999). INSIGNIA is a per-flow based soft-state reservation protocol supporting adaptive services in MANET. It uses In-band Signalling by encoding protocol commands in the IP option field of the IP packet header. This is called the INSIGNIA option. The soft-state resources reserved for a particular traffic flow on a path are refreshed upon receiving data packets belonging to that traffic flow.

Destination nodes continuously keep track of the received flows as well as measure the QoS statistics. These are sent back to the source nodes periodically for managing end-to-end adaptations.

Advantages and Disadvantages

INSIGNIA reduces the overhead of QoS reservation set-up as it is an in-band signalling protocol. However, soft-state maintenance and periodic QoS reports sent to the source node increase the overhead.

MANET Qos Routing

QoS routing is required to find network paths, if they exist, which can meet the QoS required by a traffic flow. Although it is quite difficult to discover QoS routes in MANETs which can have highly dynamic network topology, there have been some QoS routing protocols for MANETs that attain satisfactory QoS performance. This Section presents some of the important QoS routing protocols (Perkins, 2000; Chen 1999 & De, 2002). Unlike wired networks, MANET QoS routing protocols often piggyback QoS signalling and admission control information for establishing QoS reservations in parallel with the route discovery process.

QoS over AODV

QoS over AODV (QAODV) protocol (Perkins, 2000) proposes extending AODV's (Perkins, 1999) Route Request (RREQ) and Route Reply (RREP) messages to support QoS in MANET. Source nodes using QAODV may specify a maximum delay or minimum bandwidth in the RREQ message. An intermediate node rebroadcasts a route discovery message, only if it can meet the QoS requirements. If the QoS cannot be supported at an intermediate node after the QoS route has been set up, then that node sends an ICMP QoS_LOST message to the source.

Advantages and Disadvantages

QAODV is based on reactive routing (Perkins, 1999) and generally incurs less control overhead compared to proactive routing approaches. Being based on IntServ type QoS model, the scalability of QAODV poses difficulty as the network size, rate of change of topology and the number of traffic flows increase.

Ticket Based Probing

Ticket-Based Probing (TBP) (Chen, 1999) probes a path for available QoS resources using tickets issued by the source where a ticket is considered as an approval to probe a path. If a probe message has multiple tickets, that probe message can divide into multiple probe messages at an intermediate node on a path. Every probe message has one ticket at least. This way the source node can control the number of paths searched. TBP assumes that a node in the network keeps up-to-date local state of all outgoing links. The nodes are required to maintain end-to-end state information for every possible destination using a distance-vector protocol.

For most critical traffic flows, TBP uses multiple paths and sends every packet on each of the paths. In the next level of redundancy for ordinary connections, multiple paths are established, however, the packets are sent only on one path, called the primary path. Secondary paths also reserve the resources but are not used. In the last level of redundancy, QoS resource reservation is performed only on the primary path. When the primary path fails, resources are reserved on one of the secondary paths, if any of the secondary paths has the required resources, else the re-routing procedure is invoked.

Advantages and Disadvantages

Using tickets for probing paths reduces the control overhead involved in path discovery in comparison to flooding based route discovery. Increased redundancy in TBP increases the QoS but decreases the resources remaining for other flows starting later. TBP may also fail to find the most optimal path as the entire set of paths are not searched, only a limited number of paths are searched, limited by the number of tickets issued.

Trigger Based Distributed QoS Routing in MANET

Trigger-based Distributed Routing (TDR) protocol (De, 2002) makes use of on-demand route discovery for MANETs. Nodes using TDR periodically transmits beacon messages to their neighbours that contain location and mobility information. Nodes in the network store this information of their neighbourhood in a neighbourhood database. Activity-based database are also kept at the source, destination and intermediate nodes participating in a session. The activity database stores such information as session identifiers and bandwidth requirements.

TDR uses Global Positioning System (GPS) based location information along with on-demand path discovery with selective forwarding if the position of the destination node is known to the source. Otherwise if the location information is not known, it uses flooding based search. The intermediate nodes only admit one route discovery packet for a session, which has the least number of hops to ensure loop free routing. Furthermore, to search for stable routes, only neighbours whose received signal strength is above a certain threshold are used for routing.

A temporary reservation with the required bandwidth (similar to RSVP protocol) is made when the path discovery packet is received at an intermediate node, if the free bandwidth at that node meets the maximum bandwidth requirements of the flow. In order to minimise the resources being locked for a long time, the nodes closer to the destination have a reservation time less compared to nodes farther away from the destination. Once the destination receives the route discovery packet and accepts that route, it sends an Acknowledgement packet back to the source along the selected route, which updates the activity databases at the intermediate and source nodes. Destination node also sends its location update through the ACK message whenever there is significant change in the location to aid in the event when re-routing is necessary. The activity database maintains reservation in a soft-state form, data packets belonging to the reserved flow are used to refresh the soft-state timer.

Path repair utilises location information of the destination and only forwarding the rerouting requests to nodes that are nearer to the destination and that meet the QoS requirement. Rerouting can be initiated by both the Source and Intermediate nodes on a path. If the intermediate node initiated re-routing fails, the source node then initiates rerouting of the whole path. To remove a session's reservation, the source node sends a deactivation message on the reserved path. However, in TDR no deactivation message is sent in case of re-routing, the unused section of the previous path refreshes the activity database after the soft-state interval.

Advantages and Disadvantages

TDR uses location information for routing and re-routing purpose. This leads to extra overhead in terms of location information update. Maintenance of location information of neighbourhood nodes increases computational overhead and memory consumption. Relying on location information may impose limitations where such information may not be available.

MANET QoS Admission Control

Admission Control is the QoS process of admitting or rejecting new flows into the network. In case the network has QoS resources, the flow is admitted otherwise not. Although MANET QoS routing protocols presented in Section 5.2 do incorporate some admission control mechanisms, there are some more specialised admission control schemes presented in this Section. There are mainly two types of admission control techniques in MANET which can be classified as state-full and stateless, depending on whether they keep the bandwidth reservation information at the intermediate nodes or not. The state-full mechanisms maintain information of remaining bandwidth available at a node and may also have such information for its neighbourhood. In contrast, the stateless admission control techniques do not keep any such information and relying on probe messages to check instantaneous bandwidth availability.

BRuIT

Bandwidth Reservation under InTerferences influence (BRuIT) (Chaudet, 2002; Chaudet, 2005) implements Admission Control with a reactive QoS routing protocol. During route discovery, intermediate nodes forward the Route Request only if the requested resources are available. The nodes performing admission control in BRuIT use information of the used and free bandwidth from other nodes present in its carrier sense range, which is collected using Hello packets exchanged between neighbouring nodes. Furthermore, as interference can happen with parallel transmissions farther than one-hop transmission radius, the Hello packets include not just one hop bandwidth information, but two hop bandwidth information.

Guaranteeing QoS resources in a wireless environment is difficult; therefore, nodes using BRuIT also specify a step (reduction) and a (minimum) threshold value in their resource reservation messages. The intermediate nodes can reduce the bandwidth allocation by a step amount each time they experience congestion and are not able to meet the bandwidth allocated earlier for a particular flow till the threshold value is reached. At this point the flow is cancelled and the source node is sent a notification asking it to discover a new route.

Advantages and Disadvantages

BRuIT considers used and free bandwidth from neighbouring nodes present in the carrier sense range of a node while performing admission control. This is a very comprehensive mechanism. However, it increases the signalling overhead entailed in exchanging HELLO messages.

DACME

Distributed Admission Control for MANET Environments (DACME) (Calafate, 2006) uses probing of the path from the source to the destination before accepting flows into the network. DACME sources send ten packets back-to-back towards the destination per probe. When the destination receives the probe message, it notifies the source of the quantity of bandwidth available on the probed path. QoS is provided by using the Type of Service (ToS) field in the IP header of each packet (Calafate, 2006).

Advantages and Disadvantages

DACME uses back-to-back packets for probing the network paths. This mechanism gives a good picture of the state of the network compared to sending just one probe packet. However, higher number of probing packets shall lead to increased control overhead. As DACME uses IP ToS field for QoS support, the nodes do not have to maintain the QoS reservation information. As it does not maintain reservation information, it may face the problem of "false admission" (Ahn, 2002) similar to SWAN.

MANET QoS MAC

This section presents MANET QoS MAC protocols. In order to provision QoS, the real-time traffic (voice and video) should get greater priority by the Medium Access Control (MAC) protocol. This involves scheduling transmissions such that the MAC layer prioritizes the real-time traffic over best effort traffic.

IEEE 802.11e MAC Protocol

IEEE 802.11e (IEEE 802.11e Draft 3.1, 2002) is one of the QoS MAC protocols that uses two channel access mechanisms: (i) Hybrid Coordination Function (HCF) Controlled Channel Access (HCCA) and (ii) Enhanced DCF Channel Access (EDCA). In HCCA mode, the controller polls the mobile stations and grants them with transmission time-slots. In EDCA mode, the nodes have multiple access categories with different transmission queues having different priority levels. Nodes wait for a specified time period before transmitting when the medium is not being used. This time, which is known as Arbitration Inter-frame Space, is less for higher priority traffic reducing the delay experienced by higher priority traffic before transmission, compared to other access categories.

Advantages and Disadvantages

IEEE 802.11e enhances the 802.11 MAC protocol with QoS support. However, it increases the complexity of the MAC layer.

DARE

Distributed End-To-End Allocation of Time-slots for Real-Time Traffic (DARE) (Carlson, 2006) protocol is a MAC layer QoS protocol for MANET which reserves time-slots at the nodes lying on the path from source to the destination. DARE does not determine multi-hop routes.

The originator or source node sends a Request-To-Reserve (RTR) message to the destination. RTR message reserves MAC layer resources (time-slots) on the path. Information about the frequency and length of a time-slot to be reserved is carried by the RTR message. If the intermediate nodes are able to meet the reservation requirement, they make an entry into their respective reservation tables and set it to "preliminary" before forwarding it to the next hop. However, if the intermediate node is unable to reserve the required resources, it does not forward the RTR message. The "preliminary" reservations on the route will be freed after a time-out period.

The destination node upon receiving the RTR message sends back towards the source a Clear-To-Reserve (CTR) message, which traverses the path taken by the corresponding RTR message. An intermediate node upon getting the CTR message modifies the reservation state from "preliminary" to "fixed". Once the source node gets the CTR message, it begins sending data on the reserved path.

When an intermediate node gets an RTR message for reserving a time-slot which is previously reserved, it sends an Update-Transmit-Reservation (UTR) message to the upstream node with some other available transmission time-slot. If the upstream node can also transmit in the new time-slot a new RTR message is created and the previously reserved time-slots are released.

Nodes nearby a QoS reserved path, which receive RTR and CTR messages, too do not transmit in the reserved time-slots to avoid interference. Reserved time-slot information is also included in each real-time data and acknowledgement packet. This tells nodes nearby to a reserved path that did not initially receive the RTR and CTR messages about the reserved time-slots.

Advantages and Disadvantages

DARE tries to avoid interference amongst nodes in a path and those in the adjoining region. This could reduce interference, collisions and retransmissions. However, accomplishing this will require higher signalling overhead involved in exchanging RTR, CTR and UTR messages in DARE.

Figure 11. Packet scheduling in ReAP

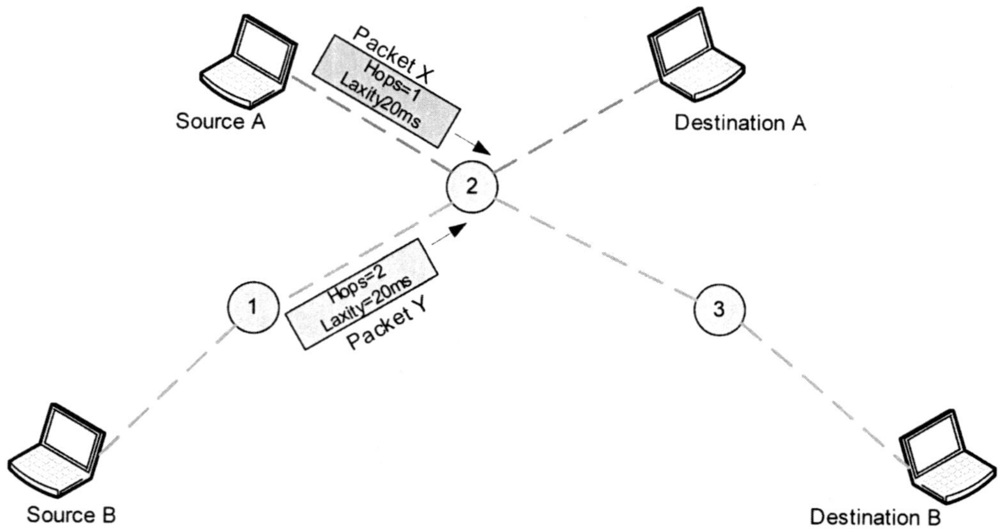

Packet Deadline Based Scheduling

Some packet scheduling schemes (e.g. Dehbi, 2008) are based on Earliest Deadline First (EDF) (Liu, 1973) approach. Another scheme dynamic ReAllocative Priority (ReAP) (Reddy, 2007) changes the priority of packet transmissions so that the packets are delivered within a specified time. ReAP utilises laxity and remaining hop count to calculate the priority of a packet in the queue. ReAP distinguishes between packets which have to travel more number of hops than those travelling on smaller number of hops.

The priority of a packet in the queue is calculated as the ratio of laxity to the remaining hop count. In ReAP a smaller ratio means higher priority. Laxity is the difference of the deadline and the current local time. For example, consider the two packets Packet X and Packet Y arriving at Node 2 from Source A and Source B respectively, as shown in Figure 11. The priority of Packet X is 20 whereas the priority of Packet Y is 10. Therefore, Packet Y is transmitted first at node 2.

In ReAP, the two queues for Voice and Video Packets also have the deadline and amount of hops left for the packets in the queue. This information is used to scan for the for the highest priority packet for transmission.

Advantages and Disadvantages

EDF based schemes consider the needs of different packets in terms of their urgency of delivery deadline. However, this may increase the complexity of the protocol as each packet entering the queue needs to be checked for its deadline and then appropriately transmitted ahead of other packets. ReAP (Reddy, 2007) enhances the basic EDF based schemes by considering not only the delivery deadline but also the amount of hops remaining. However, the use of hop count information and laxity to calculate priority of each packet can increase the complexity and overhead.

MANET CROSS-LAYER QOS FRAMEWORK

Delgado (2006) proposes a "Cross-Layer design for Video Streaming over Ad hoc networks (ViStA-

XL)" which collects information from different layers and uses all this information to dynamically adjust various parameters at the different protocol layers. ViStA-XL also uses multi-path routing for achieving QoS, focussing on a layered-coded video streaming application.

Information from all the network layers is provided to the Cross-layer Optimizer (XLO) module. For example, the Physical layer informs the Received Signal Strength from the neighbouring nodes, MAC layer informs the wireless channel utilisation, the network layers informs the various multi-hop communication routes available, as well as their quality by probing each path at regular intervals. The information about the end-to-end packet delivery and delay is provided by the transport layer to XLO and the application layer informs XLO of the bandwidth and delay requirements etc. Using multiple paths and path diversity, XLO tries to obtain required bandwidth and safeguard the most vital information packets and implement load balancing. ViStA-XL uses DSR for routing.

Advantages and Disadvantages

ViStA-XL is designed to transmit hierarchical layered-coded video and is a good step towards cross-layer optimisation in MANET QoS, however, a lot of work remains in developing a generic cross-layer optimization framework for MANET QoS.

CONCLUSION

This chapter presents the various frameworks and mechanisms for supporting Quality of Service (QoS) in MANETs. Some MANET QoS provisioning models make use of a combination of IntServ and DiffServ models for example CEQMM, while others use IntServ based on Dynamic QoS parameters such as Dynamic RSVP. QoS mechanisms in MANETs are quite different to traditional networks. A QoS routing protocol is generally needed to discover routes in MANET that can meet the necessary bandwidth and delay requirements of the traffic flows. This is due to the network capacity being inherently limited in MANETs, unlike wired networks, where paths could be over provisioned. Various QoS Routing protocols for MANET have been presented in Section 5.2 of this chapter. In addition to QoS routing, having time-slot reservations and transmission priority at the MAC layer is quite important for QoS traffic. Many MANET MAC protocols have been proposed to support QoS such as time-slot reservations based DARE protocol and packet deadline based ReAP protocol as well as others such as IEEE 802.11e. Admission control in MANET is mostly carried out in a distributed fashion at each intermediate node on a path, along with the rout discovery process. Route discovery messages also carry admission control and QoS Signalling information. This reduces the extra overhead of QoS approaches based on IntServ model. Finally, cross-layer QoS protocols such as ViStA-XL (Delgado, 2006) for MANET, combine QoS mechanisms and protocols at various layers. Given the dynamic nature of MANET networks and the resource limited nodes forming MANET, it is difficult to support hard QoS guarantees in MANET. Many promising QoS protocols for MANET have been proposed in the literature. However, more work is needed to further investigate QoS mechanisms for MANET in particular cross-layer approaches to optimise QoS mechanisms.

ACKNOWLEDGMENT

NICTA is funded by the Australian Government as represented by the Department of Broadband, Communications and the Digital Economy and the Australian Research Council through the ICT Centre of Excellence program.

REFERENCES

Ahn, G.S., Campbell, A.T., Lee, S.B., & Zhang, X. (1999). INSIGNIA. IETF MANET WG Internet Draft: draft-ietf-manet-insignia-01.

Ahn, G.-S., Campbell, A. T., Veres, A., & Sun, L. H. (2002). Supporting Service Differentiation for Real-Time and Best Effort Traffic in Stateless Wireless Ad Hoc Networks (SWAN). *IEEE Transactions on Mobile Computing, 1*(3), 197–207.

Alena, R. L., & Lee, C. (2005). Adaptive bio-inspired wireless network routing for planetary surface exploration. IEEE Aerospace Conference (pp.1438 – 1443).

Badis, H., & Agha, K. A. (2004). QOLSR multi-path routing for mobile ad hoc networks based on multiple metrics: bandwidth and delay. IEEE Vehicular Technology Conference, (Vol. 4, pp. 2181-2184).

Badis, H., & Agha, K. A. (2006). CEQMM: a complete and efficient quality of service model for MANETs. ACM Intlernational workshop on Performance Evaluation of wireless ad hoc, sensor & ubiquitous networks (pp. 25–32).

Blake, S., Black, D., Carlson, M., Davies, E., Wang, Z. & Weiss, W. (1998). An Architecture for Differentiated Service. IETF RFC: 2475.

Braden, R. (Ed.). (1997). Resource ReSerVation Protocol (RSVP) - Version 1 Functional Specification. IETF RFC 2205.

Braden, R., Clark, D., & Shenker, S. (1994). Integrated Services in the Internet Architecture: an Overview. IETF RFC: 1633.

Calafate, C. T., Manzoni, P., & Malumbres, M. P. (2006). A Novel QoS Framework for Medium-Sized MANETs Supporting Multipath Routing Protocols. In 11th IEEE Symposium on Computers and Communications (pp. 213- 219).

Carlson, E., Karl, H., Wolisz, A., & Prehofer, C. (2006). Distributed allocation of time-slots for real-time traffic in a wireless multi-hop network. *IEEE JSAC, 24*(11), 2018–2027.

Chaudet, C., & Lassous, I. G. (2002). BRuIT: Bandwidth Reservation under InTerferences influence. Paper presented at the European Wireless, Florence, Italy.

Chaudet, C., & Lassous, I. G. (2005). Evaluation of the BRuIT protocol. IEEE 61st Vehicular Technology Conference, (Vol. 4, pp. 2493 – 2497).

Chen, S., & Nahrstedt, K. (1999). Distributed quality of service routing in ad hoc networks. *IEEE Journal on Selected Areas in Communications, 17*(8), 1488–1505. doi:10.1109/49.780354

Conti, M., Giordano, S., Maselli, G., & Turi, G. (2003). MobileMAN: Mobile Metropolitan Ad Hoc Networks. [). Berlin: Springer.]. *Lecture Notes in Computer Science, 2775*, 169–174.

Crawley, E., Nair, R., Rajagopalan, B., & Sandick, H. (1998). A Framework for QoS-based Routing in the Internet. IETF RFC: 2386.

De, S., Das, S. K., Wu, H., & Qiao, C. (2002). Trigger-based distributed QoS routing in mobile ad hoc networks. *ACM SIGMOBILE Mobile Computing and Communications Review, 6*(3), 22–35. doi:10.1145/581291.581298

Dehbi, Y., & Mikou, N. (2008). Priority Assignment for Multimedia Packets Scheduling in MANET. IEEE International Conference on Signal Image Technology and Internet Based Systems (pp. 32-37).

Delgado, G. D., Frias, V. C., & Igartua, M. A. (2006). Video-streaming Transmission with QoS over Cross-Layered Ad hoc Networks. International Conference on Software in Telecommunications and Computer Networks, SoftCOM, (pp.102 – 106).

Deng, J., & Haas, Z. (1998). Dual Busy Tone Multiple Access (DBTMA), A New Medium Access Control for Packet Radio Networks. IEEE International Conference on Universal Personal Communications, (Vol. 2, pp. 973-977).

Fullmer, C. L., & Garcia-Luna-Aceves, J. J. (1995). Floor Acquisition Multiple Access (FAMA) for Packet-Radio Networks. Conference on Applications, Technologies, Architectures, and Protocols for Computer Communication (SIGCOMM), (pp.262-273).

IEEE 802.11 Standard. (1999). Wireless LAN MAC and PHY specifications.

IEEE 802.11e Draft 3.1. (2002). Wireless LAN Medium Access Control (MAC) and Physical Layer (PHY) Specifications: Medium Access Control (MAC) Enhancements for Quality of Service (QoS).

Karn, P. (1990). MACA - A New Channel Access Protocol for Packet Radio. Proceedings of the ARRL/CRRL Amateur Radio Ninth Computer Networking Conference (pp. 134.140).

Lee, B., Ahn, G. S., Zhang, X., & Campbell, A. T. (2000). INSIGNIA: an IP-based quality of service framework for mobile ad hoc networks. *Journal of Parallel and Distributed Computing*, *60*(4), 374–406. doi:10.1006/jpdc.1999.1613

Liu, C. L., & Layland, J. W. (1973). Scheduling algorithms for multiprogramming in hard real-time environment. *Journal of the ACM*, *20*(1), 40–61. doi:10.1145/321738.321743

Marwaha, S., Indulska, J., & Portmann, M. (2008). Challenges and Recent Advances in QoS Provisioning, Signaling, Routing and MAC protocols for MANETs. Australasian Telecommunication Networks and Applications Conference (ATNAC) (pp.97-102).

Miller, L. E. (2005). *Wireless Technologies and the SAFECOM SoR for Public Safety Communications, Leonard E. Miller, Wireless Communication Technologies Group. National Institute of Standards and Technology*. Report, Maryland, USA: NIST.

Mirhakkak, M., Schult, N., & Thomson, D. (2000). Dynamic quality-of-service for mobile ad hoc networks. In ACM International Symposium on Mobile ad hoc networking & computing (pp. 137 – 138).

Perkins, C. E. (2001). *Ad hoc Networking*. Boston: Addison Wesley.

Perkins, C. E., & Bhagwat, P. (1994). Highly Dynamic Destination-Sequenced Distance-Vector Routing (DSDV) for Mobile Computers. ACM Special Interest Group on Data Communications (SIGCOMM) Conference, 24(4), 234-244.

Perkins, C. E., & Royer, E. M. (1999). Ad hoc On-Demand Distance Vector Routing. IEEE Workshop on Mobile Computing Systems and Applications (pp. 90-100).

Perkins, C.E., Royer, E.M. & Das, S.R. (2000). Quality of Service for Ad hoc On-Demand Distance-vector Routing. IETF MANET WG Draft: draft-ietf-manet-aodvqos-00.txt

Ramakrishnan K., Floyd S. & Black D. (2001). The Addition of Explicit Congestion Notification (ECN) to IP. IETF RFC: 3168.

Reddy, T. B., John, J. P., & Murthy, C. S. R. (2007). Providing MAC QoS for multimedia traffic in 802.11e based multi-hop ad hoc wireless networks. Computer Networks. *The International Journal of Computer and Telecommunications Networking*, *51*(1), 153–176.

Reinisch, C., Kastner, W., Neugschwandtner, G., & Granzer, W. (2007). Wireless Technologies in Home and Building Automation. In Fifth IEEE Industrial Informatics International Conference, (Vol. 1, pp. 93-98).

Rosen E., Viswanathan A., & Callon R. (2001). Multi-Protocol Label Switching Architecture. IETF RFC: 3031.

Sekhar, A., Manoj, B. S., & Murthy, C. S. R. (2004). MARVIN: movement-aware routing over interplanetary networks. IEEE Sensor and Ad Hoc Communications and Networks conference (pp. 245- 254).

Shen, C. C., Rajagopalan, S., Borkar, G., & Jaikaeo, C. (2004). A flexible routing architecture for ad hoc space networks. *International Journal of Computer and Telecommunications Networking*, *46*(3), 389–410.

Toh, C.-K. (2007). Future Application Scenarios for MANET-Based Intelligent Transportation Systems. In Future Generation Communications and Networking International Conference: (Vol. 2, pp. 414-417). Washington, DC: IEEE Computer Society Press.

Tzamaloukas, A., & Garcia-Luna-Aceves, J. J. (2001). A Receiver-Initiated Collision-Avoidance Protocol for Multi-Channel Networks. IEEE INFOCOM, Twentieth Annual Joint Conference of the IEEE Computer and Communications Societies, (Vol.1, pp. 189-198).

Vladimirova, T., Wu, X., & Bridges, C. P. (2008). Development of a Satellite Sensor Network for Future Space Missions. IEEE Aerospace Conference (pp.1 – 10).

Wolff, R. S., Dunkle, D., Nugent, P., & Overcast, M. (2005, July). Ad-hoc Networking in Rugged and Remote Areas: Intermittently Connected Networking. Paper presented at the 17th International Conference on Wireless Communications, Calgary, Canada.

Section 2

Network Management Model

Chapter 6
Traffic Controller for Handling Service Quality in Multimedia Network

Manjunath Ramachandra
Philips - Bangalore, India

Vikas Jain
Philips - Bangalore, India

ABSTRACT

The present day Internet traffic largely caters for the multimedia traffic throwing open new and unthinkable applications such as tele-surgery. The complexity of data transactions increases with a demand for in time and real time data transfers, demanding the limited resources of the network beyond their capabilities. It requires a prioritization of data transfers, controlled dumping of data over the network etc. To make the matter worse, the data from different origin combine together imparting long lasting detrimental features such as self similarity and long range dependency in to the traffic. The multimedia data fortunately is associated with redundancies that may be removed through efficient compression techniques. There exists a provision to control the compression or bitrates based on the availability of resources in the network. The traffic controller or shaper has to optimize the quality of the transferred multimedia data depending up on the state of the network. In this chapter, a novel traffic shaper is introduced considering the adverse properties of the network and counteract with the same.

INTRODUCTION

The multimedia traffic over the Internet has characteristic requirements and features such as large buffers, real time data transfers, user interaction and monitoring, bursty traffic etc. The traffic has a few Predictable parameters in statistical sense that should be made use for effective control. The traffic pattern obeys poisson distribution. The multimedia traffic is inherently bursty and time varying due to different degree of compression for the data of a unit time. The burstiness of one flow affects other adaptive flows. This property is used in traffic control.

The multimedia data sources are often modeled as on-off sources. The overlapping of independent on-off sources leads to arrival pattern distribution with heavy-tailed autocorrelation function.

DOI: 10.4018/978-1-61520-791-6.ch006

Figure 1. Traffic controller

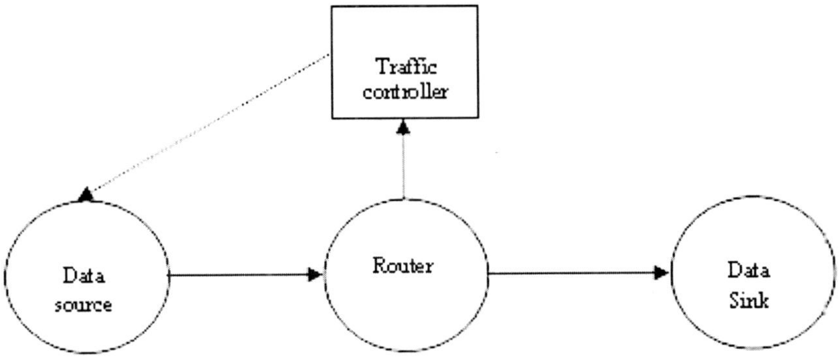

This heavy tail distribution imparts long range dependency to the traffic. As a result, there is no flattening of the distribution towards a mean when zoomed out in time scale.

As a result of burstiness or Long-range dependency, the resources would get flooded resulting in packet losses for a long duration. The other problems of long range dependency include jitter, Delay, large buffer requirements, congestion etc. As a fall out of these issues, it would be nearly impossible to meet the committed quality of service.

In a home network scenario, there will be limited support to overcome congestion. The best way to fix this issue is to avoid the congestion to happen. So, a proactive control algorithm is required than an active one (Hollot,C., Misra,V., Towsley,D., & Gong,W, 2001). A good controller has to foresee the trends in the network traffic variations and provide inputs to the traffic source well in advance as shown in Figure 1.

The source would get sufficient time to adjust the traffic rate or provide sufficient redundancies with the appropriate channel coding schemes so that it would not flood the channel when it is disturbed. In this chapter, the proactive queue management model GREEN (Wu-chun Feng; Kapadia, A., & Thulasidasan, S) together with a neural network is considered.

BACKGROUND

Meeting stringent constraints on the delay is very important in the networks supporting multimedia traffic for seamless user experience. In addition to the delay and packet losses, the variable delay suffered by the packets i.e. jitter is to be given due weightage. Analysis shows that the jitter degrades the perceptual quality as much as the packet loss (Mark Claypool, Jonathan Tanner, 1999).

To support the QoS in the Internet, the IETF has defined two architectures:

- The Integrated Services (Intserv) and
- Differentiated Services (Diffserv).

They have important differences in both the service definition and the implementation architectures. At the service definition level, the Intserv provides end-to-end guarantees or controlled load service (El-Haddadeh, R., Taylor, G.A., & Watts, S.J, 2004) on a per flow basis, while the Diffserv provides a coarser level of service differentiation among a small number of traffic classes.

Intserv

In an Intserv (Shioda, S., Mase, K, 2005), all transactions happen on per flow basis. The routers generate and process the signals for forwarding the data and maintaining the QoS in each flow.

The activities such as classification, scheduling and buffer management happens for each flow. Performing the per-flow management inside the network affects the network scalability and the performance. The IntServ although provides the agreed QoS guarantees, it results in under utilization of the resources. The scheme poses scalability issues.

Diffserv

In Diffserv (Stiliadis, D., & Varma,A., 1998), the transactions happen on per hop basis. Here, each data packet is assigned with some priority levels. The popularly used protocols support up to eight levels of priority, or equivalently eight classes of traffic. During a contention for the resources, the packets of lower priority will be discarded in preference for the packets with a higher priority.

The Diffserv needs an active resource management mechanism to provide the services with an assurance level of service comparable to those provided by the Intserv. Here a traffic shaper or a packet dropper controls the dynamics of the packet forwarding. Thus, the effective design of the dropping mechanism is important in congestion avoidance and rendering a rich class of services. In this chapter, a novel feedback mechanism called random early prediction (REP) (Manjunath,R., & Gurumurthy,K.S., 2004) based on the prediction of the status notification is proposed. First, the packet drop probability is computed using conventional tools such as random early detection (RED) (Floyd, S., & Jacobson, V, 1993). This signal is predicted in time, shifted and used as the feedback signal. Although the proposed mechanism may be used in the same way with IntServ to reserve the resources dynamically, it is not discussed as the objective here is to bring out the mechanism of dynamic sharing of the network resources.

The proposed scheme is scalable because it can provide QoS mechanism without maintaining the per flow states. It is legacy because it can be easily deployed in the current routers by adding predictors and shifters to the existing software.

Characteristics of Multimedia Traffic

The simulation study shows that the proposed method can maintain an average queue length and its variations small irrespective of the congestion control methods in end systems. Therefore the proposed method is best suit for real-time multimedia services which have stringent requirements on the delay and jitter. It is verified that the proposed active queue management scheme does not have bias against the bursty flows although it can protect well-behaving flows.

The present day home network predominantly supports multimedia traffic over the wireless medium. In a wireless network, the reflections and multi path result in increased self similarity (Willinger, W., Taqqu, M.S., Sherman, R., & D.V. Wilson, 1997) for the signal at the receiving end. The self similarity of the network refers to the invariance of the shape of the autocorrelation function when observed over multiple time scales. The self similarity imparts long range dependency in to the traffic. As a result of long range dependency, the traffic turns bursty resulting in under or over utilization of the resources, increased cell loss etc.

In order to reduce the loss of multimedia data over the wireless medium, it is required to pump in less data by controlling the degree of compression (and improving channel coding) when the channel is more noisy. To make it possible, a feedback on the channel status in terms of % loss of the data packets over the channel is required to be transferred to the source. Based on this input, a decision has to be taken on the data transmission rate.

For a perfect synergy between the feed forward (FF) and the feedback (FB) path, the properties of forward path that impart aberrations to the signal have to be annulled by generating appropriate signals in the feedback path. Ideally, the controller generating the feedback signal should have the same characteristics of the network. i.e, it should be a network in its own sense.

Round Trip Time Control

The neural network model that satisfies the aforementioned requirements of the controller is provided here. The properties of the network are reflected in to this model. Model of the controller provides a mechanism to control the behavior of the network. Performance improvement as a result of this controller model is evident from the simulation results. In a network, reduction of RTT effectively puts a higher bound on the bandwidth supported for a given loss. Thus the throughput can be increased if RTT can be made small. In order to make it happen, a feedback control signal indicating the status of the network is provide to the data sources.

In Random early detection (RED) the probability of packet loss (Christiansen,M., Jeffay, K., Ott, D., & Smith,F.D., 2001), is used as the feedback signal. In the proposed scheme, a predicted version this signal is taken with time shifts as the feedback signal. It is as though the RTT is reduced.

As the RTT gets reduced or probability of cell loss decreases, the throughput increases. With the usage of predicted packet drop as the control signal, both RTT as well as the cell loss get reduced, resulting in an increased throughput. The predictor works within the source and controls the transmission rate efficiently.

The RTT is an important state variable in this system. This includes the delay around the feedback loop, as well. The RTT varies primarily as a function of the buffer fill levels in the network path, along which the data travels. The longer the packets must wait in buffers, the longer it takes for them to traverse that path. A significant increase in RTT indicates the network congestion.

The importance of limits on RTT is highlighted here. The performance with the proposed controller is demonstrated with simulation experiments. The integration of mobile, computing and consumer electronic devices in the home network and the support for multimedia content has put burden over the available resources such as bandwidth, buffer space etc. Unlike an enterprise network, the home network provides limited infrastructure. With the addition of every device in to the network, the contention for the resources increases.

The increased contention takes a toll on the performance of the devices. Meeting the agreed quality of service (QoS) such as packet delay and cell loss would be difficult. It calls for the usage of an efficient traffic shaper at the consumer end. The traffic shaper fairly distributes the available resources for the different devices considering their real time performance requirements. It also takes care of the scalability of the network where new devices are added occasionally.

Characteristics of Internet Traffic

Today the Internet carries a variety of data. There is much experimental evidence that the network traffic exhibit the properties of self similarity and long range dependency (LRD) of correlations over a wide range of time scales. The traffic looks statistically similar on all the time scales. As a result of the self similarity, the traffic turns bursty demanding a huge buffer to maintain the agreed limits of cell loss and delay bounds. Although the bursty component constitutes a small fraction of the total traffic, it significantly affects the queuing behavior, in particular at large queue sizes. The conventional traffic models such as Poisson or Markovian (Bruckner, D., Sallans, B., & Russ, G., 2007) fail to describe this behavior.

The Internet traffic is composed of the Gaussian part and the bursty part. The Gaussian part originates due to the aggregation of the data flow from multiple connections. The bursty part is a result of a few dominant connections holding the resources momentarily blocking the other connections. It makes the traffic spiky. The self-similarity of the signal is reflected in the power law behavior of the power spectrum $S(f) = 1/f\alpha$, which lacks the characteristic time scales.

The self similarity of the traffic is associated with long range dependency leading to slowly decaying variances and heavy-tailed distributions.

In a second-order self-similar process, the variance of the aggregated packet count process, $X^{(m)}$ obeys the following rule for large m (Kihong Park, Tsunyi Tuan, 2000).

$$Var(X^{(m)}) \approx \frac{Var(X)}{m^{\beta}} \quad (1)$$

where $H = 1 - (\beta / 2)$ is called as Hurst parameter and represents the degree of self similarity. The equation (1) may be rewritten as (Kihong Park, Tsunyi Tuan, 2000).

$$\log[Var(X^{(m)})] \approx \log[Var(X)] - \beta \log(m) \quad (2)$$

The traffic shaper has to counter the self similarity in the home network to make the traffic less bursty.

The Traffic Shaper

In an IP network, the packets are transferred independently resulting in variable delay and even a possible interchange in their arrival order at the receiver, In an IPTV wherein the multimedia traffic gets streamed, the interchange in the arrival order leads to jitter. Stringent bounds are to be imposed on these parameters to put them in an acceptable range to render a better user experience. Here, a feedback based technique has been explored to achieve the same.

Impact of Shift Given to Feedback Signal on QoS Parameters

In the implementation of the scheduling algorithm, the resource allocation for different classes is dynamically made proportional to the priorities as well as the backlog of these classes at the scheduler. Here, when two classes with backlogs $B_1(t)$ and $B_2(t)$ over a link capacity C are contending, the first class is assigned with the service rate

$$r_1(t) = \frac{B_1(t)}{B_1(t) + \alpha B_2(t)} C \quad (3)$$

The value $0<\alpha<1$ represents the proportional factor and based up on the priorities. It is the ratio of the proportional differentiation factors. It represents the ratio of priorities in delay, packet loss of the first class to the priorities of the second class. Generalizing the same over several classes of priority, the service rate of class i becomes

$$r_i(t) = \frac{B_i(t)}{\sum_j \frac{s_j}{s_i} B_j(t)} C \quad (4)$$

I.e., the resources available are shared according to the priorities as well as the proportional queue lengths. Here the ratio S_j to S_i represents the relative service rate ratio. The issue with this method is, it results in more absolute delays in spite of the relative delay constraints being satisfied. This problem is addressed with a reduced backlog or queue length. With a reduced queue, the absolute delay constraints are easily met along with the relative delay constraints. It will be shown here that the shifted or predicted feedback signal actually reduces the queue size.

The settling time of delay is reduced with feedback i.e. the time taken to stabilize the ratios of delays get reduced. This is because the Queue flush time reduces as the Queue size reduces with shift. The average delay also gets reduced. With higher orders of the feedback or the larger shifts, the constraint on the absolute delay is more easily satisfied as the instantaneous delay falls off with shifts.

The shift also helps in reducing the absolute delay of the packets. The absolute delay constraint (ADC) is the sum of service delay and the stranding time in the queue. With shift given to feedback signal, the queue length gets reduced while the input rate increases. Hence, the ADC is met easily with shifted feedback signal.

IMPACT OF ROUND TRIP TIME (RTT) ON THE DESIGN OF MULTIMEDIA NETWORK

With the rollout of IPTVs the demand for live multimedia over the network has increased multifold, throwing open the challenge of meeting the stringent quality of service(QoS) parameters such as delay, loss rate etc. In interactive applications involving IPTVs, the in-time response is very important to render a pleasant user experience. In such scenarios, the Round trip time (RTT) represents the lower bound on the response time and directly affects the performance. RTT plays a crucial role in shaping the network traffic as it encompasses all the parameters such as buffer dynamics and transmission window. The traffic shaper essentially controls this parameter directly or indirectly. Here, a method has been suggested to reduce the RTT.

Importance of Limits on RTT

The roundtrip delay of packets in a network comprises of the delay in the forward path, delay in the feedback path and the associated minimal packet processing time after which the response originates from the feedback path. Thus reduction in the packet delays attribute to the reduction in RTT straightaway. In a conventional controller, RTT is small; the source transmission rate quickly increases to its former level and increases the congestion (Floyd,S., 2003). This calls for a new contrasting approach where the loss probability does not increase with the fall in RTT. It is achieved with shifts given to the predicted version of the loss probability or the feedback signal (Manjunath,R., & Gurumurthy,K.S., 2004). A new class of neural networks called differentially fed artificial neural networks (DANN) is used for the prediction of the signal (Manjunath,R., & Gurumurthy,K.S., 2002).

At a given arrival rate, the streams with different RTTs may be in different phases. i.e. increase or decrease the transmission rates. The number of packets a data source pump in to the network is smaller if the other streams that compete with the source have shorter RTTs. This makes the frequency of limit cycles more and amplitude lesser. It reduces the variance. The variance of the aggregate traffic, on the other hand, is a function of the variance of all the individual streams and is dominated by the stream with the highest variance.

Impact of Shifted Feedback on RTT and Stability

The higher order differentials translate in to linear shifts in the predicted signals. The predicted feedback signal is generated at the traffic source. The source can conveniently make use of the predicted signal to compute the window size for the subsequent transmissions. Hence, as seen by the source, it is as though the RTT is reduced. Such a reduction in RTT has profound impact on the stability of the feedback control system. The small signal fluid model for the feedback control signal gives the closed-loop system transfer function as (Hollot,C., Misra,V., Towsley,D., & Gong, W.,2002).

$$T(s) = \frac{\frac{1}{s}.k}{1 + \frac{e^{-s.t_d}}{s}.k} \tag{5}$$

where s=σ+jω and k is the system gain. The characteristic equation of this system is

$$s + e^{-st_d}k = 0\,. \tag{6}$$

$$\sigma + ke^{-\sigma t_d}\cos(\omega t_d) = 0 \tag{7}$$

$$\omega - ke^{-\sigma t_d}\sin(\omega t_d) = 0 \tag{8}$$

As the parameters K and td are increased, at some point, the right-most pole will travel from the left hand plane into the right-hand plane, resulting in an unstable system. At the point at which this pole is on the imaginary axis, $\sigma = 0, \omega = \pm k$

$$t_d = \frac{\pi}{2k}\,.$$

The system is stable when

$$k - t_d < \frac{\pi}{2} \tag{9}$$

As the delay or the gain is increased, the system can become unstable. For a stable congestion-control, it is important for the stability of this feedback system to be invariant to the delay, and the gains in the loop, due to different network topologies. The time shift given to the predicted version of the feedback signal is equivalent to reducing the delay value. Hence, shifts improve the stability and achieve it quickly.

As RTT gets reduced, they become more negative and driven well inside the s-plane making the system more stable. It is for the same reason, the amplitude of transients of the queue i.e. Q fluctuations get reduced with increase in the shift or reduction in RTT. Also, the settling time gets reduced and stability is achieved faster since the poles move farther from the imaginary axis.

The settling time is then $1/\omega$ and increases with reduction in RTT or increase in the shift. Thus, effective decrease of RTT due to prediction of the feedback signal increases the frequency of the congestion avoidance cycle giving enough scope for immediate corrections. The shifts provide the appropriate feedback matching with the characteristics of the network.

With shifts the RTT reduces giving high frequency components to the spectrum. The same is observed with the increase in the order of differential feedback in a DANN where the spectrum becomes more flat with the inclusion of more high frequency components as the order of differential increases (Manjunath,R., & Gurumurthy,K.S., 2003).

This keeps the autocorrelation small making the variance of the queue or delay constant most of the time. The shifts given to predicted feedback signal should reduce the variance. Alternative interpretation is that the higher shifts are equivalent to giving higher order feedback.

The RTT may be written as (Q/C)+rt_o, rt_o being the propagation delay and C being the rate of output that is by and large a constant unless the Q is empty(in which case output rate is the same as the input rate). It has two parts- a variable part and a fixed part with respect to the shift. Hence the three signals-Q, p and RTT behave similarly with shift.

Experiment

In a normal scenario, for RED, the RTT increases quickly with load. However the reverse happens with the proposed method. This is possible again with shifts. It is reflected in the simulation results. Figure 2 and figure 3 show the reduction in the delay with increase in the time shift provided to the feedback signal. The feedback signal has been generated with a RED controller and provides input for the data sources about the status of the congestion and an implicit advice to adjust the data transmission rates accordingly. The simulation has been carried out in MATLAB version 6. 40 FTP sources that exist as background traffic and 20 HTTP sources that start at t=0 and go off at t=70 are considered. The transient response

Figure 2. Delay for a shift=1. Load =20. Delay without shift – delay with shift

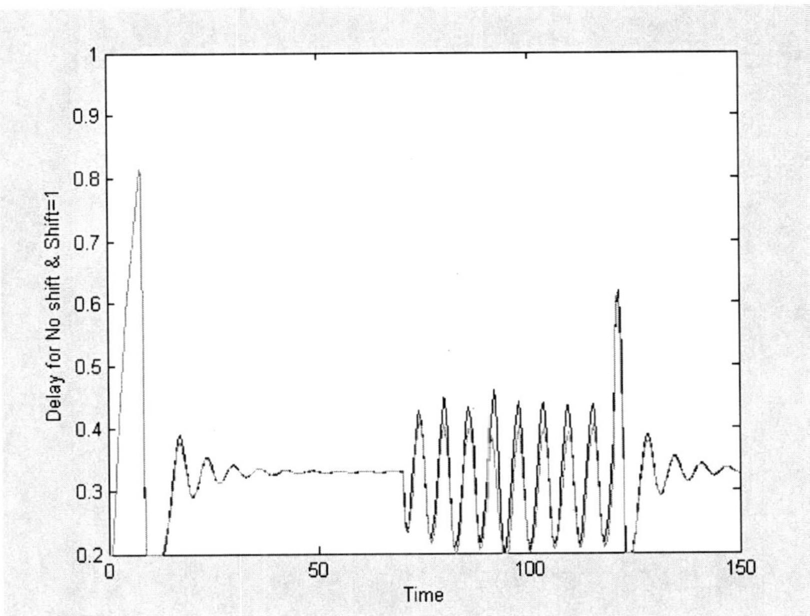

gets advanced with increase in order of shift. After some time the average delay again starts increasing. However, in any case it will be less than the delay without prediction.

Realization of the Controller

In the proposed scheme, an average input traffic rate for the next interval is predicted at a large time scale based on the history of the traffic activity. The expected average input traffic rate is used to detect the congestion. If the congestion is detected, the primary packet marking probability is calculated considering the predicted average input rate and the link capacity. By doing so, the proposed scheme can react fast to the large variation in the input traffic level.

Since the congestion is detected at a time scale longer than the round trip time (RTT) of a flow, sources can react to the congestion signal before the queue size exceeds a certain threshold value. Therefore, compared to the other schemes of the congestion control, the propose scheme does not need a large buffer space. This means that average delay and the delay jitter can be reduced when the REP is used.

Because the proposed scheme detects the congestion at a large time scale, senders can react to the network conditions more rapidly. They can receive the congestion signal and reduce their sending rates before the network goes into severe congestion. With this, the aggregated input rate at a congested router will be below the service rate. So, the amount of buffer space required accommodating an applied load greater than the link capacity gets reduced. It also reduces the end-to-end delay and the delay jitter.

The proposed active queue management scheme is superior to RED in that it can maintain the average queue length and the variation of the average queue length small. In general, as the RTT decreases, the response time of the sources to the network congestion becomes short. Therefore, the amplitude of the queue length variation gets reduced. If the gateway uses the active queue management scheme proposed here, the average queue length and the variance of the average queue length increases as the RTT increases. But the amount of increment is negligible. This is because

Figure 3. Delay for a shift=2. Load =20. Delay without shift – delay with shift

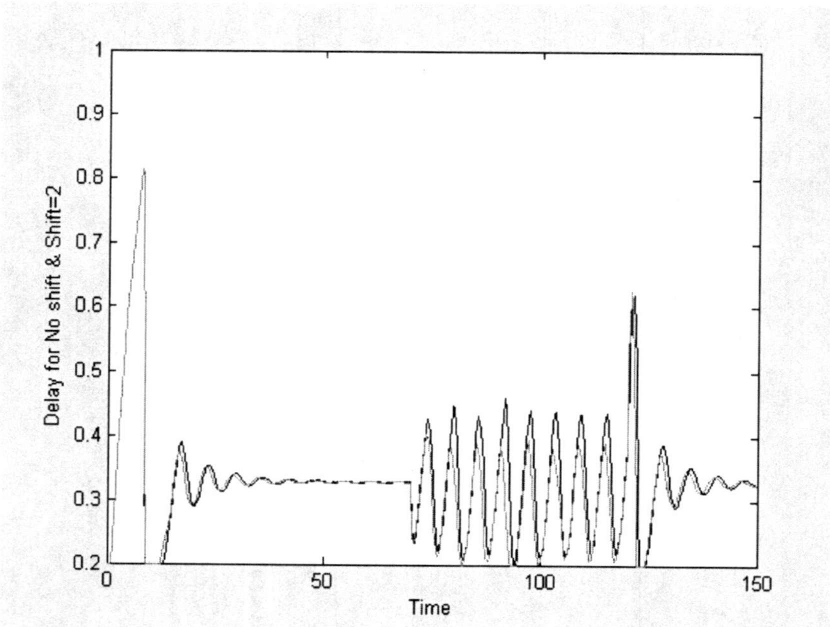

the congestion is detected by using the estimated input rate at a larger timescale. The sources can detect the network congestion before it really happens. Because sources reduce their sending rate before network goes into congestion, the average queue length fluctuations are minimized. Therefore, the amount of fluctuation of the variance of the average queue length is much smaller when the gateway uses the proposed scheme than when the gateway uses the RED.

The longer the RTT of a flow or the smaller the window size of a flow is, the burstier the flow becomes. When a gateway uses random drop queue, packet drop occurs due to the packet overflow. Therefore, the packets of flows with small RTT and large window size are more likely to occupy the buffer space. So, the probability of packet drop for a bursty flow becomes higher compared to a non-bursty flow.

Figure 4 shows the effect of shifts on the relative delay. From the simulation, it is evident that the shifts help in attaining the relative delay ratio faster. The simulation has been carried out on MATLAB version 6. For the simulation, the capacity C is set to 1Gbps, Buffer size of 8000 packets is considered.

Home Network Performance Modeling and Control through Prediction Feedback

Performance modeling of a network is very important especially when it involves multimedia traffic. The present day home network makes uses of Internet for multimedia content transfer on to the devices in real time. In such a communication system, reliability and in time data transfer is crucial. The system has to support the streaming of multimedia and entertainment data from mobile devices to the infrastructure and vice versa. Here a novel performance model is provided.

The Model

Artificial Neural Networks (ANN) are increasingly used for learning non linear functions and the mapping rules. They provide the appropriate output when they encounter an input pattern to

Figure 4. Relative delay for shift =10.: -- with out shift,. with a shift of 10

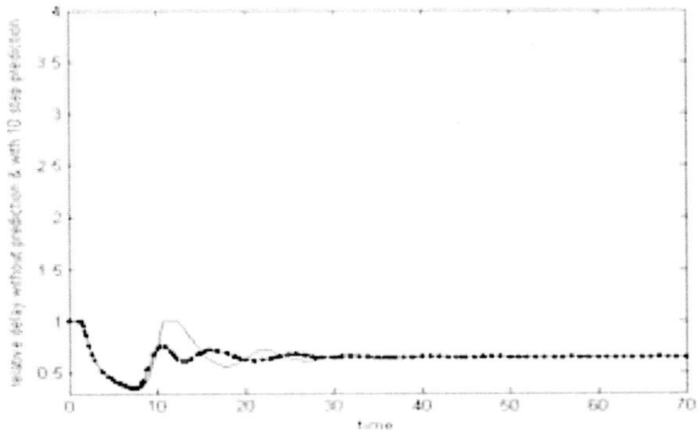

which they are not trained. They however require lengthy training sets and the performance degrades when they encounter an input pattern very much different from the training data. These issues are solved by making it auto regressive with a closed loop feedback from the output to the input as shown in figure 5.

A differentially fed neural network (DANN) (Manjunath,R., & Gurumurthy,K.S., 2002) has all the characteristics required for a controller. It is interesting to note that, a neural network exhibits these properties only when differential feedback of different orders is provided from the output to the input of the network. The resulting structure would have its output self similar, long range dependant (on the historical data), autoregressive with its spectrum obeying the power law and the output forming a space of Bayesian estimators for different orders of differential feedback (Manjunath,R., & Gurumurthy,K.S., 2003) etc.

Figure 5. Model of the DANN

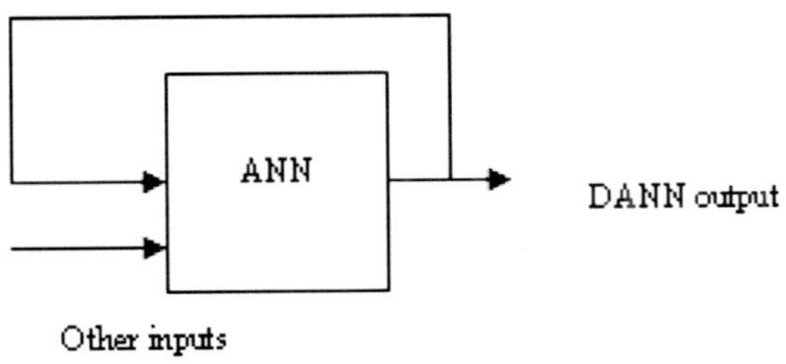

If the network is congested, data packets cannot be transmitted. So FB packets need to be slowed down. However, if the network is free, data packets can be easily transmitted calling for faster FB packet transmission. Here the sources maintain their transmission rate (which otherwise gets slowed down). The constraint is intermediate storage. Therefore, if transmitted, both are transmitted. Else, none are transmitted. Generally the feedback traffic is very small compared to the feed forward traffic. At any point of time, some weightage has to be given for the transmission of FF and FB packets. It depends up on available resources, transmission rate queue and the number of FB packets in the queue etc. The feedback packets may be intercepted and processed by the intermediate switches to control the rate of transmission.

A small change in the traffic over a small time scale will have a profound impact on the traffic envelop over a longer time. With this idea, a traffic controller has been tried in the feedback path over feedback packets. The rate of transmission depends up on the resource allotted. But the allotment of resources itself depends up on the transmission rate. This criss-cross dependency is as though two ANNs (or models) connected back to back as shown in figure 6. It reduces to DANN as shown in figure 7.

Figure 6. Resource allotment

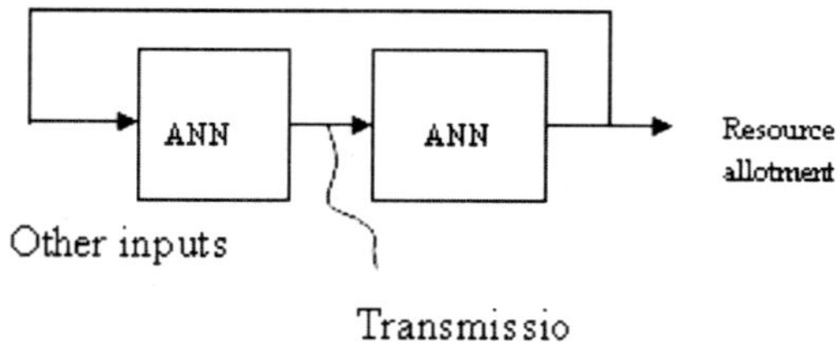

The dependency is a result of pileup due to previous transmission rates and previous allotments. This architecture implies a differential (delayed) feedback from the output. Thus the proposed architecture better catches this type of dependencies. The feedback on the status of the network resources controls the transmission rate. A shifted feedback has a strong influence on the resources as well as the characteristics of the network.

Performance Evaluation of the Model

To generate self-similar input traffic, the superposition of the ON/OFF sources with heavy-tailed distribution is used. In this simulation study, we verify that the proposed active queue management scheme can keep an average queue length and the variation of queue length small when the input traffic is generated by self similar traffic sources. Figure 9 shows the simulation network. Here both the network and the control model may be seen. The DANN gets the training data from the background GREEN algorithm. GREEN is taken as the controller for comparison. For some time, the DANN will be in learning phase. Then it predicts the data k steps in advance. This is given as the feedback to the source (Manjunath,R., & Gurumurthy,K.S., 2004). The source then recomputes the transmission rate. It may be seen that the cell loss ratio has been reduced with feedback. In each case, 42 data points computed with GREEN are used for training. The Input consists of 20 sources supporting FTP that exist over the entire simulation time. The maximum buffer size is taken as 8000 with the packet size of 512.

Figure 7. Simplified DANN architecture

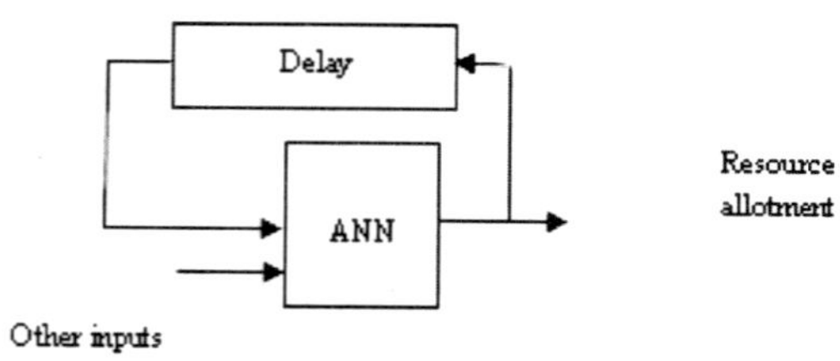

The total cell loss ratio of an ordinary GREEN scheme is found to be 7.4%. With a neural network prediction, it has been reduced to 6% and with first order differentially fed neural network, it is reduced further to 0.55%. A 6 step prediction has been used in the experiment.

Simulation time is set to 40 sec and 180 samples are taken. Matlab version 6 and Simulink have been used to carry out the simulation. The table in figure 8 shows the loss rate reduction with increase in shift.

PERFORMANCE ANALYSIS AND ENHANCEMENT IN SCALABLE NETWORKS

With the inclusion of new devices in to the home network, the size and shape of the networks increases exponentially with time throwing open the challenge of its effective maintenance. Here, the scaling is linked to the time shifts of the feedback signal provided to the content source through active control mechanism such as Random early detection RED (Floyd, S., & Jacobson, V., 1993). Simulation results indicate that, by controlling the shifts given to the predicted version of the feedback signal, the performance of the scaled network may be implemented.

Prediction Feedback Based Controller

The equation of the packet flow used for the traffic shaping is (Marco Ajmone Marsan *et.al,* 2005)

$$\dot{w}(t) = \frac{1}{R(t)} - \frac{w(t)w(t-R(t))}{2R(t-R(t))}p(t-R(t)) \quad (10)$$

Figure 8. Table of Performance

Performance with the proposed running over GREEN

Sl.No.	Shift	Loss. probability	Queue variance
1	0	7.4%	136.8258
2	1	6%	133.3290
3	2	5%	133.9068
4	4	0.725%	135.5478
5	6	0.55%	136.1364

Figure 9. Simulation model

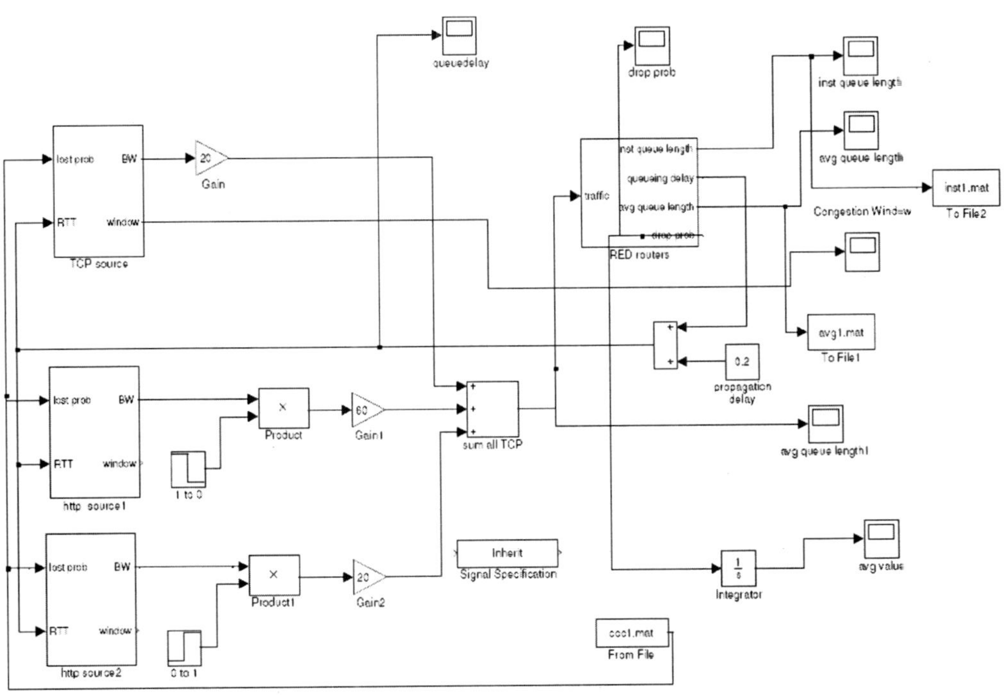

And $\dot{q}(t) = \frac{w(t)}{R(t)}N(t) - C \quad (11)$

Where $\dot{w}$ is the Data window size, q is the queue length, R is the round trip time, C is the Link capacity, N is the Load and p is the packet drop probability. The drawback with this equation is that the status of the network will be known only after the duration of the round trip time (RTT). By then, the characteristics of the network would have been changed making the feedback signal less effective. So, a time shift or prediction is proposed for the feedback signal (Manjunath,R., & Gurumurthy,K.S., 2004) to be used in the controller. In addition, if the status of the network is made known several steps ahead of time, there would be ample time for the data sources and the devices to take the appropriate steps. Bigger the network more would be the traffic and the time required to control. The scalability of the network is linked to its performance. The traffic shaper is blended with the predictor.

Effect of Scaling the Network

In the proposed method, instead of present values of the marking probability, its predicted value is used. This predicted value is generated with the help of a differentially fed neural network (DANN) (Manjunath,R., & Gurumurthy,K.S., 2002), and makes use of several previous values. The usage of these previous values is equivalent to sieving the traffic through multiple time scales. Hence, when DANN is used, it is equivalent to scale the time by a factor that is a function of the order of the feedback. DANN produces same results of scaling. Replace p(t-R(t)) with p(t). The equation may be thought of as the backward prediction starting from p(t) and up to p(t-RTT). ANN works the same way for the backward prediction. The time shift provided for the predicted samples amounts to generating samples with future and past values. Derivative action generally reduces the oscillations .So proportional derivative with prediction may be used to reduce q variance. The idea here is to use the shifted versions of the near future prediction of loss probability as the control signal that is fed back to the input. Shift in the feedback signal amounts to scaling the network.

As N, the size of the network increases, the time slot allocated for each device to share the common bandwidth decreases. This leads to the traffic control at different timescales. Let N denote the number of flows sharing a path with fixed link of capacity C and T be the propagation delay of the path.

At a time instant t, let q(t) and p(t) be the queue length and the packet dropping probability of the link. Let $W_i(t)$ and $R_i(t)$ denote, respectively, the window size and the round trip time of flow i at time t. Then (10) and (11) reduce to

$$R_i(t) = T + \frac{q(t)}{C} \tag{12}$$

$$\frac{dq}{dt} = \sum_{i=1}^{N} \frac{W_i(t)}{R_i(\tau_i)} - C \tag{13}$$

$$\frac{dW_i(t)}{dt} = \frac{1}{R_i(t)} - \beta . W_i(t) . \frac{W_i(\tau_i)}{R_i(t)} . p(\tau_i) \tag{14}$$

where β is the multiplicative parameter, $p(.)$ is the packet dropping probability, and $\tau_i = t_i - R_i(t)$.

The rescaling or the equivalent shift given to the feedback signal increases the link bandwidth and reduces the link delay by the scaling parameter, α. since each packet is served at α times larger bandwidth (which reduces its transmission time by 1/ α) and experiences 1/ α times larger delay. The time instants at which packet events occur are also advanced by 1/ α. The delay reaches the stable value faster. Specifically, a packet event that occurs at time t in the original network is advances to (1/ α)t in the scaled network .

Effect of Scaling on the Queue

The delay gets scaled as the available bandwidth reduces and it increases with increase in N.

$$\frac{dq'}{dt} = \alpha \sum_{i=1}^{N} \frac{P'_{i,BDP}(t)}{D_i(t)} - C \tag{15}$$

$$= \alpha \frac{dq}{dt} - (1 - \alpha)C \tag{16}$$

This shows that $\frac{dq'}{dt} \geq \frac{dq}{dt}$. The effect of scaling is that all events get advanced by the factor of 1/ α. Here it is shown that shifts amount to scaling and by appropriately shifting the feedback signal, it is possible to achieve a better performance in the scaled network compared to the original network.

Performance Evaluation with Scaling

The queue and delay are shown in the simulation for different loads. The total number of data sources activated in each of the 120s simulation period ranged from 40 to 120. To see the effect of the shift, the no of sources changed to 40 & 120 respectively. The results are taken for the shifts of 4. As the load increases, the advantage due to shifts gets reduced. However, the delay with shifts is always less than the one without shifts. Figure 10 shows a packet delay for 40 sources with a shift of 4 steps given to the output of the traffic shaper. One can see that the delay reduces significantly as a result of using time shifted version of the feedback signal generated from the RED controller. Figure 11 shows a similar graph for the queue size with a shift of 8 steps provided to the feedback signal. Reduction in the queue size may be seen when shifted signals are used for traffic shaping.

The loss rates are found to be 5.2% and 4.6% respectively. This makes the throughput with shift 1.2 times larger. The factor is 1.06 for a shift of 1. The higher gain 5.32 of throughput factor may be observed when the load is low i.e. 20 and a shift of 1 is given.

Handling the Issue of Self Similar of Video Traffic over Multimedia Home Network

While streaming the digital content over the home network, the different flows tend to superpose, imparting a kind of long range dependency for the traffic (Kihong Park, Tsunyi Tuan, 2000). The routers in between are subjected to self similarity in the traffic. The Self similarity of traffic (Kihong Park, Walter Willinger, 2000) in a home network results in burstyness of the traffic. To handle the same, the mobile and CE devices such as TV, Mobile PDA attached to

Figure 10. Packet delay for 40 sources with a shift of 4. -- without shift, - with a shift

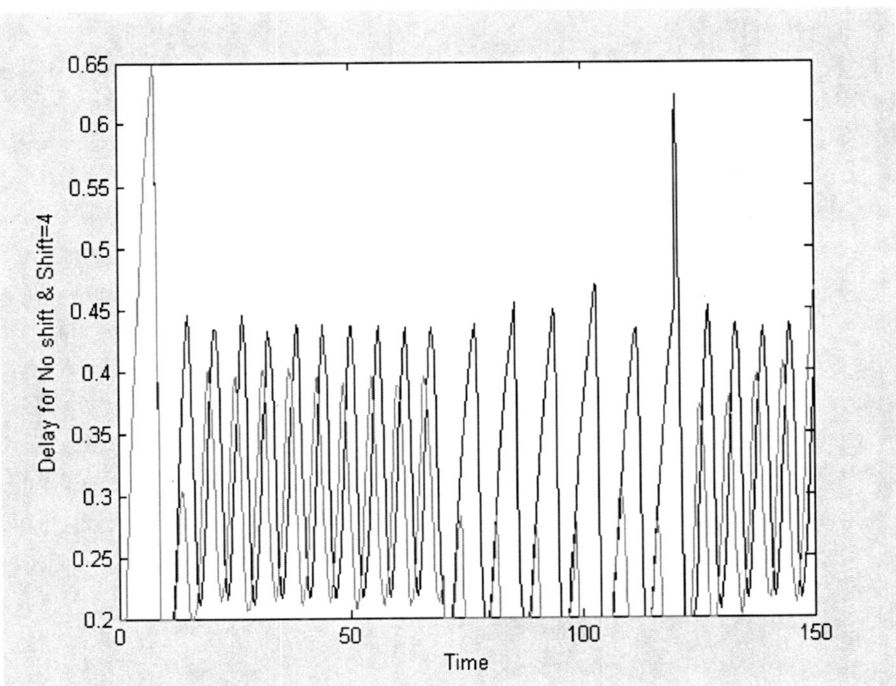

Figure 11. Queue size for 40 sources with a shift of 8 -- without shift, - with a shift

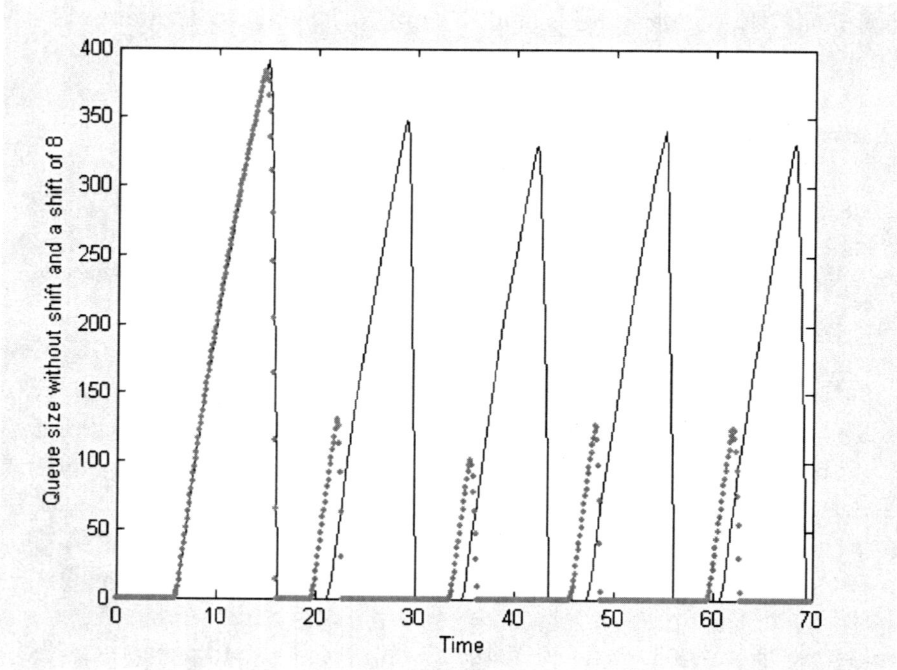

the network and the home gateways supporting them are required to maintain large buffers. The impact is severe in portable handheld devices. The traffic prediction counters the impact of the self similarity in the traffic.

Countering the Self Similarity in the Network Traffic

In order to reduce the impact of the self similarity, various active queue management schemes have been suggested (Floyd, S., and Jacobson, V., 1993). The schemes provide a feedback to the content source to reduce the transmission rate when the buffers are about to get flooded. The congestion is detected at a larger time scale.

The feedback signal is the packet drop probability that is calculated with algorithms such as Random early detection (RED) and predicted before being sent as the feedback signal. Because the congestion is detected at a large time scale, which is longer than typical round trip time of a flow, sources can react to congestion signal before queue size exceeds the threshold value. Therefore, compared to the other schemes, the propose scheme does not need large buffer space. As a result, the average queue length, delay and delay jitter can be reduced. Therefore it is best suited for the real-time multimedia services which have stringent requirements on the delay and jitter. Here, the prediction of the packet drop probability is done using a differentially fed neural network (Manjunath, R., & Gurumurthy, K.S.,2002). The output of a differentially fed neural network exhibits self similarity having Gaussian and bursty components and power law behavior (Manjunath, R., & Gurumurthy, K.S.,2004). The degree of self similarity is controlled by the step or order of the feedback. Presence of this self similar signal in the feedback path counters the self similarity of the network traffic.

CONCLUSION

Internet is evolving into a multi service network. To make it happen, Internet has to support various kinds of services efficiently, each demanding a different data rate. In order to provide enhanced user experience over real time interactive devices such as IPTV, it is required to put constraints on the jitter. A controller is required to maintain the agreed quality of services for the data pumped in to the devices. For constructing QoS enabled next generation Internet, It is crucial to know the traffic characteristics of services that Internet must support, and to develop efficient traffic control mechanisms.

Modeling and controlling the multimedia traffic is challenging. Here, the characteristics of a typical home network are listed and related to the properties of a neural network. The neural network is then inserted in to the network in the feedback path to indicate the congestion status and adjust the transmission rate of the content sources. Presence of the controller in the feedback path ultimately leaves a well behaved network.

Packet roundtrip time plays a significant role in dictating the performance of interactive applications involving IPTV. The two components of RTT–forward data packet delay and the feedback congestion notification delay are to be controlled separately. A controller is required to shape this value within the safe margins. By using the predicted signal rather than the actual one for the congestion notification in a network, the stability improves. The degree of improvement is linked to the amount of time shift provided to the feedback signal.

With the addition of every device in to the home network, the performance of rest of the devices gets affected. Through advance prediction of the status of the network, it should be possible to overcome the issues with loading the network. The delay as well as the loss rate gets reduced which otherwise would be substantial.

The aggregation of traffic over the Internet results in self similarity in the statistical properties of the traffic due to which there will be a substantial loss of packets and the flow turns bursty. Such traffic demands a large buffer that is difficult for the portable devices to afford. The cheapest solution is to use a controller to predict the traffic in advance and use the shifted version of this predicted signal to shape the source characteristics and thereby reduce the degree of self- similarity as well as its impact. The predicted signal is time shifted to different steps to correspond to different degree of the prediction.

REFERENCES

Bruckner, D., Sallans, B., & Russ, G. (2007). Hidden Markov Models for Traffic Observation. In *5th IEEE International Conference on Industrial Informatics*, (pp. 23-27).

Christiansen, M., Jeffay, K., Ott, D. & Smith, F.D. (2001 June). Tuning RED for Web Traffic. *IEEE/ACM Transactions on Networking*.

Claypool, M., & Tanner, J. (1999). The Effects of Jitter on the Perceptual Quality of Video. In *Proc. ACM Multimedia*, (pp. 115-118).

El-Haddadeh, R., Taylor, G. A., & Watts, S. J. (2004). Towards scalable end-to-end QoS provision for VoIP applications. Telecommunications Quality of Services: The Business of Success, (pp.132-135).

Feng, W-C., Kapadia, A. & Thulasidasan, S. (n.d.). GREEN: proactive queue management over a best-effort network. *IEEE GLOBECOM*, (pp 1774 - 1778).

Floyd, S. (2003). *High Speed TCP for Large Congestion Windows*, RFC 3649.

Floyd, S. & Jacobson, V. (1993). Random Early Detection gateways for Congestion Avoidance. *IEEE/ACM Transactions on Networking, 1*(4), 397-413.

Hollot, C., Misra, V., Towsley, D., & Gong, W. (2001). *A Control Theoretic Analysis of RED*. INFOCOMM.

Hollot, C., Misra, V., Towsley, D., & Gong, W. (2002). Analysis and design of controllers for AQM routers supporting TCP flows. *IEEE Transactions on Automatic Control, 47*(6). doi:10.1109/TAC.2002.1008360

Manjunath, R., & Gurumurthy, K. S. (2002). *Information geometry of differentially fed artificial neural networks* (*Vol. 3*, pp. 1521–1525). TENCON.

Manjunath, R. & Gurumurthy, K.S. (2003), Bayesian decision on differentially fed hyperplanes. *ITSim2003.*

Manjunath, R. & Gurumurthy, K.S. (2003). System Design using differentially fed Artificial Neural Network. *ICAAI'03.*

Manjunath, R. & Gurumurthy, K.S. (2004) Maintaining Long-range dependency of traffic in a network. *CODEC'04.*

Marsan, M. A., et.al. (2005). Using Partial Differential Equations to Model TCP Mice and Elephants in Large IP Networks. *IEEE/ACM Transactions on Networking, 13*(6), 1289-1301.

Park, K., & Tuan, T. (2000). Performance evaluation of multiple time scale TCP under self-similar traffic conditions. *ACM Transactions on Modeling and Computer Simulation, 10*(2), 152–177. doi:10.1145/364996.365005

Park, K., & Willinger, W. (2000). *Self-Similar Network Traffic and Performance Evaluation*. New York: John Wiley & Sons, Inc. doi:10.1002/047120644X

Shioda, S. & Mase, K. (2005). Performance comparison between IntServ-based and DiffServ-based networks. *GLOBECOM,* 2005

Stiliadis, D. & Varma, A. (1998, April). Rate-Proportional Servers: A Design Methodology Fair Queuing Algorithms. *IEEE/ ACM Trans. on Networking.*

Willinger, W., Taqqu, M.S., Sherman, R. & Wilson, D.V. (1997). Self-similarity through high Variability: Statistical analysis of Ethernet LAN traffic at the source level. *IEEE/ACM transaction on networking, 5*, 71-86.

Chapter 7
Multiple Optimization of Network Carrier and Traffic Flow Goals Using a Heuristic Routing Decision System

Wayne S. Goodridge
University of West Indies, Trinidad and Tobago

Shyamala C Sivakumar
Saint Mary's University, Canada

William Robertson
Dalhousie University, Canada

William J. Phillips
Dalhousie University, Canada

ABSTRACT

This chapter presents a multiple constraint optimization algorithm called routing decision system (RDS) that uses the concept of preference functions to address the problem of selecting paths in core networks that satisfy traffic-oriented QoS requirements while simultaneously satisfying network resource-oriented performance goals. The original contribution lies in the use of strong scales employed for constructing a multiple criteria preference function in an affine space. The use of preference functions makes it possible for paths that match both traffic-oriented and resource-oriented goals to be selected by the algorithm. The RDS algorithm is used in conjunction with a heuristic path finding algorithm called Constraint Path Heuristic (CP-H) algorithm which is a novel approach to finding a set of constraint paths between source and destination nodes in a network. The CP-H algorithm finds multiple paths for each metric and then passes all the paths to the RDS algorithm. Simulation results showed that the CP-H/RDS algorithm has a success rate of between 93 and 96% when used in Waxman graph topologies, and is shown to be significantly better than other heuristic based algorithms under strict constraints. In addition, it is shown that the associated execution time of the CP-H/RDS algorithm is slightly higher than other heuristic based algorithms but good enough for use in an online traffic engineering (TE) ap-

DOI: 10.4018/978-1-61520-791-6.ch007

plication. Simulations to assess the performance of CP-H/RDS algorithm in a TE environment show that the algorithms has lower call block rates than other TE algorithms. It is also shown that the CP-H/RDS has a 96% probability of providing at least two distinct feasible backup paths in addition to the main QoS path. A framework for implementing the CP-H/RDS as a routing server is proposed. The routing decision system server (RDSS) framework is novel in that the complexity introduced by QoS awareness remains outside the network.

INTRODUCTION

Finding the best path to route packets for a traffic flow in IP networks is extremely important for providing quality of service to multimedia applications. Traffic transmitted through communication networks is characterized by five primary metrics, namely packet loss, delay, jitter, bandwidth and security. Since the flow QoS requirements have to be mapped onto path metrics this means that metrics define the types of QoS guarantees the network can support. Depending on the nature of the metric, metrics can be classified into three types: additive, concave and multiplicative metrics. Delay and jitter are additive metrics. Bandwidth is a concave metric, while packet loss is a multiplicative metric. Metrics can also be classified as path-constrained or link constrained. Concave metrics are link-constrained because the metric for a path depends on the link's bottleneck value. Additive and multiplicative metrics are path-constrained because the metric for a path depends on all the values along the path. Many routing protocols including Open Shortest Path First (OSPF) and Routing Information Protocol (RIP) use routing that is optimized for a single arbitrary metric (shortest path routing). Other routing algorithms use the bandwidth metric to calculate optimal paths which may not satisfy other QoS requirements such as delay, jitter and packet loss. Hence, routing algorithms using one metric to calculate the path cannot satisfy the diverse QoS requirements needed by multimedia applications. When QoS algorithms attempt to find multi-metric optimal paths also known as multi-constraint optimization problem (MCOP), most do so only for additive metrics. When a concave metric such as bandwidth is involved in the optimization process, no QoS algorithm, in the work reported here, offers a solution where bandwidth can be optimized. Typically, QoS algorithms deal with the problem of meeting the requested bandwidth by pruning the network of all links that do not satisfy the bandwidth request. A cost function that is typically based on additive metrics is used to find an optimal path from the pruned network. Hence, an optimal path selection algorithm that finds feasible paths for all requests while minimizing the total network resource usage is required. Although single metric algorithms such as the Constraint Shortest Path First provide a mechanism for finding optimal bandwidth paths, the existing MCOP solutions do not provide a mechanism where a pareto-optimal path can be found that includes both bandwidth and additive metrics in the optimization process.

There are two dimensions to the problem of providing QoS to applications in an IP network. The first is finding the best path to route packets for a given connection and the second is to reserve network resources on that path. Traffic Engineering (TE) is the technique of mapping network traffic flows with a given set of user QoS constraints onto an existing network topology in such a way that the goals of the user traffic flows and maximizing resource utilization are simultaneously met (Marzo, Calle, Scoglio, & Anjah, 2003). Performance objectives can be traffic-oriented and/or resource-oriented. Traffic-oriented performance objectives relate to the improvement of the user's QoS and can be measured by the packet loss, delay, jitter, and throughput (Awduche,

1999). On the other hand, resource-oriented objectives relate to the optimization of the bandwidth asset (Mitra, & Wang, 2003), a revenue source for the network carrier. When core networks use multi-metric QoS routing algorithms in traffic engineering (TE), meeting the traffic oriented QoS goals is just part of the problem. The other is to select paths that also satisfy the network carrier goals such as maximizing bandwidth usage, maximizing the number of flows in the network and meeting administrative policies. There are two main ways that traffic engineering algorithms can be executed; offline (pre-computation) and online (on demand). Traffic engineering is usually associated with offline routing and assumes that all the traffic requests are known *apriori*. With an offline algorithm this objective is possible since algorithms have a longer time frame to execute and all the requests are known upfront. In online routing algorithms path requests are attended to in a one by one fashion. The major difficulty of using QoS algorithms in a TE application is that global optimization is difficult to achieve since the flow sequence and therefore allocation of resources is random. In addition, most TE online algorithms do not consider user constraints apart from the concave bandwidth metric mainly due to the fact that routing with multiple additive metrics is an NP-complete problem. Online traffic engineering is more desirable than offline traffic engineering because it is dynamic and reacts in real time to changes in the network and user requests. Also, online optimization approaches take into account traffic paths in the sequence in which traffic flows request network resources may result in traffic being blocked because of the inefficient allocation of network resources.

Several researchers have investigated the constraint-based path selection problem also known as multi constraint optimization problem (MCOP) and proposed various algorithms, both exact and heuristic. Exact QoS routing algorithms including SAMCRA and TAMCRA involving multiple QoS metrics are NP-complete problems, and paths that satisfy all traffic QoS requirements may not be found in polynomial time (Kuipers, Korkmaz, Krunz, & Mieghem, 2004). Hence, the majority of past efforts have concentrated on finding various heuristics that simplify the MCOP problem (Jaffe, 1984). Heuristic solutions have been shown to have low performance in terms of finding a constraint path based on the user QoS constraints. On the other hand, exact solutions have 100% success rates but perform poorly in terms of running times. To address these problems we decouple the path finding mechanism from the optimization mechanism. This modular approach makes it possible to employ heuristic techniques to find a set of constraint paths that satisfy multiple QoS constraints. We propose a novel heuristic path finding algorithm called the constraint-path finding heuristic algorithm (CP-H) that finds a set of paths from source to destination that satisfy multiple QoS metrics including bandwidth. Next, we propose an optimal path selection algorithm called the routing decision system (RDS) for selecting an optimal path based on traffic and network resource optimization goals. This optimization strategy is novel in that both network resource and individual user requirements can influence the path selection process. The RDS algorithm selects a path that best matches the user QoS constraints and the network resource optimization requests as closely as possible. To achieve this, the RDS algorithm employs a preference function that has a preference scale for each metric on each constraint path connecting the source and destination node in the network. This provides a framework where all metrics including bandwidth can participate in the path selection process.

Typically, network carriers use differentiated services to implement QoS routing on the internet. Their QoS routing models use class type to control the maximum and minimum bandwidth guarantees for traffic classes. Assigning applications to different classes of service and marking the traffic appropriately allows for scheduling, queuing, and drop behavior based on application type. A disadvantage of class based QoS routing is that any incremental changes to QoS routing policies would mean updating every router on the Internet. A solution to these limitations is to move the routing decision functionality to the management plane, thereby reducing the need for updating router software (Hui-Lan, & Faynberg, 2003). The key advantages for making routing decisions in the management plane are that the complexity introduced by QoS awareness remains outside the network layer, and it is now possible to use state-of-the-art hardware with sufficient memory and CPU power for QoS routing. In this paper we implement QoS routing policies in the management plane by employing a centralized server called the routing decision system server (RDSS) with paths calculated based on a global view of all the network trunks. The proposed routing decision system server (RDSS) framework is novel in that it allows both concave and additive metrics to be used in a TE environment. Also, the RDSS integrates the per-class approach of the DiffServ model and the intelligent path finding mechanism of the CP-H algorithm to offer a unique solution that meets the end-to-end QoS needs of individual traffic flows. The key to our online traffic engineering solution is how the traffic mappings are created. The RDS path selection algorithm selects a pareto-optimal path subject to a set of user QoS requirements and network resource utilization criteria, and does so based on a complete picture of the network topology and link state information (Goodridge, Robertson, Phillips, & Sivakumar, 2004a, 2004b, 2005). An efficient way to deploy the RDS algorithm is to use a centralized approach similar to the one proposed in (Aukia, Kodialam, Koppol, Lakshman, Sarin, & Suter, 2000), where a routing decision system server (RDSS) stores the traffic engineering database consisting of customer flow needs and network topology information, and makes optimal path selection decisions. Traffic engineering solutions are also concerned with improving the reliability of the network and protecting the network against failures. Hence, provision must be made for the installation of backup paths. The novel feature of the CP-H algorithm is that it employs techniques to find a subset of *disjoint* constraint paths connecting source and destination that satisfy the user QoS requirements. This feature makes it easy for the RDS server to select and install back up paths in case of link failure anywhere along the path.

This paper is organized as follows. The following section discusses the common exact and heuristic routing algorithms proposed for QoS management and how they have influenced the design of the CP-H and RDS algorithms proposed in this paper. The next section discusses the QoS routing algorithms used in traffic engineering, their benefits and drawbacks and how they have influenced the design of the novel routing decision system server framework presented. Next we present our solution to the QoS routing problem namely, the CP-H/RDS algorithm. Next we discuss how the CP-H/RDS algorithm can be adapted for use in a traffic engineering environment. We show the CP-H/RDS can use existing protocols including OSPF, COPS and MPLS in a Routing Decision System Server (RDSS) framework to achieve online traffic engineering goals. We provide performance analysis of the CP-H/RDS algorithm with respect to success rates, execution times, the probability of finding distinct-disjoint paths and the call blocking rate.

ROUTING ALGORITHMS RELATED TO QOS MANAGEMENT

This section discusses existing routing algorithms used in QoS management and the problems associated with them. The QoS routing problem can be categorized as the Multi-constraint path problem and the Multi-constraint optimal path problem. The goal of a MCP algorithm is to find feasible paths from source to destination that satisfies all the QoS constraints. Computation becomes more difficult as multiple constraints are introduced into the path calculation problem. In a typical network, multiple feasible paths can be found that satisfy the user's multiple QoS constraints. Hence, it may be necessary to define optimization criteria to select a path from the set of feasible paths. The inclusion of optimizing QoS constraints to the MCP problem is described as the Multi-constraint optimal path problem. QoS routing involving multiple optimizing metrics is NP-complete, which means that suitable paths satisfying the user QoS requirements may not be found in polynomial time. Solutions proposed for the MCP and MCOP can be classified as either generic or non-generic. Non-generic algorithms focus on specific QoS parameters and, since they are restricted to a predefined set of metrics, are not able to solve the general MCP problem. On the other hand, generic algorithms are able to compute a path from source to destination based on an arbitrary set of QoS constraints.

Generic algorithms can be sub-classified into exact and heuristic algorithms. Exact algorithms guarantee that a path satisfying the design goals of the algorithm will be returned, providing that at least one such path exists in the network. Some researchers propose exact solutions to the MCP/MCOP problem in light of the fact that the NP-complete character of graphs is not common in real networks. This fact has driven approaches like the Self Adaptive Multiple Constraints Routing Algorithm (SAMCRA) (Van Mieghem, De Neve, and Kuipers, 2001), Tunable Accuracy Multiple Constraints Routing Algorithm (TAMCRA) algorithm (De Neve, and Van Mieghem, 2000) and A*prune (Liu and Ramakrishnan, 2001) algorithms. However, exact algorithms have very high running times relative to heuristic approaches. Hence, the majority of recent research efforts have concentrated on finding various heuristics that simplify the MCP/MCOP problem including (Chen, and Nahrstedt, 1998a; Chen, and Nahrstedt, 1998b; Jaffe, 1984; Iwata, and Fujita, 2000). This paper focuses on designing a generic heuristic constraint path algorithm that satisfies multiple arbitrary user QoS constraints. In the following sections we review generic-exact and generic- heuristic algorithms that have influenced our work.

Generic-Exact Algorithms for QoS Management

The Tunable Accuracy Multiple Constraints Routing Algorithm (TAMCRA) algorithm (De Neve, and Van Mieghem, (2000), and its successor the Self Adaptive Multiple Constraints Routing Algorithm SAMCRA (Van Mieghem, De Neve, and Kuipers, 2001) are generic exact algorithms for the MCP problem and use a non-linear function to calculate path lengths. The combined path weight $L(P)$ is given in Equation 1

$$L(P) = \max_{1 \le j \le m} \left(\frac{w_j(P)}{L_j} \right) \qquad (1)$$

where $w_j(P)$ is the jth metric for path P and L_j is the user requested constraint. The TAMCRA and the SAMCRA use the k-shortest path algorithm to find the shortest path from a list of k-constraint paths. However, because k, the number of paths that exists between source and destination nodes can be large, this means that to find the shortest path among k paths can be time consuming. The use of a k-shortest path algorithm forces the algorithm to exhaustive searches in order to find an optimal path. This practice can lead to exponential running times. To overcome this problem, in TAMCRA, k is pre-selected, while the SAMCRA algorithm controls the value of k self-adaptively. The selection of k in TAMCRA is a trade-off between performance and complexity; a small k implies that the algorithm will have polynomial running times but poor performance in terms of returning optimal paths while a large k means that the algorithm returns optimal paths at the expense of long running times. SAMCRA, on the other hand, guarantees to find a feasible path, if one exists, at the expense of exponential running times. The SAMCRA algorithm offers many advantages in its approach to solving the MCP/MCOP problem. The major difficulty is that the optimization strategy of the SAMCRA algorithm is fixed for a given network and cannot be influenced by individual user flows. Hence, we separate the heuristic constraint paths finding algorithm (CP-H) from the optimal path selection algorithm the RDS. Additionally, the proposed CP-H algorithm introduces tuning parameters and techniques that assist with the reduction of actual execution times involved in finding constraint paths. In the RDS algorithm, we solve the multi-metric optimization problem by employing a preference function to indicate user and network carrier optimization requests. The preference function employs a preference scale for each metric on each constraint route connecting the source and destination node in the network. This provides a framework where by all metrics can participate in the path selection process. This paper uses the SAMCRA algorithm to gauge the performance of the proposed CP-H/RDS algorithm. It is shown that the CP-H/RDS algorithm achieves high success rates under strict user constraints.

Generic-Heuristic Algorithms for QoS Management

Many heuristic solutions have been proposed for solving the MCP and MCOP problems. A path that reflects the user constraints and network optimization goals may not necessarily found by such algorithms.

The Chen and Nahrstedt algorithm in (Chen, and Nahrstedt, 1998a; Chen, and Nahrstedt, 1998b) proposed a technique for solving the MCP problem for two additive metrics. Suppose that MCP($G; s; t; w_1; w_2; C_1; C_2$) represents the original problem, where G is the network, s and t are the source and destination nodes respectively, w_1 and w_2 are the metrics, and C_1 and C_2 are the user specified metric values for w_1 and w_2 respectively. The technique involves reducing the original problem to a simpler problem MCP($G; s; t; w_1; w'_2; C_1; x$) where x is some predetermined integer and

$$w_2 = \left\lceil \frac{w_2 x}{C_2} \right\rceil \quad (2)$$

(Chen and Nahrstedt 1998a) proved that a solution to the new problem is also a solution to the original problem. This is a heuristic approach since finding a feasible path is a function of x. The success rates and running times of the algorithm are heavily influenced by the value of x. To obtain high success rates a high value of x is required. However, using high values for x can result in very high running times. In a similar fashion, the proposed CP-H algorithm employs a parameter λ (the threshold used in the CP-H algorithm to determine the number of optimized paths considered for each metric), that impacts the trade-off between execution times and success rates of the algorithm. Simulations show that in the CP-H algorithm high values of λ results in high success rates but poor execution times. Simulation results indicate that when $\lambda = 3$ success rates of between 90-93% are obtained even under strict user constraints. However, results in (Jaffe, 1984) suggest that the Chen and Nahrstedt algorithm does not exceed a success rate of 50% under strict user constraints.

The Jaffe algorithm in (Jaffe, 1984) is a method for solving the MCP problem for two metrics. Consider a graph $G(N, E)$, where N is a set of vertices and E is a set of edges, and $(u, v) \in E$. Suppose that link is characterized by weight functions $w_1(u, v)$ and $w_2(u, v)$. The Jaffe algorithm replaces the two link values of each link by a single link value which is a linear combination of the original link values as given in the equation 3

$$w(u,v) = d_1.w_1(u,v) + d_2.w_2(u,v) \quad (3)$$

where d_1 and d_2 are constraints. The problem with the combined weight as a metric is solvable by a shortest path algorithm. The solution is then checked to determine whether the constraints are satisfied. However, the shortest path of the converted graph consisting of single weights may not satisfy user constraints L_1 or L_2. Jaffe argued that the values for d_1 and d_2 should be chosen based on equation 4. This implies that in the worst-case scenario, one of the constraints can be violated.

$$\frac{d_2}{d_2} = \sqrt{\frac{d_2}{d_2}} \tag{4}$$

The key issue now is to determine the appropriate d_1 and d_2 such that an optimal path with respect to the new single weighted graph is likely to satisfy the individual constraints. The Jaffe algorithm is heavily influenced by the nature of the user constraints and the link correlation structure of the network. Hence the performance of the algorithm in terms of success rates is unpredictable. In addition, the optimization strategy of the algorithm is fixed and cannot be influenced by individual user flows. The CP-H route searching algorithm is tailored to satisfy individual user QoS requirements, while the RDS algorithm, selects a path that best matches the user and network carrier optimization requests as closely as possible. The optimal path selection strategy based on multiple optimization requirements is achieved by employing a preference function that has a preference scale for each optimization metric on each constraint path connecting the source and destination node in the network. This provides a framework where by all optimization metrics can participate in the optimal path selection process.

The Iwata algorithm presented in (Iwata, and Fujita, 2000) attempts to find a path optimized for one of the metrics, instead of being optimized for a single cost of weighted QoS parameters. The algorithm finds a shortest path, or paths, based on one metric and then checks if all the constraints are met. If not, it finds a shortest path for another metric and again checks if the other constraints are met. The Iwata algorithm provides a straightforward approach to solving the MCP problem. However, results in (Kuipers, Korkmaz, Krunz, & Mieghem, 2004) suggest that the Iwata algorithm has very low success rates under strict user constraints. The CP-H introduced in this paper has similarities to the Iwata algorithm. However, rather than testing only one path for each metric, the CP-H algorithm tests λ paths for each metric. Simulation results indicate that this approach leads to a significant increase in success rates over the Iwata algorithm.

The routing paradigm presented in this paper attempts to rectify the problems associated with existing generic-exact and generic-heuristic algorithms above, by separating the path searching mechanism from the optimization mechanism. This modular approach makes it possible to design more flexible constraint path searching and optimal path selection techniques. Since the path selection process is decoupled from the path search process, the associated expense that comes with the search for *k*-constraint paths is reduced. Instead, the designer of the path searching algorithm is free to use a wide range of techniques to find a set of constraint paths connecting source and destination. In addition, decoupling the optimal path selection mechanism from the constraint path search algorithm makes it possible for optimization techniques (such as the use of preference functions) from other areas of Mathematics including utility theory to be used. The results presented in this paper will show that the CP-H/RDS provides the best success rate /execution time trade-off relative to current generic-exact and generic-heuristic algorithms.

APPLICATION OF QOS ROUTING TO TRAFFIC ENGINEERING

This section discusses existing work that has studied QoS algorithms used in traffic engineering and the problems associated with them. QoS routing algorithms can be broadly classified into two categories class based and flow based. Some network carriers offer services tailored for each customer by using the DiffServ model that involves assigning a Per-Hop Behavior (PHB) code to each class (Sanjay, & Hassan, 2002). DiffServ routers in the core network use this code to sort packets into their corresponding treatment classes, without having to know to which flows or what types of applications the packets belong to. However, this approach has a major drawback in that the desired behavior of an application is typically specified by end-to-end parameters, while the DiffServ mechanisms define per hop behavior.

Flow based QoS algorithms that are used in online TE include Minimum Interference Routing Algorithm (MIRA), and Least Interference Optimization Algorithm (LIOA) and Minimal Hop Algorithm. The MIRA is a flow-based routing algorithm proposed in the context of MPLS networks to set up bandwidth-guaranteed label switched paths (Figueiredo, da Fonseca, & Monteiro, 2006). MIRA selects a path for a traffic flow request by maximizing the minimum available capacity between all ingress-egress pairs. This routing strategy helps to reduce blocking rate and prevents the creation of bottlenecks for flows.

A variation of MIRA is the Light Minimum Interference Routing Algorithm (LMIR) which attempts to find *K* paths with the lowest capacity from among all possible paths between two nodes, and then selects the path which minimizes the interference between the two nodes. It has been shown that the LMIR has significant improvements over the MIRA algorithm (Figueiredo, da Fonseca, & Monteiro, 2006).

The Least Interference Optimization Algorithm (LIOA) (Bagula, Botha, & Krzesinki, 2004) reduces the interference among competing flows by balancing the number and quantity of flows carried by a link to achieve efficient routing of label switched paths (LSPs). The algorithm uses the current bandwidth availability and the traffic flow distribution to achieve traffic engineering in IP networks. The link cost function employed is given in Equation 5.

$$Cost_1 = \frac{1^a}{\left(R^l - r^l\right)_{1-a}} \tag{5}$$

where *I* is the is the number of flows on link *l*, R_l is the maximum reserve-able bandwidth on link *l*, r_l is the total bandwidth reserved by the LSPs traversing the link, α is a parameter representing the trade-off between the number and the magnitude of the LSPs traversing the link *l*.

The main advantage of the CP-H/RDS over current traffic engineering QoS algorithms is that it is designed to satisfy multiple QoS constraints including bandwidth. Most current traffic engineering QoS algorithms only allow for the bandwidth user constraint to be used (Awduche, 1999). Hence network carriers can only find paths that satisfy the bandwidth constraint which in turn forces bandwidth to be sold as a commodity (Mitra and Wang, 2003). This causes a situation where network carriers that have the lowest price per unit bandwidth get the most business. Our solution is unique in that the optimal path selection process can be influenced by any optimization constraint including bandwidth.

Problems Associated with QoS Routing

The problems associated with QoS routing in core networks include the problem of routing with imprecise state information and stability of paths found by the QoS routing algorithm. In large networks, maintaining precise global network state information in a dynamic environment is extremely challenging. QoS routing with imprecise state information may result in suboptimal paths or may result in increased call blocking rates (Guerin, & Orda, 1999). The three main factors that contribute to imprecise state information are infrequent link state update due to state update policy of the routing protocol; propagation delay of the link state update packets; and hierarchical state aggregation (Guerin, & Orda, 1999). A number of QoS routing methods that tolerate imprecise state information have been proposed. These method include safety-based routing (Apostolopoulos, Guerin, Kamat and Tripathi,1999), localized routing (Nelakuditi, Zhang, Tsang, and Du, 2002) and centralized server based QoS routing (Kim and Lee, 2001). The Safety-Based Routing (SBR) approach infers a range of the actual link state values from the link state updates, and finds the path that has the highest probability to satisfy a connection request. SBR assumes routing with bandwidth constraints and on-demand path computation. SBR computes the probability that a path can support an incoming bandwidth request. Assuming that links are mutually independent, the safety of a path can be determined as a product of the safety of the links in the path. Path safety can then be handled in exactly the same way as other path metrics. Localized routing totally eliminates the impact of the imprecise global network state information by making routing decisions based on the information maintained locally at each router. Instead, source nodes infer the network QoS state based on flow blocking statistics collected locally, and perform flow routing using this localized view of the network state. In (Aukia, Kodialam, Koppol, Lakshman, Sarin, & Suter, 2000) a centralized server based QoS routing scheme is proposed in which routers are clients of the route server and send routing queries for each one of the incoming requests. This paper proposes the RDS server framework that uses a centralized server based QoS routing model. In addition, SBR can be implemented by including an additional metric in the RDS algorithm that tracks the safety factor for each link.

QoS routing is also sensitive to changes in link state information which could lead to the problem of oscillation of traffic between paths. For example, if path selection relies on link state information about available bandwidth, it can easily lead to a situation where all the traffic is routed to a path with a lot of available bandwidth. This path will then be congested and the traffic will be routed through another path. To help rectify this problem a reservation protocol can be used in conjunction with QoS routing to pin the network paths. In this way, even if some other path becomes a better choice, the connections already routed through a given path will not switch to the better path. The proposed RDSS framework uses the MPLS protocol which supports route pinning for setting up explicit paths for flows.

A large percentage of the traffic flows in core networks is still best effort traffic. Since best effort traffic share paths with QoS traffic, whose priority is higher than best effort traffic, the performance of best effort traffic can be significantly affected. The routing objectives in an environment with both QoS guaranteed traffic and best-effort traffic are minimizing the call-blocking ratio of QoS flows; and optimizing the throughput and fairness for best-effort flows. Since the first objective only considers QoS traffic and the second objective only best-effort traffic, this could lead to a contradiction. The proposed RDS algorithm searches for a QoS path that optimizes individual traffic flow optimization requirements. As a result, this approach tends to reserve paths that have a lot of resources for QoS flows, while best effort flows are routed along paths that have less network resources.

A QOS AWARE HEURISTIC CONSTRAINT PATH FINDING ALGORITHM AND ROUTING DECISION SYSTEM FOR OPTIMAL PATH SELECTION

In the Constraint Paths Heuristic Routing Decision System (CP-H/RDS) presented in this paper, the mechanism for finding multiple constraint paths

(MCP) is decoupled from the mechanism employed for network resource optimization. There are two main components to this algorithm:

1. The heuristic constraint path (CP-H) algorithm finds a set of paths connecting source and destination nodes that meet the user traffic flow constraints.
2. The routing decision system (RDS) algorithm uses a multi-criteria preference function to always select a pareto-optimal path provided such a path exists in the set of constraint paths output by the CP-H based on user traffic flow needs and network operator optimization goals.

Figures 1a and 1b, show how the CP-H and RDS algorithms can be used to find a QoS route from a communication network graph given a set of user specified metrics, and a set of policy based metrics from the network provider. The first step is to eliminate or prune all links not satisfying the concave bandwidth metric. The second step is to find a set of constraint paths that are feasible with respect to the user specified traffic flow additive metrics such as delay, packet loss and jitter. The final step executes the RDS algorithm with the specified traffic flow and resource utilization policy metrics, along with the constrained paths found by the CP-H. The RDS algorithm calculates a preference ranking for each CP-H path based on the QoS and network carrier traffic engineering requirements. Traffic engineering policy metrics include network resource utilization, and path protection for the duration of the traffic flow.

The Constraint Path - Heuristic (CP-H) Algorithm

The proposed heuristic constraint path (CP-H) algorithm finds $\lambda x m$ paths between source and destination nodes, where λ is a small positive integer and m is the number of QoS metrics under consideration. For a given metric, say m_l, the Dijkstra's algorithm is executed to produce a shortest path P_l with respect to metric m_l. A pruning procedure is executed that attempts to prevent path P_l from being selected the next time the Dijkstra's algorithm is executed for metric m_l to ensure that distinct paths result from successive runs of the Dijkstra's algorithm which in turn increases the chance that one of the λ paths would satisfy all QoS constraints. Thus, a set of λ shortest paths $\{P_\lambda\}$ is chosen for each metric m. The $\lambda x m$ paths constitute the set of constraint paths C produced by the algorithm. The pseudo code for the constraint path – heuristics algorithm is given below:

CP-H Algorithm: CP-H(G,s,t,C,L, λ,m)

```
1)  {j ←1
2)  while (j≤m) {
3)     i ←1
4)     while (i≤ λ) {
5)        Pi ← Dijkstra(G, s, t, j)
6)        PrunePath(P_i, j)
7)        C← C U Pi
8)        i ←i+1
9)          }
10)    j ←j+1
11)       }
12)    }
13) PrunePath (P,j)
14) { For each link l in P
15)    { τ = max_j(P)
16)    l_j ← τ+ l_j
17)    }
18) }
```

Lines 15 and 16 sets the link weight for the jth metric, where τ is the largest value for the jth metric in path P.

The Routing Decision System (RDS) Algorithm for Optimal Path Selection

First, for each metric in the constraint path set C, a preference function is used to scale the network metric value x to lie between -1 and 1. The scaled

Figure 1. (a) Overview of the CP-H/RDS algorithm for satisfying user constraints (b) Inputs to and outputs of the routing decision system

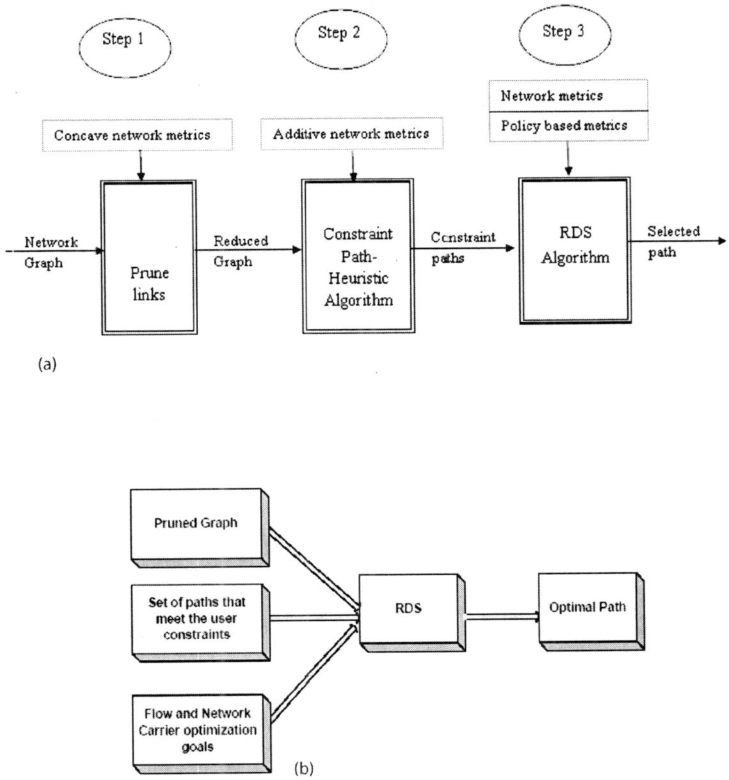

metric value represents the preference value of x relative to all the network values for this metric. Next, the user QoS requirement metrics are scaled by using the preference functions for each metric to arrive at the user traffic flow demand vector v. The RDS algorithm decides which path in set C best satisfies the traffic flow demand vector v. The RDS algorithm returns a path P that is pareto optimal with respect to at least one QoS metric, and satisfies the traffic flow and network carrier resource utilization goals. The steps in the RDS algorithm is given below.

RDS (C,P,V) {

```
k ← C.size()
if k=1 then
   Return P ← C.get(0)
For j← 0 to m Do {
   a_j ← BEST(C,j)
   b_j ← worse(C,j)
   For i ← 0 to k Do {
      If a_j ≠b_j then
         s_j(x_i,j) ← 2((x_j.b_j)/(a_j-b_j)) - 1
      Else
         S_j(x_i,j) ← 1
         }
      }
Let s_j(d_j) ← -1, for all j ∈ [1,m]
Let sum_i ← 0, for all i ∈ [1,k]
For j ← 0 to m Do {
   If (v[j] = 1) then
   s_j(d_j) ← 1
   Else
   If (v[j] = 2) then
      s_j(d_j) ← 0
```

Figure 2. Illustration of the CP-H/RDS algorithm (a) Network with delay, cost and jitter values (b) constraint path set C (c) Constraint path set C after preference function scaling

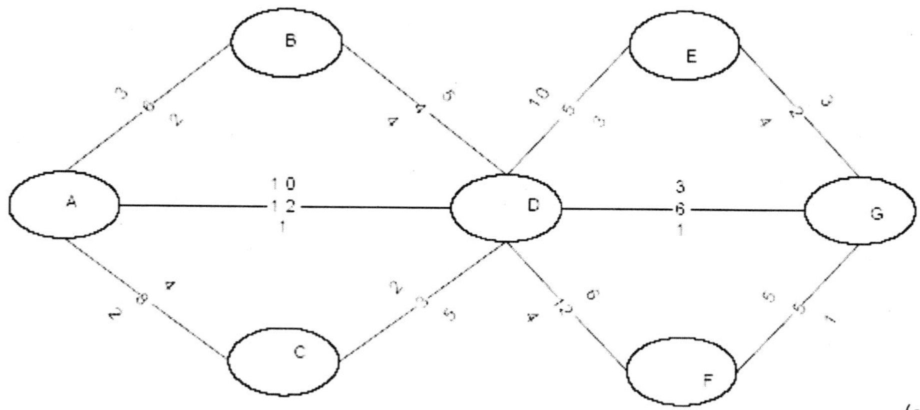

(a)

(b)

$$A' = \begin{bmatrix} 13 & 18 & 2 & 2 \\ 10 & 16 & 7 & 3 \\ 9 & 17 & 8 & 3 \\ 23 & 19 & 8 & 3 \\ 20 & 17 & 13 & 4 \\ 19 & 18 & 14 & 4 \end{bmatrix}$$

Path	Delay	Cost	Jitter	HopCount
A-D-G	13	18	2	2
A-B-D-G	10	16	7	3
A-C-D-G	9	17	8	3
A-D-E-G	23	19	8	3
A-B-D-E-G	20	17	13	4
A-C-B-E-G	19	18	14	4

(c)

$$A = \begin{bmatrix} 0.43 & -0.33 & 1.00 & 1.00 \\ 0.86 & 1.00 & 0.17 & 0.00 \\ 1.00 & 0.33 & 0.00 & 0.00 \\ -1.00 & -1.00 & 0.00 & 0.00 \\ -0.57 & 0.33 & -0.83 & -1.00 \\ -0.43 & -0.33 & -1.00 & -1.00 \end{bmatrix}$$

Figure 3. Summary of tasks performed by RDS server and ingress router when flows request admission into the network

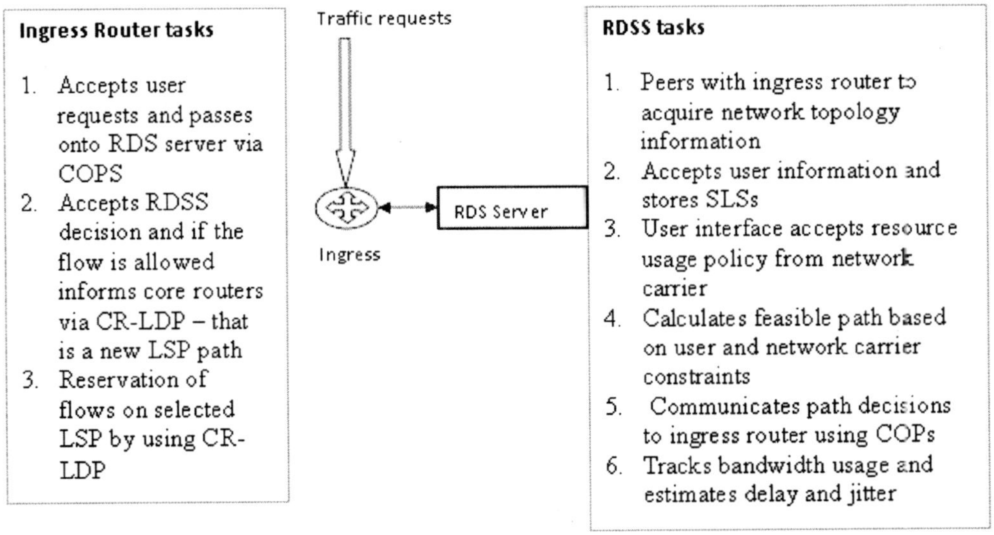


```
    For j ← 0 to m Do {
        sum_i ← sum_i + s_j(d_j) x s_j(x_i,j)
    }
y ← LARGEST(sum)
return P← C.get(y)
        }
```

Figure 2 illustrates how the CP-H/RDS algorithm works. Let the user flow request a cost of no more than 22 units that minimizes delay, jitter and hop count. This can be modeled by the vector $v = (1, -1, 1, 1)$. Path A-D-G is chosen since it is the only path for which at least one metric, hop count, is minimum with all the other metric values being relatively small.

FRAMEWORK FOR USING CP-H/RDS IN TRAFFIC ENGINEERING

Online Traffic Engineering (TE) provides a means of controlling traffic through a network, offering services tailored to traffic flow requirements while ensuring economical use of network resources. On the other hand, QoS routing is concerned with satisfying user traffic flow requirements. In this section a framework under which the CP-H/RDS algorithm can be used in the context of a traffic engineering environment is presented. A set of protocols and procedures are proposed that allows the CP-H/RDS algorithm to function in the management plane. The most important advantage in this approach is that there is opportunity for graceful migration to the CP-H/RDS algorithm with little disruption to existing layer 3 operations. Equally important the complexity introduced by QoS awareness remains outside the network. A major advantage is that a provider need not over-provision resources when the CP-H/RDS algorithm is deployed. In order for Traffic Engineering to take advantage of multiple constraint-based routing algorithms like the CP-H/RDS, it must make use of mechanisms already in place to a) distribute/ acquire information about the network topology (including link characteristics); b) capture the constraint information of user traffic flows; c) install explicit routes in the core network; and d) setup traffic flow priorities in routers and switches. These goals are achieved by adopting a centralized route server approach similar to the RATES server (Aukia, Kodialam, Koppol, Lakshman, Sarin, & Suter, 2000) where a centralized routing server is used to make routing decisions on behalf of ingress routers.

The Routing Decision System Server

Figure 3 shows a summary of the tasks involved in the relationship between the ingress router and the proposed RDS server.

Maintenance of Topology Information

RDSS assumes that a link state protocol like OSPF is implemented in the core. Topology information about the core network can be obtained and maintained by peering with other nodes in the network and using a link state protocol. An advantage of using link state peering is that, in the case of a link failure, the routing server will learn about the failure in the same time frame that the link state protocol takes to converge.

User Constraint Information

User constraint information may be provided to the RDSS by means of a user interface. Typically a user communicates their expectations of the network via the use of a Service Level Specification (SLS) which describes the technical details of how the user traffic will be treated (Sanjay, & Hassan, 2002). SLS configuration parameters stored by the RDSS are given in Table 1. Extensions to the Common Open Policy Service protocol (COPS) can be used so that the RDSS can communicate policy decisions to the ingress routers.

Calculating and Installing Explicit Paths

Explicit paths can be installed using the multi protocol label switching (MPLS) protocol after route calculation by RDSS. When an egress node receives customer traffic requesting use of the network, these requests are passed onto the RDSS via COPS. The RDSS then uses information in the traffic engineering database (TED) and the CP-H/RDS algorithm calculates a label switched path that the user traffic flow should use. This information is communicated to the ingress node by COPS. The ingress node then uses the MPLS explicit option to install the LSP in the core network.

Table 1. Contents of the service level specification

Content	Description	Information stored
Scope	The area of the network where the policies outlined for traffic in a given direction within the SLS will be enforced.	ingress - egress {interface identifier (s)}
Flow identification (ID)	Indicates which IP packets in a stream will be given a particular treatment	source, destination, application information, - Differentiated Services, information Per-Hop-Behavior (PHB)
Traffic parameters	Traffic parameters indicate what should be done with in- & out-of-profile packets	Token bucket algorithm (b, r) - Token bucket rate (r) - Bucket depth = b
Performance guarantees	Service guarantees that the network offers to the customer for the packet stream identified by Flow ID over the geographical region defined by Scope	Bandwidth, packet loss, delay (optional), jitter (optional), cost, minimum hop count

Estimating Delay and Jitter

Metrics like delay and jitter require extensions of the routing protocol. In order for the TED to ascertain delay and jitter from network topology information it is proposed that these values be based on the estimates for link residue bandwidth, link propagation delay and token bucket parameters from routers and switches that use rate proportional policing. The queuing delay and jitter bounds are those given in (Ma and Steenkiste, 1997)

Setting up Reservations

Calculating an appropriate path for a given user traffic flow in the core network helps achieve QoS and resource optimization for the flow. The requested resources can be reserved or pinned so that the flow is guaranteed consistent QoS. This can be done if network managers specify the treatment of packets at each node, also known as PHB (per-hop behavior), for each class of differentiated service. This information can be stored in the SLS as indicated in Table 1. PHB and traffic conditioning information can be passed to the ingress router after the LSP path calculation is done by the RDSS. The ingress node could then use the Constraint-based Routing Label Distribution Protocol (CR-LDP) to enable the specification of QoS and traffic parameters. This includes the specification of service class and traffic descriptors such as bandwidth requirements for all routers/switches on the LSP. In addition, CR-LDP facilitates state management, path-tear-down and maintenance of LSPs.

Path Protection

The CP-H/RDS by design has a high probability of returning disjoint paths that are ranked in a preference ordering that conforms to the optimization goals of the user flow and network carrier. Sharing protection capacity that is assumed to be exempt from simultaneous failure is an efficient solution for providing failed primary paths with backup paths.

EVALUATION RESULTS AND ANALYSIS

The feasibility of the proposed CP-H/RDS approach for simultaneously satisfying user traffic flow constraints and network resource utilization goals in traffic engineering is illustrated with simulations. All algorithms used in simulations have been implemented in Java and have used the Binary Heap data structure. The BRITE (Medina, Matta, and Byers, 2000) graph generator tool is used to generate Waxman graphs. In a real network, two nodes close to each other are, likely to be connected by a link. The Waxman graph (Waxman,

Table 2. Configuration of Brite tool employed to generate waxman graphs used in simulations

Parameter name	**Value**
Network size	N
Size of main plane	1000
Size of inner plane	100
Node placement	Random
Growth type	Incremental
Number of neighboring nodes each new node connects to	3
α (Waxman parameter)	0.10
β (Waxman parameter)	0.70

1988) is a variation of the random graph where the probability of there being a link between two nodes decreases as the distance between the nodes increases. The Waxman's method starts by placing the nodes of the network randomly on a two-dimensional grid. Then, a link between any pair of two distinct nodes *u* and *v* is added according to the following probability function:

$$p(u,v) = a\ \mathrm{e}\frac{-d(u,v)}{\beta L}$$

where $0 \leq \alpha, \beta \leq 1$, $d(u, v)$ is the Euclidian distance between *u* and *v*, and *L* is the maximum Euclidean distance between any two nodes. The configuration parameters used for generating the Waxman graphs are given in Table 2. The value for both α and β are in [0.0, 1.0] range. Note that the larger the value of α, the greater the number of edges in the graph, while the larger the value of β the larger the ratio of long edges to short edges. The value of α and β were chosen so that graphs containing chain like topologies are likely to be generated. (Kuipers, Korkmaz, Krunz, and Mieghem, 2004) state that under loose constraints most MCP algorithms have small execution time and high success rates (i.e.,find a feasible path if it exists). Hence, all results presented with respect to success rate, normalized execution times, and number of distinct feasible paths is under strict constraints.

Success Rate of the CP-H/RDS Algorithm

The success rate is defined as the ratio of the number of user requests satisfied using a given algorithm divided by the total number of requests generated (Kuipers, Korkmaz, Krunz, & Mieghem, 2004). To study the success rate of the CP-H/RDS algorithm, simulations were performed comparing the CP-H/RDS with well known heuristic QoS algorithms including the Iwata (Iwata, and Fujita, 2000) and the Jaffe (Jaffe, 1984). Four sets of graphs were generated, each set containing 2000 Waxman graphs consisting of 100, 200, 300, and 400 nodes. Two independent QoS link metrics (m = 2) were considered. Also 500 random sets of strict user requests for each graph in each set were generated and used for simulations comparing the CP-H, Iwata and Jaffe algorithms.

The results in Figure 4a indicate that the CP-H/RDS algorithm performs consistently better than the heuristic Jaffe and Iwata algorithms in terms of success rates. The success rate of the CP-H/RDS ranges between 93% and 96% when strict constraints and 2 additive metrics are used with a Waxman graph topology. Figure 4b shows that as the number of additive metrics increase the success rate of the CP-H/RDS remains constant. The Iwata algorithm success rate decreases with an increase in the number additive metrics. This may be explained by the fact that for both the CP-H/RDS and the IWATA algorithms the number of paths considered in the search process increases as the number of additive metrics increases. However, in the case of the CP-H/RDS, the number of paths drastically decreases as the number of additive metrics increases as is further illustrated from Figure 7a in the following subsection.

Normalized Execution Time of the CP-H/RDS Algorithm

The CP-H/RDS algorithm's execution time was compared with a well known exact algorithm SAMCRA, and the heuristic IWATA. The choice of user constraints can heavily influence how many feasible paths exist and therefore will affect the execution time needed to find an optimal path.

The normalized execution time can be used as a measure of how well the given algorithm will perform online to accomplish QoS routing and implement dynamic TE goals. We compared the CP-H/RDS with the SAMCRA algorithm as the SAMCRA is an exact QoS routing algorithm that guarantees to find a feasible path if such a path exists (Van Mieghem, De Neve, and Kuipers, 2001).

Figure 4. Success rates for the class of Waxman graphs (N=200) for strict constraints (a) as a function of number of nodes with additive metrics m = 2; (b) as a function of the number of additive metrics m

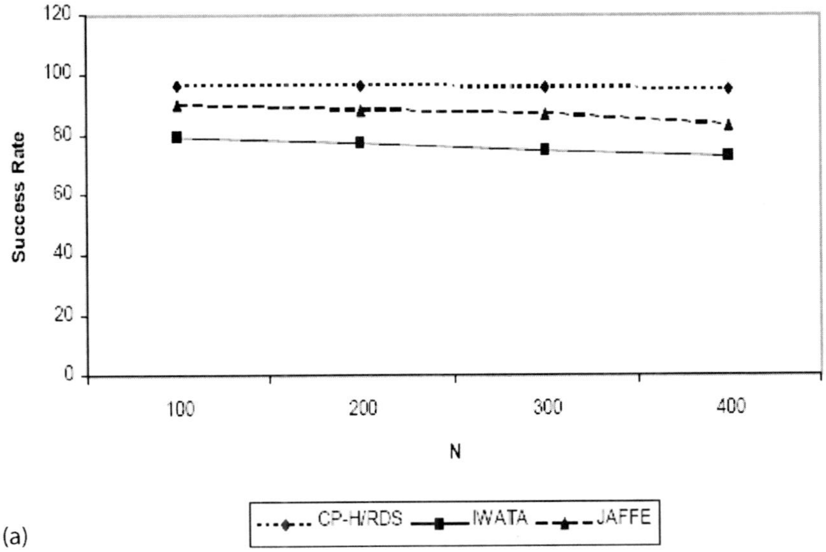

(a)

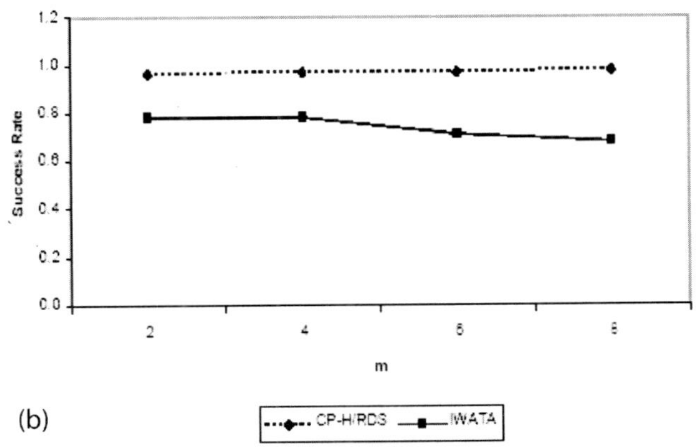

(b)

Figure 5 shows that, under strict constraints, the normalized execution time of the CP-H/RDS is better than the SAMCRA and marginally worse than the Iwata for 2 additive QoS metrics. The execution times of the CP-H/RDS algorithm increases proportionally with the number of additive metrics. Also, the CP-H/RDS algorithm has lower running times than the SAMCRA algorithm as the number of metrics increases.

Figure 6 shows, under strict user constraints, the normalized execution times for the CP-H/RDS, SAMCRA, Iwata and Jaffe algorithms as a function of the size of the network for strict constraints. Under strict constraints the CP-H/RDS algorithm has significantly lower running times than the SAMCRA algorithm. However, the CP-H/RDS algorithm has higher running times than its heuristic counterparts. The average execution time

Figure 5. Normalized execution time as a function of the number of additive metrics m under strict constraints

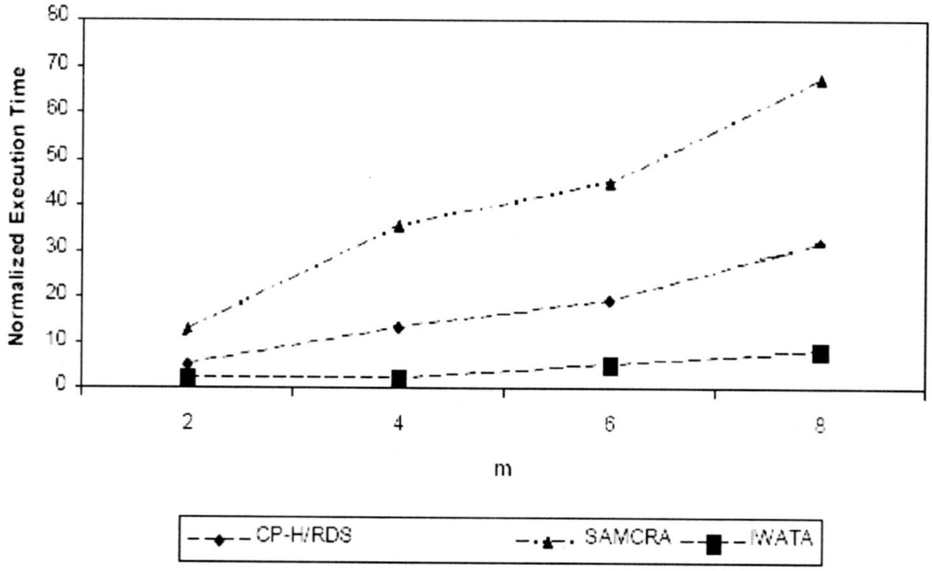

Figure 6. Normalized execution time for the class of Waxman graphs as a function of number of nodes N (strict constraints, and number of additive metrics m =2)

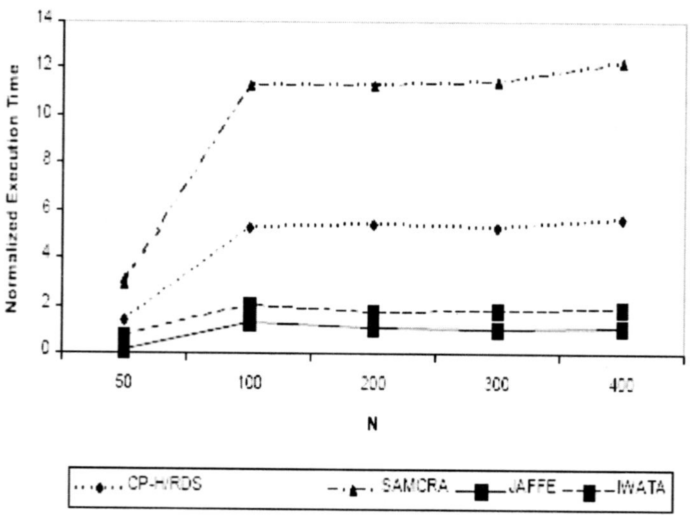

of the CP-H/RDS algorithm is about 5 times the Dijkstra's algorithm.

The CP-H/RDS algorithm is fast relative to exact algorithms and has higher success rates than other heuristic algorithms. The results in this chapter suggest that there is a trade-off between execution time of algorithms and their ability to find feasible paths. However, from the set of

Figure 7. Constraint path selection in the CP-H algorithm for Waxman graphs (m = 2, strict constraints, 100 - 400 nodes) (a) Number of constraint paths selected as a function of the number of additive metrics (b) Probability of the number of distinct feasible paths

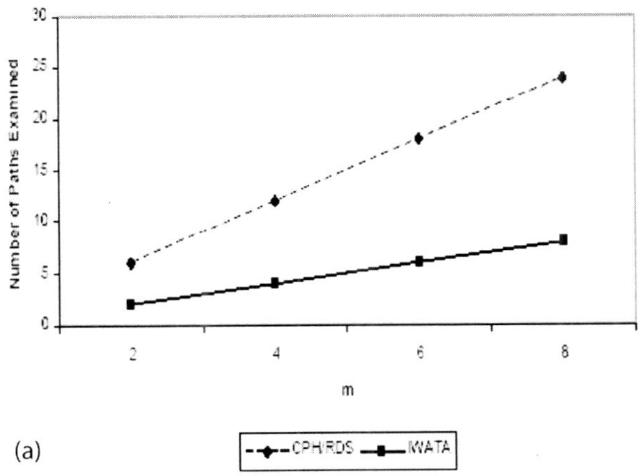

(a)

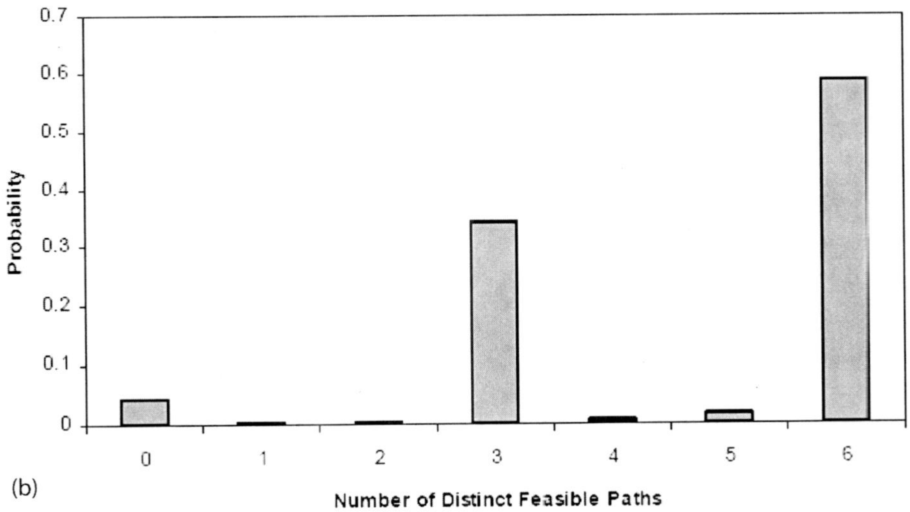

(b)

algorithms considered the CP-H/RDS algorithm offers the best trade-off between execution time and success rates. This makes it a good candidate for use in online routing where there are high demands for fast processing of multiple network and policy criteria.

Distinct Feasible Paths Finding Capability of the CP-H Algorithm

Finding more than one distinct feasible path ensures providing a back up path in case of failure of the primary QoS path, and is a measure of the path protection metric used in TE. From Figure 7a, it is seen that as the number of additive metrics increases the paths considered in the search process for both the CP-H/RDS and Iwata increase. However, in the case of the CP-H/RDS algorithm, the number of paths drastically increases as the number of additive metrics increases. A larger path search space implies a better chance of finding a path satisfying all metrics. In the case of the Iwata algorithm, although the search space increases, only one path per metric is being examined as a candidate for satisfying all metrics which can lead to an overall reduction in success rate since the selected path must satisfy an increased number of constraints. However, in the case of the CP-H/RDS algorithm λ paths are considered for each metric.

Figure 7b shows the probability of the CP-H algorithm returning a number of distinct feasible paths for Waxman graphs under strict user constraints. The probability that at least two distinct feasible paths are returned by the CP-H algorithm is 0.96. In addition, the probability that at least five distinct feasible paths are returned by the CP-H algorithm is 0.60. By design the CP-H algorithm has a high probability of returning disjoint paths and thereby supports the technique of sharing protection capacity.

The RDS algorithm depends on distinct feasible paths being passed from the constraint path algorithm in order to find the most suitable paths that match the optimization goals of both the user application and policy objectives of the network carrier. The CP-H algorithm has a very high probability of returning three or more distinct paths and therefore is very suitable for use with the RDS algorithm.

Call Blocking Rate for the CP-H/RDS Algorithm

The main goal of TE is to maximize network resource utilization. This objective can also be seen in terms of reducing call blocking rates as the number of traffic flows entering the network increases. To study the call blocking rate of the CP-H/RDS algorithm, simulations done in (Figueiredo, da Fonseca, & Monteiro, J., 2006) were reproduced with the main goal of comparing the CP-H/RDS with existing TE QoS algorithms such as the Minimum Hop Algorithm (MHA), the Least Interference Optimization routing Algorithm (LIOA) and the SAMCRA algorithms. The Minimum Interference Routing Algorithm (MIRA) and its improvement L-MIRA are not considered since results in (Bagula, Botha, & Krzesinki, 2004) suggests that the LIOA has significantly reduced blocking rates and resource utilization over these algorithms. Bandwidth (concave metric) is the only user constraint that MHA and LIOA employed. Figure 9 shows the test network employed which consists of 15 nodes and 28 links. Links are bi-directional, representing two links with the same capacity in opposite directions. Lighter links have a capacity of 1200 bandwidth units, whilst the darker ones have 4800 bandwidth units, representing OC-12 and OC-48 rates respectively. In addition, each link has a delay value uniformly generated in the interval (0.02, 0.04). Bandwidth requests are generated using a uniform distribution in the interval (1, 4) and a delay request is derived by first generating a value in the range (0.02, 0.04) and then multiplying this value by a hop count value generated using a uniform distribution in the interval (6, 8). The CP-H and SAMCRA algorithms primarily use additive metrics after pruning links not meeting the requested bandwidth. Therefore, for comparison purposes only delay is used as a metric for the CP-H algorithm while delay, cost, bandwidth and hop count are used as metrics for the RDS algorithm. The CP-H/RDS is implemented to address user and network carrier goals with the elimination of jitter from the model. Note that in the case of the SAMCRA algorithm, delay and cost (same as LIOA) metrics are used. Three simulations were performed corresponding to permanent, short and long lived flows respectively. Parameter values associated with each simulation are given in Table 3. The mean request rate is μ_1 and the mean service rate is μ_2. The requests are assumed to follow a Poisson distribution and the departures an exponential distribution. *T* denotes

Table 3. Simulation parameters for call blocking rate analysis: permanent, long and short flows

Connection Type	Permanent	Long	Short
μ_1 (mean request service)	3	3	3
μ_2 (mean service rate)	∞	5000	50
T (number of simulation trials)	20	20	20
N (number of requests per trial)	8000	8000	8000

the number of simulation trials and N the number of requests per trial.

The simulation results for permanent flows (no link failures) are shown in Figure 9a. The number of requests rejected is plotted as a function of the number of requests arriving at the network. The SAMCRA algorithm rejects highest number of requests followed by the MHA and then the CP-H/RDS. The SAMCRA algorithm chooses an optimal path based on a length function that involves both delay and cost. This strategy proves very expensive in terms of wastage of the bandwidth resource. On the other hand, the MHA algorithm always chooses the shortest path which causes links of this path to rapidly saturate. SAMCRA started rejecting requests from around 2800 requests, MHA around 3200 requests, CP-H/RDS around 3300 requests and LIOA started around 3600 requests. However, the rate of rejected requests for SAMCRA is higher than the MHA, LIOA and CP-H/RDS algorithms.

The simulation results for short lived and long lived flows (no link failures) are shown in Figure 9b and Figure 9c respectively. Figures 9b and 9c indicate a significant improvement in the number of requests allowed into the network. This is expected since the bandwidth resource is constantly being consumed and returned to the network. The CP-H/RDS performs very well in terms of maintaining a low call blocking rate considering that its path selection process considers more than one user and network resource constraint.

Figure 8. Topology simulated for studying the call blocking rate

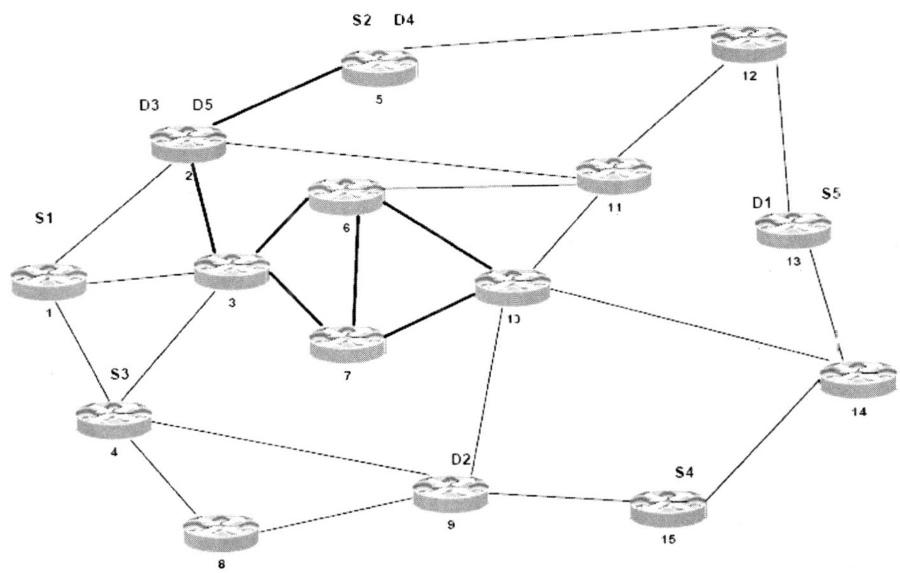

Figure 9. (a) Permanent flows: Number of requests vs. blocking rate (b) Short lived flows: Number of requests vs. blocking rate(c) Long lived flows: Number of requests vs. blocking rate

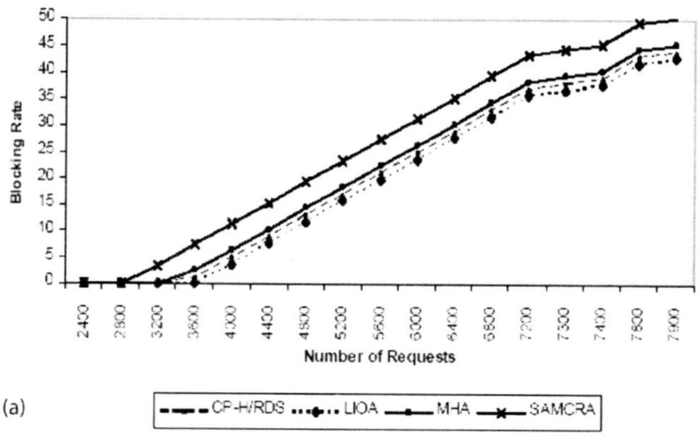

(a)

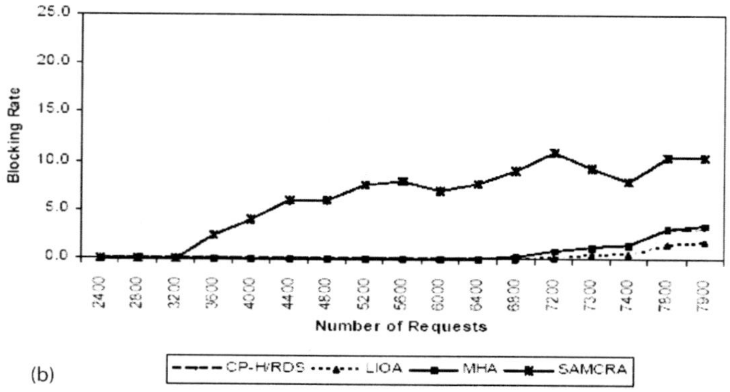

(b)

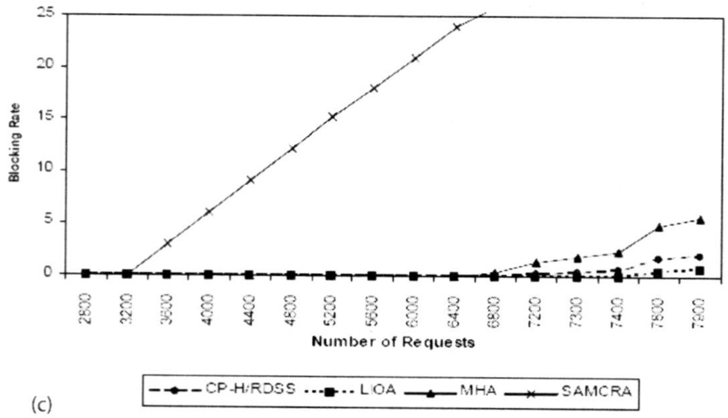

(c)

The SAMCRA algorithm like the CP-H/RDS algorithm finds optimal paths based on delay and cost. However, the important advantage that the CP-H/RDS has over the SAMCRA algorithm is that it is able to find optimal paths that minimize the bandwidth resource as well as the number of hops between source and destination nodes. Also, the call blocking rate of the CP-H/RDS algorithm is comparable to TE algorithms like MHA and LIOA. This means that the network carrier can achieve high resource usage as a result of using the CP-H/RDS algorithm.

CONCLUSION

The contribution of this paper is the use of a preference function modeling approach to solve the multiple-criteria optimization problem associated with choosing paths that meet traffic-oriented and resource-oriented objectives. The main contribution is the novel approach used to solve the multiple optimization problem associated with the traffic-oriented and resource-oriented optimization objectives. The use of strong scales provided the basis for constructing a multiple criteria preference function in an affine space. The use of preference functions in turn made it possible for paths that match traffic-oriented and resource-oriented goals to be selected by the algorithm. The heuristic constraint-path (CP-H) algorithm has a very high probability of returning three or more distinct paths that satisfy each of the QoS metrics under consideration. The routing decision system (RDS) algorithm finds a pareto optimal path that best matches the optimization goals of both the user traffic and network carrier policy objectives. The CP-H/RDS algorithm is much faster and has higher success rates than exact QoS algorithms such as the SAMCRA. Also, the CP-H/RDS algorithm is fast relative to and has higher success rates than comparable heuristic algorithms including the Jaffe, and Iwata. This makes the CP-H/RDS ideal for use in online TE requiring fast processing of multiple user QoS constraints and network carrier policy criteria. The call blocking rate of the CP-H/RDS algorithm is comparable to online traffic engineering algorithms like MHA and LIOA. Hence, network carriers employing the CP-H/RDS algorithm can achieve high resource utilization. The proposed routing decision system server (RDSS) framework is implemented in the CP-H/RDS's management plane rather than the network (control) layer. This enables dynamic admission control to admit user flows into the network, and creates a management environment in which it is easy to deploy network policies that benefit both network carrier and user traffic flows. Future work will investigate how pricing and billing can be incorporated into the routing decision system server framework.

REFERENCES

Apostolopoulos, G., Guerin, R., Kamat, S., & Tripathi, S. (1999). Improving QoS routing performance under inaccurate link state information. In *16th International Teletraffic Congress* (ITC. 16).

Aukia, P., Kodialam, M., Koppol, P., Lakshman, T., Sarin, H., & Suter, B. (2000). Rates: a server for MPLS traffic engineering. *IEEE Network*, *14*, 34–41. doi:10.1109/65.826370

Awduche, D. (1999). MPLS and traffic engineering in IP networks. *IEEE Communications Magazine*, *37*, 42–47. doi:10.1109/35.809383

Bagula, A., Botha, M., & Krzesinki, A. (2004). The least interference optimization algorithm. In. *Proceedings of the IEEE International Conference on Communications*, *2*, 1232–1236.

Chen, S., & Nahrstedt, K. (1998). On finding multi-constrained paths. *IEEE International Conference on Communications*, (vol. 2, pp. 874-879).

Chen, S. & Nahrstedt, K. (1998-2). An overview of quality-of-service routing for the next generation high- speed networks: Problems and solutions. *IEEE Network, Nov/Dec, 12*(6), 64-79.

Crawley, E., Nair, R., Rajagopalan, B., & Sandick, H. (1998). *A framework for QoS- based routing in the internet. In Internet Engineering Task Force Request for Comment – IETF RFC2386.* Retrieved from http://www.ietf.org/rfc/rfc2386.txt

De Neve, H., & Van Mieghem, P. (2000). Tamcra: A tunable accuracy multiple constraints routing algorithm. *Computer Communications*, *23*, 667–679. doi:10.1016/S0140-3664(99)00225-X

Figueiredo, G., da Fonseca, N., & Monteiro, J. (2006). A minimum interference routing algorithm with reduced computational complexity. *Computer Networks: The International Journal of Computer and Telecommunications Networking*, *50*(11), 1710–1732.

Goodridge, W., Robertson, W., Phillips, W. J., & Sivakumar, S. (2004a). *Multiple metric QoS in differentiated services networks using preference functions measurement concepts. Lecture Notes in Computer Science* (pp. 390–399). Berlin: Springer Verlag.

Goodridge, W., Robertson, W., Phillips, W. J., & Sivakumar, S. (2004b). Over-constraint QoS routing in large networks. In. *Proceedings of the London Communications Symposium*, *2*, 61–64.

Goodridge, W., Robertson, W., Phillips, W. J., & Sivakumar, S. (2005). Traffic driven multiple constraint-optimization for QoS routing. *International Journal of Internet Protocol Technology*, *1*, 1–11. doi:10.1504/IJIPT.2005.007555

Guerin, R. & Orda, A. (1999). QoS-based routing in networks with inaccurate information: Theory and algorithms. *IEEE/ACM Transactions on Networking*, *7*(6), 350-364.

Hui-Lan, L., & Faynberg, I. (2003). An architectural framework for support of quality of service in packet networks. *IEEE Communications Magazine*, *41*, 98–105. doi:10.1109/MCOM.2003.1204754

Iwata, A., & Fujita, N. (2000). A hierarchical multilayer QoS routing system with dynamic SLA management. *IEEE Journal on Selected Areas in Communications*, *18*(12), 2603–2616. doi:10.1109/49.898740

Jaffe, J. (1984). Algorithms for finding paths with multi constraints. *Networks*, 95–116. doi:10.1002/net.3230140109

Kim, S., & Lee, M. (2001). Server based QoS routing with implicit network state updates. *IEEE GLOBECOM*, *4*, 2182–2187.

Kuipers, F., Korkmaz, T., Krunz, M., & Mieghem, P. V. (2004). Performance evaluation of constraint-based path selection algorithms. *IEEE Network*, *18*, 16–23. doi:10.1109/MNET.2004.1337731

Liu, G., & Ramakrishnan, K. (2001). A*prune: An algorithm for finding k shortest paths subject to multiple constraints. In *Twentieth Annual Joint Conference of the IEEE Computer and Communications Societies (INFOCOM)*, (vol. 2, pp. 743-749).

Ma, Q., & Steenkiste, P. (1997). Quality of service routing with performance guarantees. *4th International IFIP Workshop on QoS*, (pp. 1-12). Boca Raton, FL: Chapman & Hall.

Marzo, J., Calle, E., Scoglio, C., & Anjah, T. (2003). QoS online routing and MPLS multilevel protection: a survey. *IEEE Communications Magazine*, *41*, 126–132. doi:10.1109/MCOM.2003.1235604

Medina, A., Matta, I., & Byers, J. (2000). *Brite: A flexible generator of internet topologies. Technical Report: 2000-005*. Boston: Boston University.

Mitra, D., & Wang, Q. (2003). Stochastic traffic engineering with applications to network revenue management. In *Twenty-Second Annual Joint Conference of the IEEE Computer and Communications Societies (INFOCOM)*, (vol. 1, pp. 396-405).

Nelakuditi, S., Zhang, Z., Tsang, R., and Du, D.H.C, (2002). Adaptive proportional routing: A localized QoS routing approach. *IEEE/ACM Transactions on Networking, 10*(6), 790 - 804.

Sanjay, S., & Hassan, M. (2002). *Engineering Internet QoS*. Norwood, MA: Artech House.

Van Mieghem, P., De Neve, H., & Kuipers, F. A. (2001). Hop-by-hop Quality of Service Routing. *Computer Networks*, *37*(3-4), 407–423. doi:10.1016/S1389-1286(01)00222-5

Waxman, B. (1988). Routing of multipoint connections. *IEEE Journal on Selected Areas in Communications*, *6*(9), 1617–1622. doi:10.1109/49.12889

Chapter 8
QoS Routing and Management in Backbone Networks

Gilles Bertrand
Institut Telecom, France

Samer Lahoud
IRISA-University of Rennes I, France

Miklós Molnár
IRISA-INSA , France

Géraldine Texier
Institut Telecom, France

ABSTRACT

The Internet relies on the cooperation of competitive network operators that typically administrate their networks unilaterally and autonomously to interconnect people and companies in different locations. Recent work calls for extending this organizational model with augmented interactions between network operators, to provide a higher level of end-to-end quality of service and to ease certain aspects of traffic management in backbone networks. This chapter presents the emerging collaborative network management models as well as related technologies. In particular, it describes recent techniques for interdomain traffic engineering and for qualityofservice aware routing. The detailed methods are of great interest for network operators and permit the development of new types of commercial relationships between them, ranging from simple interconnection agreements to collaborative traffic management and automated provisioning.

INTRODUCTION

The Internet supports a growing number of services ranging from legacy web browsing to the more recent online gaming or voice over IP. Among these services, some emerging network applications, such as IP television or video on demand, have stringent requirements in terms of guaranteed endtoend performance. These requirements translate into multiple quality of service (QoS) constraints related to, for example, delay, jitter, bandwidth, and packet loss. Network operators use several QoS mechanisms to protect critical applications and to ensure that proper

DOI: 10.4018/978-1-61520-791-6.ch008

resources are allocated for each service. Soldatos et al. (2005) classify these mechanisms depending on their operation level. For example, scheduling and queue management operate at packet scale in the Differentiated Services (DiffServ) architecture described in (Blake et al., 1998), whereas resource reservation and signaling operate at flow scale in the Integrated Services (IntServ) architecture standardized in (Braden, Clark, & Shenker, 1994), and Traffic Engineering (TE) operates at network scale. In particular, QoS aware routing is essential when ensuring that each flow follows a path with appropriate performance. For instance, delay- and losssensitive traffic should typically be routed on paths with short delays and low packetloss rates.

The level of QoS experienced by end-users depends on the performance of the endto-end path traversed by service flows. Thus, the successful delivery of services with stringent QoS requirements, like realtime multimedia services, requires QoS to be enforced on all the network segments crossed by service flows. However, varied problems must be addressed depending on the considered segment, and thus, network operators deploy diverse QoS techniques. For example, bandwidth is usually a scarce resource in access networks; hence QoS mechanisms are required in this segment to guarantee that appropriate resources are available for every service. In backbone networks, network operators commonly favor practices related to overprovisioning over sophisticated QoS techniques. However, overprovisioning requires a continuous increase in network capacity in order to cope with traffic evolution or the required level of QoS. As a result, network operators are increasingly interested in efficient network management techniques in backbone networks to delay their investments while maintaining QoS. The present chapter describes such techniques and their application in inter-domain networking.

An Autonomous System (AS) is a set of routers and hosts administrated with homogeneous policies by a network operator. An operator can divide its network into several ASes for administrative reasons. ASes and smaller routing areas are often named domains. The Internet relies on the interconnection of operator's backbone networks, that is, of their domains. The endtoend QoS performance experienced by flows crossing several domains depends on how the packets are processed inside each traversed domain. In particular, efficient traffic management is required inside every domain to protect critical services as well as to control network costs. Numerous studies propose solutions for QoS routing and management inside a single domain, based on enhancements of IP routing or on the MultiProtocol Label Switching (MPLS) architecture. Wang et al. (2008) present a good overview of these solutions.

It is important to note that, in the Internet, connectivity for flows crossing several domains usually relies on the cooperation of interconnected entities with competing interests. In particular, QoS policies often differ from one AS to another and every AS typically takes unilateral routing and networkmanagement decisions, even though these decisions may directly affect other domains. This absence of coordination complicates the provision by an operator of performance guarantees for packets once they leave its own network. Therefore, interdomain traffic flows require mechanisms for QoS routing and traffic management that involve several domains. Specifically, recent work calls for more collaboration among domains, for example in (Mahajan, Wetherall, & Anderson, 2004; J. P. Vasseur, Zhang, Bitar, & Le Roux, 2009), to enhance network performance and to provide support for delivering endtoend QoS. Therefore, the main purpose of this chapter is to describe the emerging management models for the future Internet and, in particular, their application for interdomain traffic management.

Two main technical possibilities have been proposed for the future Internet to provide performance guarantees across AS boundaries. The first consists of adding QoS capabilities to the Border

Gateway Protocol (BGP), the de facto standard interdomain routing protocol of the Internet, as in (Boucadair, 2005; Benmohamed, Liang, Naber, & Terzis, 2006; Knoll, 2009). The second consists of deploying the MPLS architecture at the interdomain level and is developed in (Douville, Le Roux, Rougier, & Secci, 2008; J. P. Vasseur et al., 2009). In relation to the second possibility we have recently proposed collaborative methods for multiconstrained QoS routing in multidomain MPLSTE networks in (Bertrand, Lahoud, Molnár, & Texier, 2009).

The remainder of the chapter is organized as follows. We first describe emerging management models for multidomain QoS and their impact on the policies of network operators. Network operators rely on two main technologies to implement these traffic management models: IP and MPLS. Thus, on one hand, we describe QoS management techniques based on IP routing, and on the other we present recent advances in MPLS-based techniques for inter-domain traffic engineering. We analyze the strengths and weaknesses of independent and collaborative network management models and highlight the tradeoffs between IP and MPLS based QoS management solutions. In particular our analysis covers the support of multiple constraints in QoS routing solutions. The conclusion of this chapter presents the applications and possibilities of multidomain QoS and network management techniques.

MANAGEMENT MODELS FOR MULTI-DOMAIN QOS

The Internet is a federation of autonomous domains without central authority, where the management of each domain is performed solely by the network operator responsible for the domain. Network management functions are numerous and can be classified into the following areas: network configuration management, user management and administration, security management, fault management, and performance management, which includes quality of service provisioning, network throughput and resource utilization management. Despite the independent management of the domains, the Internet enables worldwide services based on the establishment of communications traversing multiple domains. For instance, Internet users can initiate a voice over IP communication that uses the network resources of multiple domains. Typical multidomain services necessitate a minimal collaboration between the network operators: this collaboration consists of establishing an agreement for exchanging routing information with the BGP (Rekhter, Li, & Hares, 2006). However, this management model presents serious limitations when considering emerging services that require stringent performance guarantees. Applications such as IP Television or videoconferencing require QoS guarantees in terms of bandwidth, delay or jitter, across the domains. These guarantees should be coherently implemented by the management policies of each domain. Therefore, the legacy management models used by the network operators need to evolve in order to enable the establishment and maintenance of multidomain communications with QoS requirements.

Emerging management models for multidomain QoS should always consider that network operators have their own policies and are subject to various regulations. Therefore, QoS management schemes should permit the cooperation of different policies within the confines of typical policybased network management. In policybased network management, the different policies are defined as rules that guide the overall behavior of the network through high-level, declarative directives. The IETF policy-framework working-group has defined a manageragent reference model for managing IPbased multiservice networks with quality of service guarantees (Strassner, 2003). This model distinguishes Policy Decision Points (PDPs) and Policy Enforcement Points (PEPs). The PDP is the point where the policy decisions

Figure 1. Taxonomy of the main network management models

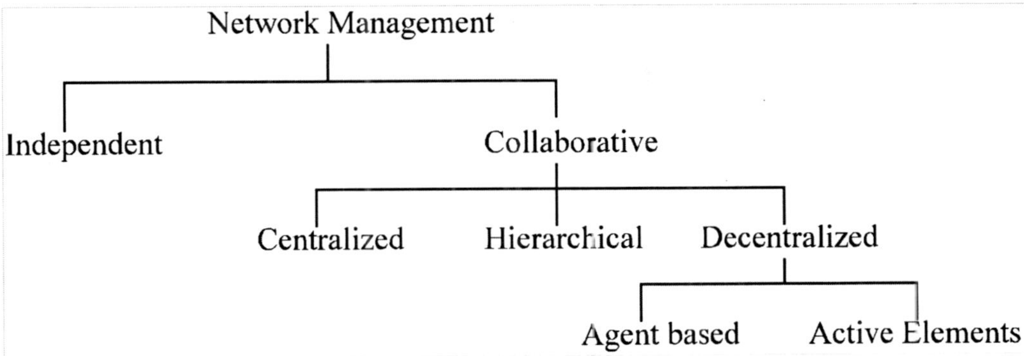

are made and the PEP is the point where they are permanently enforced. The major benefit of policy based network management is that it enables operators to automate the establishment of management level objectives using different underlying models and technologies. Thus, network administrators can interact with the network by providing highlevel abstract policies (Boutaba & Xiao, 2002).

Network management models can be based on independent decisions of autonomous operators or on the collaboration of these actors. In particular, Figure 1 classifies various independent and collaborative network management models that we describe in subsequent sections. Both types of network management model should always guarantee a high level of autonomy for operators and support the coexistence of heterogeneous network technologies.

Independent Management

Independent management is a network management model in which the operators of interconnected networks take unilateral decisions corresponding to their own interests and policy. As the result of isolated decision making techniques, this model is also named selfish management.

In this chapter, we examine network management from the point of view of routing decisions. Routing is an essential tool for network operators to enforce their management policies. For instance, network technologies detailed in subsequent sections (based on IP or MPLS protocols) allow operators to adapt the routing of certain traffic flows depending on their QoS requirement or to select particular paths for transit traffic coming from neighboring domains.

Currently, interdomain routing is based on BGP, which selects domain-level routes according to operator policies. A domain-level route refers to the sequence of domains that the traffic traverses, whereas a router-level route refers to the sequence of routers inside the domains. Consequently, two management levels can be identified in the context of routing, namely domain-level and router-level management. In particular, at the domain level, each domain border router makes local decisions that determine the next hop for the traffic. Therefore, BGP enables domain operators to apply any selfish routing strategy according to their local policies.

An alternative to BGP based routing uses the MPLS technology. Particularly, per-domain path computation, as proposed in (J. Vasseur, Ayyangar, & Zhang, 2008), enables the establishment of MPLS tunnels across domain borders. Management in the aforementioned proposal is performed in a perdomain manner, where each operator independently manages the tunnel segment that crosses its network. In this approach, each domain determines the best routing inside the domain and the different segments are concatenated to perform endtoend routing.

Network operators need to gain finer control over the quality of multidomain routes. Thus, many solutions have been proposed to replace current network architecture practices. For instance, Yang et al. (2007) propose an Internet routing architecture that gives a user the ability to choose the sequence of providers that their traffic crosses. This ability fosters competition between service providers and may lead to enhanced service levels and improved endtoend performance guarantees and reliability.

Unfortunately, selfish routing decisions can not always guarantee the required QoS for users and optimal load-balancing in the network. Without cooperation between the concerned domains, the routes obtained become nonoptimal from the point of view of QoS because the unilateral decisions of the domains may negatively impact transit traffic (Teixeira, Shaikh, Griffin, & Rexford, 2008). Consequently, improved cooperation between autonomous domains could efficiently resolve the QoS routing problem. For instance, we explain in the next section that cooperative methods can find winwin configurations in which all operators benefit: these solutions may be Pareto optimal (Mahajan et al., 2004).

Collaborative Management

Collaborative management is a model in which entities operating interconnected networks interact in order to take mutually beneficial network management decisions. Many forms of cooperation are possible, ranging from bilateral Service Level Agreements (SLAs) between two domains (interprovider QoS) to full architectural solutions enabling the collaboration of multiple domains (Griffin et al., 2007). Similarly, the level of cooperation between the domains ranges from a minimal exchange of information and simple interconnection agreements to full collaboration in a domain alliance and cooperative network engineering (Torab et al., 2006). For instance, Mahajan, Wetherall, & Anderson (2005) explain that specific cooperation mechanisms enable optimal solutions for management to be found and relieve operators of certain time-consuming and errorprone network management tasks.

Emerging architectures that support collaborative management models are being standardized. For instance, the Path Computation Element framework (Farrel, Vasseur, & Ash, 2006) is a good candidate to enable collaborative route computation. A PCE is an entity that receives a path computation request and replies with a solution. It is capable of computing an endtoend path given enough information. Alternatively, it may collaborate with other PCEs, potentially responsible for other domains. Cooperation between different operators could be efficiently aided by the formation of alliances to exchange management information and mutually support management decisions (Douville et al., 2008).

As illustrated in Figure 1, collaborative management schemes can be classified into three typical categories: centralized, hierarchical and decentralized management (Leinwand & Fang, 1993; Boutaba & Xiao, 2002). The centralized management scheme is not adequate for increasingly large networks with complex management and service requirements and should be replaced by distributed management models. Several technologies have been proposed to implement such decentralized management models. Specifically, cooperation between intelligent agents and active networks represent two interesting proposals, described in subsequent paragraphs.

In the intelligent agent approach, dedicated manager entities are no longer needed, as intelligent agents can perform pre-defined highlevel management tasks in a distributed and coordinated fashion. Moreover, agent based systems can be organized in a hierarchical manner. In a hierarchy, each agent could accomplish a limited function in its local environment. For instance, the work in

(Gavalas, Greenwood, Ghanbari, & O'Mahony, 2002; Flegkas, Trimintzios, Pavlou, Andrikopoulos, & Cavalcanti, 2001) presents a mobile agent based hierarchical management system and a hierarchical policy based network management scheme. Finally, distributed agent-based network management systems are robust and dependable, because the outage of some agents has limited negative consequences for the overall network management. When the entire network management system is autonomous, network administrators need to provide only servicelevel directives to the system (Boutaba & Xiao, 2002).

Network management can also be solved by using active networks. In this type of network, network entities such as routers and switches are programmable and run customized services. These networks present an effective enabling technology for distributing management tasks to device level, as illustrated in (Raz & Shavitt, 1999). The active engines run programs received from the (centralized or distributed) network management. They can monitor the network and the traffic and control the local processes. Such a solution provides good adaptability and interoperability between different platforms and could accelerate the deployment of new services and technologies.

IP-BASED ROUTING FOR QOS MANAGEMENT

QoS Features of the Internet Protocol

IP level communications are based on datagram routing; IP datagrams, also called packets, are routed independently in the network according to their destination address. Each router forwards packets to the next hop that is best able to bring them closer to their destination. Forwarding is based on routing tables and typically does not take the current network load into consideration. The path to reach a destination may change (due to a link failure for example) during a transfer, necessitating packet-reordering operations at arrival, and thus preventing an estimation of transfer delays. Furthermore, the network offers a best-effort delivery and packets toward the same destination are aggregated on the same path. Therefore, the performance of a packet transfer is conditioned by the concurrent traffic in the network. Due to flow aggregation in the routers, the time that packets spend in the succession of routers on the path cannot be accurately predicted. When arriving at a router, the packet is first stored in the appropriate queue before being served by the scheduler. If the network load is low, the queue may be quite empty and the packet will be treated quickly before being sent to the output queue. Thus, the packet will benefit from a low transfer delay. On the contrary, if it arrives during a heavy load phase the queue will be rather full, the packet will need more time to be served and will then be delayed. During congestion, if the router tries to store the packet in a queue that is already full the packet will be discarded. Therefore, the datagram paradigm in a best effort network does not provide any guarantee on packet delivery or transfer delays.

QoS mechanisms based on resource reservation (IntServ, DiffServ) or on introducing QoS concerns in routing management have been designed to offer more guarantees for identified flows that need to be protected or given preferential treatment. QoS routing is performed by both intra-domain and inter-domain routing protocols. Figure 2 illustrates the distinction between these two levels of operations for the routing protocols: intra-domain routing facilitates network connectivity within a particular domain, whereas inter-domain routing is responsible for determining the sequence of domains and the border nodes that enable a destination to be reached outside a particular domain.

Figure 2. Division of routing operations into two levels: intra-domain and inter-domain

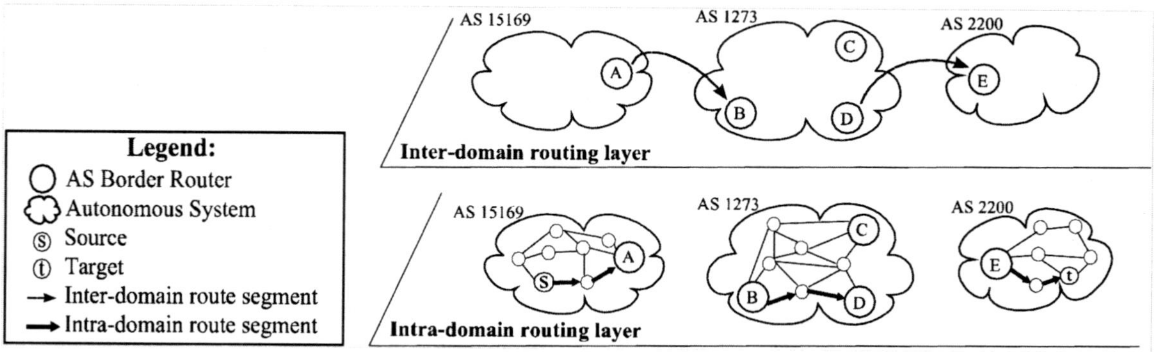

QoS Management with Intra-Domain Routing

Intra-domain routing is performed by Interior Gateway Protocols (IGP) such as OSPF, ISIS, and RIP. Intra-domain routing facilitates network connectivity within a particular domain. Information on node interconnections is exchanged in a cooperative fashion. The goal of intra-domain routing protocols is to maximize the knowledge of the routers within the domain while minimizing the information exchange overhead. Routing protocols employ various routing algorithms. For instance, RIP relies on a distance-vector algorithm that selects the suitable next hop for each destination by attempting to minimize the number of traversed links (hop count). OSPF and ISIS use Dijkstra's algorithm to compute the shortest path tree for each router, based on a link cost. The shortest path tree feeds the next-hop field of the routing table.

The link cost used for shortest path computation can be set administratively or can depend on the nominal capacity of the network interfaces. Typically, link cost is based on relatively static information about the network which doesn't integrate any knowledge of current network performance. Network operators improve their routing strategy by selecting appropriate path computation link weights. In particular, a common strategy is to introduce QoS considerations in the IGP weights to influence the path taken in the network. For OSPF, Cisco (1997) recommends the use of link costs inversely proportional to the nominal link capacity to favor the use of the links with the largest capacity. Note, nevertheless, that it is hardly possible to consider the currently available link bandwidth in the cost computation. Alternatively, the routing protocol EIGRP introduces QoS by using composite metrics that combine delay and bandwidth by default, with possible extension to load, reliability, and maximum transmission unit (MTU).

Another well-known strategy for improving the performance of the network is to optimize the link weights considered by the IGP to influence the path taken in the network. However, Fortz and Thorup (2004) have proven that finding an optimal setting of OSPF weights for an arbitrary network is NPhard even for an approximation. Furthermore, changing the weight of a link implies an update of OSPF variables, a set of update advertisement between routers, and a recomputation of the routing tables. Dynamically changing link weights may also affect the route stability and the traffic continuity, as packets will not necessarily follow the same path and reordering may be needed. Therefore, changing IGP weights is neither a flexible nor a harmless way to introduce QoS in the network.

RFC 2676 (Apostolopoulos et al., 1999) defines QoS routing mechanisms and OSPF extensions

Figure 3. Basic principle of IP interdomain routing with BGP

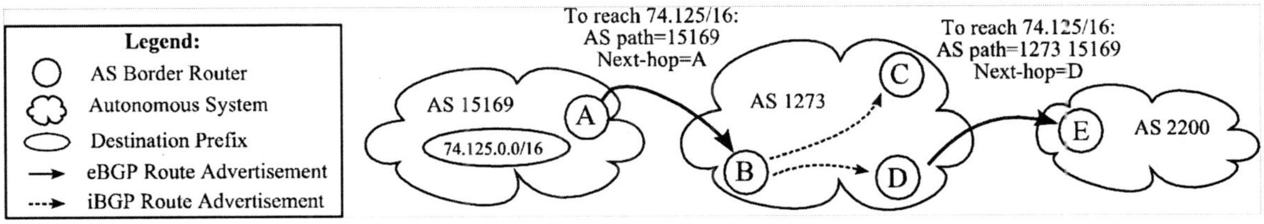

that consider the available bandwidth and the hop count as metrics for the shortest path first (SPF) algorithm. However, this approach is limited by the destination-based forwarding paradigm of IP, the result of which is that flows destined to the same node are not differentiated. Finally, QoS routing requires not only the integration of QoS concerns in the computation of the path, but also a consideration of the flow level to achieve a fine-grained treatment of the traffic transferred within the domain.

QoS Management with Inter-Domain Routing

Presentation of BGP

Rekhter et al. (2006) describe BGP, the de facto standard interdomain routing protocol of the Internet. BGP uses a pathvector routing algorithm to allow communications between hosts in different ASes, as illustrated in Figure 3. Concretely, this means that every AS advertises network reachability information, which includes a list of ASes that can be followed to reach a particular destination network (a network prefix), as well as several path attributes.

BGP relies on two different mechanisms named iBGP (internal) and eBGP (external) to convey the routes advertisement inside an AS or to neighboring ASes. With these mechanisms, a BGP router can receive several routes for the same destination prefix. Therefore, BGP routers use a sophisticated decision process supporting complex routing policies to select the routes that will be introduced into the routing table and that will be advertised to neighboring BGP routers. This bestpath selection process is based on the calculation of a degree of preference for each route and can take some path attributes into account.

Rekhter et al. (2006) describe multiple tie-breaking rules, which are applied successively to decide which route should be advertised when several equivalent routes for the same destination exist. These rules begin by considering all equally preferable routes to the same destination, and then select routes to be removed from consideration. The tie-breaking algorithm terminates as soon as only one route remains in consideration. For example, one rule specifies that the AS paths which do not have the lowest number of hops must be removed from consideration. Another rule states that the routes which do not have the lowest value of the MultiExit Discriminator (MED) attribute must be discarded. The lowest MED rule enables network operators to control how traffic leaves their networks (McPherson & Gill, 2006).

QoS Capabilities of BGP

Even if IP routing is traditionally best effort, BGP provides some QoS routing and network management features. For example, an operator can favor the forwarding of its transit traffic through a domain A rather than through another domain B by allocating a higher degree of preference to the routes received from A than to those received from B. This ability is particularly important to enforce commercial relationships with adjacent Internet Service Providers (ISPs). Furthermore, an appropriate configuration of BGP enables operators to perform traffic engineering. Specifically, Quoitin et al. (2005) describe the path prepending technique, which uses the shortest ASpath tie-breaking rule to divert incoming traffic: it artificially increases the length of the ASPath of certain routes to make them less preferable.

Although the reduction of routing information is desirable to preserve the scalability of interdomain routing, it limits the QoS routing and traffic engineering capabilities of BGP. The route advertisements include minimal information about the QoS level of the paths. In addition, each router typically advertises only a single route to a particular destination network and this route can differ from the one that best fulfills the QoS constraints for a given traffic class. Furthermore, the flow of routing information goes in only one direction: from the destination domain of the data traffic toward the source domain. However, bidirectional information exchanges are required in order for operators to take mutually beneficial routing decisions, as observed by Mahajan et al. (2004).

Numerous solutions have been proposed in the past few years to extend the QoS and network management capabilities of BGP. Fonte and others (2008) present an overview of the limitations of BGP and of possible solutions to these limitations. In this paragraph, we review two interesting aspects of existing proposals. First, Boucadair (2005) proposes that QoSenabled reachability information between service providers should be advertised to enable the use of an enhanced route selection process that takes the QoS performance of the paths into account. Second, the traffic could be separated into multiple classes and different configurations could be applied for different types of traffic so that service flows follow paths with appropriate QoS performance (Griffin et al., 2007). However, modifying BGP is difficult because this protocol is widely deployed and its behavior is complex. In particular, the proposed extensions of BGP must preserve the scalability, stability, and convergence time of this protocol. Thus, currently, there is no deployment plan for BGP QoS extensions.

Although intra- and interdomain routing are conceptually separated, they interact in the Internet. In particular, the MED attribute used in the BGP decision process often represents an IGP path cost, which introduces a relationship between the weight settings of the IGP and the route choices of BGP, as described by McPherson and Gill (2006). Thus, traffic management in backbone networks necessitates a complex coordination between intra- and interdomain routing decisions. In particular, a fine tuning of IP routing protocols is necessary. These problems could be avoided by robust traffic management methods or by cooperative network engineering, and facilitated by the introduction of MPLS technology.

MPLS TRAFFIC ENGINEERING FOR QOS MANAGEMENT

Traffic Engineering with MPLS

The current trend in networking involves integrating legacy heterogeneous technologies, simplifying the layering in order to ease network control and management, and further optimizing resource usage. The MPLS architecture (Rosen, Viswanathan, & Callon, 2001) is a promising approach to the aforementioned integration. Particularly, MPLS achieves the basic objective of protocol simplification and integration and adds the concept of a unified control plane.

The initial goal for MPLS was to improve router packet-switching performance by forwarding packets with a label lookup instead of the legacy longest-prefix match algorithm. The label is an integer value that is transmitted inside the packet itself and is used by devices called Label Switching Routers (LSR) to determine the interface to which the packet should be forwarded. In MPLS networks, traffic is routed along Label Switched

Figure 4. Basic principle of the MPLS packet forwarding mechanisms

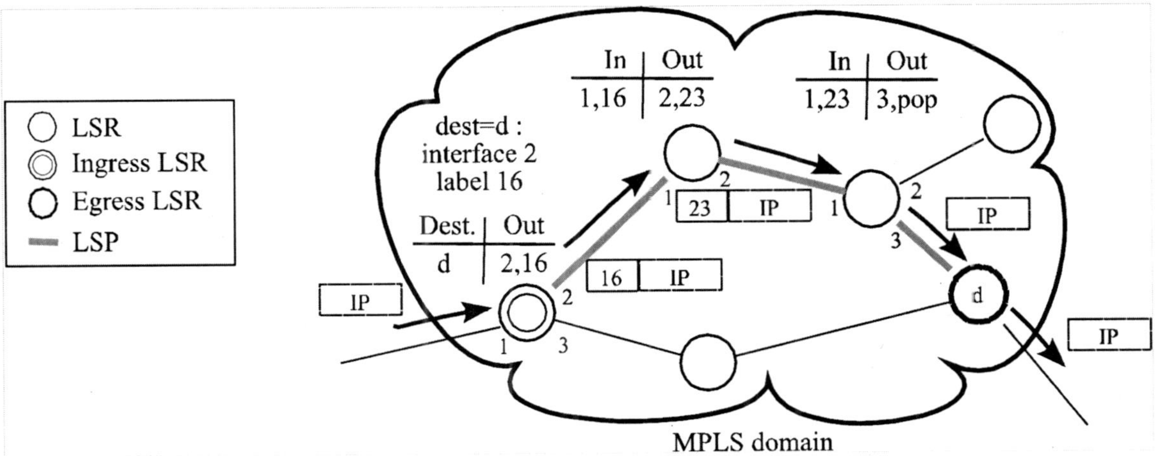

Paths (LSP), which consist of unidirectional paths between an ingress LSR and an egress LSR. The ingress LSR classifies IP packets into forwarding equivalence classes (FECs) and appends different labels for packet forwarding within the MPLS domain. A signaling protocol such as LDP (Andersson, Minei, & Thomas, 2007) distributes the label bindings, which populate the label forwarding tables and enable the packet switching.

Figure 4 illustrates these mechanisms. In the figure, an IP packet arrives in an ingress LSR. The ingress LSR determines that it must forward the packet to the egress router *d*. It searches the outgoing interface and the label corresponding to this destination in its MPLS switching table, the label Forwarding Information Base (FIB), and determines the relevant outgoing interface (2) and the new label (16). Then, the ingress LSR forwards the labeled packet to the next LSR, which receives the packet with label 16 on interface 1 and performs the label switching operations. In the example, the penultimate LSR removes the MPLS header and forwards an IP packet to the egress LSR. This action, called penultimate hop popping, reduces the load on the egress LSR.

The MPLS architecture provides a solution for implementing QoS routing and Traffic Engineering in backbone networks (Awduche, Malcolm, Agogbua, O'Dell, & McManus, 1999). Traffic engineering consists of the set of strategies deployed by network operators in order to facilitate efficient and reliable network operations while simultaneously optimizing network resource utilization and traffic performance (Awduche, Chiu, Elwalid, Widjaja, & Xiao, 2002). As detailed in the previous section, IPbased traffic engineering and QoS management present serious limitations. Consequently, network operators increasingly use MPLS for traffic engineering and QoS management. MPLS is able to configure data tunnels through the network. The tunnels, also called TE tunnels, can be placed according to explicit routes calculated offline or online and modified in real time. These routes may not necessarily follow the shortest path computed by conventional IP routing schemes: they are computed to optimize operator objectives and to satisfy traffic QoS constraints.

To compute the path for a TE tunnel, LSRs use extended information about the current state of the network, such as total link bandwidth, reserved link bandwidth, available link bandwidth, and link color. This information is flooded by the TE extensions of the internal routing protocols, for example OSPFTE (Katz, Kompella, & Yeung, 2003) or ISISTE (Li & Smit, 2008). Each LSR maintains information on the network-link attributes and the network topology in a specialized TE database (TED), which is used exclusively for calculating explicit paths for TE tunnels. Moreover, extended signaling protocols such as RSVPTE (Awduche et al., 2001) are used for the placement of TE tunnels along the explicit path across the physical topology. Note that the legacy forwarding protocols such as frame relay and ATM provide tunneling similar to that in MPLS. However, MPLS brings a unified IP control plane umbrella that eases the management and the construction of heterogeneous networks (Vázquez, Álvarez-Campana, & García, 2004).

Two different interaction models exist between the MPLS control plane (signaling and routing) and the management plane. In many systems, the Network Management Station (NMS) can select network paths for LSPs based on its knowledge of the network topology and of available resources. In this case, the NMS invokes its path computation function to determine a path that satisfies the service request, and then, commands the control plane to provision the LSP. Alternatively, the NMS can simply pass the service request to the control plane on the first traversed (or head-end) LSR and let the control plane select a path by invoking a path computation function on this LSR.

Online Traffic Engineering with MPLS

Online traffic engineering consists of enabling the path computation and path selection tasks at each LSR in a distributed manner. These tasks are performed on the fly with no a priori knowledge of the upcoming requests. The main objectives of online traffic engineering algorithms for QoS routing include reducing the blocking probability of flows, minimizing network costs and distributing network load. Moreover, online traffic engineering algorithms consider a set of QoS constraints and requirements that typically include bandwidth, delay, and policy rules, such as resource class attributes. Online traffic engineering algorithms are generally referred to as ConstraintBased Routing (CBR) (Younis & Fahmy, 2003).

A basic version of CBR uses an adaptation of the shortest path algorithm named Constrained Shortest Path First (CSPF). In order to improve routing efficiency (e.g., to reduce blocking probability and network costs), CBR algorithms integrate additional information in the computation process: for example, they can consider the residual bandwidth (Ma & Steenkiste, 1997; Guerin, Orda, & Williams, 1997), the location of ingress and egress routers (Kodialam & Lakshman, 2000), or the traffic profile (Suri, Waldvogel, & Warkhede, 2001; Capone, Fratta, & Martignon, 2003). CBR problems subject to multiple additive metrics such as link delay and link cost have a higher complexity and they are specifically studied in (Kuipers, Van Mieghem, Korkmaz, & Krunz, 2002) and (Avallone, Kuipers, Ventre, & Mieghem, 2006).

Online traffic engineering provides fast and dynamic provisioning and necessitates reduced management effort. However, online optimization considers traffic trunks in sequence, as they are proposed to the network. In particular, the order in which the trunks are set up influences their placement in the network and does not necessarily lead to an optimal solution. Network operators can overcome the limitations of online traffic engineering by combining online traffic engineering with a more global reoptimization of the network called offline centralized traffic engineering.

Offline Traffic Engineering with MPLS

Offline traffic engineering consists of examining each link's resource constraints and the requirements of each ingresstoegress demand in order to compute a set of LSPs that optimizes the use of all network resources. The offline approach performs global calculations, and thus, necessitates a longer running time than online traffic engineering. This global optimization can be achieved through the use of linear programming based algorithms. A generalized MPLS routing optimization is typically formulated as a multicommodity flow problem (Mitra & Ramakrishnan, 1999). The common objectives for the optimization problem include minimizing network costs and load balancing. In (Erbas & Erbas, 2003) and (Mirrokni, Thottan, Uzunalioglu, & Paul, 2004), a multi-objective approach tackles the tradeoff between load balancing, network costs, and the number of active LSPs. Typical QoS constraints include bandwidth and endtoend delay guarantees (Beker, Puech, & Friderikos, 2004), maximum hop count, and preferred node/link list (Lee et al., 2002), or protection level (Srivastava, S.R.Thirumalasetty, & Medhi, 2005).

InterDomain MPLSTE

A key issue is the provision of the same level of QoS across domain boundaries. Some traffic engineering features, as defined in (Awduche et al., 2002), may be required to offer QoS guarantees for interdomain connections. In particular, interdomain traffic engineering should allow the optimization of interdomain link utilization, deliver strict interdomain QoS guarantees (bandwidth, delay, and jitter) and should support fast recovery following interdomain link or node failure.

A promising solution to support interdomain traffic engineering relies on deploying MPLSTE at interdomain level (Zhang & Vasseur, 2005), which enables operators to setup TE LSPs that go beyond domain boundaries. The interdomain MPLSTE approach enables interdomain constraint based routing, admission control and resource reservation. Consequently, it can be used to ensure resource optimization, strict QoS delivery and fast protection across domain boundaries.

The RSVPTE protocol is used as a signaling protocol to exchange MPLS labels and to reserve bandwidth between service domains. There are currently three interdomain TE LSP types defined for interdomain MPLSTE (Farrel, Vasseur, & Ayyangar, 2006): a contiguous LSP is a single endtoend LSP signaled from ingress LSR to egress LSR, across domain boundaries. The management of a contiguous LSP is entirely under the control of the domain containing the headend LSR. In the LSP hierarchy approach, an endtoend interdomain LSP is nested, in each domain, into an intradomain LSP. Each intradomain LSP may nest multiple interdomain LSPs and is fully managed by the domain owner. In the LSP Stitching approach, an endtoend interdomain LSP is stitched, in each domain, with an intradomain LSP, which is also known as an LSPsegment.

The key interdomain MPLSTE challenges lie in path computation. The ingress LSR can no longer perform this operation, as its topological view is limited to its domain. There are currently two interdomain path computation methods that have been defined by the IETF. We detail them in the following sections.

QoS Management with the MPLS PerDomain Model

In the MPLS perdomain path computation approach (J. Vasseur et al., 2008), the endtoend path relies on a sequence of intra-domain path computations performed during the signaling process. With this model, every intermediate domain computes a QoS path segment independently, without using any information shared by other domains. The complete QoS path is obtained by concatenating the path segments that are computed for every domain. The ingress LSR computes an intradomain path to a selected downstream border node (BN), and starts LSP signaling to this downstream node. Then, each BN along the path expands the explicit route by computing the path to a downstream BN. The downstream BN can be selected statically or dynamically, for instance with the help of a BGPbased selection procedure.

The MPLS perdomain model applies where the interdomain path cannot or is not determined at the source node. This situation is most likely to arise owing to visibility limitations. As the segments are computed without collaboration between the domains, their concatenation is not necessarily an optimal or a feasible endtoend path. Moreover, the per-domain computation model can be quite slow. For instance, in some cases, there is no route from a selected downstream BN to the destination, and another downstream BN has to be selected, which leads to signaling crankbacks.

QoS Management with the PCE-Based Model

As standardized in (Farrel, Vasseur, & Ash, 2006), the PCE is an entity responsible for computing an interdomain path upon receiving a request from a path computation client (PCC). In most cases, the source node serves as the PCC. When a new path computation request arrives, the PCC forwards this request to a selected PCE using PCCtoPCE communication (J. P. Vasseur & Le Roux, 2009). A PCE may compute the endtoend path itself, if enough topology and resource information is available to it. Furthermore, the PCE architecture provides mechanisms for the resolution of path computation requests when an individual PCE does not have sufficient visibility. For example, a PCE may cooperate with other PCEs to determine a full explicit path or intermediate loose hops: path components that rely on the routing table of an LSR or on path computation operations to determine the next-hop.

The IETF has standardized the Backward Recursive PCEbased Computation (BRPC) procedure (J. P. Vasseur et al., 2009). BRPC utilizes multiple PCEs to compute the shortest interdomain constrained path along a determined sequence of domains. Figure 5 describes its operations on a simple example. In the figure, we compute the shortest path from **s** to **t** along the domain sequence AS_1-AS_2-AS_3. Starting from the destination domain, each domain computes a shortest path tree rooted at the destination node and terminating on the entry BNs of this domain. This tree is forwarded to the previous domain, which uses it in order to compute a similar shortest path tree from its BNs towards the destination. This process is repeated until the source node is reached. This kind of PCE based interAS path computation method allows an optimal path with a single additive metric to be found, along a given ASpath, while avoiding signaling crankbacks. The case with multiple additive metrics is studied in (Bertrand et al., 2008) where an extension of the exchanged tree structure is introduced together with an algorithmic solution to the multiconstrained problem.

Figure 5. Operations of BRPC for computing a path from s to t with the minimum number of traversed links along the domain sequence AS_1-AS_2-AS_3

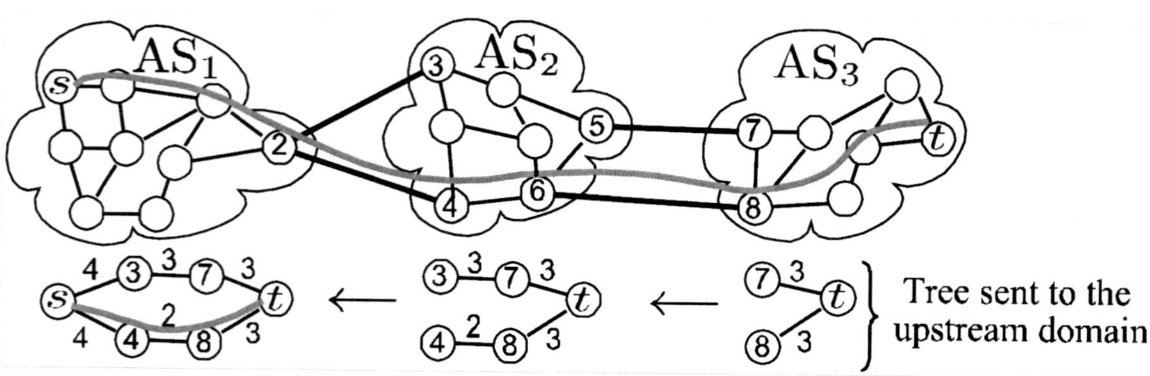

ANALYSIS

Comparison of Management Models

The present section compares the different network management models and is summarized in Table 1. We review the status of the independent network management model and highlight its limitations. Moreover, we describe how collaborative management overcomes these limitations.

In the Internet, the commonly deployed selfish routing strategy leads to limited information exchanges, and thus, is well suited for security and scalability constraints. This strategy and the corresponding independent management model guarantee a high degree of flexibility and full autonomy for the domains as a result of the limited relational constraints. However, these benefits are associated with significantly increased congestion on certain network links. Particularly, the unilateral decisions of one domain may affect the transit traffic of other domains and lead to a service degradation for all domains (Teixeira et al., 2008).

Interdomain routing in the Internet is largely based on an independent management model implemented by BGP, which necessitates a limited form of cooperation and reduced information exchange between domains. The route selected by BGP is largely influenced by local decision criteria, and thus may not always be optimal in terms of performance and reliability. Moreover, BGP does not support routing policies based on performance and load balancing criteria, therefore, complementary mechanisms are required to enforce performance guarantees. Furthermore, network management needs to guess the routing decisions of other operators in order to anticipate the consequences of changes in its policy and to protect against unpredictable traffic shifts. For this purpose, the network operators typically use a "trial and error" method, which generally results in frequent network instabilities (Mahajan et al., 2004), to manage traffic.

Alternatively, an independent management model can be implemented with MPLS technology. For example, TE tunnels can be established for the routing of interdomain traffic from endtoend through the networks of different domains. These TE tunnels are managed on a perdomain level and each domain has full control over the LSP segment that crosses its network. A perdomain computation model is particularly adapted to independent management; however it presents severe limitations and leads to sub-optimal results. Moreover, the limited information exchange in independent management induces blocking situations (Aslam, Uzmi, & Farrel, 2007): during the establishment phase, a TE tunnel may not find sufficient resources in one domain. This implies crankbacks in the signaling process and consequently higher establishment delays.

The collaborative management model is a promising alternative to the widely deployed

Table 1. Comparison of independent and collaborative management models

	Independent	Collaborative
Advantages	• Domain autonomy • Model simplicity • Security • Scalability	• Optimal performance • Simplified tasks
Drawbacks and risks	• Service degradation • Instability	• Novel model (modified relationships) • Scalability concerns • Security concerns
Compatible technologies	• IP • MPLS per-domain	• PCE

independent management approach. Collaborative management extends the traffic engineering possibilities for network operators and enables them to implement performance guarantees for inter-domain services. This management model supports collaborative path computation based for instance on PCEs. Used in conjunction with a BRPC mechanism, PCE-based computation enhances the quality of the computed routes, and thus, enforces the multi-domain QoS guarantees. Moreover, collaboration between domains relieves operators of certain time-consuming and errorprone network management tasks (Mahajan et al., 2005).

Recently, different mechanisms for the collaboration of autonomous domains have been investigated: the work in (Hu, Zou, Zhu, & Liu, 2008) presents a study of cooperation for interdomain routing. It highlights the required elements for fostering interdomain cooperation: information sharing, reputation management, and incentives. The criteria that must be satisfied so that two neighboring domains cooperate are presented in (Shrimali, Akella, & Mutapcic, 2007). These criteria include minimum information revealed, efficiency, and fairness.

A number of challenges remain before collaborative management can be implemented at a large scale. Collaborative management necessitates modifications of interprovider relationships as well as an evolution of their business models. Moreover, the increase of information exchange raises a scalability concern and security issues, which should be resolved in order to encourage the adoption of the new management paradigm.

Comparison of IP and MPLS Based Solutions

This section compares network management techniques based on IP and on MPLS, and is summarized in Table 2. We detail the scope of IP-based network management functionalities as well as their limitations. Moreover, we describe how MPLS based technologies resolve these limitations.

A first important consideration is that, in the best-effort Internet, the path used to forward data packets can vary during a session, which can introduce outoforder packet arrivals, as well as unpredictable delay variations. This property inherently limits the QoS capabilities of IPbased solutions. Connection-oriented solutions allowing route "pinning" and based, for example, on interdomain MPLS TE can solve these problems.

Typically, IPbased solutions rely on destinationbased hopbyhop forwarding, which implies that the route followed by a packet depends only on its destination. The coarse granularity of this paradigm does not permit QoS aware routing, as all packets for the same destination are forwarded along the same path without regard to their service requirements.

The most common IP-based TE methods optimize the calculation of the path for every destination. These methods, for example adjustments of IGP weights or BGP tuning, are somewhat limited and introduce instability in the network. In addition, they must take potential interactions between intra- and interdomain routing into account.

Table 2. Comparison of IP- and MPLS-based traffic management

	IP-based	**MPLS-based**
Advantages	• Well known • Scalable	• Support of advanced traffic management strategies • Extensions for inter-domain TE
Drawbacks and risks	• Unpredictable path variations • Destination based forwarding • Limited TE capabilities	• More complicated than IP

Figure 6. Synthesis of the tradeoffs between the management models and related corresponding technologies

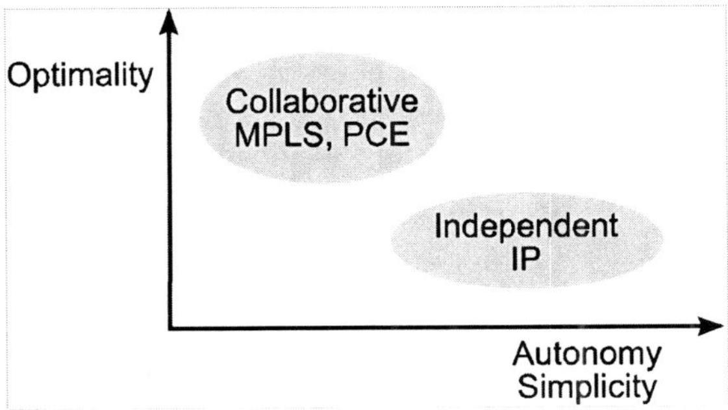

On the contrary, MPLS TE networks support explicit routing and enable network operators to classify traffic into multiple forwarding equivalence classes. The classification depends, for example, on both the destination address and the class of service of the packets, which makes it possible to forward packets belonging to certain classes along specific routes that can be different from the default IP routes. In addition, the classification can include protection and restoration considerations, so that losses on sensitive traffic can be avoided in case of failure. These mechanisms enable operators of MPLS networks to implement advanced traffic management strategies.

In IP networks, the path used for a destination is typically computed without regard to the current traffic load on the links and routers. This restriction improves the scalability of the routing protocols as less information is advertised, but complicates load balancing. On the contrary, MPLS supports both TE enabled routing protocols that can advertise information related to the bandwidth usage on the links in the network, and the required functionalities for balancing the traffic load on the links of a network.

To conclude this comparison, Figure 6 summarizes the advantages of the studied management models and of the related networking technologies. The principle advantage of IPbased techniques rests in their relative simplicity. In particular, IP networks rely on a well-known business model requiring only limited cooperation from competitive entities, which keep their autonomy and take independent decisions. Despite this simplicity, sophisticated policies can be used in IP networks to select the route for a particular destination, which allows operators to classify paths according to their own objectives. Nevertheless, MPLS networks provide superior QoS routing and TE capabilities due to explicit routing, route pinning, and collaborative path computation mechanisms. These abilities provide network operators with a high level of flexibility in their management strategies and allow them to select optimal paths with respect to their network management objectives. In addition, these functionalities play an increasingly important role in providing QoS guarantees in multiservice networks that carry both data traffic and congestion sensitive traffic, such as telephony. In addition, they permit the development of new types of commercial relationships between domains, ranging from simple interconnection agreements to collaborative TE and automated provisioning.

APPLICATION AND PERSPECTIVES

Various collaborative management models are emerging and the required technologies to support them are being standardized. This section presents the relevant applications and perspectives of the previously described network management techniques, addressing the problem of collaborative and endtoend QoS provisioning.

Today, the Internet is recognized as the unifying architecture for multiservice networks transporting telephony as well as data traffic; however, it is paradoxically confronted with new unresolved challenges. The Internet architecture was initially conceived to provide best-effort connectivity; however, the need for end-to-end QoS becomes more acute as service requirements become more stringent. In particular, the deployment of

IP television creates large flows with strict QoS requirements. In addition, some limitations of the current organizational model of the Internet have become apparent: the large autonomy of the domains and their unilateral routing and traffic management choices limit the scope of the QoS guarantees that can be provided. In particular, this organization complicates the provision of end-toend QoS guarantees for flows crossing several domains in the current Internet.

Consequently, a first important application of the techniques described in the present chapter is to extend the scope of the QoS guarantees that can be provided for the flows and ultimately to provide endtoend QoS guarantees. For example, interdomain MPLS mechanisms permit resource reservations for interdomain flows in a set of cooperative operators. This feature enables operators to route premium traffic on MPLS tunnels with guaranteed performance and to use default IP routing based on BGP for best-effort traffic. The traffic management techniques described in the present chapter can also be used to extend some of the QoS management functions defined in novel network architectures, such as the Resource and Admission Control Subsystem (RACS) defined for next generation networks (TISPAN, 2008), for interdomain resource management.

A second important application of the new methods for interdomain traffic management is to automate route optimization tasks. For example, Quoitin et al. (2003) report that traffic engineering with BGP is often done in a trialanderror fashion. In fact, the lack of information about the configuration of the neighboring domains prevents an operator from predicting the exact impact of BGP configuration changes on the routing. However, more cooperation among the domains would enable the automation of this process. In addition, researchers are investigating innovative solutions for the automation of network provisioning tasks based on novel overlay architectures and enhanced interprovider interactions (Douville et al., 2008).

It is too early to evaluate the impact of the nascent paradigms described in the present chapter on network operator's policies. Nevertheless, we expect that interdomain TE will be based on explicit coordination mechanisms between network operators, to manage the interdomain traffic in a stable, efficient, and predictable manner, as argued by Shrimali et al. (2007). New protocols and mechanisms will be required for negotiating the interdomain routes and the level of QoS for interdomain flows (Mahajan et al., 2005), and for resolving policy conflicts (Fu, Wang, Zhou, & Song, 2006). Network operators will need to adapt their business models to consider the current evolutions of the Internet toward more cooperation among competitors. In particular, network operators will probably be bound by more complex interdomain SLAs. These agreements will involve two or potentially more collaborating operators to enable the provision of performance guarantees for traffic flows, not only in their own network, but also in the networks of collaborating domains. However, Mahajan et al. (2004) note that most network operators appear reluctant to provide endtoend guarantees for traffic transiting through domains belonging to other network operators. The partnership strategies of the network operators will involve even more important stakes than today, notably if the level of QoS that network operators are able to provide to their clients becomes a key market differentiator. In particular, network operators will eventually collaborate in one or more types of alliance, as proposed in (Fonte, Monteiro, Yannuzzi, MasipBruin, & DomingoPascual, 2005; Kumar & Saraph, 2006; Hu, Li, Mao, Steenkiste, & Wang, 2004).

CONCLUSION

This chapter has described novel network management techniques in backbone networks, based on optimized routing and traffic engineering, for providing a higher level of endtoend QoS. These techniques provide key elements for future multiservice networks that will carry realtime multimedia services with stringent QoS requirements.

We first classified network management models depending on the level of cooperation between the domains and their impact on the policies of network operators. Two main types of management models exist: the legacy independent management model, which gives a large autonomy to the domains, and the emerging collaborative management models, in which domains have more complex interactions. Network operators derive their network management objectives from these models and adapt the routing of the traffic in their network to implement these objectives. In particular, they use the features of IP routing or the more extended traffic-control functionalities of the MPLS architecture.

We have underlined the limitations of IPbased technologies for multidomain QoS and presented recent advances of MPLS technologies that open interesting perspectives for interdomain traffic management. The chapter has analyzed the strengths and weaknesses of the presented management models, as well as of the technologies used to implement these models. The main conclusions that can be drawn from this study are the following. Firstly, that collaborative management models seem extremely promising, although they introduce some modifications in the network operator's business models. Secondly, that recent extensions of MPLS based techniques have created interesting possibilities for providing guaranteed QoS levels for interdomain flows and engineering interdomain traffic more efficiently.

The techniques described in the present chapter may have a large impact on operator's policies. For instance, we expect that the interconnection agreements between network operators will evolve toward new management models and that some forms of network operator alliance will appear. These evolutions will enable network operators to guarantee a higher level of endtoend QoS for sensitive flows, as well as to manage their network more efficiently.

REFERENCES

Andersson, L., Minei, I. & Thomas, B. (2007, October). *LDP Specification.* RFC 5036. IETF.

Apostolopoulos, G., Kama, S., Williams, D., Guerin, R., Orda, A. & Przygienda, T. (1999, August). *QoS Routing Mechanisms and OSPF Extensions.* RFC 2676. IETF.

Aslam, F., Uzmi, Z. A., & Farrel, A. (2007). Interdomain Path Computation: Challenges and Solutions for Label Switched Networks. *IEEE Communications Magazine*, *45*(10), 94–101. doi:10.1109/MCOM.2007.4342830

Avallone, S., Kuipers, F., Ventre, G., & Mieghem, P. V. (2006). Dynamic Routing in QoSaware Traffic Engineered Networks. In *EUNICE 2005: Networks and applications towards a ubiquitously connected world* (pp. 45–58). Boston: Springer. doi:10.1007/0-387-31170-X_4

Awduche, D., Berger, L., Gan, D., Li, T., Srinivasan, V. & Swallow, G. (2001, December). *RSVP-TE: Extensions to RSVP for LSP Tunnels.* RFC 3209. IETF.

Awduche, D., Chiu, A., Elwalid, A., Widjaja, I. & Xiao, X. (2002, May). *Overview and Principles of Internet traffic Engineering.* RFC 3272. IETF.

Awduche, D., Malcolm, J., Agogbua, J., O'Dell, M. & McManus, J. (1999, September). *Requirements for traffic Engineering Over MPLS.* RFC 2702. IETF.

Beker, S., Puech, N., & Friderikos, V. (2004). A Tabu Search Heuristic for the Offline MPLS Reduced Complexity Layout Design Problem. In *Networking* (p. 514525). Berlin, Germany: Springer.

Benmohamed, L., Liang, C., Naber, E. & Terzis, A. (2006). *QoS Enhancements to BGP in Support of Multiple Classes of Service.* draftliangbgpqos00. txt, work in progress, IETF.

Bertrand, G., Lahoud, S., Molnár, M., & Texier, G. (2008). *InterDomain Path Computation with Multiple Constraints* (Tech. Rep. No. 1902). IRISA Campus de Beaulieu 35042 Rennes Cedex: IRISA. Retrieved from http://hal.inria.fr

Bertrand, G., Lahoud, S., Texier, G., & Molnár, M. (2009). Computation of Multi-Constrained Paths in Multi-Domain MPLS-TE Networks. In *NGI 2009: Fifth EuroNGI Conference on Next Generation Internet Networks* (to appear). Piscataway, NJ: IEEE Computer Society.

Blake, S., Black, D., Carlson, M., Davies, E., Wang, Z. & Weiss, W. (1998, December). *An Architecture for Differentiated Service.* RFC 2475. IETF.

Boucadair, M. (2005). *QoSEnhanced Border Gateway Protocol.* draftboucadairqosbgpspec01, work in progress, IETF.

Boutaba, R., & Xiao, J. (2002). Network management: state of the art. In Communication systems: The state of the art IFIP world computer congress (pp. 127-146). Deventer, Netherlands: Kluwer, B.V.

Braden, R., Clark, D. & Shenker, S. (1994, June). *Integrated Services in the Internet architecture: an Overview.* RFC 1633. IETF.

Capone, A., Fratta, L., & Martignon, F. (2003). Virtual Flow Deviation: Dynamic Routing of Bandwidth Guaranteed Connections. In *QoSIP 2003: Proceedings of the second international workshop on quality of service in multiservice IP networks* (pp. 592-605). London: SpringerVerlag.

Cisco. (1997). *Configuring OSPF.* Documentation at http://www.cisco.com/en/US/docs/ios/ 12_0/np1/configuration/guide/1cospf.pdf

Douville, R., Le Roux, J. L., Rougier, J. L., & Secci, S. (2008, June). A Service Plane over the PCE Architecture for Automatic Multidomain ConnectionOriented Services. *IEEE Communications Magazine, 46*(6), 94–101. doi:10.1109/MCOM.2008.4539472

Erbas, S. C., & Erbas, C. (2003, Aug.Sep.). A Multiobjective Offline Routing Model for MPLS Networks. In J. Charzinski, R. Lehnert, & P. TranGia (Eds.), Providing quality of service in heterogeneous environments, 5, proceedings of the 18th international teletraffic congress. Amsterdam, Netherlands: Elsevier B.V.

Farrel, A., Vasseur, J.P. & Ash, J. (2006, August). *A Path Computation Element (PCE)Based Architecture.* RFC 4655. IETF.

Farrel, A., Vasseur, J.P. & Ayyangar, A. (2006, November). *A Framework for InterDomain Multiprotocol Label Switching traffic Engineering.* RFC 4726. IETF.

Flegkas, P., Trimintzios, P., Pavlou, G., Andrikopoulos, I., & Cavalcanti, C. F. (2001). On Policy Based Extensible Hierarchical Network Management in QoSEnabled IP Networks. In *Policy '01: Proceedings of the international workshop on policies for distributed systems and networks* (pp. 230-246). London: SpringerVerlag.

Fonte, A., Curado, M., & Monteiro, E. (2008, December). Interdomai quality of service routing: setting the grounds for the way ahead. *Annales des Télécommunications, 63*(1), 683–695. doi:10.1007/s12243-008-0065-y

Fonte, A., Monteiro, E., & Yannuzzi, M. Masip-Bruin, X. & DomingoPascual, J. (2005). A Framework for Cooperative InterDomain QoS Routing. In EUNICE (pp. 91104). Secaucus, NJ: SpringerVerlag, Inc.

Fortz, B., & Thorup, M. (2004). Increasing Internet Capacity Using Local Search. *Computational Optimization and Applications*, *29*(1), 13–48. doi:10.1023/B:COAP.0000039487.35027.02

Fu, X., Wang, J., Zhou, W., & Song, J. (2006, Nov.). EndtoEnd QoS Architecture and Interdomain QoS Model across Multiple Domains. In *International Conference on Communication Technology. (ICCT)* (p. 14). New York: IEEE Communications Society.

Gavalas, D., Greenwood, D., Ghanbari, M., & O'Mahony, M. (2002). Hierarchical network management: a scalable and dynamic mobile agentbased approach. *Computer Networks*, *38*(6), 693–711. doi:10.1016/S1389-1286(01)00277-8

Griffin, D., Spencer, J., Griem, J., Boucadair, M., Morand, P., & Howarth, M. (2007, Feb.). Interdomain routing through QoSclass planes [QualityofServiceBased Routing Algorithms for Heterogeneous Networks]. *IEEE Communications Magazine*, *45*(2), 8895.

Guerin, R. A., Orda, A., & Williams, D. (1997, November). QoS routing mechanisms and OSPF extensions. In *IEEE Global Telecommunications Conference (GLOBECOM)* (Vol. 3, pp. 1903-1908). Piscataway, NJ: IEEE Computer Society.

Hu, N., Li, L. E., Mao, Z. M., Steenkiste, P., & Wang, J. (2004). Locating internet bottlenecks: algorithms, measurements, and implications. *SIGCOMM Computer Communication Review*, *34*(4), 41–54. doi:10.1145/1030194.1015474

Hu, N., Zou, P., Zhu, P., & Liu, X. (2008). Cooperative Management Framework for interdomain Routing System. In *ATC '08: Proceedings of the 5th international conference on autonomic and trusted computing* (pp. 567-576). Berlin: SpringerVerlag.

Katz, D., Kompella, K., & Yeung, D. (2003, September). *Traffic Engineering (TE) Extensions to OSPF Version 2*. RFC 3630. IETF.

Knoll, T. (2009). *BGP Extended Community Attribute for QoS Marking*. draftknollidrqos-attribute02, work in progress, IETF.

Kodialam, M., & Lakshman, T. V. (2000). Minimum interference routing with applications to MPLS traffic engineering. In *IEEE INFOCOM* (*Vol. 2*, pp. 884–893). Piscataway, NJ: IEEE Computer Society.

Kuipers, F., Van Mieghem, P., Korkmaz, T., & Krunz, M. (2002). An overview of constraint-based path selection algorithms for QoS routing. *IEEE Communications Magazine*, *40*(12), 50–55. doi:10.1109/MCOM.2002.1106159

Kumar, N., & Saraph, G. (2006). EndtoEnd QoS in Interdomain Routing. In *ICNS '06: Proceedings of the international conference on networking and services* (pp. 82). Washington, DC: IEEE Computer Society.

Lee, Y., et al. (2002, April). A Constrained Multipath traffic Engineering Scheme for MPLS Networks. In International conference on communications (ICC). New York: IEEE Communications Society.

Leinwand, A., & Fang, K. (1993). *Network management: a practical perspective*. Boston: AddisonWesley Longman Publishing Co., Inc.

Li, T. & Smit, H. (2008, October). *ISIS Extensions for traffic Engineering*. RFC 5305. IETF.

Ma, Q., & Steenkiste, P. (1997). On path selection for traffic with bandwidth guarantees. In *Proceedings of IEEE International Conference on Network Protocols* (pp. 191-202). Washington, DC: IEEE Computer Society.

Mahajan, R., Wetherall, D., & Anderson, T. (2004). Towards coordinated interdomain traffic engineering. In SIGCOMM workshop on hot topics in networking (HotNets). New York: ACM.

Mahajan, R., Wetherall, D., & Anderson, T. (2005). Negotiationbased routing between neighboring ISPs. In *NSDI'05: Proceedings of the 2nd conference on symposium on networked systems design & implementation,* (pp. 29-42). Berkeley, CA: USENIX Association.

McPherson, D. & Gill, V. (2006, March). *BGP MULTI_EXIT_DISC (MED) Considerations.* RFC 4451. IETF.

Mirrokni, V. S., Thottan, M., Uzunalioglu, H., & Paul, S. (2004, March). A Simple Polynomial Time Framework For ReducedPath Decomposition in MultiPath Routing. In *IEEE INFOCOM* (*Vol. 1*, p. 739749). Washington, DC: IEEE Computer Society.

Mitra, D., & Ramakrishnan, K. (1999). A case study of multiservice, multipriority traffic engineering design for data networks. *IEEE Global Telecommunications Conference, 1999. GLOBECOM '99*, 1B, 10771083.

Quoitin, B., Pelsser, C., Bonaventure, O., & Uhlig, S. (2005). A performance evaluation of BGP based traffic engineering. *International Journal of Network Management, 15*, 177–191. doi:10.1002/nem.559

Quoitin, B., Pelsser, C., Swinnen, L., Bonaventure, O., & Uhlig, S. (2003, May). Interdomain traffic engineering with BGP. *IEEE Communications Magazine*, *41*(5), 122–128. doi:10.1109/MCOM.2003.1200112

Raz, D., & Shavitt, Y. (1999). An Active Network Approach to Efficient Network Management. In *IWAN'99: Proceedings of the first international working conference on active networks* (pp. 220-231). London: SpringerVerlag.

Rekhter, Y., Li, T. & Hares, S. (2006, January). *A Border Gateway Protocol 4 (BGP4).* RFC 4271. IETF.

Rosen, E., Viswanathan, A. & Callon, R. (2001, January). *Multiprotocol Label Switching Architecture.* RFC 3031. IETF.

Shrimali, G., Akella, A., & Mutapcic, A. (2007, May). Cooperative InterDomain traffic Engineering Using Nash Bargaining and Decomposition. In *IEEE INFOCOM* (p. 330338). Piscataway, NJ: IEEE Computer Society.

Soldatos, J., Vayias, E., & Kormentzas, G. (2005). First Quarter). On the building blocks of quality of service in heterogeneous IP networks. *IEEE Communications Surveys and Tutorials*, *7*(1), 69–88. doi:10.1109/COMST.2005.1423335

Srivastava, S., Thirumalasetty, S. R., & Medhi, D. (2005). Network traffic Engineering with varied levels of Protection in Next Generation Internet. In A. Girard, B. Sanso, & F. VazquezAbad (Eds.), Performance evaluations and planning methods for the next generation internet (pp. 99-124). New York: Springer US.

Strassner, J. C. (2003). *Policybased network management.* San Francisco, CA: Morgan Kaufmann Publisher.

Suri, S., Waldvogel, M., & Warkhede, P. R. (2001, September). ProfileBased Routing: A New Framework for MPLS traffic Engineering. In F. Boavida (Ed.), Quality of future internet services (Vol. 2156, pp. 138–157). Berlin: Springer Verlag.

Teixeira, R., Shaikh, A., Griffin, T. G., & Rexford, J. (2008, Dec.). Impact of HotPotato Routing Changes in IP Networks. *IEEE/ACM Transactions on Networking, 16*(6), 12951307.

TISPAN. (2008, May). *Resource and Admission Control SubSystem (RACS): Functional Architecture.* ETSI ES 282 003 v2.0.0.

Torab, P., Jabbari, B., Xu, Q., Gong, S., Yang, X., Lehman, T., et al. (2006). On Cooperative InterDomain Path Computation. In *ISCC '06: Proceedings of the 11th IEEE symposium on computers and communications* (pp. 511-518). Washington, DC: IEEE Computer Society.

Vasseur, J., Ayyangar, A., & Zhang, R. (2008, February). *A PerDomain Path Computation Method for Establishing InterDomain traffic Engineering (TE) Label Switched Paths (LSPs)*. RFC 5152. IETF.

Vasseur, J. P. & Le Roux, J. L. (2009, March). *Path Computation Element (PCE) Communication Protocol (PCEP)*. RFC 5440, IETF.

Vasseur, J. P., Zhang, R., Bitar, N., & Le Roux, J. L. (2009, April). *A Backward Recursive PCE-based Computation (BRPC) Procedure to Compute Shortest Constrained Interdomain traffic Engineering Label Switched Paths*. RFC 5441, IETF.

Vázquez, E., Álvarez-Campana, M., & García, A. B. (2004). Network Convergence over MPLS. In *High Speed Networks and Multimedia Communications* (*Vol. 3079*, pp. 290–300). Berlin: Springer Verlag.

Wang, N., Ho, K., Pavlou, G., & Howarth, M. (2008). First Quarter). An overview of routing optimization for Internet traffic engineering. *IEEE Communications Surveys and Tutorials, 10*(1), 3656. doi:10.1109/COMST.2008.4483669

Yang, X., Clark, D. & Berger, A. W. (2007). NIRA: a new interdomain routing architecture. *IEEE/ACM Transactions on Networking, 15*(4), 775-788.

Younis, O., & Fahmy, S. (2003). Constraint-Based Routing in the Internet: Basic Principles and Recent Research. *IEEE Communications Surveys and Tutorials, 5*, 2–13. doi:10.1109/COMST.2003.5342226

Zhang, R. & Vasseur, J.P. (2005, November). *MPLS InterAutonomous System (AS) traffic Engineering (TE) Requirements.* RFC 4216. IETF.

Chapter 9
Providing Quality of Service to Computer Networks through Traffic Modeling:
Improving the Estimation of Bandwidth and Data Loss Probability

Flávio Henrique Teles Vieira
Federal University of Goiás (UFG), Brazil

George E. Bozinis
Federal University of Goiás (UFG), Brazil

ABSTRACT

In this chapter, the authors examine two important network traffic issues: estimation of effective bandwidth and data loss probability in communication networks. They focus on estimation approaches based on network traffic modeling. Initially, they review some concepts related to network traffic modeling such as monofractal and multifractal properties. Further, they address the issue of estimating the effective bandwidth for network traffic flows. Besides effective bandwidth, the knowledge of the loss probability explicitly allows us to guarantee some QoS parameters required by the traffic flows, for example, by discarding flows with intolerable byte loss rate. In this sense, the authors present an overview of loss probability estimation methods including an approach that considers multifractal characteristics of network traffic. That is, given the model parameters, the data loss probability for network traffic can be directly computed. They conclude that both the multifractal based effective bandwidth and loss probability estimation methods can be powerful tools for really providing QoS to network flows.

INTRODUCTION

The seminal paper published by Leland et al. triggered a new direction on traffic modeling research, by unveiling the fractal nature of network traffic processes (Leland, Taqqu, Willinger, Wilson, & Bellcore, 1994). These authors experimentally demonstrated that the LAN Ethernet traffic collected in Bellcore Morristown Research and Engineering Center exhibits self-similar properties and burstiness in a wide range of time scales.

DOI: 10.4018/978-1-61520-791-6.ch009

After that, many research papers have shown that such self-similar behavior, unable to be faithfully represented through most classic Markovian stochastic models, is not restricted solely to the Ethernet LAN environment (Willinger, Taqqu, & Erramilli, 1996), and in fact, strongly impacts on the network performance (Park & Willinger, 2000). Among many different fractal modeling approaches, the fractional Brownian motion (fBm) or its incremental process, called fractional Gaussian noise (fGn), has become popular for modern traffic modeling because of its simplicity. However, such a self-similar traffic model is capable of capturing the traffic correlation property only over large time scales.

A more sophisticated description of network traffic behavior based on multifractal analysis was introduced by Lévy Véhel et al. (J. Lévy Véhel & R. H. Riedi, 1997), and latter by Feldmann et al. (Feldmann, Gilbert, Willinger, & Kurtz, 1998). The multifractal analysis generalizes the self-similar behavior observed in the network traffic in a natural way.

Self-similar processes, or more generically speaking, monofractal processes are characterized by a single time-invariant parameter, the Hurst parameter (Garrett & Willinger, 1994). Contrary to monofractal processes, multifractal processes allow such characteristics to vary in time, therefore, increasing the flexibility in describing irregular phenomena that arise in real signals.

Statistical models derived from multifractal processes are capable of representing the actual network traffic behavior in a more complete and accurate manner. Although the research carried out on multifractals is not quite recent, few multifractal models in fact have been developed up to now. Among them, we cite the following: the Multifractal Wavelet Model (MWM) proposed by Riedi et al (Riedi, Crouse, Ribeiro, & Baraniuk, 1999), the Variable Variance Gaussian Multiplier Model (VVGMM) proposed by Krishna et al (Krishna P, Gadre, & Desai, 2003), and the multifractional Brownian model (mBm) in (Peltier & Lévy Véhel, 1995). The definition of the mBm process generalizes the fractional Brownian motion, a monofractal process with a constant exponent H (global scaling parameter) to the case where H is no longer a constant, but a time-varying function (Peltier & Lévy Véhel, 1995).

The explanations for the origins of monofractal and multifractal characteristics of network traffic processes have physical interpretations. The self-similarity observed in Web traffic can be related to the underlying heavy tailed distribution of file sizes (Crovella & Bestavros, 1997). Some researches about the probability distributions of ON and OFF times lead to the conclusion that ON times are heavier tailed than OFF times and are hence more significant in determining Web traffic self-similarity. The flow of packets over fine time scales is shaped mainly by protocols and end-to-end congestion control schemes (e.g., TCP/IP) that regulate the complex interactions between different flows on a network. This small-scale behavior of traffic can be modeled by a multiplicative cascade that is a multifractal model. According to this theory, the effects of some network mechanisms and protocols at different time scales causes this multiplicative behavior (Feldmann, Gilbert, & Willinger, 1998).

In this chapter, we discuss about estimation of effective bandwidth and data loss probability considering different network traffic modeling approaches. We focus on works involving self-similar and multifractal concepts, presenting some recent developments on these issues. We also briefly point out the importance and influence of such traffic modeling concepts to algorithms and tools developed to provide QoS guarantees to network traffic flows. Furthermore, we present results of traffic modeling, effective bandwidth and loss probability estimation considering real Ethernet and Internet traffic traces. Concerning the underlying network, we assume a simplified model. That is, we consider a single server queue model for the verification of the proposed effective bandwidth and loss probability estimation approaches. However, the equations and algorithms presented in this chapter can be applied in various QoS-network architecture types such as ATM, Intserv, Difserv networks, etc.

NETWORK TRAFFIC MODELING: MULTIFRACTAL PROCESSES

Analysis of measured traffic streams taken from a wide range of sources has indicated that many traffic sources present correlation structure that decays much more slowly than exponentially. These slowly decaying correlation structures have been shown in VBR video (Fitzek & Reisslein, 2001), Ethernet LAN traffic (Leland, et al., 1994), MAN traffic (Addie, Zukerman, & Neame, 1995) and general Internet WAN traffic (Paxson & Floyd, 1995). Such a slow decay property in autocorrelation has been related to the concept of self-similarity and long-range dependence (LRD).

While the short-range dependent (SRD) traffic models are significant for their tractability, they cannot capture the long-range dependencies present in real packet data traffic. Many studies have revealed high variability of today's Internet traffic, i.e., traffic is bursty over a wide range of time scales in contrast to the assumption that traffic burstiness exists only at short time scales while traffic is smooth at large time scales (Leland, et al., 1994; Paxson & Floyd, 1995). This multiscale burstiness has been shown to make a significant impact on network performance (Erramilli, Narayan, & Willinger, 1996; Leland, et al., 1994; Paxson & Floyd, 1995).

Most LRD traffic models are based on self-similar processes. Precisely, asymptotically second order self-similarity implies LRD and vice versa. In traffic modeling, the term self-similarity is usually used to refer to the asymptotically second order self-similar or monofractal processes (Park & Willinger, 2000). The Hurst parameter H is used to measure the degree of 'self-similarity'. For random processes suitable for network traffic modeling, the Hurst parameter is basically a measure of the tail decaying rate of the autocorrelation function. However, it is known that distinct long-range dependent processes with the same measured Hurst parameter value can produce vastly different queueing behavior (Grossglauser & Bolot, 1999). In addition, as argued in (Erramilli, et al., 1996), the queueing performance mostly depends on the traffic's variability over certain time scales rather than on the value of H.

For many real network traffic processes, the variance-time plots usually do not tend to straight lines. Instead, these processes have piecewise fractal behavior with varying Hurst parameter over some small ranges of time scales (Li & Mills, 1999). Processes with such fractal behavior are usually referred to as multifractal processes. It has been observed that queueing performance greatly depends on the degree of traffic irregularities at small time scales which are believed to be due to the complex dynamics of data networks (Grossglauser & Bolot, 1999). Feldmann, et al. claimed that this combination of scaling behaviors is best represented via a multifractal process (Feldmann, Gilbert, & Willinger, 1998). In (Erramilli, Narayan, Neidhardt, Saniee, & Qnetworx, 2000), Erramilli et al. confirmed this finding of multifractal behavior on fine time scales, and indicated that this behavior can have a significant impact on queueing performance when utilizations are low. In (J. Lévy Véhel & R. Riedi, 1997), Lévy Véhel and Riedi showed that a multifractal version of fractional Brownian motion (fBm) may better reflect the properties of measured network traffic than the fBm itself.

In (Riedi, et al., 1999), the authors presented a multifractal wavelet model (MWM) and argued that this model better predicted the behavior of both a TCP trace (Paxson & Floyd, 1995) and an Ethernet trace (Leland, et al., 1994) when compared to the fractional Brownian motion. The MWM can closely match the properties of the original traffic stream in both marginal distribution and correlation structure. In (Gao

& Rubin, 1999), Gao and Rubin showed that both packet inter-arrival times and packet length sequences could be modeled by multifractal processes. In (Krishna P, Gadre, & Desai, 2001), for packet inter-arrival time modeling, Krishna et al. proposed a multiplicative cascade with the multiplier distribution being assumed Gaussian (VVGM- Variable Variance Gaussian Model). The VVGM model assumes that the multiplier distribution has a constant mean value in every stage of the cascade.

In order to mathematically represent the self-similarity detected in the network traffic, a variety of stochastic models were proposed (Leland, et al., 1994; Norros, 1994). Particularly, the fractional Brownian motion is pointed as possibly the simplest mathematical model capable of taking account of the monofractal characteristics observed in traffic data. However, investigations into WAN TCP/IP traffic traces (Feldmann, Gilbert, Willinger, et al., 1998; J. Lévy Véhel & R. H. Riedi, 1997) concluded that there are properties observed in short time scales that are better described through multifractal analysis. Such multifractal traffic properties are consequences of the action of some network layer protocols that impose certain end-to-end traffic control mechanisms in order to control the information flow behavior between different layers in, for example, the TCP/IP protocol stack (Feldmann, Gilbert, & Willinger, 1998).

We can define multifractals through the scaling properties of process moments over different time increments.

Definition 1: A stochastic process *Z(t)* is called multifractal if it satisfies the following condition:

$$E(|Z(t)|^q) = c(q)t^{\tau(q)+1}, \forall t \in T, q \in Q \qquad (1)$$

where *T* and *Q* are intervals on the real line, and τ(q) and c(q) are functions with domain *Q*. The function τ(q) is called the scaling function of multifractal processes or the partition function (B B Mandelbrot & Van Ness, 1968; B B Mandelbrot & Wallis, 1969).

The multifractal analysis is regarded as a generalization of the monofractal analysis, allowing different traffic behavior to be observed in various time scales, and therefore, providing a better description of irregularities (or singularities) for the traffic process.

In the following subsections, we describe some multifractal models and other advances on network traffic modeling.

DETERMINISTIC MULTIPLICATIVE CASCADE AND BINOMIAL MEASURE

The simplest multifractal is the binomial measure defined on the compact interval *[0,1]*, built from an iterative procedure called "Multiplicative Cascade" that iteratively divide a interval into two equal length subintervals, however, the left one receiving the *r* fraction of the original interval while right one *(1-r)* fraction mesure. Let $m_0 = r$ and $m_1 = 1-r$. At stage $k=0$ of the cascade, the unit uniform measure is defined on the interval *[0,1]*. At stage $k=1$, by division, two equal length subintervals, $\left[0,\frac{1}{2}\right]$ and $\left[\frac{1}{2},1\right]$ are generated, with the mass m_0 and m_1 uniformly distributed, respectively. That is, we have measure $\mu_1\left[0,\frac{1}{2}\right] = m_0$ and $\mu_1\left[\frac{1}{2},1\right] = m_1$. At stage k=2, further divisions will result in 4 subintervals with the following measures: $\mu_1\left[0,\frac{1}{4}\right] = m_0 m_1$, $\mu_1\left[\frac{1}{4},\frac{1}{2}\right] = m_1 m_0$, $\mu_1\left[\frac{1}{2},\frac{3}{4}\right] = m_0 m_0$ and $\mu_1\left[\frac{3}{4},1\right] = m_1 m_1$.

This process is iterated for k levels, and at each stage it can be seen that the total measure is preserved. Consider the *kth* stage of the cascade and a dyadic interval $[t,t+2^{-k}]$ where $t = \sum_{i=1}^{k} \eta_i 2^{-i}$ (or in its binomial format $t=0.\eta_1 ...\eta_k$). Let φ_0 and φ_1 be the relative frequencies of 's and 's in the binary development of t. The measure on the dyadic interval $[t,t+2^{-k}]$ is equal to:

$$\mu\lfloor t, t + 2^{-k} \rfloor = m_0^{\ k\varphi_0} m_1^{\ k\varphi_1}. \tag{2}$$

Since the cascade preserves at each stage the mass of the split dyadic intervals, so the process is said to be conservative or microcanonical. If, at each stage of the cascade, each interval is split up $t\ b>2$ subintervals of equal size, this defines a class of multinomial measures. For $b=2$ and a fixed m_0, we have a binomial multiplicative cascade (Benoit B. Mandelbrot, Fisher, & Calvet, 1997). Such a deterministic cascade process has its scaling function $\tau(q) = -log(m_0 + m_1^{\ q}) + 1$.

STOCHASTIC MULTIPLICATIVE CASCADES

Allowing the multipliers of a cascade to be random variables, we get a stochastic multiplicative cascade. For a binomial multiplicative cascade, the multiplier r is a sample of random variable R defined on $[0,1]$ with a probability distribution function $f_R(r)$. The measure of the dyadic interval $[t,t+2^{-k}]$ with $t = \sum_{i=1}^{k} \eta_i 2^{-i}$ is given by:

$$\mu(\Delta t) = R(\eta_1).R(\eta_1.\eta_2).....R(\eta_1....\eta_k) \tag{3}$$

where $R(\eta_1 ... \eta i)$ is a multiplier at stage i. Since the multipliers at distinct stages are i.i.d., it can be shown that the measure μ in (3) satisfies the following scaling relationship (Molnár, Dang, & Maricza, 2002):

$$E\left(\mu(\Delta t)^q\right) = \left(E(R)^q\right)^k = \Delta\tau_k^{\ -log_2 E(R^Q)} \tag{4}$$

which defines a multifractal process with scaling function $\tau(q) = \ -log_2 E(R^q)$.

MULTIFRACTAL WAVELET MODEL

R. Riedi et al. proposed an important multifractal model, namely the Multifractal Wavelet Model (MWM). The MWM is based on the Haar wavelet to characterize network traffic (Riedi, et al., 1999). This model can be viewed as a multiplicative cascade in the Haar wavelet domain that aims to capture the decay of wavelet energy on scale (Chui, 1992).

Discrete wavelet transforms can be used for multi-scale representation of a process X(t) through the wavelet $\psi(t)$ and scaling $\phi(t)$ functions as the following (Chui, 1992):

$$X(t) = \sum_k U_{J_{0.k}} \phi_{J_{0.k}}(t) + \sum_{j=J_0}^{n} \sum_k W_{j.k} \phi_{j.k}(t) \tag{5}$$

Where $W_{j.k}$ and $U_{j.k}$ are respectively the wavelet and the scaling coefficients at scale index j and translation index k, given by:

$$W_{j.k} = \int X(t) \varphi_{j.k}(t)\,dt \tag{6}$$

And

$$U_{j.k} = \int X(t) \phi_{j.k}(t)\,dt \tag{7}$$

Multiplicative cascades in the wavelet domain can be used to characterize network traffic by computing the corresponding wavelet coefficients as (Riedi, et al., 1999):

$$W_{j.k} = U_{j.k} A_{j.k} \tag{8}$$

where $A_{j.k}$ is a random variable in the range[-1,1]. Further, some additional conditions are frequently assumed: the multipliers $A_{j.k}$ are statistically independent and identically distributed (i.i.d) within each scale, independent of $U_{j.k}$ and symmetric at the origin. A traffic model can capture multifractal characteristics by choosing the multipliers $A_{j.k}$ in order to control the wavelet coefficient energy $E\left(W^2{}_{j.k}\right)$ (Ribeiro, Riedi, Crouse, & Baraniuk, 2000).

In the MWM synthesis process, one needs to apply the Haar DWT (Discrete Wavelet Transform) to network traffic, to calculate the second order moments of the wavelet coefficients at each scale, and to estimate the mean and the variance of the scaling coefficient at the coarsest scale (Riedi, et al., 1999). The MWM model efficiently approximates the network traffic properties in terms of marginal distribution (it produces approximately lognormal distribution) and correlation structure (Ribeiro, et al., 2000). However, the MWM requires the determination of a large number of model parameters. Such a drawback of the MWM, make it unsuitable for on-line traffic characterization since it requires the knowledge of all traffic process samples. Next, we present a multifractal network traffic model suitable for on-line traffic modeling.

ADAPTIVE WAVELET BASED MULTIFRACTAL MODEL

In this section, we introduce a traffic model based on some properties of the Haar wavelet and multiplicative cascades. This multifractal model, namely Adaptive Wavelet based Model (AWMM), has some advantages over some existing models in terms of few input parameters and on-line updating capability.

Our proposal consists of estimating the second order moment of the Haar wavelet coefficient of the pairwise product of a cascade and i.i.d. samples of a positive random variable and then generating the model multipliers $A_{j.k}$ in order to capture the wavelet coefficient energy decay. That is, we introduce a model with a novel characteristic; the model is able to simultaneously capture the functions τ(q) and c(q) of multifractal processes and also the wavelet coefficient energy decay. To this end, we derived explicit equations that allow direct computation of the variance of the aggregated process and the second moment of the wavelet coefficients at any time instance.

Let *X(k)* be a discrete time process corresponding to the network traffic volume per unit time interval. When the representation of a process is done in the Haar wavelet domain, the scaling coefficient $U_{j.k}$ can be recursively computed as (Riedi, et al., 1999; Vieira & Ling, 2009):

$$U_{j.2.k} = 2^{-\frac{1}{2}}\left(U_{j-1.k} + W_{j-1.k}\right) \tag{9}$$

$$U_{j.2.k+1} = 2^{-\frac{1}{2}}\left(U_{j-1.k} + W_{j-1.k}\right) \tag{10}$$

In this case, the scaling coefficient $U_{j.k}$ represents the local mean of the process at different scales and time shifts. The shift k_j of scaling coefficients is related to the shift of one of its two direct descendents in a dyadic cascade as the following (Riedi, et al., 1999):

$$k_j + 1 = 2k_j + k_j \tag{11}$$

where k_j=0 corresponds to the left-hand side descendent and k_l=1 to the right-hand side descendent. Two general relations for the coefficients can be stated as follows:

$$U_{j,k_j} = 2^{\frac{1}{2}} U_{0,0} \prod_{t=0}^{j-1}\left[1 + \left(-1\right)^{k_t} A_{i,k_j}\right] \tag{12}$$

$$W_{j,k_j} = 2^{\frac{1}{2}} U_{0,0} \prod_{t-0}^{j-1}\left[1 + \left(-1\right)^{k_i} A_{i,k_i}\right] A_{i,k_i} \tag{13}$$

where here $U_{0,0}$ is assumed to be a Gaussian random variable.

It can be easily demonstrated that the discrete time traffic process X(k) is related to the scaling coefficients $U_{j,k}$ at the finest scale, scaled by a factor, i.e.:

$$X\left(k\right) = 2^{\frac{1}{2}} U_{j,k} \tag{14}$$

The scaling function τ(q)can be accurately modeled by choosing the cascade multipliers $A_{j,k}$ as a symmetric *Beta* random variable with *Beta(a,a)* distribution for a>0 and the random variable Y as a lognormal process whose moment function is $E\left(Y^q\right) = e^{pq+\frac{y^2q^2}{2}}$, defined by the parameters ρ and *y*. Thus, the scaling function $\tau_0(q)$ and the moment factor *c(q)* can be respectively written as the following (Molnár, et al., 2002):

$$\tau_0\left(q\right) = log_2\left(\frac{\Gamma\left(a\right)\Gamma\left(2a+q\right)}{\Gamma\left(2a\right)\Gamma\left(a+q\right)}\right) \tag{15}$$

and

$$c\left(q\right) = e^{pq+\frac{y^2-q^2}{2}} \tag{16}$$

where $\Gamma\left(.\right)$ is the Gamma function.

Assuming that *X(k)* is a pairwise product process and through Haar wavelet properties, we can derive an analytical expression for the second moment $E\left(W_j^2\right)$ of the wavelet coefficients that can be adaptively computed. We will use this analytical expression to generate the multipliers $A_{j,k}$ so that the model captures the wavelet energy decay.

The variance of the aggregated process $var\left[X^m\right]$ and the second moment of the wavelet coefficients $E\left(W_j^2\right)$ that are used in the AWMM model synthesis procedure can be given respectively by (Vieira & Ling, 2009):

$$var\left[X^{2^j}\right] = 2^{-4j}\left(e^{2p+2y^2}\left(\frac{a+1}{a+\frac{1}{2}}\right)^j - e^{2p+y^2}\right) \tag{17}$$

$$E\left(W_j^2\right) = e^{2p+2y^2}\left(\frac{a+1}{a+\frac{1}{2}}\right)2^{-3j} - 2Z_j \tag{18}$$

where:

$$Z_j = 2^{j-1}\left[\sigma^2_{x^{(2j)}} - e^{2p+2y^2}\left(\frac{a+1}{a+\frac{1}{2}}\right)2^{-3j} + \left(e^{2p+y^2}\right)2^{-2j}\right] \tag{19}$$

Moreover, the mean and variance of the scaling coefficients $U_{j,k}$ at the coarsest scale j=N are respectively given by (Vieira & Ling, 2009):

$$E\left\{U_{N,k}\right\} = 2^{\frac{N}{2}}\left(e^{p+\frac{y^2}{2}}\right) \tag{20}$$

$$\sigma^2_{U_{N,k}} = -e^{2p+2y'^2}\left(\frac{a+1}{a+\frac{1}{2}}\right)2^{-3j} + 2Z_N - \left(2^{-N}e^{2p+y^2}\right) \tag{21}$$

Equations (18) and (19) allow the model parameters to be updated without computing the DWT (Discrete Wavelet Transform) for the entire traffic trace. In other words, we do not need to store all the past traffic data in order to update the model parameters as required by the MWM and other traffic models (Molnár, et al., 2002). This property is especially desirable for real-time applications that demand on-line updating of the traffic model multipliers. Besides, the knowledge of the parameters *(a,y,p)* is enough for the AWMM traffic synthesis procedure.

In order to make our model fully adaptive, we need to periodically update the triple *(a,y,p)* parameters obtained through the scaling function τ(q) and the moment factor *c(q)*. A method for estimating these functions based on equation (1) is as the following: Given the process increments $X_1, X_2, \ldots, X_k$, we build the corresponding *m*-level aggregated sequence X^m defined as:

$$X_m^k = X_{(k-1)m+1} + X_{(k-1)m+2} + \ldots + X_{(k)m}, \qquad m = 1,2\ldots \tag{22}$$

If the sequence $\{X_k\}$ has scaling properties, then the absolute moments $E\left(| X |^q\right)$ versus m on a log-log plot should be a straight line as follows (Molnár, et al., 2002):

$$\log\ E\left(| X |^q\right) = \tau_0\left(q\right) \log\ m + \log\ c\left(q\right) \tag{23}$$

The slope of this straight line provides an estimate of $\tau_0(q)$ and its interception point on the vertical axis is the numerical value of *log c(q)*. The proposed AWMM traffic synthesis algorithm includes a recursive least squares algorithm (Hayes, 1996) to adaptively obtain the updated values of $\tau_0(q)$ and *log c(q)* based on equation (23).

In the AWMM traffic synthesis algorithm, after obtaining the values for $\tau_0(q)$ and *log c(q)*, the Levenberg-Marquardt algorithm is applied to estimate the parameters a, p and y of functions $\tau_0(q)$ and *log c(q)* (Marquardt, 1963). The Levenberg-Marquardt algorithm allows us to accomplish this estimation through the minimization of a quadratic function ϕ (Marquardt, 1963):

$$\phi = \frac{1}{2}\sum_{i=1}^{n} r_i\left(x\right) \tag{24}$$

where $r_t(x)$ corresponds to the error between the measured function value and the analytical function value using parameter x.

Figure 1 compares the correlation coefficients computed from the Bellcore Ethernet Bc-Aug traffic trace and the synthetic traces of the AWMM and MWM models. The AWMM generated series presents correlation coefficients closely matching to those computed directly from the network traffic, even for higher values of k. The decay of autocorrelation function reveals the long-range dependent characteristics of the synthetic AWMM process.

Figure 2 presents the byte loss ratio in function of the buffer utilization for a buffer of finite size equal to 65Kbytes for the 10-7-S-1 TCP/IP Petrobrás multifractal traffic trace at the 100ms time scale. The byte loss ratio was verified by using the average of 100 realizations of the corresponding AWMM and MWM processes. The simulation results validate the proposed AWMM approach which faithfully models the considered real Internet traffic traces by providing similar queueing behaviors. Different from the MWM, the AWMM achieves these byte loss ratio values through an adaptive modeling. That is, the parameters of the traffic model are updated at each corresponding time instant to generate the desired synthetic trace.

Figure 1. Comparison of correlation coefficients

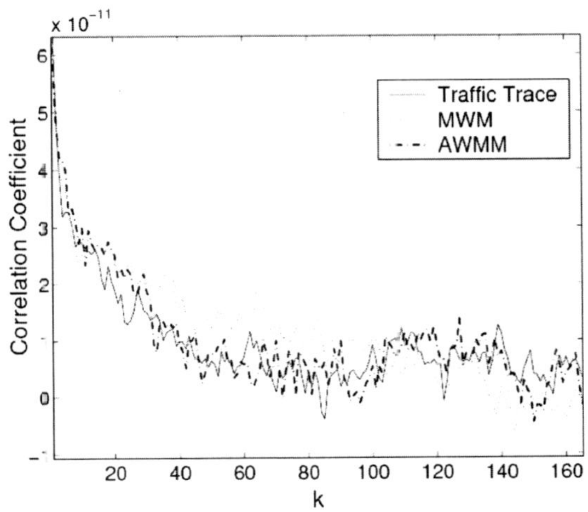

Figure 2. Byte percentual loss

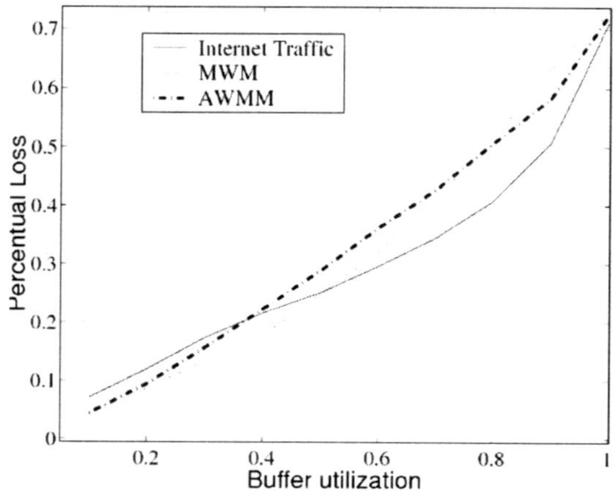

Further, the obtained AWMM synthetic trace is used in the queueing simulation test.

OTHER NETWORK TRAFFIC MODELS

In (Bianchi, Vieira, & Ling, 2004; Vieira, Bianchi, & Ling, 2008), the authors extended the notion of the widely mentioned and used fractional Brownian traffic model (Norros, 1994). Extensive experimental investigations indicate that the proposed traffic model, named extended fractional Brownian traffic (efBt), can capture not only the self-similar properties, but also the inherent multifractal characteristics of those traffic flows found in modern communication networks. Additionally, the structure of this traffic model is taken into account in a traffic prediction algorithm that benefits from the more accurate traffic modeling. The experimental results clearly point out the advantages of using the proposed model in traffic modeling as well as in traffic prediction.

A multifractal traffic model that consists of a multiplicative cascade with generalized multiplier distributions (CGMD) is presented in (Vieira & Ling, 2006). The multipliers are determined through their probability densities estimated from real network traffic flows by using Kernel and Acceptance/Rejection methods. Network performance bounds are computed by relating the CGMD based effective bandwidth to statistical network calculus concepts. The results demonstrate that the CGMD is efficient in describing the byte loss probability and mean buffer occupation for real TCP/IP network traffic flows assuming FIFO queues.

ESTIMATION OF EFFECTIVE BANDWIDTH OF NETWORK TRAFFIC FLOWS

In order to provide quality of service (QoS) guarantees to users, such as byte loss and delay, traffic flows need to be controlled. The concept of effective bandwidth associates a bandwidth value for a connection, independent of other flows in a switch simplifying resource allocation. The effective bandwidth of traffic flows is the rate greater than the mean value rate but less than the peak rate of a flow, that can be used to estimate the link capacity required to support the flow at the required QoS, given the amount of available buffer space.

The concept of effective bandwidth for high speed networks was first presented independently in (Gibbens & Hunt, 1991; Guérin, Ahmadi, & Naghshineh, 1991; Kelly, 1991) where it was tested for i.i.d and On-Off sources. The computation of effective bandwidths for Markov and other processes was carried out in (Chang, 1994; Elwalid & Mitra, 1993). Further development of the theory for admission control, traffic regulation, and other applications can be found in (Veciana, Courcoubetis, & Walrand, 1994; Veciana, Kesidis, & Walrand, 1995) and many others.

Bursts of traffic may arrive at a switch faster than they can be served on output links. Thus, switches are provided with buffers and a basic question is how small buffers can be while keeping byte loss small. The simplest model of a switch is a single server queue with service time fixed at a rate c (bits per second). If δN_k is the number of bits arrivals in the time $k \left(N_k = \sum_{r=1}^{k} \delta N_r \right)$, the buffer content (queue length) is given by:

$$Q_n \overset{d}{=} \sup_{1 \le k \le n} E_k \tag{25}$$

$$E_k = N_k - kc \tag{26}$$

The byte loss measured by the probability of buffer overflow can be stated for large buffer b as:

$$P = \sup_{kE_k} \left(> b \right) \sup_{kP\left(E_k > b\right)} \approx = \sup_{1 \le k \le n} P\left(N_k > b + kc\right) \tag{27}$$

Supposing that δN_k is stationary, the Gartner Ellis theorem allows us to use the large deviation approximation (Bucklew, 1990):

$$P\left(Q_n > b\right) \approx \sup_{1 \le k \le n} e^{-kI_N\left(c + \frac{b}{k}\right)} = e^{-\inf_k kI_N\left(c + \frac{b}{k}\right)} \tag{28}$$

where $I_n\left(x\right)$ is the rate function and $K_n\left(\theta\right)$ is the pseudo-cumulant function:

$$I_N\left(x\right) = \sup_{\theta}\left(x\theta - K_N\left(\theta\right)\right) \tag{29}$$

$$K_N\left(\theta\right) = \lim \frac{1}{n} \log E\left(e^{\theta \Sigma_{k=1}^{n} \delta N_k}\right) \tag{30}$$

The service rate c that attains a QoS requirement specified by $P\left(Q_n > b\right) \le e^{-\gamma} = e^{-b\delta}$ for large buffers is the effective bandwidth $a\left(\delta\right)$ given by:

$$a\left(\delta\right) = \frac{K_N\left(\delta\right)}{\delta} \tag{31}$$

The effective bandwidth is affected by the correlation structure of the source and a loss parameter that is chosen to match the QoS demands of that source. In addition if several sources are serviced simultaneously at one switch and all are serviced at their effective bandwidths, then their QoS demands will not be violated (Duffield & O'Connell, 1995).

It is generally know that effective bandwidths assigned to independent flows being multiplexed behave additively (Chang & Thomas, 1995). Furthermore, it has been shown that under many sources limiting regime, i.e., the number of independent inputs to a switch increases and the service rate and buffer size per input stays fixed, an effective bandwidth assigned to a flow passing through a switch is not changed, and inductively a flow has the same effective bandwidth through the entire network (Wischik, 1999).

The effective bandwidth may be modeled parametrically, but this requires to choose an analytical form of the source's effective bandwidth. Some analytical effective bandwidth (AEB) are known for example for Poisson, On-Off, and fractional Gaussian noise (fGn) processes (Kelly, 1996). On the other hand, we have the 'measured effective bandwidth' (MEB), i.e., for the effective bandwidth it is not assumed a model and by direct measuring the source computes the effective bandwidth: a direct estimator, a block estimator, an estimator based on Kullback-Leibler distance and based on linear regression (Tartarelli, Falkner, Devetsikiotis, Lambadaris, & Giordano, 2000). In the following sections, we will describe some analytical and measured effective bandwidth estimators, as well as an approach for multifractal processes.

EMPIRICAL EFFECTIVE BANDWIDTHS

The empirical effective bandwidth of a traffic stream can be defined as (Tartarelli, et al., 2000):

$$a\left(\theta,t,N\right)=\frac{1}{\theta t}\log\tilde{E}_{N}\left[e^{\theta X(0,\,t)}\right]\quad 0<\theta;\ 0<\mathrm{t}<\mathrm{N} \tag{32}$$

where $X(0,t)$ indicates the aggregate number of cell or packet arrivals in an interval of length t and $\tilde{E}_N\left[e^{\theta X(0,\,t)}\right]$ is the measured log moment generating function over a trace consisting of N samples. For Poisson and On-Off traffic the empirical effective bandwidth is very close to their analytical effective bandwidths (Tartarelli, et al., 2000).

COURCOUBETIS EFFECTIVE BANDWIDTH ALLOCATION

The method described in (Courcoubetis & Weber, 1996) is based on large deviation theory and a large buffer assumption. The effective bandwidth is given by:

$$a=m+\frac{ID\ \mathrm{s}}{2b} \tag{33}$$

The parameters m, b, s and ID are the mean rate, buffer size, space parameter and index of dispersion, respectively. The space parameter s is given by $P\left(\mathrm{Q}_n>b\right)\le e^{-y}=e^{-bs}$. This equation is a generic loss probability expression. It is simple but it still does not address long-range dependent traffic.

NORROS EFFECTIVE BANDWIDTH ALLOCATION

Norros introduced a Gaussian self-similar model (fBm) for modeling of real network traffic (Norros, 1995). After this, an effective bandwidth formula for fBm was also derived:

$$a=m+K\left(H\right)\sqrt{-2\ \ln\left(P_{loss}\right)}^{\frac{1}{H}}a^{\frac{1}{2H}}b^{-\frac{1-H}{H}}m^{\frac{1}{2H}} \tag{34}$$

where $K\left(H\right)=H^{H}\left(1-H\right)^{1-H}$. The parameters m, H, P_{loss}, x and a are respectively the mean, Hurst parameter, buffer overflow probability, buffer size and coefficient of variation. When the traffic is short-range dependent the parameter a is approximated by the index of dispersion (Norros, 1995). The self-similarity and long-range dependence are addressed by this effective bandwidth formula.

EFFECTIVE BANDWIDTH FOR THE AWMM TRAFFIC PROCESS

In this section, we present an effective bandwidth expression for AWMM based traffic processes. The effective bandwidth of the adaptive wavelet based multifractal modeled process $X(k)$ can be expressed in terms of its corresponding multipliers $A_{j,k}$ as (Vieira & Ling, 2009):

$$a\left(s,k\right)=\frac{1}{s2^{k}}\left(\log\frac{\sum_{k=1}^{2^N}\left|\odot_{j,k}\right|}{2^{N}}\right) \tag{35}$$

where:

$$\odot_{j,k}=2^{\frac{1}{2}}\left[e^{sv_1}-e^{sv_2}\right] \tag{36}$$

$$v_1 = 2^{\frac{1}{2}} U_{0,0} \prod_{t=0}^{j-1} \left[1 + \left(-1\right)^{k_i^t} A_{i,2k_i} \right] \tag{37}$$

$$v_1 = 2^{\frac{1}{2}} U_{0,0} \prod_{t=0}^{j-1} \left[1 + \left(-1\right)^{k_i^t} A_{i,2k_i+1} \right] \tag{38}$$

and N is the number of AWMM cascade stages.

Notice that since the AWMM can be seen as a random binomial cascade, the effective bandwidth of a multifractal cascade process can also be estimated by (35) through the knowledge of the cascade multipliers.

Figure 3 shows the effective bandwidths computed through (35) as well as those given by the measured effective bandwidth (MEB) (Tartarelli, et al., 2000) and NEB (Norros Effective Bandwidth) (Norros, 1995) approaches versus the buffer size, under the target byte loss probability set to 10^{-6}. The TCP/IP traffic trace dec-pkt-2 was used here on purpose because it is monofractal with $H = 0,8$, and as consequence, its effective bandwidth can be appropriately determined via the NEB approach, which corresponds to a monofractal based effective bandwidth formulation (Norros, 1995). The MEB and our effective bandwidth method show similar results. For small buffer size, the NEB granted a high effective bandwidth estimate value; evidently is different from the AWMM based effective bandwidth and the MEB estimates that were less sensitive to the buffer size variation.

We also simulated a link serving the 10-7-S-1 Petrobrás traffic trace at time scale of 100ms with the server capacity equal to the effective bandwidth given by (35) and a target QoS loss ratio of 10^{-4}. Figure 4 shows how the packet loss ratio varies with buffer size. Evidently, it can be seen that the effective bandwidths given by the proposed approach attain the loss probability requirement 10^{-4}. We found that Norros' approach is more conservative than ours, also achieving the target loss probability ratio but at the expense of more waste of bandwidth.

Figure 3. Effective bandwidth versus buffer size

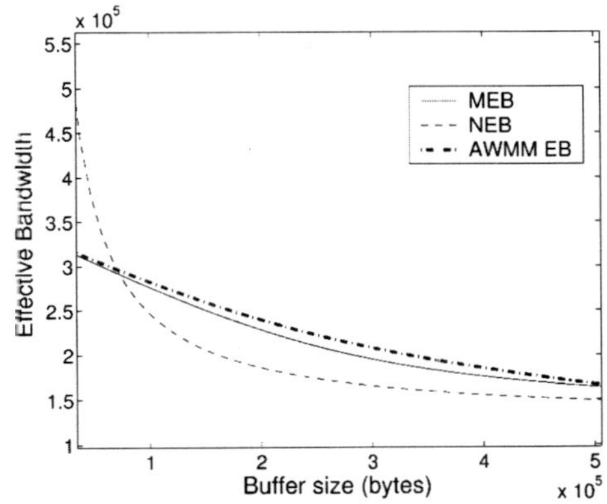

DATA LOSS PROBABILITY

Packet loss in switch buffers is one of the fundamental performance measures associated with the QoS of modern broadband networks. Loss Probability being an important quality of service measure in communication networks has led to efforts to characterize and study the queue length distribution, the distribution of the number of packets or the number of information in the buffer.

Let A(t) be the cumulative packet arrival process on a server in the continuous time interval $\left[0,t\right)$ with stationary increments, C be the server capacity and I(t) be the data arrival process at the network input for arrivals within the time interval $\left[0,t\right)$ given by:

$$I\left(t\right) = A\left(t\right) - Ct \tag{39}$$

The process W that corresponds to the queue size in continuous time is represented by (40) and (41):

$$W\left(0\right) = 0 \tag{40}$$

and

Figure 4. Loss ratio obtained through the AWMM based effective bandwidth versus buffer size

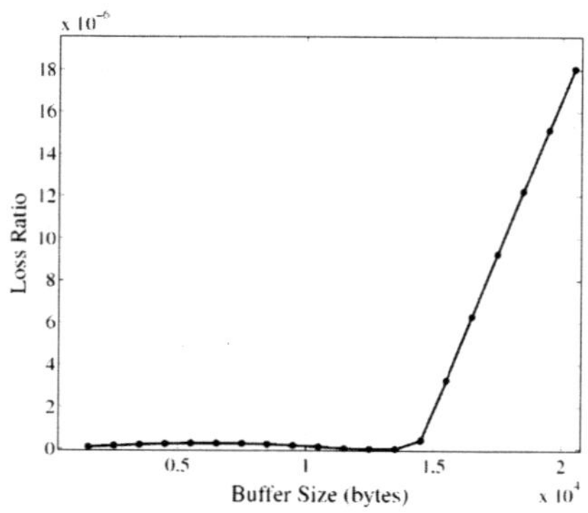

$$W(t) = \sup_{s \le t} \{ I(t) - I(s) \} \tag{41}$$

For the queue to be stable it is required that $E[A(t) - Ct] < 0$. Therefore, the queue size process in the steady-state regime can be expressed as a generalization of Lindley's equation (Rolls, Michailidis, & Hernández-Campos, 2005) as:

$$Q \overset{d}{=} \sup_{t \le 0} \{ A(t) - Ct \} \tag{42}$$

where $\overset{d}{=}$ denotes distribution equality.

LOSS PROBABILITY FOR LRD PROCESSES

An important question is to quantify the impact of long-range dependence (LRD) on queueing. Several engineering issues, such as buffer dimensioning and traffic control, are related to this question. There are two opposing viewpoints on this problem. One claim is that the queueing performance is determined by the time scale of busy periods of the queues and there is no practical impact of correlations above this time scale (Grossglauser & Bolot, 1999; Heyman & Lakshman, 1996; Kobayashi & Takahashi, 1997; Ryu & Elwalid, 1996). The contradicting claim is based on several studies (Erramilli, et al., 1996; Leland, et al., 1994) and states that LRD is one of the main characteristics of the traffic with significant impact on queueing behavior.

The works of Norros (Norros, 1994) and Duffield and O'Connell (Duffield & O'Connell, 1995) study queueing system with self-similar input such as the fBm process. A lower-bound on the probability of buffer occupancy exceeding a threshold in both transient and steady-state regime has been obtained by Norros, while Duffield and O'Connell present an asymptotic expression for the same performance measure at steady-state by applying a Large Deviation Principle (LDP). The latter result verifies that the lower-bound of Norros is asymptotically tight in the steady-state regime, however its availability is questionable for moderate values of buffer threshold. Norros demonstrated that the behavior of a queueing system is remarkably different from that of a system with traditional traffic models (with SRD) as inputs. The lower-bound for $P(\mathrm{Q} > b)$ decays asymptotically (for *b* very large) in a Weibullian fashion. The tail distribution of the queue occupancy in this case is much heavier than the exponential distribution predicted by traditional traffic models. The result of Duffield an O'Connell (Duffield & O'Connell, 1995) shows that $P(\mathrm{Q} > b)$ when scaled properly, will satisfy the following large deviation principle:

Lemma 1: For $H \in (0,5,1)$ it holds that:

$$\lim_{b \to \infty} b^{-2(1-H)} \ln \mathrm{P}(\mathrm{Q} > b) = -a^{-2(1-H)} \frac{(a + C)^2}{2} \tag{43}$$

where $a = \frac{C}{H} - C$.

We can use the result by Duffield and O'Connell to approximate $P\left(Q > b\right)$ by:

$$P\left(Q > b\right) \approx e^{-\gamma b^{2(1-H)}} \tag{44}$$

where $\gamma = a^{-2(1-H)} \dfrac{\left(a + C\right)^2}{2}$. This approximation is accurate for very large b, but it is not guaranteed for all values of b, in many cases, this approximation can underestimate $P\left(Q < b\right)$.

The probability of buffer overflow for short-range dependent traffic presents an exponential decay relative to the buffer size; contrary to that result, such probability has a Weibullian tail for Fractional Brownian Motion, while the corresponding tail is hyperbolic for the general alfa-stable case. The discrepancy between this result and the probability of buffer overflow predicted with traditional traffic models is even more remarkable than that obtained for the Gaussian case (Norros, 1994).

LOSS PROBABILITY FOR MULTIFRACTAL TRAFFIC PROCESSES

Few works deal with queueing problems in which the input traffic *A* has a more complex scale behavior, such as multifractal traffic input (Gao & Rubin, 1999; Molnár, et al., 2002; Vieira & Lee, 2006; Vieira, Lee, & Jorge, 2008). For many traffic models, the only available analysis is that of the asymptotic behavior of queue *Q*. The asymptotic approximation usually yields an simplified vision of network traffic and generally is not applicable to finite buffer cases. For multifractal input traffic the traditional and classic queue analysis such as M/M/1, M/G/1 and G/G/1 are not helpful. In this case, the power laws and behaviors of different orders of the traffic flow statistics in several scales are more important and relevant aspects.

Among the asymptotic estimation studies of loss probability for multifractal traffic, Gao et al. simulated queues with multifractal multiplicative input processes but they did not present analytical results (Gao & Rubin, 1999, 2000). Meanwhile, Molnár et al, proposed an approximate analytical expression for the queueing tail asymptotic behavior, i.e., they determined a mathematical expression for the tail loss probability for a server having a multifractal process as input. In particular, when the input traffic is monofractal, this asymptotic loss probability has a Weibull decay which is consistent with other results (Molnár, et al., 2002; Norros, 1994).

Regarding multifractal input traffic, we can cite the work of Ribeiro et al. (Ribeiro, et al., 2000) where a multiscale queueing analysis for cascade-based multifractal models via a non-asymptotic method has been developed and is valid for any buffer size. This approximation called Multiscale Queueing Analysis incorporates the traffic data distributions in multiple time resolutions (and not only second order statistics) (Ribeiro, et al., 2000). Considering that the discrete random process L_i represents the traffic load (volume) that enters into a server with an infinite buffer and constant service capacity *c*, assuming as well that Q_i represents the queue size at time instant *i* and that K_r is the aggregate number of packets that arrives between instants *i* and r, it is possible to write the following:

$$K_r = \sum_{i=0}^{r} L_i. \tag{45}$$

The process K_r refers to the traffic data for the time scale r. Multiplicative cascade based models provide explicit and simple formulas for K_r in dyadic time scales, i.e. $r=2^n$ $\left(n = 1, 2, \ldots, \infty\right)$. The Multiscale Queueing Analysis states that the loss probability $P_l(x)$ may be estimated as:

$$P\left[Q > b\right] \approx 1 - \prod_{t=0}^{n} P\left[K_{2^{n-1}} < b + c2^{n-i}\right] \quad (46)$$

In the next subsection we will describe another approach for estimating loss probability for multifractal input traffic where the buffer does not need to be large.

LOSS PROBABILITY FOR MULTIFRACTAL TRAFFIC BY MANY SOURCES ASSUMPTION

Given an effective bandwidth estimator $a_n(s, t)$ of $a(s, t)$ for a traffic trace length T=nt, the operating point, i.e. the values of time and space parameters in which the effective bandwidth is related to the asymptotic overflow probability, can be accurately estimated. The parameters *s* and *t* referred to the effective bandwidth depend not only on the source itself but on the context on which this source is involved, the capacity, buffer size, scheduling policy of the multiplexer, QoS parameters, etc.

The so called large buffer asymptotic takes an infinite buffer and studies its filling above some large threshold. On the other hand, effective bandwidth can be estimated using the assumption of many sources instead of large buffer assumption to solve the problem of estimating the space and time parameters s and t (Courcoubetis, Siris, & Stamoulis, 1999). The effective bandwidth is related to the stationary buffer overflow probability $\psi \approx logP\left(Q_n > b\right)$ under the many sources asymptotic regime by the formula:

$$\psi = \inf_{t\geq 0} \sup_{s\geq 0} \left(\left(b + ct\right)s - Nsta\left(s,t\right)\right) \quad (47)$$

Where *c* is the link capacity, *b* is the buffer size and *N* is the number of incoming sources of effective bandwidth.

The values of $s^{\bullet}$ and $t^{\bullet}$ in which the inf sup□ is attained are called the link's operating point. They are found from a non-linear and implicit function. Rewriting equation (47) on a per source basis and using $a_n\left(s,t\right)$:

$$\psi = \inf_{t\geq 0} \sup_{s\geq 0} \left(\left(b + ct\right)s - sta_n\left(s,t\right)\right) \quad (48)$$

Now, let $\Lambda_n\left(s,t\right)$ be an estimator of $\Lambda_n\left(s,t\right) = E\left(e^{sX}\right)$, the moment generating function, $\left(s_n^{\bullet}, t_n^{\bullet}\right)$ are consistent estimators of $\left(s^{\bullet}, t^{\bullet}\right)$ given by the system of equations (Aspirot, et al., 2005):

$$b + ct_n^{\bullet} = \frac{\left(\frac{\partial}{\partial s}\right)\Lambda_n\left(s_n^{\bullet}, t_n^{\bullet}\right)}{\Lambda_n\left(s_n^{\bullet}, t_n^{\bullet}\right)} \quad (49)$$

$$cs_n^{\bullet} = \frac{\left(\frac{\partial}{\partial s}\right)\Lambda_n\left(s_n^{\bullet}, t_n^{\bullet}\right)}{\Lambda_n\left(s_n^{\bullet}, t_n^{\bullet}\right)} \quad (50)$$

It can be demonstrated that multifractal processes possesses global scaling parameter H_g (Vieira & Ling, 2007). Notice that the global scaling parameter H_g is related to the multifractal scaling function t(q).

Solving the system of equations (49) and (50), we can find that (Vieira & Ling, 2007):

$$t^{\bullet} = \frac{H_g b}{\left(c - u\right)\left(1 - H_g\right)} \quad (51)$$

$$s^{\bullet} = \frac{b\left(t^{\bullet}\right) - 2H_g}{\sigma^2\left(1 - H_g\right)} \quad (52)$$

Substituting equations (51) and (52) into equation (48), we get an analytic expression for the loss probability based on the following equation:

$$\log P\left(Q_n > b\right) \approx \left(b + ct_n^{\bullet}\right)s_n^{\bullet} - \Lambda_n\left(s_n^{\bullet}, t_n^{\bullet}\right) \quad (53)$$

This approximation applies equally to traditional teletraffic models and to long range dependent models. Additionally, if we consider that the density probability of the network traffic tends to be lognormal in small time scales, the loss probability in a single queue server with capacity c and buffer size b can be written as (Vieira, Garcez, & Miranda, 2008):

$$P_l\left(x\right) = e^{\left(xs^{\bullet}\right)-\left(p+\frac{y^2}{2}\right)} \int_c^{\infty} \left(r - c\right) \frac{1}{r\theta\sqrt{2\pi}} e^{\frac{-\left(\ln\left(r\right)-\varpi\right)^2}{2\theta^2}} dr \quad (54)$$

In Figure 5, we compare the loss probabilities in terms of buffer size given by equation (54), using the multiscale queueing approach and through the single server link simulation for the dec-pkt-3 traffic flow at the 512ms time scale. The server capacity was set to 120 percent of the mean rate of the traffic trace, considering a FIFO single server simulation fed by the dec-pkt-3 real TCP/IP traffic trace. The simulations were carried out using the Matlab program.

Therefore, the knowledge of some parameters allows us to analytically compute loss probabilities for multifractal processes. The proposed method provides a closer decay rate of the loss probability than the multiscale queueing approach to the real one.

Figure 5. Loss probability for the DEC-pkt-2 traffic trace

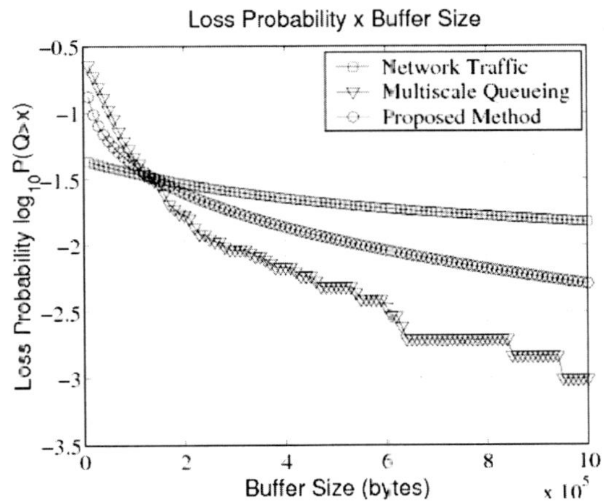

CONCLUSION

Network Traffic has characteristics that are described more adequately by multifractal models (J. Lévy Véhel & R. H. Riedi, 1997; Ribeiro, et al., 2000). It is known that some of the multifractal process properties have a direct impact on the network performance (Erramilli, et al., 1996; Grossglauser & Bolot, 1999). Therefore, more efficient resource allocation methods can be obtained when such models are considered.

In this chapter, we firstly reviewed some important multifractal traffic model concepts. Then, we presented an adaptive wavelet based model through the wavelet coefficients of multifractal processes for network traffic characterization. Statistical and performance tests showed that the AWMM matched closely to the MWM (non-adaptive parameter updating) as well as to real network traffic in simulations. Besides, AWMM requires fewer input parameters and possesses on-line parameter updating.

One of the main issues focused in this chapter is the estimation of effective bandwidth. Initially, we discuss about the existing methods of effective bandwidth estimation. Related to multifractal processes, we have introduced an effective bandwidth function for the AWMM, extendable to other cascade processes. The experimental results showed that the AWMM based effective bandwidth estimate is much more realistic than the Norros' monofractal one, not only guaranteeing the required loss probability for network traffic processes, but also achieving higher link utilization.

In this chapter, we also presented a mathematical expression for the loss probability in a queue server with a finite buffer assuming a multifractal model for the input traffic. Through simulations it was shown that the proposed equation results are continuously more precise regarding the buffer size and/or the server capacity variation than the Multiscale Queueing Analysis.

The packet or byte loss rate is one of the main parameters used to evaluate the quality of service offered to a traffic flow. In this study, the queueing behavior described by the loss probability, was analytically characterized through multifractal traffic parameters. The results obtained with the non-asymptotic analysis proposal for the packet loss probability estimation make it a promising analytical alternative for network design and performance analysis.

It can be concluded that some approaches involving multifractal characteristics can enhance QoS provisioning techniques. Network traffic control algorithms can benefit from the tools for estimation of multifractal parameters. Such estimating tools can be used in a great number of applications and technologies involving QoS provisioning, for example, in WiMAX networks. In future researches, we envision to apply these concepts and techniques in different real scenarios and technologies in order to increase network performance.

REFERENCES

Addie, R. G., Zukerman, M., & Neame, T. (1995). Fractal traffic: measurements, modelling and performance evaluation. In *Proceedings of the Fourteenth Annual Joint Conference of the IEEE Computer and Communication Societies Infocom '95, 3,* (pp. 977-984).

Aspirot, L., Belzarena, P., Bermolen, P., Ferragut, A., Perera, G., & Simon, M. (2005). Quality of service parameters and link operating point estimation based on effective bandwidths. *Performance Evaluation, 59*(2-3), 103–120. doi:10.1016/j.peva.2004.07.006

Bianchi, G. R., Vieira, F. H. T., & Ling, L. L. (2004). A novel network traffic predictor based on multifractal traffic characteristic. In *Proceedings of the IEEE Global Telecommunications Conference, 2004. GLOBECOM'04, 2,* (pp. 680-684).

Bucklew, J. (1990). *Large deviation techniques in decision, simulation, and estimation*. New York: John Wiley & Sons.

Chang, C. S. (1994). Stability, Queue Length and Delay of Deterministic and Stochastic Queueing Networks. *IEEE Transactions on Automatic Control, 39*(5), 913–931. doi:10.1109/9.284868

Chang, C. S., & Thomas, J. A. (1995). Effective bandwidth in high-speed digital networks. *IEEE Journal on Selected Areas in Communications, 13*(6), 1091–1100. doi:10.1109/49.400664

Chui, C. K. (1992). *An introduction to wavelets.* San Diego, CA: Academic Press Professional, Inc.

Courcoubetis, C., Siris, V. A., & Stamoulis, G. D. (1999). Application of the many sources asymptotic and effective bandwidths to traffic engineering. *Telecommunication Systems, 12,* 167–191. doi:10.1023/A:1019194628625

Courcoubetis, C., & Weber, R. (1996). Buffer overflow asymptotics for a buffer handling many traffic sources. *Journal of Applied Probability, 33*, 886–903. doi:10.2307/3215366

Crovella, M. E., & Bestavros, A. (1997). Self-similarity in World Wide Web traffic: evidence and possiblecauses. *IEEE/ACM Transactions on networking, 5*(6), 835-846.

Duffield, N. G., & O'Connell, N. (1995). Large deviations and overflow probabilities for the general single-server queue, with applications. *Mathematical Proceedings of the Cambridge Philosophical Society, 118*, 363–374. doi:10.1017/S0305004100073709

Elwalid, A. & Mitra, D. (1993). Effective bandwidth of general Markovian traffic sources and admission control of high speed networks. *IEEE/ACM Transactions on networking, 1*(3), 329-343.

Erramilli, A., Narayan, O., Neidhardt, A., Saniee, I., & Qnetworx, M. (2000). Performance impacts of multi-scaling in wide area TCP/IP traffic. In *Proceedings of the Nineteenth Annual Joint Conference of the IEEE Computer and Communications Societies (INFOCOM 2000), 1,* (pp. 352-359).

Erramilli, A., Narayan, O., & Willinger, W. (1996). Experimental queueing analysis with long-range dependent packet traffic. *IEEE/ACM Transactions on Networking, 4*(2), 209-223.

Feldmann, A., Gilbert, A. A., & Willinger, W. (1998). Data networks as cascades: investigating the multifractal nature of Internet WAN traffic. In *Proceedings of the ACM SIGCOMM '98 conference on Applications, technologies, architectures, and protocols for computer communication,* (pp. 42-55).

Feldmann, A., Gilbert, A. C., Willinger, W., & Kurtz, T. G. (1998). The changing nature of network traffic: Scaling phenomena. *ACM SIGCOMM Computer Communication Review, 28*(2), 5–29. doi:10.1145/279345.279346

Fitzek, F. H. P., & Reisslein, M. (2001). MPEG-4 and H. 263 video traces for network performance evaluation. *Network, IEEE, 15*(6), 40–54. doi:10.1109/65.967596

Gao, J., & Rubin, I. (1999). Multifractal analysis and modeling of long-range-dependent traffic. *Proceedings of the IEEE International Conference on Communications, 1999, (ICC '99). 1,* 382-386.

Gao, J., & Rubin, I. (2000). Superposition of multiplicative multifractal traffic streams. In *Proceedings of the IEEE International Conference on Communications, 2000 (ICC 2000), 2,* (pp. 816-820).

Garrett, M. W., & Willinger, W. (1994). Analysis, modeling and generation of self-similar VBR video traffic. *Computer Communication Review, ACM SIGCOMM, 24*(4), 269–280. doi:10.1145/190809.190339

Gibbens, R. J., & Hunt, P. J. (1991). Effective bandwidths for the multi-type UAS channel. *Queueing Systems, 9*(1-2), 17–28. doi:10.1007/BF01158790

Grossglauser, M., & Bolot, J. C. (1999). On the relevance of long-range dependence in network traffic. *IEEE/ACM Transactions on Networking, 7*(5), 629-640.

Guérin, R., Ahmadi, H., & Naghshineh, M. (1991). Equivalent capacity and its application to bandwidth allocation in high-speed networks. *IEEE Journal on Selected Areas in Communications, 9*(7), 968–981. doi:10.1109/49.103545

Hayes, M. H. (1996). *Statistical digital signal processing and modeling*. New York: John Wiley & Sons, Inc.

Heyman, D. P. & Lakshman, T. V. (1996). What are the implications of long-range dependence for VBR-video traffic engineering? *IEEE/ACM Transactions on Networking (TON), 4*(3), 301-317.

Kelly, F. P. (1991). Effective bandwidths at multi-class queues. *Queueing Systems, 9*(1-2), 5–16. doi:10.1007/BF01158789

Kelly, F. P. (1996). Notes on effective bandwidths. In Kelly, F. P., Zachary, S., & Ziedins, I. (Eds.), *Stochastic Networks: Theory and Applications* (pp. 141–168). Oxford, UK: Oxford University Press.

Kobayashi, K., & Takahashi, Y. (1997). Tail probability of a Gaussian fluid queue under finite measurement of input processes. In *Proceedings of the IFIP TC6 / WG6.3 & WG7.3 International Conference on the Performance and Management of Complex Communication Networks,* (pp. 43-58).

Krishna, P. M., Gadre, V. M., & Desai, U. B. (2001). Global Scaling Exponent for Variable Variance Gaussian Multiplicative (VVGM) Multifractal Cascades. In *Proceedings of the Sixth Biennial Conference on Signal Processing and Communications (SPCOM'01),* (pp. 19-25).

Krishna, P. M., Gadre, V. M. & Desai, U. B. (2003). Multifractal based network traffic modeling. Boston: Kluwer Academic Publishers.

Leland, W. E., Taqqu, M. S., Willinger, W., Wilson, D. V., & Bellcore, M. (1994). On the self-similar nature of Ethernet traffic (extended version). *Networking, IEEE/ACM Transactions on, 2*(1), 1-15.

Lévy Véhel, J., & Riedi, R. (1997). Fractional Brownian motion and data traffic modeling: The other end of the spectrum. In Lévy Véhel, J., Lutton, E., & Tricot, C. (Eds.), *Fractals in engineering: from theory to industrial applications* (pp. 185–202). Berlin: Springer.

Lévy Véhel, J., & Riedi, R. H. (1997). *TCP traffic is multifractal: a numerical study. INRIA research report No. 3129.* INRIA - Institut National de Recherche en Informatique et en Automatique.

Li, Q., & Mills, D. L. (1999). Investigating the scaling behavior, crossover and anti-persistence of Internet packet delay dynamics. In *Proceedings of the Global Telecommunications Conference, 1999 (GLOBECOM '99), 3,* (pp. 1843-1852).

Mandelbrot, B. B., Fisher, A. J., & Calvet, L. E. (1997). *A Multifractal Model of Asset Returns.* Cowles Foundation Discussion Paper No. 1164. Cowles Foundation for Research in Economics at Yale University, New Haven, CT.

Mandelbrot, B. B., & Van Ness, J. W. (1968). Fractional Brownian motions, fractional noises and applications. *SIAM Review, 10*(4), 422–437. doi:10.1137/1010093

Mandelbrot, B. B., & Wallis, J. R. (1969). Computer experiments with fractional Gaussian noises, parts 1, 2 and 3. *Water Resources Research, 5*(1), 228–267. doi:10.1029/WR005i001p00228

Marquardt, D. W. (1963). An Algorithm for Least-Squares Estimation of Nonlinear Parameters. *SIAM Journal on Applied Mathematics, 11*(2), 431–441. doi:10.1137/0111030

Molnár, S., Dang, T. D., & Maricza, I. (2002). On the queue tail asymptotics for general multifractal traffic. In *Proceedings of the Second International IFIP-TC6 Networking Conference on Networking Technologies, Services, and Protocols; Performance of Computer and Communication Networks; and Mobile and Wireless Communications, 2002 (IFIP Networking '02)* (Vol. LNCS 2345, pp. 105-116). Berlin: Springer-Verlag.

Norros, I. (1994). A storage model with self-similar input. *Queueing Systems, 16*(3), 387–396. doi:10.1007/BF01158964

Norros, I. (1995). On the use of fractional Brownian motion in the theory of connectionless networks. *IEEE Journal on Selected Areas in Communications, 13*(6), 953–962. doi:10.1109/49.400651

Park, K., & Willinger, W. (2000). *Self-Similar Network Traffic and Performance Evaluation*. New York: Wiley-Interscience. doi:10.1002/047120644X

Paxson, V. & Floyd, S. (1995). Wide area traffic: the failure of Poisson modeling. *Networking, IEEE/ACM Transactions on, 3*(3), 226-244.

Peltier, R. F., & Lévy Véhel, J. (1995). *Multifractional Brownian motion: definition and preliminary results. INRIA research report No. 2645*. INRIA - Institut National de Recherche en Informatique et en Automatique.

Ribeiro, V. J., Riedi, R. H., Crouse, M. S., & Baraniuk, R. G. (2000). Multiscale Queuing Analysis of Long-Range-Dependent Network Traffic. In *Proceedings of the Nineteenth Annual Joint Conference of the IEEE Computer and Communications Societies (INFOCOM 2000). 2,* (pp. 1026-1035).

Riedi, R. H., Crouse, M. S., Ribeiro, V. J., & Baraniuk, R. G. (1999). A multifractal wavelet model with application to network traffic. *IEEE Transactions on Information Theory, 45*(3), 992–1018. doi:10.1109/18.761337

Rolls, D. A., Michailidis, G., & Hernández-Campos, F. (2005). Queueing analysis of network traffic: methodology and visualization tools. *Computer Networks, 48*(3), 447–473. doi:10.1016/j.comnet.2004.11.016

Ryu, B. K., & Elwalid, A. (1996). The importance of long-range dependence of VBR video traffic in ATM traffic engineering: Myths and realities. *ACM SIGCOMM Computer Communication Review, 26*(4), 3–14. doi:10.1145/248157.248158

Tartarelli, S., Falkner, M., Devetsikiotis, M., Lambadaris, I., & Giordano, S. (2000). Empirical effective bandwidths. In *Proceedings of the IEEE Global Telecommunications Conference, 2000 (GLOBECOM '00), 1,* (pp. 672-678).

Veciana, G., Courcoubetis, C., & Walrand, J. (1994). Decoupling bandwidths for networks: a decomposition approach to resource management. In *Proceedings of the Thirteenth Annual Joint Conference of the IEEE Computer and Communications Societies (INFOCOM '94), 2,* (pp. 466-473).

Veciana, G., Kesidis, G., & Walrand, J. (1995). Resource management in wide-area ATM networks using effective bandwidths. *IEEE Journal on Selected Areas in Communications, 13*(6), 1081–1090. doi:10.1109/49.400663

Vieira, F. H. T., Bianchi, G. R., & Ling, L. L. (2008). A Network Traffic Prediction Approach Based on Multifractal Modeling. *Journal of High Speed Networks*.

Vieira, F. H. T., Garcez, S. G., & Miranda, W. F. (2008). Uma Abordagem para Estimação de Probabilidade de Perda em Redes Através da Teoria de Muitas Fontes e Modelagem Multifractal de Tráfego. In *7th International Information and Telecommunication Technologies Symposium (I2TS 2008)*.

Vieira, F. H. T., & Lee, L. L. (2006). Queueing analysis for multifractal traffic through network calculus and global scaling parameter. In *Proceedings of the IEEE International Telecommunications Symposium, 2006 (ITS 2006),* (pp. 181-186).

Vieira, F. H. T., Lee, L. L., & Jorge, C. (2008). An improved GPS scheduling discipline based on multifractal traffic characteristics. In *Proceedings of the IEEE/IFIP Network Operations and Management Symposium, 2008 (NOMS 2008),* (pp. 987-990).

Vieira, F. H. T., & Ling, L. L. (2006). Performance bounds for a cascade based multifractal traffic model with generalized multiplier distributions. *Journal of Communication and Information Systems, 21,* 1.

Vieira, F. H. T., & Ling, L. L. (2007). Limitantes de Desempenho de Fila para Tráfego Multifractal de Redes. *INFOCOMP - Journal of Computer Science, 6*(4), 100-110.

Vieira, F. H. T., & Ling, L. L. (2009). Adaptive Wavelet Based Multifractal Model Applied to the Effective Bandwidth Estimation of Network Traffic Flows. *IET Communications*, *3*(6), 906–919. doi:10.1049/iet-com.2008.0078

Willinger, W., Taqqu, M. S., & Erramilli, A. (1996). A bibliographical guide to self-similar traffic and performance modeling for modern high-speed networks. In Kelly, F. P., Zachary, S., & Ziedins, I. (Eds.), *Stochastic Networks: Theory and Applications* (*Vol. 4*, pp. 339–366). Oxford, UK: Oxford University Press.

Wischik, D. J. (1999). The output of a switch, or, effective bandwidths for networks. *Queueing Systems*, *32*(4), 383–396. doi:10.1023/A:1019107708752

Section 3
Integrations of Quality of Service and Network Management Model

Chapter 10
Disruption in the ICT-Sector: Will Former Telecommunications Monopolists Stumble across VoIP?

Justus Bross
University of Potsdam, Germany

Long Wang
University of Potsdam, Germany

Rehab AlNemr
University of Potsdam, Germany

ABSTRACT

In this chapter, the authors discuss innovations associated with the transition from the circuit-switched public telephone network to IP packet-switched networks for the provision of voice services by focusing on research findings in the area of quality of service (QoS). To give a meaningful answer on how this transition affects the telecommunications industry, we elaborate on the frequently-cited concept of disruptive innovations, pioneered by Harvard Professor Clayton M. Christensen.

INTRODUCTION

In the context of the European wire-line telecommunications industry this work elaborates on the popular claim that the data-oriented voice transmission technology Voice-over-Internet-Protocol (VoIP) does constitute a disruptive technology or innovation. The inability to anticipate new technologies, which emerge from below, has often been put forward as the main reason for the failure of established firms and the advantage for the attacker, namely the new entrant. Previously, the most dominant view in technology strategy was that the displacement of established firms and technologies by new firms and their technologies is driven by the superior performance characteristics offered by newcomers and the incumbents' difficulties in matching their performance and capabilities. Clayton M. Christensen calls all new technologies that exhibit improved performance characteristics sustaining technologies. They can be incremental, radical or discontinuous, but what they all have in common is that they improve the performance with respect to the technology used before (Christensen, 1997). However, by identifying the possibility that technologies with inferior performance can displace

DOI: 10.4018/978-1-61520-791-6.ch010

established players and their technology in a certain industry, the way in which managers and scholars alike approach technology competition has fundamentally changed, prompting a reassessment of innovation strategies in general. These technologies that, at least in the short-term, result in worse product performance are what Christensen terms disruptive technologies. They are inferior to the established products measured along the dimensions of certain performance attributes in main-stream markets.

The corresponding research identifies QoS as the most important performance attribute for telephony services in general. The comparison of VoIP to traditional telephony QoS levels and their corresponding performance development has revealed that QoS of Internet Telephony was intolerably low when first introduced, compared to the standards set by the traditional telephony. However, these shortcomings were largely factored out and optimized through numerous QoS enhancing methods, meaningful traffic engineering and network planning. This chapter will show that QoS of today's VoIP solutions is, however, absolutely satisfactory to customers.

The underlying and deductive reasoning of what Christensen calls "performance oversupply" in traditional telecommunication services, is the possibility that what does not satisfy customer needs today may be fully performance-competitive in the same market tomorrow. This performance oversupply in the mainstream market can clearly be identified on the basis of an extended QoS-comparison of both VoIP and traditional telephony by a graphical depiction of VoIP QoS performance trajectories, which represent the performance supplied by the technology and the one demanded by the mainstream market. This chapter will therefore compare the QoS levels for both transmission technologies in a way similar to Christensen's "Trajectory Performance Diagrams".

Due to the fact that QoS is a dependent variable of numerous different factors with each one having a different impact on either one of the two transmission technologies of interest, the comparison is considerably more complex and extensive than those known from Christensen's works. This research thus provides an integrated, recapitulating and straightforward depiction of QoS-differences between the transmission techniques, which ultimately show that VoIP proves to be a disruptive technology. The trend towards data-oriented networks and therefore VoIP might therefore eventually lead to the failure of former telecommunications monopolist's wire-line business; following the universal claim of Christensen's theory.

THE "INNOVATORS DILEMMA": FAILURE FRAMEWORK BY CHRISTENSEN

Why might firms be regarded as well managed, yet subsequently lose their leadership position in an industry when faced with disruptive change? Management researchers have studied the commercial potential of disruptive technologies for nearly a century. Kondratief was among the early researchers in the field, suggesting the potential of long waves of techno-logical change caused by new technologies and new skill sets in either creating or redefining firms and existing markets (Kondratief, November 1935). Creative destruction, a term coined by Joseph Schumpeter (1942) to denote a "process of industrial mutation that incessantly revolutionizes the economic structure from within, incessantly destroying the old one, incessantly creating a new one," was the basis for several follow-up studies that tried to explain why innovative entrepreneurship destroys established enterprises and simultaneously yields new ones (Schumpeter, 1942). The key hypothesis of Schumpeter's work is that large firms not only innovate more intensively than small firms do (Scherer, 1992), but are also better suited to innovations (Schumpeter, 1942).

Yet several studies on innovation suggest that new entrants regularly surpass technology leaders (Cohen, 1984; Nelson & Wright, 1992) - an assertion which stands in total contrast to Schumpeter's central hypothesis. Other scholars have similarly argued that incumbent firms may stumble when technological change destroys the value of established competencies (Tushman & Anderson, 1986) or when new architectural technologies emerge (Bower & Christensen, 1995; Henderson & Clark, 1990). Numerous explanations for technological change can be found in academic literature. They range from a firm's unwillingness to cannibalise its existing sales and, therefore, its underlying technologies (Chandy & Tellis, 1989; Kamien & Schwartz, 1982; Reinganum, 1983), managerial and organizational inertia inside the company (Christensen & Bower, 1996; Henderson, 1993), superior innovations with respect to the existing technologies (Dewar & Dutton, 1986), incompetence and under investment (Henderson, 1993), and rigidities or inabilities in dealing with competence-destroying technologies (Leonard-Barton, 1992).

However, latest research (Bower & Christensen, 1995; Christensen, 1997; Gilbert, 2002; Tripsas, 1997) doubted the general validity of these theories because, in many instances, firms that have missed important innovations suffered from none of these problems. One concept that addresses this unexplained issue is that of disruptive innovations, thoroughly explained by Christensen in numerous articles, papers and books. Christensen's articles and papers about creative destruction are mainly based on in-sights derived from an extensive study of the disk drive industry. The obvious repetitive pattern of failure in this industry allowed Christensen to develop a theoretical framework which makes it possible to shed some light on the discussion of why even good management can lead to the failure of established firms (Christensen, 1993).

The Notion of Disruption

The first main finding from this study is the distinction between what he refers to as sustaining technologies and disruptive technologies. Here, technology is broadly defined as the process by which an organization transforms labour, capital, materials, and information into products and services (Christensen, 1997). Building on this characterization, sustaining technologies are defined as technological changes that progress on an established trajectory of performance improvement. This implies that all sustaining technologies improve the performance of established products in accordance with the dimensions of performance demanded by mainstream customers in major markets (Christensen, 1997). Disruptive technologies, on the other hand, are defined as technologies which disrupt an established trajectory of performance improvement, or redefine what performance means (Christensen & Bower, 1996). They are innovations that underperform established products in the mainstream markets initially, yet have the long-term potential of substituting these sustaining technologies due to the fact that they incorporate values that a fringe, and most of the time new, customer group desires.

This distinction is fairly different from the one predominantly used by previous researches. From the earliest studies of innovation, scholars exploring the factors influencing the rate and direction of technological change have sought to distinguish between radical and incremental innovations. In this context, technologies launching in new directions in innovation were commonly referred to as radical innovations, while those making progress along established paths were often called incremental innovations (Christensen & Rosenbloom, 1995). Several authors (Dewar & Dutton, 1986; Dutton & Thomas, 1985; Sahal, 1981) suggest that the major difference captured by the labels radical and incremental is the degree of novel technological process content embodied in the innovation and hence, the degree of new knowledge embedded in the innovation. Radical innovations were therefore innovations containing a high degree of new knowledge, while incremental innovations were innovations incorporating a low degree of new knowledge (Dewar & Dutton, 1986).

Christensen, in turn, introduced a completely different concept with his distinction between sustaining versus disruptive technologies. This distinction was meant to account for the differences of performance characteristics, which clearly differs from the notion of incremental versus radical. It is therefore a more process-based concept of technology. To provide a theoretical background for understanding the behaviour and performance of firms in the realm of radical innovations (Dewar & Dutton, 1986) or disruptive innovations (Christensen, 1997) it seems worthwhile to mention the theory of S-curves. This theory suggests that technologies evolve along a series of successive S-curves that drive various new product innovations (Chandy & Tellis, 1998). The S-shaped pattern of the curve emerges because a new technology offers few consumer benefits when first introduced, offers rapidly growing consumer benefits as it develops, becoming better understood, controlled, and diffused, and finally offers again only slowly increasing benefits as it matures. In the maturing stage, the technology will asymptotically approach a natural or physical limit, which requires increasingly more effort and inputs to achieve improvements. This development is also known as the product-life-cycle theory.

It is essential for strategic management to identify when the point of inflection on the S-curve has been passed so its second derivative is negative (Christensen, 1997). At this point a new or disruptive technology may emerge to supplant the established one. The inability to anticipate new technologies, which emerge from below, has often been put forward as the main reason for the failure of established firms and the advantage for the attacker, namely the new entrant.

Previously, the most dominant view in technology strategy was that the displacement of established firms and technologies by new firms and their technologies is driven by the superior performance characteristics offered by newcomers and the incumbents' difficulties in matching their performance and capabilities. Christensen calls all new technologies that exhibit improved performance characteristics sustaining technologies. They can be incremental, radical or discontinuous, but what they all have in common is that they improve the performance with respect to the technology used before (Christensen, 1997). However, by identifying the possibility that technologies with inferior performance can displace established players and their technology in a certain industry, the way in which managers and scholars alike approach technology competition has fundamentally changed, prompting a reassessment of innovation strategies in general. These technologies that, at least in the short-term, result in worse product performance are disruptive technologies. They are inferior to the established products measured along the dimensions of performance in mainstream markets.

Unsurprisingly, the question of why exactly a customer should be interested in such a disruptive technology arises; because the most dominant impression one has regarding this new technology is the aura of inferiority. The answer to this paradox lies in different value propositions that are brought to the market by these new technologies, since products based on disruptive technologies are typically cheaper, smaller, simpler and, frequently, more convenient to use. Several authors identified rigid value networks inside the companies as the prime initiator for the above-mentioned failure framework and, subsequently, one of the main culprits for the displacement of established firms through disruptive innovation (Christensen & Bower, 1996; Christensen & Rosenbloom, 1995).

Investing in Disruptive Technologies is Not Rational

The perception of the economic value of a new technology is ultimately a logical deduction from the second main finding of Christensen, on which he builds his failure framework. His conviction that disruptive technologies are not rational investments rests on three bases; the first one being that disruptive products are simpler and cheaper. Therefore, by stemming from the low-end of the market, they generally promise lower margins, not greater profits. Second, disruptive technologies are initially only commercialised in insignificant or emerging markets. A disruptive technology is therefore initially only embraced by the least profitable customer segment (Zook & Allen, 2001). The third reason is that a firm's most profitable and therefore most important customers do not, and initially cannot, use a disruptive technology. Chesbrough (2003) supports this reasoning by finding evidence of incumbent firms delaying the sub-market entry for the same reasons as outlined above. His findings are quite consistent with the story of internal resource allocation conflicts between incumbents serving the existing markets versus pursuing new markets.

Value Networks, Resource-Allocation and -Dependence

Christensen's concept of different value propositions, or value networks, as he calls it, builds on Giovanni Dosi's concept of technological paradigms, which he defines as a "pattern of solution of selected technological problems, based on selected principles derived from natural sciences and on selected material technologies" (Dosi, 1982). Within such a value network, each firm's competitive strategy determines its own subjective perceptions of the economic value of a new technology (Christensen, 1997). It is these particular perceptions that shape the respective rewards each firm expects to retain through the pursuit of sustaining and disruptive innovation (Christensen & Rosenbloom, 1994, 1995).

There are two concepts that underline the power of value networks to influence firm behaviour and therefore their importance in explaining the emergence of different value networks: *resource dependence and resource allocation*. To explain the interrelationship between value networks, resource allocation and resource dependence, the definition of value networks by Pfeffer et al. must be examined. According to Pfeffer et al., value networks consist of linkages that relate different interest groups with the firm and its management, effectively constraining managerial independence. These interest groups, whether customers, suppliers, investors, intermediaries, or other managers, create resource dependence (Pfeffer & Salancik, 1978; Ulrich & Barney, 1984), and therefore ultimately control the allocation of resources and the innovative decision-making within the firms (Christensen & Bower, 1996). This infers that sufficient impetus to successfully execute difficult technological innovations may be developed only when the most significant customers of a company demand it. Conversely, when a proposed innovation "only" addresses the needs of small customers in remote or emerging markets who do not supply a significant share of the resources that are important for a firm, this firm will find it enormously difficult to succeed, even with innovations that are technologically straightforward (Christensen & Rosenbloom, 1995).

The notions of value networks, resource dependence and resource allocation thus view the reason for firm's failure as an issue of misinvestments or strategic decisions, rather than technological incompetence. Christensen and Bower (1996), for instance, used the theories of resource allocations and resource dependence to highlight that the allocation of resources to some product developments and commercialisation programs, and the denial to others, is a key decision in the implementation of strategy. This suggests a causal relationship between the resource allocation processes, as modelled by Bower (1970a, 1970b) and Burgelman (1983a, 1983b), and the phenomenon of resource dependence, as argued by Pfeffer and Salancik (1978). In this way the concept of value networks and the related notions of resource dependence and the resource allocation process help to explain the mechanisms through which independent and induced strategic behaviour (Burgelman, 1983a) can affect, or fail to affect, a company's course (Foster, 1986; Cooper & Schendel, 1976).

The Pace of Technological Progress Often Outstrips Market Needs

The exact effect of value networks on a firm's behaviour and the corresponding action taken by customers is as follows: established and incumbent firms initially reject disruptive technologies when confronted with a low-end market segment. A small and, to the incumbent firm initially unattractive, set of customers however gets attracted to these new technologies. The customers most of the time use these disruptive technologies in new or low-end applications (Christensen, 2002). According to Christensen, incumbent firms facing this poorly defined and unattractive market tend to move upwards, away from this segment, to satisfy premium customer segments that promise higher margins and superior profits. Through the developing vacuum, or "asymmetric motivation," that is left behind by established firms focusing on the more profitable market segments, there is sufficient room for new entrants to enter these markets. The new entrants can serve the needs of this new group of consumers, therefore competing against the incumbent firm in its own market. Zook and Allen (2001) support this notion by stating that up-market movements give low-price competitors a flank to attack. Generalizing the approach employed by Henderson and Clark (1990), established firms were defined as firms that had previously manufactured certain products which employed an older, established technology, whereas entrant firms were those whose initial product upon entry into the industry employed the new component or architectural technology being analysed.

In the case of the disruptive technology, the new market, which has been created by the attack of the new entrants into the incumbent's markets, has enough growth potential for the initially inferior technology to be further developed by start-up firms. This is achieved by sustaining improvements in their own value network up to a level that might be sufficient to satisfy performance attributes as required by the mainstream customers of the incumbent firms (Christensen & Rosenbloom, 1995). Although the performance of the disruptive technology remains inferior to the performance supplied by the established technology, as measured according to the performance attributes demanded in the mainstream market of the incumbent, it starts to attract the less-demanding mainstream customers in the incumbent's market. At this point the rate of improvement of the disruptive technology's performance exceeds the rate of improvement expected in less demanding customer segments of the incum-bent's market. This enables new entrants or start-ups to attack the established firm in its own market by creating a sub-market. To explain the differences of the impact of certain kinds of technological innovations on a given industry, the concept of performance trajectories is help-ful. Almost every industry has a critical performance trajectory (Bower & Christensen, 1995).

Performance Trajectories and Performance Oversupply

By extending Dosi's (1982) notion of a "technological trajectory" associated with each technological paradigm, Christensen and Rosenbloom (1995) suggest that two distinct trajectories can be identified – one that defines the performance demanded over time within a given value network and another one that exhibits the performance that companies are able to provide within that value network. In the context of disruptive innovations, these two trajectories frequently graphically depict what several authors identified as one of the main culprits for the displacement of established firms and their technologies: the notion of performance oversupply (Adner, 2002; Christensen & Bower, 1996).

The underlying and deductive reasoning of this performance oversupply, is the possibility that what does not satisfy customer needs today may be fully performance-competitive in the same market tomorrow. When the slopes of two trajectories are similar, Christensen et al. (1995) expect the technology to remain relatively contained within the value network in which it is initially used. In case these two slopes differ, however, new technologies may migrate into other networks, thus offering a chance for innovators to attack established players in those new networks. Technologies that disrupt an established trajectory of performance improvement, or redefine what performance means, are disruptive technologies (Christensen & Bower, 1996) and ultimately trigger a change in the basis of competition. The reasoning for such a performance oversupply to happen is that once the demand for a certain performance attribute is satiated, other attributes whose performance has not yet satisfied market demands are valued more highly and therefore have the potential to catch the customer's interest.

A scholar who confirms this notion is Chesbrough in his work "Environmental Influences upon firm entry into new sub-markets." He analysed the hard disk industry and ultimately came to the conclusion that, although disruptive technologies offer inferior performance attributes, they ultimately fulfil the requirements of a specialized consumer group and are consequently suited for a sub-market (Chesbrough, 2003). Chesbrough defines sub-markets as markets in which a new technology offering causes one group of customers (some of whom may be new arrivals to that market) within an existing market to behave similarly to one another and differently from other customers in that market. Different terms used in academic literature to denote a sub-market are "market segments," as used by economists (Kamien & Schwartz, 1982), and "niches," as used by organizational ecologists (Carroll, 1985). In many cases of the prior inferior disruptive technology, many start-ups of-fering this technology proved Christensen and his reasoning right by becoming fully performance-competitive and capturing significant shares of the incumbent firm's established market.

QUANTIFICATION AND COMPARISON OF QOS

Value Network in Telecommunication

The assessment of a product or service by the customer is of central importance to the above-mentioned failure framework and is therefore of special importance in this chapter. Christensen's distinction between disruptive or non-disruptive technologies accounts for the differences of performance characteristics.

The most important service performance attributes in the voice arena of both the traditional telecommunications industry and Internet Telephony is Quality of Service (QoS). QoS is the only real technical performance characteristic of voice transmission services and is therefore attributed special importance in this chapter. Furthermore, it is used for the development of the so-called "Performance Trajectory Diagram". According to Hein et al. (2002), QoS could be defined as the capability of offering the guarantee to accomplish certain service requirements like comprehensibility, absence of echo, etc. Regarding voice quality in general, it could be defined along the subsequent requirements for a sufficient comprehensibility of voice:

1. Sufficient bandwidth
2. Time conditions like delay and jitter
3. Low data loss and good voice encoders

These requirements count equally for circuit switched GSTN networks, like traditional wire line telephony, as well as for packet-oriented data networks and consequently for Internet Telephony respectively. QoS should always be available on an end-to-end basis between two communicating parties, meaning that QoS should be supported by all network elements throughout the complete path travelled inside the network. The topic of QoS is extensively discussed in several recommendations of the International Telecommunications Union (ITU), workshops of the European Telecommunications Standards Institute (ETSI), proposals of the Internet Engineering Task Force (ITEF) and several other exploratory projects.

QoS in Circuit-Switched Networks

Scholars and researchers alike agree on one issue when it comes to quality performance in communication networks: the PSTN is the ultimate benchmark for voice quality (Doshi et al., 2003; Hein et al., 2002; Houck & Yang, 2004; Pracht, Newman, & Douskalis, 2000). Due to the fact that the PSTN was from the start designed to provide optimal service for real-time sensitive voice applications requiring low delay, echo, and jitter, today's digital wire line networks are a synonym for outstanding quality performance what voice transmission is concerned. Until the introduction of mobile communication networks, this high quality standard was taken for granted, even though a certain loss of quality was tolerated for calls forwarded through a satellite connection and for long-distance calls. In the following, we will apply the requirements for a sufficient comprehensibility of voice as outlined with the three points in the introduction of this section:

1. **Bandwidth:** The requirement of sufficient bandwidth in today's circuit-switched networks is satisfied through the reservation of a 64 Kbit/s channel, since it not only provides a constant bandwidth, which is optimized especially for the transmission of speech, but furthermore is at the disposal of the communicating parties throughout the duration of the call.
2. **Delay and Jitter:** Delay and latency are similar terms that refer to the amount of time it takes a bit to be transmitted from the source to the destination. Jitter is delay that varies over time. In circuit switched networks however, this effect is negligibly small, due to the fact that there is no variation of transmission paths. Delay of voice signals from the sender to the recipient has a substantial effect on the quality of a conversation. To quantify this effect, the ITU-T recommendations G.114 and G.131 specify the tolerable mouth-to-ear delay bounds for undistorted (analogue or G.711; 64kBit/s) voice with (hybrid or acoustic) echo. Communication is increasingly disturbed by the loss of speech interactivity when the 150 ms bound is exceeded. Even though there is a minority of sensitive customers who perceive delays bigger than 90 ms, a 150 ms delay should be targeted as the maximum for network planners. The higher the delay and jitter, the worse a conversation gets through distortion, echo effects and pauses. The limit of 150ms, however, postulates that above a delay of 20-30ms echo compensation should be implemented. In circuit-switched networks end-to-end delay is somewhere below 10 ms for local calls. Due to the fact that delay has a positive relationship with geographic transmission distances, delay is higher for long-distance calls or connections forwarded over satellites, in which case the delay can sum up to around 250 ms, which is only conditionally acceptable. In GSM networks in turn, end-to-end delay is somewhere around 100 ms -well inside the acceptable level.
3. **Loss of voice data:** The loss of voice data in circuit-switched networks lies somewhere within 0,1% one tenth of a percent (Hein et

al., 2002) and is therefore neglected in this paper.

Quantification of Traditional Telephony Voice Quality

The first standard for measuring voice quality was specified by the ITU recommendation P.800 in 1996 and is commonly referred to as the Mean Opinion Score or, simply, "MOS" (ITU-T, 1996). It defines a method to derive a mean opinion score of voice quality between 1 (bad) and 5 (excellent) from human listeners. It is a subjective measure of how individual users perceive the speech quality and ease of conversing. An MOS factor of 4 corresponds to today's long-distance call quality (also known, and hereafter referred to, as "Toll Quality") and 3-4 an acceptable quality. The G.711 codec, which is exclusively used in the PSTN for ordinary calls, scores a MOS factor of 4,3, while codecs used in the GSM achieve a score between 3.7 and 4 (Hein et al., 2002; Houck & Yang, 2004; ITU-T, 1988). Other user-perceived and equally subjective quality indexes similar to the MOB are the "good or better" (GOB) index, the "poor or worse" (POB) index and the "Terminate Early" (TME) (Janssen, de Vleeschauwer, & Petit, 2000; Johannesson, 1997; Minacom, 2003), which are not of primary interest to this paper and are therefore not further discussed. The above-mentioned tests are on a subjective basis, in which factors like gender, language and age play an important role. A more objective method to measure voice quality was therefore indispensably required.

The ITU has developed such a class of a more objective measure, which is known as the E-Model and specified in ITU-T Recommendation G.107. It is a tool for predicting how an "average" user would rate voice quality of a phone call with known characterizing transmission parameters. Originally, the E-model was developed for network planners analyzing narrowband-telephony like POTS, ISDN and GSM (Hein et al., 2002; ITU-T, 2003), but is now widely accepted to measure the key metric voice quality in a VoIP network (Houck & Yang, 2004). It includes a multiplicity of input parameters like, for instance, the Quality of Voice-codecs as well as psychological factors, which incorporate a higher acceptance of lower voice quality in mobile networks when compared to the wire line network. The output parameter of the E-model is the so-called "Rating Factor R", which accords to a db-value between 0 and 100. R-values between 0 and 50 are not defined. A breakdown of the Rating Factor R in tenners according to the G.109 recommendation of the ITU (ITU-T, 1999) adds up to 5 different quality classes as the following table depicts:

Due to the fact that we are only interested in the voice quality of today's traditional wire line telephony services, we should only focus on the respective application, namely the PSTN/ISDN services and their corresponding quality value, whether the R-value or the MOS factor. All the wire line connections possible in the traditional telephony that can be considered equivalent to recent ISDN services what the quality level is concerned score an R-value of at least 80 or an MOS factor of no less than 4,03 respectively (ETSI, 2001). Quality rating factors of less than 80 can already be found in mobile networks and should therefore not be included to represent wire line PSTN/ISDN service quality. The lower "borderline" in the table above depicts this partition graphically. To give the reader a clearer understanding of the following comparison between traditional telephony and Internet Telephony quality, we will refer to all applications that score an R-value above the borderline ("Toll Quality") as PSTN applications.

Figure 1 depicts the relationship between R and the one-way-delay with the example of a G.711 codec, the codec used exclusively in the GSTN (Britt, 2000; Gardner, Frost, & Petr, 2003; Hein et al., 2002; Houck & Yang, 2004). Originally, the E-model was developed for network planners of narrow band telephony (330 till 3.400 Hz) to measure the maximum achievable Voice quality

Figure 1. Table of own visualization (Bross, 2008), according to ITU-T recommendation G.109 (ITU-T, 1999)

Rating factor	Quality class	Customer satisafaction	MOS-factor *	Application
90 <= R < 100	Best	Absolutly satisfactory	4,34 <= MOS	all local PSTN calls
80 <= R < 90	High	Satisfactory	4,03 <= MOS < 4,34	all national calls
70 <= R < 80	Medium	Some insatisfied	3,60 <= MOS < 4,03	international calls without compression, national wireline to wireless calls
60 <= R <70	Low	Not Satisfactory	3,10 <= MOS < 3,60	international wireline to wireless calls, national wireless calls, satellite connections without compression
50 <= R < 60	Poor	Absolutly Insatisfactory	2,58 <= MOS < 3,10	international wireless to wireless calls, satelite connections with compression

in the POTS, ISDN and GSM with respect to a so-called reference connection. R = 94,15 is the maximum value that PSTN telephony could score with a delay of zero ms and an I_e factor of zero. As outlined before in, the curve exhibits a kink at 150 ms, the point at which one-way-delay significantly negatively influences the quality-rating factor R.

Existing PSTN quality, as indicated by the "Existing PSTN" labelled area in figure 1, was derived from the fact that the speech codec used in traditional telephony, was, and still is, the G.711 codec. The required network bandwidth capacity is provided at all times in the PSTN due to the exclusive reservation of a 64kBit/s channel for the duration of the call (Hein et al., 2002).

According to the TIPHON recommendation of the ETSI, an end-to-end or one-way delay of up to 100 ms corresponds with today's POTS and ISDN services respectively (ETSI, 2001). This limit was consequently taken as the boundary on the x-axis for one-way delay in today's traditional telephony. For local calls, circuit-switched networks even incorporate a one-way delay of only 10 ms (Hein et al., 2002). Therefore, due to the TIPHON suggestion and the fact that GSM network delay is said to begin at around 100 ms (Hein et al., 2002), this paper will take this very limit as the boundary for one-way delay for existing PSTN and ISDN services respectively. The lower boundary on the y-axis (R=80) is set according to ITU-T's recommendations G.107 (ITU-T, 2003) and G.109 (ITU-T, 1999), as well as the ETSI publication TS 101 329-2 (2001). Concordantly they state that existing PSTN/ISDN services would never score below a Quality Rating Factor of 80. As a conclusion, the resulting field within the above-specified boundaries represents the quality one can expect when making a phone call in the PSTN.

QoS of Internet Telephony

The possibility of combining data, voice and multimedia services into one facility assures huge benefits in added value to companies and users deploying the service of VoIP. However, the IP telephony market has not expanded as expected. It is a common belief that the reason for this development is VoIP systems struggling to reach the levels of voice transmitting quality standards set by the PSTN for over a century (Andersson, 2002). The future of VoIP networks is like most fields of business determined by the end-user demand. If a potential customer expects the advantages to be larger than the drawbacks, the total service may be considered as value-adding to the company. The public opinion that identifies a lack of satisfactory quality within the IP telephony is therefore a very important issue for developers and standardization organizations, since the perceived end-to-end quality is definitely a factor that will determine the future success of VoIP networks.

One reason for a real qualitative disadvantage on the side of Voice over IP technology might be the fact that in the original design of TCP/IP networks and systems, QoS was only attributed minor importance. TCP/IP was optimized for the transport of data for applications like email and Internet and not for voice or video applications this was consequently not necessary. QoS therefore concentrates on the circumvention of data loss and/or data falsification, main occurrences which negatively influence voice quality stemming from the initial conception of TCP/IP. Today QoS is a main issue in the field of Internet Telephony, due to the fact that not all issues related to the continuous transmission capabilities of packet-oriented networks have been solved:

1. **Bandwidth:** In contrast to circuit switched transmission, in which 64kBit/s are reserved for every single conversation, several different customers making distinct phone calls by using packet-oriented technologies share the bandwidth. In case this bandwidth is not constantly and sufficiently provided, traffic blockages can lead to a higher delay and packet loss. There are three alternatives through which sufficient bandwidth can be provided at all times in packet oriented networks: Over dimensioning of the network (therefore over-provisioning bandwidth), bandwidth reservation and traffic prioritization, or traffic engineering:
2. **Delay and Jitter:** While in circuit-switched networks end-to-end-delay only adds up to about 10 ms and therefore does not constitute a problem for voice quality in these networks at all, it is significantly higher when carried over packet-oriented networks (since there are additional sources of delay). Since the minimal delay in circuit switched networks is only induced by network- and geographic delay, the following three components are equally capable of lowering the voice quality in packet-oriented networks significantly: (1) the Input delay, which comprises encoding-, packetizing- and serialization delay, (2) the network delay that consists of the serialization- the routing-, the queuing-, the traffic shaping and the propagation delay and ultimately (3) the output delay in the gateway and IP-terminal, which is determined by the sum of jitter buffer-, Decoding-, Packet Loss- and Concealment delay.
3. **Loss of data packets:** Loss of data packets is an absolutely normal occurrence in TCP/IP networks and occurs for two reasons; the first one being traffic blockages in the network that result in a rising number of queues and consequently in the rejection of data packets. Due to the nature of the TCP/IP protocol, any packet loss leads to a request for a repeated sending of the respective data package. For real-time applications like the transmission of voice packet loss should be avoided, which can be pursued through the application of the already mentioned Diff-Serve, for instance. They are necessary to ensure a guaranteed flow-rate with a minimum packet-loss and delay rate.

The second reason for the loss of data packets is high delay, through which packets arrive behind schedule in the jitter buffers and consequently get discarded. One solution is the appliance of large buffers that can balance out delay and therefore the loss of data packages. Due to the fact that a

5-10% loss rate of voice packages already significantly lowers voice quality, a 2% rate should therefore be aimed at by network planners (Hein et al., 2002). For the sake of an improved quality, lost data packages can be reconstructed or simply hidden by the so-called Packet Loss Concealment (PLC) method. This method, however, requires additional processing power and storage and may consequently result in higher delay times, which in turn has a negative impact on voice quality.

Quantification of VoIP Quality

There are plenty of methods that were already used to assess the voice quality of Internet Telephony systems. The Mean Opinion Score (MOS) built upon ITUs recommendation P.800 and used for the evaluation of voice quality in circuit-switched networks is one method that can also be used for Internet Telephony. Another one is the Perceptual Speech-Quality-Measure method (PSQM), which was originally developed by the Research department of the former Dutch telecommunications monopolist and taken over by the ITU-T in 1996. Other examples are the Perceptual Analysis Measurement System (PAMS) (Rix & Hollier, 2000) introduced in 1998 by British Telecom (BT) and its successor, Perceptual Evaluation of Speech Quality (PESQ), which was jointly developed by BT and the KPN in 2001 and later suggested as a standard by the ITU (ITU-T, 2001).

The model of interest, however, is the already introduced E-model, which can be equally applied to evaluate traditional telephony as well as Internet Telephony. To account for the impairment factors that are only relevant in Internet Telephony (Jitter, Echo, Voice-encoding and packet loss), factor I_e was introduced. While this factor is zero for the G.711 codec (used in the traditional telephony), it already adds up to 11 for the G.729 and 15 for the G.723 codec (both used for VoIP), as specified in ITU's recommendation G.113 (ITU-T, 2001). According to the E-model formula as depicted in Figure 1, this linear expression lowers the overall Quality Rating Factor R for these codecs significantly.

For the sake of straightforwardness, this chapter will limit itself to three codecs (G.711, G.729A and G.723.1) in order to exemplify the characteristics of voice codecs in the presence of delay and packet loss in voice transmission. Using the information from the preceding sections, one can use the E-model to plan new VoIP networks or predict the impact of various potential changes resulting from the network design, certain router configurations, a VoIP traffic model, and the call routing. Thus, trade-offs can be explored between equipment/codec choices and network configurations to deliver good voice quality. Figure 1 also depicts the R factor of the E-model as a function of delay for our codec choices G.711 (64kBit/s), G.729A (8kBit/s) and G.723.1 (6.3kBit/s). It should be kept in mind, however, that in this figure only the different delay requirements depending on our respective codecs of choice were included. All other factors were assumed to be at their nominal ideal factors. With other additional impairments, the voice quality of the codecs used predominantly for VoIP could be worse than depicted. This paper will, however, limit itself to only showing the delay requirements depending on the respective codecs of choice to allow a meaningful comparison of quality levels. After all, the inclusion of additional impairment factors would only make our final point clearer, namely the fact that Internet Telephony Quality can only reach, in very limited cases, the quality benchmark of PSTN telephony.

APPLICATION OF THE BASIC FAILURE FRAMEWORK – PROVING QOS PERFORMANCE OVERSUPPLY

We argue that the notion of performance oversupply can be clearly identified by the graphical depiction of VoIP QoS performance trajectories, which represent the performance supplied by the

Figure 2. QoS of PSTN and VoIP (Bross, 2008)

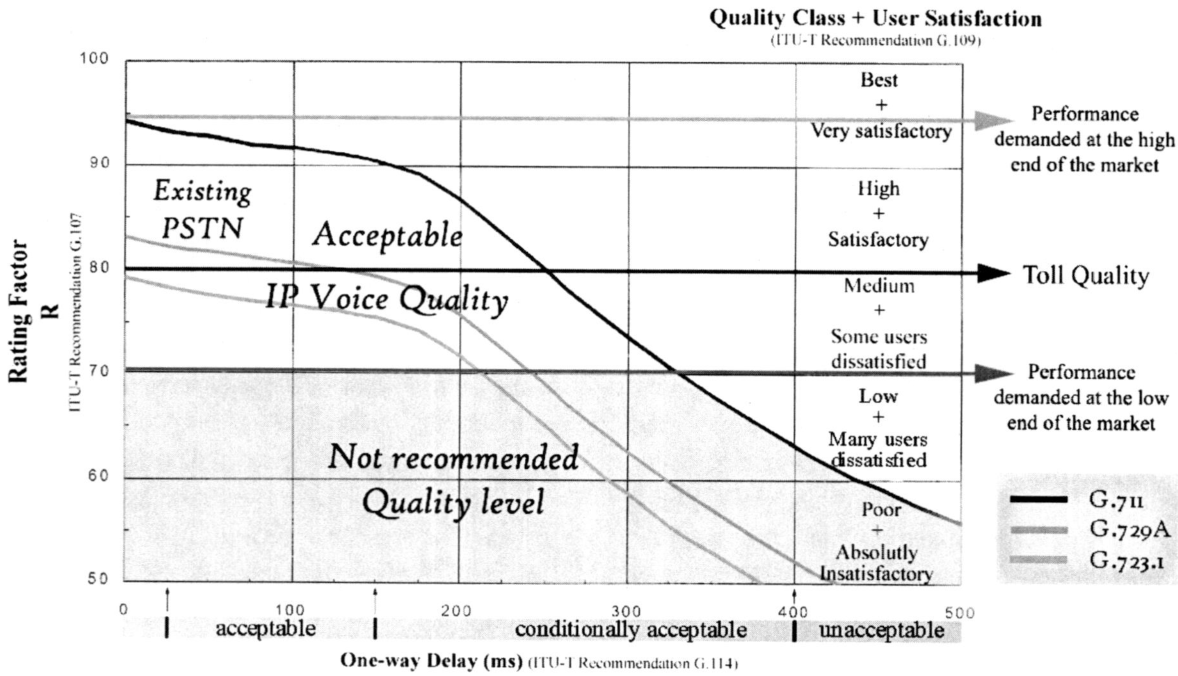

technology and the one demanded by the mainstream market. It can, as a result, be noted that the second basis of Christensen's failure framework could be identified in the telecommunications industry.

In circuit-switched networks, good voice quality for those calls admitted into the network was generally given. IP networks, however, introduce many new sources of distortion. The subsequent section will graphically compare the QoS levels for both transmission technologies in a way similar to Christensen's "Trajectory Performance Diagrams". Due to the fact that QoS is a dependent variable of numerous different factors with each one having a different impact on either one of the two transmission technologies of interest, the comparison was considerably more complex and extensive than those known from Christensen's works. Figure 2 summarizes all information obtained throughout this paper. It was developed to spare the reader a technical and detailed discussion about the factors that exert influence on QoS. It thus provides an integrated, recapitulating and straightforward depiction of quality differences between the transmission techniques.

While Christensen, to adhere to performance changes over time, depicts the performance development of attributes along a time line of several years on the x-axis, this approach would not make sense when depicting QoS as the most important performance variable of wire-line telecommunications. This is due to the fact that VoIP QoS is constructed from numerous variables adding up to certain QoS levels (as outlined in the appendix). Figure 2 is furthermore more suitable to account for the trade-off decisions that need to be made between the resources and technical possibilities available, the need to satisfy certain different quality demands, and the costs associated with each decision. This trade-off is of absolute importance in the QoS context and could not be graphically depicted by using Christensen's conception of a performance trajectory diagram. Figure 2 below is therefore a more meaningful graphical depiction to compare QoS performance differences than the original Performance Trajectory Diagram proposed by Christensen.

The conclusions that can be drawn from this graph are similar to the ones that can be obtained through Christensen's graphical depiction; therefore, both are considered equally useful for their respective areas of application. The coloured areas within figure 2 depict the different market demands, while the curves represent the performance provided by the different voice transmission technologies.

The area labelled "Existing PSTN" marks the quality level a customer can expect when making a phone call in the PSTN. The upper arrow ("*Performance demanded at the high end of the market*") set at the quality maximum quality level depicts the maximum QoS market demand traditional telephony can provide within the PSTN. The area marked "*Acceptable IP Voice Quality*" depicts the quality levels that today's VoIP technology is capable of providing. QoS performance of IP Voice transmission cannot reach the QoS levels of traditional transmission technology, but this is unnecessary, as the following section will demonstrate.

While "Toll Quality" was commonly perceived by network planners to be the minimal QoS level to provide, the analysis actually uncovered that minimum QoS market demand for the end-customer is actually substantially lower. To be precise, it is 10 points lower on the quality rating scale "R" of the E-model chosen by this paper. Consequently, the lower arrow ("*Performance demanded at the low end of the market*") in figure 1 should graphically depict minimum market demand. The area labelled "*Not recommended Quality level,*" therefore represents quality levels below the minimum market demand that could be accepted neither by customers using traditional telephony nor by those using VoIP. The actual performance development of the two transmission technologies is depicted by the three curves in Figure 1: G.711, rep-resenting the traditional voice transmission, and G.729A and G.723.1, both representing VoIP transmission technology. The two codecs chosen to both represent VoIP technology underline the importance the trade-off decisions mentioned earlier. Correspondingly we see that VoIP transmission technology reaches well into the acceptable quality area. It even meets quality standards set by the traditional transmission technologies within the PSTN under optimal conditions and trade-off decisions.

Christensen's reasoning for performance oversupply is that once the demand for a certain performance attribute is satiated, other attributes whose performance has not yet satisfied market demands are valued more highly. They now have the potential to catch the customer's interest. QoS performance provided by traditional telephony in the PSTN absolutely over-shoots market demand. Even though VoIP QoS performance should be considered as under-performing with respect to the traditional telephony, it fully satisfies market demands from all customer segments. This thesis correspondingly suggests that the sustaining technology was over-supplying its customers with QoS performance. According to Christensen (1997), performance oversupply of an attribute perceived to be important by the customer within the value network of the sustaining technology is a fundamental reason for a disruptive technology to emerge.

Underlining Christensen's and Bower's (1996) beliefs, performance oversupply, as identified on the example of QoS, triggered a change in the basis of competition. Other attributes, whose performance have not yet satisfied market demands, are valued more highly and, therefore, have the potential to catch the customer's interest. For the case of VoIP these "other attributes" include the value-adding services of mobility, flexibility and convergent applications, as well as functionality and pricing variables.

This ultimately supports Christensen et al's conviction that disruptive technologies can generally redefine what performance means (Christensen & Bower, 1996). This chapter therefore argues that the QoS performance oversupply in the traditional telecommunications market, underlines the disruptive aura of VoIP. The shift of the importance attributed by the customer to the different performance variables and the corresponding rank ordering ultimately defines the boundaries between the distinct value networks of traditional as well as Internet Telephony. This supports Christensen's conviction that different value networks might very well exist within the same broadly defined industry (Christensen, 1997), as in this case the German wire-line voice telecommunications market.

VOIP STATUS REPORT

Internet Telephony first broke into public view in 1996, with the Israeli firm VocalTec offering the first solution for the transmission of voice signals through the public Internet using IP. While the initial "greenfield" solution by VocalTec was limited to PC-to-PC calls, companies like Net2Phone and Deltathree expanded upon this technical development in the middle of the 1990's by installing gateways into the public telephone network. This allowed them to offer low-priced overseas calls in the traditional telephone networks, thus enabling both PC-to-Telephone and Telephone-to-PC calls. During the following years however, this story became a moot point, since telecommunication carriers dramatically lowered the costs of national and international calls.

VoIP development has accordingly shifted from providing the price sensitive Internet community with cheap calls over the public Internet, to providing telephony services over IP-based networks as a real alternative to traditional telephony services for both business users and the private mass market alike. The ongoing success story of the improved VoIP technology (50% of all global telecoms traffic is already done over IP) and respective service provider pioneers such as Skype or Vonage, which have been quietly generating huge user bases, is confirmed in updated market reports (BuddeComm, 2007):

While there were twice as much residential VoIP subscribers in 2006 compared to the previous year with a total of 40 million, the numbers more than tripled in 2007 to approximately 135 million residential subscribers. On top of the increasing popularity among private customers, market reports also monitored an increasing importance of IP networks for corporate telecommunication needs. The true value of IP here is that it is becoming the core of the next generation public networks (NGNs), in which it facilitates "triple play" business models by seamlessly integrating voice, data and video (DTAG, 2004). Hence, there seems to be no end in sight to the success story of VoIP and IP telecommunication in general at this moment.

CONCLUSION

Based upon the fundamentals of the disruptive technology concept pioneered by Christensen, this paper intended to analyse the popular claim that VoIP is a disruptive technology. By applying the discussion to the context of the wire-line telecommunications industry, it was of specific interest to uncover if VoIP, as a consequence of being a disruptive technology, does indeed pose a threat to the traditional telephony business.

The existence of what Christensen calls performance oversupply – the most crucial characteristic proving the existence of disruption - could as a consequence be confirmed by this chapter on the example of the QoS performance attribute. It was demonstrated that traditional telephony oversupplied its customers regarding QoS performance. Customers subsequently recognized that the potentially disruptive technology VoIP provided quality levels that, although lower than those in the PSTN, were absolutely satisfying. Because of this, customer's attentions shifted to other attributes whose performance had not yet satisfied market demands. They correspondingly started to put increased importance on pricing variables, the possibility of increased mobility, and the use of convergent applications - attributes in which VoIP increasingly became competitive in the course of its product life cycle regarding the established service offerings.

LIMITATIONS AND SUGGESTIONS FOR FURTHER RESEARCH

Even though the notion of performance oversupply is the most important of Christensen's failure framework in the opinion of the authors, there are additional characteristics and trends of VoIP incorporating the disruptive aura of initial inferiority and subsequent performance improvement. This does furthermore count for performance attributes like branding, security, compatibility, functionality, usability, as well as availability. Focussing on all of these variables would have been out of scope for this research, they should however be kept in mind in future research. It is furthermore Christensen's conviction that a disruptive technology usually has an absolute price competitive advantage to the traditional product or service. A corresponding research should be undertaken accordingly. It might furthermore be of interest to include more traffic and network variables that may degrade quality of VoIP. This is however out of scope for this paper.

REFERENCES

Adner, R. (2002). When are technologies disruptive? A demand-based view of the emergence of competition. *Strategic Management Journal, 23*, 667–668. doi:10.1002/smj.246

Andersson, J. (2002). *Addressing voip speech quality with non-intrusive measurements*. Retrieved January 02, 2005 from http://www.techonline.com/community/tech_group/comm/tech_paper/21663

Bower, J. (1970a). Planing within the firm. *The American Economic Review, 60*(2), 186–194.

Bower, J. L. (1970b). *Managing the resource allocation process*. Homewood, IL: Richard D. Irwin, Inc.

Bower, J. L., & Christensen, C. M. (1995, January-February). Diusruptive technologies: Catching the wave. *Harvard Business Review*, 43–53.

Britt, R. (2000, 5.12). *Ip-telephony.* Paper presented at the FCC Industry Meeting.

Bross, J. F. M., & Meinel, C. (2008), Can VoIP Live up to the QoS Standards of Traditional Wireline Telephony? *AICT, Fourth Advanced International Conference on Telecommunications,* (pp.126-132).

BuddeComm. (2007). *June 2007 Global NGN IP VoIP – Analyses Statistics and Forecasts*. BuddeComm.

Burgelman, R. (1983a). A model of the interaction of strategic behaviour, corporate context, and the concept of strategy. *Academy of Management Review, 3*(1), 61–69. doi:10.2307/257168

Burgelman, R. (1983b). A process model of internal corporate venturing in teh diversified major firm. *Administrative Science Quarterly, 28*(2), 223–244. doi:10.2307/2392619

Carroll, G. R. (1985). Concentration and specialization: Dynamics of niche width in populations of organizations. *American Journal of Sociology, 90*, 1262–1283. doi:10.1086/228210

Chandy, R. K., & Tellis, G. J. (1998, November). Organizing for radical product innovation: The overlooked role of willingness to cannibalize. *JMR, Journal of Marketing Research, 35*, 474–487. doi:10.2307/3152166

Chesbrough, H. W. (2003). Environmental influences upon firm ebtry into new sub-markets: Evidence from the worldwqide hard disk drive industry conditionally. *Research Policy, 32*, 659–678. doi:10.1016/S0048-7333(02)00033-1

Christensen, C. M. (1993). The rigid disk drive industry: A history of commercial and technological turbulence. *Business History Review*, (67): 531–588. doi:10.2307/3116804

Christensen, C. M. (1997). *The innovator's dilemma: When new technologies cause great firms to fail*. Boston: Harvard Business School Press.

Christensen, C. M. (2002). The rules of innovation. *Technology Review, 105*, 32–38.

Christensen, C. M., & Bower, J. (1996). Customer power, strategic investment, and the failure of leading firms. *Strategic Management Journal, 17*, 197–218. doi:10.1002/(SICI)1097-0266(199603)17:3<197::AID-SMJ804>3.0.CO;2-U

Christensen, C. M., & Rosenbloom, R. S. (1994). Technological discontinuities, organizational capabilities, and strategic commitments. *Industrial and Corporate Change*, (3): 655–685.

Christensen, C. M., & Rosenbloom, R. S. (1995). Explaining the attacker's advantage: The technological paradigms, organizational dynamics, and the value network. *Research Policy, 24*, 233–257. doi:10.1016/0048-7333(93)00764-K

Cohen, A. J. (1984). Technological change as historical process: The case of the U.S. Pulp and paper industry, 1915-1940. *The Journal of Economic History, 44*(3), 775–799. doi:10.1017/S0022050700032368

Cooper, A., & Schendel, D. (1976, Feb.). Strategic responses to technological threats. *Business Horizons, 19*, 61–69. doi:10.1016/0007-6813(76)90024-0

Dewar, R. D., & Dutton, J. E. (1986). The adoption of radical and incremental innovations: An empirical analysis. *Management Science, 32*(11), 1422–1433. doi:10.1287/mnsc.32.11.1422

Doshi, B. T., Eggenschwiler, D., Rao, A., Samadi, B., Wang, Y. T., & Wolfson, J. (2003). Voip network architectures and qos strategy. *Bell Labs Technical Journal, 7*(4), 41–59. doi:10.1002/bltj.10033

Dosi, G. (1982). Technological paradigms and technological trajectories. *Research Policy, 11*, 147–162. doi:10.1016/0048-7333(82)90016-6

DTAG. (2004). *Vendor market report - insights into the telecommunication and information technology equipment and software markets (internal paper)*. Deutsche Telekom AG - Zentralbereich Technologie und Plattformen.

Dutton, J., & Thomas, A. (1985). Relating technological change and learnign by doing. *Research on Technological innovation. Management and Policy, 2*, 187–224.

ETSI. (2001). *Telecommunications and internet protocol harmonization over networks (tiphon) release 3; end-to-end quality of service in tiphon systems; part 2: Definition of speech quality of service (qos) classes*. ETSI.

Foster, R. N. (1986). *Innovation: The attacker's advantage*. New York: Summit Books.

Gardner, M. T., Frost, V. S., & Petr, D. W. (2003). *Using optimization to achieve efficient quality of service in voice over ip networks*. Retrieved January 03, 2009 from http://www.ittc.ku.edu/publications/documents/Gardner2003_ipc31-Todd-Gardner-VoIP-Optimization.pdf

Gilbert, C. G., & Bower, J. (2002). Disruptive change - when trying harder is part of the problem. *Harvard Business Review*, 94–101.

Hein, M., Reisner, M., & Voß, A. (2002). *Voice over ip: Sprach-daten-konvergenz richtig nutzen*. Berlin: Franzis Verlag GmbH.

Henderson, R. M. (1993). Underinvestment and incompetence as responses to radical innovation: Evidence from the photolithographic alignment equipment industry. *The Rand Journal of Economics*, *24*(2), 248–270. doi:10.2307/2555761

Henderson, R. M., & Clark, K. B. (1990). Architectural innovation: The reconfiguration of existing systems abd the failure of established firms. *Administrative Science Quarterly*, *35*, 9–30. doi:10.2307/2393549

Houck, D. J., & Yang, W. (2004). *Voicer over internet protocol - voice quality of service*. White Paper, Lucent Technologies - Bell Labs Innovators, Murray Hill, NJ.

ITU-T. (1988). *Itu-t recommendation g.711: Pulse code modulation (pcm) of voice frequencies*. ITU.

ITU-T. (1996). Itu-t recommendation p.800: Methods for objective and subjective assessment of quality:ITU.

ITU-T. (1999). *Itu-t recommendation g.109: Definition of categories of speech transmission quality*. ITU.

ITU-T. (2001). *Itu-t recommendation g.113: Transmission impairments due to speech processing*. Telecommunications and Standardization Sector of the ITU.

ITU-T. (2001). Itu-t recommendation p.862: Methods for objective and subjective assessment of quality:ITU.

ITU-T. (2003). *Itu-t recommondation g.107: Definition of categories of speech transmission quality*. Telecommunications and Standardization Sector of the ITU.

Janssen, J., de Vleeschauwer, D., & Petit, G. H. (2000). Delay and distortion bounds for packetized voice calls of traditional pstn quality. In *IPtel 2000*. Berlin: Alcatel.

Johannesson, N. O. (1997). *The etsi computation model: A tool for transmission planning of telephone networks. IEEE Communications* (pp. 1–10). Washington, DC: IEEE.

Kamien, M., & Schwartz, N. (1982). *Market structure and innovation*. Cambridge, UK: Cambridge University Press.

Kondratief, N. D. (1935, November). The long waves in economic life. *The Review of Economics and Statistics*, *17*(6), 105–115. doi:10.2307/1928486

Leonard-Barton, K. (1992). Core capabilities and core rigidities: A paradox in managing new product development. *Strategic Management Journal*, *28*(2), 228–247.

Minacom. (2003). *Extended e-model solution.* Retrieved January 22, 2005 from http://www.minacom.com/products/pp6000_files/Extended%20E-Model%20Solution%20Sheet%20001-000104-101_A.pdf

Nelson, R. R., & Wright, G. (1992). The rise and fall of american technological leadership: The postwar era in historical perspective. *Journal of Economic Literature*, *30*(4), 1931–1964.

Pfeffer, J., & Salancik, G. R. (1978). *The external control of organizations: A resource dependence perspective*. New York: Harper & Row.

Pracht, S., Newman, D., & Douskalis, B. (2000). Now hear this. *Telephony*, *239*(6), 58–65.

Reinganum, J. (1983). Uncertain innovation and the persistence of monopoly. *The American Economic Review*, *73*(4), 741–748.

Rix, A. W., & Hollier, M. P. (2000). The perceptual analysis measurement system for robust end-to-end speech quality assessment. In *IEEE ICASSP*. BT Advanced Communications Research.

Sahal, D. (1981). *Patterns of technological innovation*. London: Addison-Wesley.

Scherer, F. M. (1992). Schumpeter and plausible capitalism. *Journal of Economic Literature*, *30*(3), 1416–1433.

Schumpeter, J. A. (1942). *Capitalism, socialism and democracy*. New York: Harper & Row.

Tripsas, M. (1997). Unraveling the process of creative destruction: Complementary assets and incumbent survival in teh typesetter industry. *Strategic Management Journal*, *18*(6), 119–142. doi:10.1002/(SICI)1097-0266(199707)18:1+<119::AID-SMJ921>3.3.CO;2-S

Tushman, M. L., & Anderson, P. (1986). Technological discontinuities and organizational environments. *Administrative Science Quarterly*, *31*, 439–465. doi:10.2307/2392832

Ulrich, D., & Barney, J. (1984). Perspectives in organizations: Resource dependence, eficiency, and population. *The Academy of Management Review*, *9*(3), 471–481. doi:10.2307/258287

Zook, C., & Allen, J. (2001). *Profit from the core*. Boston: Harvard Business School.

Chapter 11
Traffic and Network Performance Monitoring for Effective Quality of Service and Network Management

P. Papantoni-Kazakos
University of Colorado Denver, USA

A.T. Burrell
Oklahoma State University, USA

ABSTRACT

The authors consider distributed mobile networks carrying time-varying heterogeneous traffics. To deal effectively with the mobile and time-varying distributed environment, the deployment of traffic and network performance monitoring techniques is necessary for the identification of traffic changes, network failures, and also for the facilitation of protocol adaptations and topological modifications. Concurrently, the heterogeneous traffic environment necessitates the deployment of hybrid information transport techniques. This chapter discusses the design, analysis, and evaluation of distributed and dynamic techniques which manage the traffic and monitor the network performance effectively, while capturing the dynamics inherent in the mobile heterogeneous environments. Specifically, the design of a monitoring sub-network is sought, where the arising research tasks include: the adoption of a core sequential algorithm which monitors both the variations in the rates of the information data flows and the dynamics of the network performance. The identification of the specific operational and performance characteristics of the monitoring systems, when the core algorithm is implemented in a distributed environment; for a given network topology, it is important to identify the minimum size monitoring sub-network for complete "visibility" of data flows and network functions. Dynamically changing monitoring sub-network architectures, as functions of time-varying network topologies. The deployment of Artificial Intelligence learning techniques, in the presence of dynamically changing network and information flow environments, to appropriately adapt crucial operational parameters of the data monitoring algorithms.

DOI: 10.4018/978-1-61520-791-6.ch011

INTRODUCTION

Distributed mobile networks are of high interest in this information technology era, where efficient bandwidth utilization is a key issue due to its limited availability. These networks aim at the satisfaction of the Quality of Service (QOS) of heterogeneous information data traffics (e.g., image, audio, data, graphics, text), with simultaneous high utilization of network resources and bandwidths. The performance demands imposed on mobile networks carrying heterogeneous connections are challenging and can be satisfied via the deployment of highly dynamic statistical multiplexing protocols which honor the traffic QOS, while utilizing the network resources efficiently. While the successful design of high-performance traffic multiplexing protocols requires accurate modeling of traffic statistical characteristics and QOS, variations in the latter characteristics, topological network changes (some due to mobility) and/or failures in the response of network components, affect directly, and frequently dramatically, their performance characteristics. It is thus crucial that traffic and network performance monitoring techniques be deployed, first for the identification of traffic changes and network failures, and then for the subsequent adaptation of the protocol operations, the pertinent recovery of failures, and the appropriate reconfiguration of network topologies; such are the fundamental components towards the successful information management.

The main theme of this chapter is the effective traffic and performance monitoring of mobile heterogeneous networks, via the deployment of distributed and dynamic information management and network performance monitoring techniques. These techniques are implemented by statistically sound algorithms and are placed at key network locations, to accurately and efficiently track the dynamics of the system. The locations change as the network topology does; thus the traffic management and network performance monitoring system is mobile, where mobility induces time-varying network topologies.

This chapter suggests a systematic and comprehensive approach for the design of the distributed and mobile sub-network that monitors network and traffic dynamics, to subsequently dictate appropriate changes in accessing protocols (including bandwidth allocation), routing, and network topologies, and to also identify network failures.

We seek to develop and evaluate a mobile and distributed sub-network whose objective is to manage information traffic and to monitor network performance, in mobile heterogeneous networks. The fundamental issues addressed are:

- Characterization and modeling of the fundamental environment in which traffic and network performance monitoring operate, towards the development of a core monitoring algorithm.
- Identification of performance metrics and exploitation of algorithmic characteristics of the traffic and network performance monitoring techniques, as implemented by a mobile and distributed system.
- For given network topologies, identification of the minimum-size monitoring sub-network and its optimal topology, for complete traffic and network "visibility". Exploitation of tradeoffs between computational load and bandwidth for information exchange within the monitoring sub-network.
- Investigation of mobility and the time-varying topology for the monitoring sub-network, as functions of dynamically changing network topologies.
- Consideration of Artificial Intelligence (AI) learning techniques for the adaptation of key monitoring operational parameters in the presence of dynamically changing traffic and network environments.

BACKGROUND

The connectivity of mobile networks is secured via interconnected base stations. The interconnection network of the latter is generally broadband and may be either wireless or wire-line, such as the B-ISDN (Acampora, 1994; Pados, 1994; Paterakis, 1989). For heterogeneous mobile networks deploying the Asynchronous Transfer Mode (ATM), the base stations must include signaling detectors, pagers, and ATM switches which implement protocols for transmission.

It is desired that mobile networks support a wide range of services such as voice, low- and high-priority/speed data, image, audio, graphics, and text (Bar-Noy & Kessler, 1993; Burrell, 1994; Burrell & Papantoni-Kazakos, 1998; EIA/TIA, 1990; EIA/TIA, 1991; Meier-Hellstern, Pollini & Goodman, 1991; Special Issue on Asynchronous Transfer Mode, 1988; Special Issue on Portable and Mobile Communications, 1987). In existing networks, the medium access protocol is ALOHA-based and the protocols for transmission are hybrid TDMA/CDMA configurations. None of these protocols are directly suitable for the high demands placed on large scale mobile networks. The services offered by such networks produce an increased number of messages and cause the ALOHA-based medium access protocol to collapse. Additionally, the hybrid TDMA/ CDMA transmission protocols configurations may not, on their own, provide the flexibility required by the variety of traffic characteristics and QOS present in mobile heterogeneous environments (Burrell, 1994; Burrell & Papantoni-Kazakos, 1998; Raychaudhuri & Wilson, 1993; Ross, Gottschalck & Harrington, 1980).

Existing literature for mobile networks focuses on protocols for transmission (Acampora & Naghshineh, 1994; Berruto, Eynard, Fiorina & Napolitano, 1993; Chlamtac & Farago, 1994; Coviello & Vena, 1975; Goodman, Valenzuela, Gayliard, & Ramamurthi, 1989; Goodman & Wei, 1991; Kummerle, 1974; Liu & Papantoni-Kazakos, 1992; Liu & Papantoni-Kazakos, 1993; Nanda, Goodman, & Timor, 1991; Papantoni-Kazakos, 1992; Papantoni-Kazakos, Delic, Paterakis, & Liu, 1993; Papantoni-Kazakos, Likhanov, & Tsybakov, 1995; Paterakis, Georgiadis & Papantoni-Kazakos, 1989; Paterakis & Papantoni-Kazakos, 1989; Rozenbaum, Papantoni-Kazakos & Kazakos, 1995; Schwartz 1987; Tsybakov & Mikhailov, 1979); and on some system issues (Acampora, to appear; Bar-Noy & Kessler, 1993; Basagni, Chlamtac, Syrotiuk & Woodward, 1998; Chandler, Hulburt & McTiffin, 1991; Chlamtac & Farago, 1994; Coviello & Vena, 1975; Cox, 1992; Cox, 1991; EIA/TIA, 1990; EIA/TIA, 1991; Fischetti, 1993; Gejji, 1992; Gilhousen, Jacobs, Padovani, Viterbi, Weaver & Wheatley III, 1991; Goodman & Wei, 1991; Goodman, 1991; Goodman, Pollini & Meier-Hellstern, 1992; Gruber, 1982; Guo & Morgera, 1993; Jain, Lin, Lo & Mohan, 1994; Jakes, 1974; Karn, 1990; Lee, 1982; Lee, 1989; Lee, 1991; Lin, 1994; Liu & Papantoni-Kazakos, 1992; Meier-Hellstern, Pollini & Goodman, 1991; Meier-Hellstern, G.P. Pollini, and D.J. Goodman; Mermelstein, Jalali & Leib, 1993; Mohan & Jain, 1994; Prakash, Shivaratrai & Singhal, 1995; Raychaudhuri & Wilson, 1993; Raychaudhuri, 1994; Ross, Gottschalck & Harrington, 1980; Special Issue on Asynchronous Transfer Mode, 1988; Special Issue on Portable and Mobile Communications, 1987; Wang, 1993; Winters, 1993; Woodruff and R. Kositpaiboon, 1990; Zhang, Hafez & Falconer, 1994). The proposed protocols consist mainly of TDMA, CDMA and an integration of both; they mainly address only voice or sometimes voice and data. As an exception, for environments with dynamically changing heterogeneous traffics, dynamic transmission protocols have been proposed and analyzed in (Burrell & Papantoni-Kazakos, 1998; Burrell & Papantoni-Kazakos, 1996; Burrell, Makrakis & Papantoni-Kazakos, 1998); in (Burrell & Papantoni-Kazakos, 1996), a stable medium access protocol is proposed as well. The system issues addressed are either partially architectural or focus on user locations and they do not include the larger and comprehensive traffic and network management issues. The issues of traffic and network performance monitoring, implemented by a mobile and distributed sub-network, have been completely ignored. Some isolated views on loss performance monitoring can be found in (Moa, 2005; IEEE Communications Magazine, 2008).

APPROACH OUTLINE

Mobile networks consist of two parts — mobile users and base stations interconnected via a generally broadband wire-line or wireless backbone network. The base stations provide connectivity between mobile users and can also access network data banks. The base stations may also be mobile and the backbone network they form may be dynamically re-configurable.

Three stages are necessary in establishing a communication path between either two mobile users or a mobile user and a data bank:

1) *Signaling or Medium Access* from the initiating user to the base station,
2) *Paging* from the base station to either other users (addressed via broadcasting) or to the data bank sought, and
3) *Transmission* via a path established by the base station and announced to the involved users.

The signaling/medium access and transmission stages require careful design of the corresponding protocols and of the pertinent architectural connectivity, so that the time-varying multimedia traffic QOS be satisfied and the overall system performance be satisfactory and controllable. This can only be accomplished with the assistance of high-level traffic and performance monitoring protocols that track the system dynamics effectively, and subsequently dictate time-varying capacity allocations to heterogeneous traffics, as well as possible reconfigurations of network topologies.

In this chapter, we present an approach towards the development of a mobile and distributed system that implements the traffic and performance monitoring techniques in an efficient and accurate fashion. We first present the fundamental characterizations and modeling of the traffic and network performance environments, and subsequently propose a core sequential monitoring algorithm. We then identify the metrics monitored and discuss the corresponding algorithmic characteristics of the core algorithm, as implemented by a distributed sub-network. Subsequently, we discuss the issue of the minimal size of a distributed monitoring sub-network for complete network and traffic "visibility" in given network topologies, and the resulting tradeoffs between computational load and information exchange within the sub-network. Consequently, we present and discuss the issue of sub-network mobility and structural variation as a function of dynamically varying network topologies. Finally, we present the consideration of AI learning techniques for the adaptation of key monitoring operational parameters in the presence of dynamically changing network environments.

CHARACTERIZATIONS AND MODELING – A CORE MONITORING ALGORITHM

In heterogeneous mobile environments, various traffic classes are present (i.e., voice, image, high-speed data, etc.) and the statistical characteristics per class are time-varying. In some cases, the traffic variations consist of changes solely in traffic rates, while the statistical characteristics of the traffics remain parametrically known (traffics generated by well-characterized processes). The per traffic class time-varying traffic characteristics, in conjunction with the deployed network multiplexing protocols (for transmission, medium access, routing, etc.), induce time-varying network performance characteristics (i.e., delays, traffic blocking rates, wasted capacity rates, etc., per traffic class) as well. It is desired that traffics and network performance metrics be continuously monitored to identify, timely and accurately, changes in their statistical characteristics, for subsequent adaptation of network operations and protocols, for identification of network failures, and for possible topological reconfigurations as well. The development of statistically sound monitoring techniques requires that first the traffics and network performance metrics be effectively modeled, so that the models capture their statistical variations. We model them as sets of distinct and well-known stochastic processes (e.g., Poisson with known rates, geometric with known parameters, etc.). For example, for the k-th traffic class we consider the general scenario where the various possible arrival processes that characterize the traffic may be represented by the set $\{\mu_i^{(k)}\}_{1\le i\le M}$ where $\mu_i^{(k)}$ depicts a well-known process, such as a Poisson process with known fixed rate, and where all processes in the set are distinct (e.g., all Poisson with different and distinct rates); it is assumed that the set $\{\mu_i^{(k)}\}_{1\le i\le M}$ has been obtained via thorough traffic characterization methods. The objective of monitoring the k-th traffic class is then to identify, timely and accurately, shifts from some process $\mu_j^{(k)}$ in the set to any other process in the same set. Below, we present a core monitoring algorithm that operates on models represented by sets of distinct stochastic processes.

We first represent an initial restricted form of the algorithm and then a re-initialization extension. The latter actually represents the core monitoring algorithm that we propose. Both the initial restricted form and the re-initialization extension operate on observed data sequences $x_1, x_2, \ldots, x_n, \ldots$ that are generated by the acting processes (e.g., in the case of processes representing traffics, the x_i's may be numbers of arrivals within consecutive fixed-length time intervals). Below, we use the abbreviated form x_1^n, for the sequence $x_1, \ldots, x_n$.

Initial Restricted Algorithm

The restricted algorithm addresses the following problem.

Let the process which initially generates the data sequence be the process μ_0. Let it be possible that a shift to any one of M-1 independent processes μ_i; i=1, ..., M-1 may occur at any point in time, where if a $\mu_0 \rightarrow \mu_i$ shift occurs, then the process μ_i remains active thereafter. The objective is to detect the occurrence of a $\mu_0 \rightarrow \mu_i$ shift as accurately and as timely as possible, including the detection of the process μ_i which μ_{00} changed to. Let us denote by f_i; i=0, 1, ..., M-1 density or probability functions induced by the processes μ_i; i=0, 1, ..., M-1. Then, for the present problem, we propose the following algorithm, fully analyzed in (Burrell & Papantoni-Kazakos, 1998).

Algorithm

(a) Select a threshold $\delta_0 > 0$.

(b) Have M-1 parallel algorithms operating. The ith algorithm; i=1, ..., M-1 is monitoring a $\mu_0 \rightarrow \mu_i$ shift. $T_n^{0i}(x_1^n)$ denotes the operating value of the ith algorithm at time n, given the observation sequence x_1^n. The operating value $T_n^{0i}(x_1^n)$ is updated as follows:

$$T_0^{0i} \equiv 0$$

$$T_n^{0i}(x_1^n) = \max\left(0,\ T_{n-1}^{0i}(x_1^{n-1}) + \log \frac{f_i(x_n \mid x_1^{n-1})}{f_0(x_n \mid x_1^{n-1})}\right)$$

(c) The algorithmic system stops the first time n when either one of the M-1 parallel algorithms crosses the common threshold δ_0. If the ith algorithm is the one that first crosses the threshold, then it is declared that a $\mu_0 \rightarrow \mu_i$ shift has occurred. □

The algorithm described above is clearly sequential and thus computationally simple and efficient. Its fundamental performance characteristics are given by the Theorem and the Corollary given below, where first some quantities are defined.

Let N_{0i} denote the extended stopping variable induced by the ith algorithm in the system; that is, $N_{0i} \triangleq inf\left\{n : T_n^{0i}(x_1^n) \geq \delta_0\right\}$. Let us define the following quantities:

$$L_n^{ij}(x_1^n) \triangleq n^{-1} \log \frac{f_j(x_1^n)}{f_i(x_1^n)} \qquad ;i, j=0,\ 1,\ ..,\ M\text{-}1$$

$$I_{ij} \triangleq \lim_{n \to \infty} L_n^{ij}(x_1^n) \qquad ;i, j=0,\ 1,\ ..,\ M\text{-}1$$

$$p_n^{ij}(v) \triangleq P\ (L_n^{ij}(x_1^n) < v\,|\mu_j) \qquad ;i, j=0,\ 1,\ ..,\ M\text{-}1$$

Consider then, the following conditions:

(A) I_{ij};i,j=0,1,..,M-1 exist and
$I_{ij} = E\left\{I_{ij}|\mu_j\right\}$, a.s. (P_{μ_j})

(B) For i, j=0, 1, .., M-1 and for $v \in (0, I_{ij})$,

$$\lim_{n \to \infty} n\ p_n^{ij}(v) = 0 \text{ and } \sum_{n \geq 1} p_n^{ij}(v) < \infty$$

Conditions (A) state the existence of the generalized Kullback-Leibler information numbers $\left\{I_{ij}\right\}$ while conditions (B) ensure that the convergence of the large-deviation probabilities $\left\{p_n^{ij}(v)\right\}$ is sufficiently fast. The following theorem and corollary can now be expressed.

Theorem 1

Let the processes $\{\mu_j; j=0, 1, .., M\text{-}1\}$ be stationary, ergodic, mutually independent, and satisfying conditions (A) and (B). Then,

$$\text{As } \delta_0 \to \infty,\ \underset{\substack{j=0,1,..,M-1 \\ i=1,...,M-1}}{E\{N_{0i}|\mu_j\}} : \begin{cases} \sim \left[I_{0j} - I_{ij}\right]^{-1} \log \delta_0 & ;\text{ if } I_{0j} \geq I_{ij} \\ \geq 2^{-1}\delta_0 & ;\text{ if } I_{0j} < I_{ij} \end{cases}$$

Corollary

Given that the process μ_j; j=1, .., M-1 is acting throughout, the algorithmic system will asymptotically detect the $\mu_0 \to \mu_j$ shift correctly, in the expected stopping time sense. That is:

$$E\left\{N_{0j}\,|\,\mu_j\right\} \sim I_{0j}^{-1} \log \delta_0 : \begin{cases} < E\left\{N_{0i}\,|\,\mu_j\right\} \sim \left[I_{0j} - I_{ij}\right]^{-1} \log \delta_0 & ;\quad \forall i \neq j : I_{0j} > I_{ij} \\ < E\left\{N_{0i}\,|\,\mu_j\right\} \geq 2^{-1}\delta_0 & ;\quad \forall i \neq j : I_{0j} < I_{ij} \end{cases}$$

Given that the process μ_j ; j =1, .., M-1 is acting throughout, the asymptotic expected stopping time of the algorithmic system is: $E\left\{N_{0j}\,|\,\mu_j\right\} \sim I_{0j}^{-1} \log \delta_0$. □

We note that the performance of the algorithm depends on the values of the Kullback-Leibler numbers $\{I_{ij}\}$ which represent a measure of "closeness" between the different processes in the model. The "closer" to each other the processes are in that sense, the worst is the performance of the algorithmic system.

Re-Initialization Extension

The re-initialization extension of the restricted algorithm consists of its sequential repetitions, as dictated by its instantaneous decisions. Specifically, if the restricted algorithm above decides that the process μ_m starts acting, then a μ_m to any one of the remaining processes monitoring starts immediately, utilizing a decision threshold δ_m. This process goes on indefinitely.

Non-Asymptotic Performance

The algorithmic system described above utilizes the reflective threshold zero and a decisive threshold $\delta_m > 0$, for detecting a change from a acting

Figure 1. Time evolution of sequential algorithmic system for monitoring μ_m to any other process change

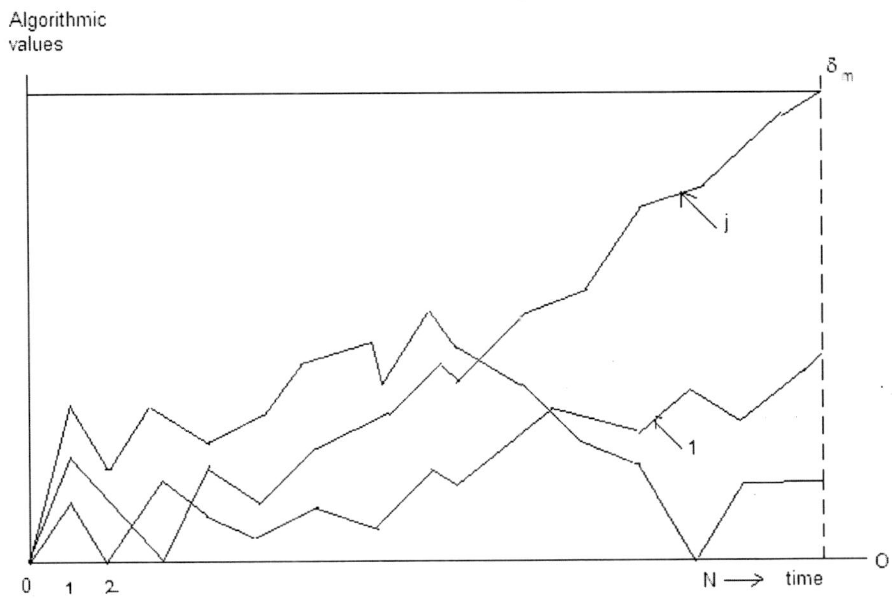

stochastic process μ_m to one of the m-1 remaining processes.. Figure 1 depicts a time evolution of the system.

We note that the M-1 parallel algorithms included in the algorithmic system are sequential with low complexity updating steps. The implementation possibility of the algorithmic system clearly depends on its non-asymptotic performance. In particular, we are interested in the performance of the system when the threshold values δ_j ; j = 0,..., M-1 are finite and when the conditional probabilities utilized by the algorithms are simply available, without any statistically qualifying conditions being imposed on them. The objective is then to determine non-asymptotic performance metrics and to subsequently utilize these metrics for the selection of the decision thresholds. After the selection of the latter thresholds is complete, the overall system performance can be predictably known.

To detect a change from the acting stochastic process μ_m to one of the remaining M-1 processes, the algorithmic system utilizes M-1 parallel algorithms and a common threshold $\delta_m > 0$. Each one of the M-1 parallel algorithms monitors then a change from process μ_m to one of the remaining M-1 processes. The algorithm, which crosses the common threshold first, dictates the global decision by the system. We now discuss performance metrics for one of the M-1 parallel algorithms, say the one that monitors a change from process μ_m to process μ_l where m differs from l. The performance of this algorithm is basically characterized by two time curves: the power and false alarm curves, denoted respectively β_{ml} (n) and α_{ml}(n), where n denotes the time instant t_n and where,

β_{ml} (n): The probability that the μ_m to μ_l change monitoring algorithm crosses its threshold before or at time t_n, given that the acting process is μ_l throughout.

α_{ml} (n): The probability that the μ_m to μ_l change monitoring algorithm crosses its threshold before or at time t_n, given that the acting process is μ_m throughout.

In Figure 2 below, we depict the β_{ml} (n) and α_{ml} (n) curves, to observe and discuss qualitative behavior. We plot these curves for two different threshold values.

From Figure 2, we note that as the value of the decision threshold increases, the false alarm curve decreases, but so does the power curve. The threshold selection for the μ_m to μ_l change monitoring algorithm may be based on a required lower bound for the power and a required upper bound for the false alarm, at a given time instant t_n. When all the M-1 algorithms that monitor change from process μ_m are considered, the common threshold δ_m may be selected based on the following principle: At given time t_n, have the powers induced by the parallel algorithms be above a predetermined lower bound, while the false alarm induced by each algorithm remains below a predetermined upper bound. After the common threshold, δ_m for the detection of change from process μ_m to one of the M-1 remaining processes has been selected, the performance of the corresponding algorithmic system needs to be evaluated. The appropriate performance metrics are the set $\{\beta^j_{ml}$ (n)$\}$; j,l = 0,..m-1; m different from l, where,

β^j_{ml} (n): Given that the process μ_j is acting throughout, the probability that the algorithmic system makes a decision in favor of process μ_l, before or at time t_n.

Clearly, it is desirable that for each given process μ_j, the power β^j_{mj}(n) be larger than each β^j_{ml}(n), for l different than j, for all n. In other words, the desirable behavior should be as that exhibited in Figure 3, where better behavior is represented by larger differences β^j_{mj}(n) - β^j_{ml}(n), for j different than l.

The performance of the algorithmic system that monitors process μ_m to any other process change is qualitatively determined by the values of the probabilities of correct decision $\{\beta^j_{mj}$(n)$\}$, at some predetermined time t_n, in conjunction with the values of incorrect decision probabilities

Figure 2. False alarm and power curves for the μ_m to μ_l change monitoring algorithm. Threshold values $\delta_m < \delta_m'$.

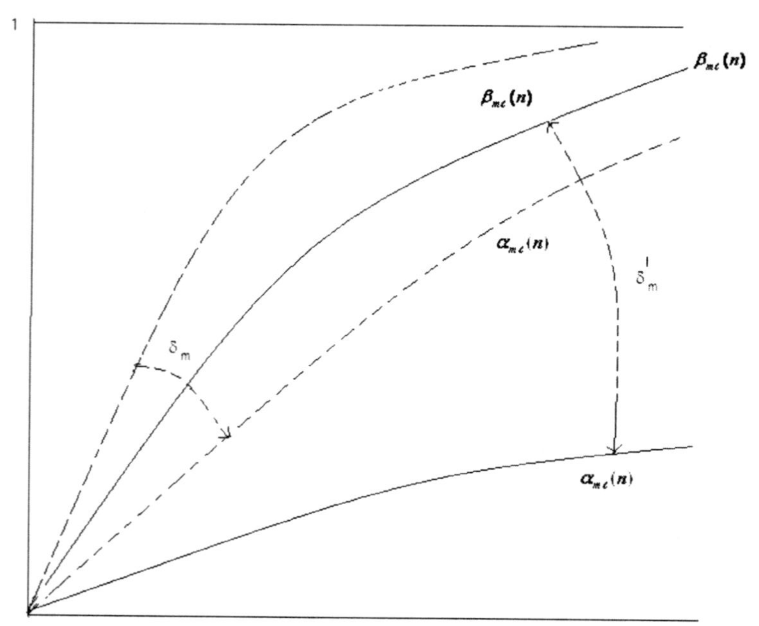

Figure 3. Given acting process μ_j, probability curves induced by the μ_m to any other process change monitoring system, where j different than l.

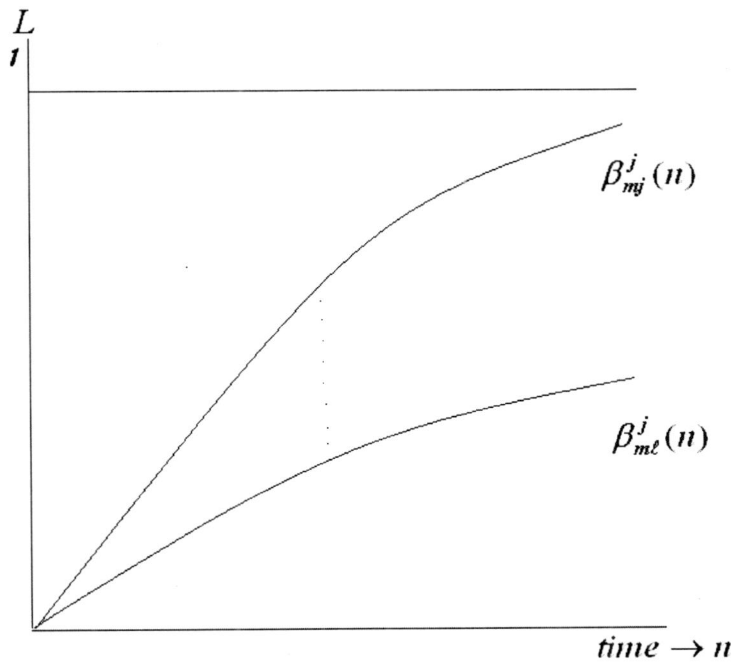

$\{\beta^j_{ml}(n)\}$. The former should be high, while the latter should be as low as possible.

THE POISSON TRAFFIC MODEL WITH GEOMETRICLY DISTRIBUTED CHANGES

In mobile network environments, the mobile units are frequently spatially randomly and independently distributed and their number is large. A least favorable scenario arises then when each unit is perceived as basically transmitting a short duration pulse and then expiring. This, gives rise to a Poisson traffic model; that is, the overall data traffic may be modeled as cumulatively comprising a homogeneous Poisson process, with rate λ bits/time unit. Due to the mobility and the possible expiring of the units, the rate of the latter Poisson process varies in real time, among a set of rates $\{\lambda_i\}$. The monitoring algorithm is deployed to continuously monitor such rate changes, where the observed data used by the algorithm are number of data arrivals within consecutive frames of fixed number of time units. The Poisson arrival process is memoryless: the conditioning in the log-ratio updating step of the restricted monitoring algorithm then drops. If d denotes the length of a frame in time units and n_r denotes the number of data arrivals within the rth frame of the algorithm's execution, the $\{\lambda_k \rightarrow \lambda_j\}$ monitoring algorithm takes the following form:

$$V_{kj}(0) \overset{\Delta}{=} 0$$

$$V_{kj}(r+1) = \max\left(0,\; V_{kj}(r) + d\left[\lambda_k - \lambda_j + n_{r+1} \log\left(\frac{\lambda_j}{\lambda_k}\right)\right]\right) \tag{1}$$

where n_{r+1} denotes the number of data arrivals within the (r+1)[th] frame from the beginning of the $\{\lambda_k \rightarrow \lambda_j\}$ monitoring algorithm.

Let us define:

$$\zeta(\lambda_k,\lambda_j) \triangleq [\lambda_k - \lambda_j][\log(\frac{\lambda_k}{\lambda_j})]^{-1} \quad (2)$$

where $\min(\lambda_k, \lambda_j) < \zeta(\lambda_k, \lambda_j) < \max(\lambda_k, \lambda_j)$. We may select $\{\lambda_i\}$ rates such that $\zeta(\lambda_k, \lambda_j)$ are rational numbers for all k and j, and we then define the integers t_{kj} and s_{kj}, $t_{kj} < s_{kj}$, as follows:

$$\zeta(\lambda_k,\lambda_j) = \frac{t_{kj}}{s_{kj}} \quad (3)$$

The algorithmic thresholds can then all be selected as positive integers, and without lack in generality, the algorithmic adaptation in (1) can be transformed as follows:

$$V_{kj}(r+1) = \max\{0, V_{kj}(r) + (-1)^{\text{ime}(k,j)}[s_{kj}n_{r+1} - dt_{kj}]\} \quad (4)$$

where:

$$\text{ime}(k,j) = \begin{cases} 0; & \text{if } \lambda_j > \lambda_k \\ 1; & \text{if } \lambda_j < \lambda_k \end{cases}$$

Considering the above per frame algorithmic adaptations, the pertinent Kullback-Leibler numbers

$\{K_d\ \{\lambda'_i / \lambda_q\}\}$, are per frame adaptations; thus,

$$K_d\ \{\lambda'_i / \lambda_q\} = d\lambda_q[1 - \frac{\lambda'_i}{\lambda_q} + \frac{\lambda'_i}{\lambda_q}\ln(\frac{\lambda'_i}{\lambda_q})] \quad (5)$$

$$K_{d,\max}(\lambda_m) = d\lambda_m \max\{1 - \frac{\lambda'_0}{\lambda_m} + \frac{\lambda'_0}{\lambda_m}\ln(\frac{\lambda'_0}{\lambda_m}),\ 1 - \frac{\lambda'_{n-1}}{\lambda_m} + \frac{\lambda'_{n-1}}{\lambda_m}\ln(\frac{\lambda'_{n-1}}{\lambda_m})\} \quad (6)$$

where the design rates monitored are $\lambda_0 < \lambda_1 < \lambda_2 < \ldots < \lambda_{n-1}$, and where $\lambda'_0 < \lambda'_1 < \ldots < \lambda'_{n-1}$ are the acting rates.

The randomness and independence of the times at which units may expire is best modeled by a geometric distribution. In particular, we may assume then that shifts from a given acting rate to either one of the remaining acting rates are equally probable and that the time period during which a given rate λ'_i is continuously acting is geometric, having the form, $Q_i(k) = (1-\rho_i)^{-1}\rho_i^{k-1}$; $k \geq 1$, where k is measured in time units. The expected time $E\{l_i\}$ during which λ'_i is continuously acting and the average fraction of time γ_i for the λ'_i activity are:

$$E\{l_i\} = (1-\rho_i)^{-1}$$

$$\gamma_i = [\sum_{k=0}^{n-1} E\{l_k\}]^{-1} E\{l_i\} = [\sum_{k=0}^{n-1}(1-\rho_k)^{-1}]^{-1}(1-\rho_i)^{-1}$$

where n is the total number of rates considered. Given n, and assuming rates ordered as $\lambda_0 < \lambda_1 < \ldots < \lambda_{n-1}$, we may select the γ_i's such that $\gamma_{n-1} < \ldots < \gamma_0$ and the γ_i 's sum to 1. Then, for some constant $C > \max\left\{\frac{1}{\gamma_0}, \ldots, \frac{1}{\gamma_{n-1}}\right\}$, the ρ_i values are determined as $\rho_i = 1 - (C\gamma_i)^{-1}$; $0 \leq i \leq n-1$. Regarding the selection of the of the γ_i's, we adopt a geometric structure, for ease of graphic representation. Specifically, for some constant α, $0 \leq \alpha \leq 1$, we may generate the γ_i's as follows:

$$\gamma_0 = \gamma_0(\alpha) = (1-\alpha^n)^{-1}(1-\alpha)$$
$$\gamma_1 = \gamma_1(\alpha) = \alpha\gamma_1(\alpha) = (1-\alpha^n)^{-1}(1-\alpha)\alpha$$
$$\vdots$$
$$\gamma_{n-1} = \gamma_{n-1}(\alpha) = \alpha^{n-1}\gamma_1(\alpha) = (1-\alpha^n)^{-1}(1-\alpha)\alpha^{n-1}$$

Thus, for any α value, the generated γ_i's are such that $\gamma_{n-1} < \ldots < \gamma_0$ and the γ_i values sum to 1. The following conclusions can be drawn:

a) $\gamma_0(\alpha)$ is a decreasing function of α.
b) For $1 \leq k \leq \frac{n-1}{2}$, there exists α_k such that $\gamma_k(\alpha)$ is an increasing function of α for $\alpha < \alpha_k$, and is a decreasing function of α for $\alpha > \alpha_k$.
c) For $k \geq \frac{n-1}{2}$, $\gamma_k(\alpha)$ is an increasing function of α.
d) In general, as α decreases, the higher rates become increasingly bursty, while the frequencies with which the lower rates occur increase monotonically; as $\alpha \rightarrow 0$, γ_0 approaches 1. As α increases, instead, the frequencies of occurrence for the different rates tend to equalization; as $\alpha \rightarrow 1$, the γ_i values all approach n^{-1}, for $0 \leq i \leq n-1$.

In the Appendix, we include recursive expressions used for the computations of the probability curves of Figures 2 and 3, as induced by the monitoring algorithm, for the Poisson-geometric model.

MONITORED METRICS AND DISTRIBUTED MONITORING SYSTEM

The metrics to be monitored in the mobile environment are determined by the objectives. The global objectives are traffic and network management.

Traffic Management — Monitoring Metrics

Traffic management refers to the development of effective signaling/medium access and transmission algorithms and protocols that, in conjunction with dynamic capacity allocation techniques, satisfy the various Quality of Service (QOS) characteristics of the time-varying heterogeneous traffics. The dynamic capacity allocation techniques (Burrell & Papantoni-Kazakos, 1998; Burrell & Papantoni-Kazakos, 1996; Burrell, Makrakis & Papantoni-Kazakos, 1998) are assisted by Traffic Monitoring Algorithms (TMA), such as those in Section 4, which track effectively changes in the statistical characteristics of the traffics (such as rates). The various characteristics of both the external and the intra-network traffics are modeled as sets of distinct stochastic processes (see Section 4) and the monitored metrics are the corresponding number of traffic arrivals.

Network Management — Functions and Monitored Metrics

Network management is a crucial issue, which has not been comprehensively addressed. It should be clear, however, that the key components of effective network management are performance monitoring, identification of network failures, and topological network reconfigurations assisted by traffic monitoring techniques. We proceed with the concretion of these concepts.

Performance Monitoring

Performance monitoring is the indispensable component in network management. The term is meaningful only if, at first, the important network performance metrics are identified, and then, statistically reliable algorithms are deployed for the continuous monitoring of these metrics. The key network performance metrics are: delays, traffic rejection rates, wasted network resource rates, and satisfaction of the various other (e.g., jittering, bit error rates, etc.) traffic QOS. Under normal network operational conditions (low error channels, fast ATM switches, etc.), the "other" traffic QOS are observed if comprehensively designed dynamic signaling and transmission multiplexing protocols are deployed, assisted by a TMA. In the latter case, the remaining key network performance metrics are delays (D), rejection rates per traffic message (MRR), and wasted capacity rates (WCR). Given normal network operational conditions, given comprehensively designed protocols for signaling and transmission, the D, MRR, and WCR metrics take predictable (via analysis and numerical evaluations) values for given statistical descriptions of the various network traffics (see [10, 62]). Thus, the reasons for the monitoring of the D, MRR, and WCR metrics are either to identify changes in traffic characterizations for normal operational network conditions, or, in conjunction with traffic monitoring, to identify failures in network components and functions. Our proposal is to:

- Deploy continuous monitoring algorithms/protocols for the D, MRR, and WCR network performance metrics, as well as the traffic monitoring protocols, as those in Section 4, for the identification of network failures.

Given the statistical descriptions of the various network traffics, given comprehensively designed and fully analyzed and evaluated protocols for signaling and transmission, complete statistical characterizations of the D, MRR, and WCR network performance metrics are feasible (see (Burrell 1994; Burrell, Papantoni-Kazakos, 1996; Burrell, Makrakis & Papantoni-Kazakos, 1998; Special Issue on Portable and Mobile Communications, 1987)). Thus, the monitoring of these metrics can be implemented by sequential algorithms as those in Section 4. To present our ideas clearly, consider one of the three metrics (D, MRR, or WCR) and complete statistical descriptions of the network traffics (provided by a priori traffic analyses in conjunction with decisions induced by the traffic monitoring protocol). Given the statistical descriptions of the network traffics, the distribution of the metric under normal operational conditions of the network is known (obtained via a priori performance analysis of the deployed signaling and transmission protocols). In addition, a set of "abnormal" distributions of the metric may be characterized then, each representing a distinct "abnormal" network state.

A performance monitoring system for the metric at hand may then include sequential algorithms, as those in Section 4, to detect shifts from the distribution of the metric under normal operational conditions of the network to any of the "abnormal" distributions (each being associated with a specific "abnormal" network state). The performance monitoring system for the metric may also include sequential estimation algorithms for some of its statistical measures and comparisons of the estimated values with those predicted by the analysis of the signaling/medium access and transmission protocols.

Identification of Failures

In consistency with our above proposal, we may consider the simultaneous deployment of specific and comprehensively designed signaling/medium access and transmission protocols, (together with their full evaluation and subsequent performance figures and tables), of traffic monitoring protocols as those in Section 4, and of the-similar to the latter-monitoring protocols of the D, MRR, and the WCR network performance metrics. The decisions performed by the traffic monitoring system dictate the distributions of the D, MRR, and WCR metrics both under normal and "abnormal" operational network conditions. These distributions can be used by the — as that in Section 4 — sequential algorithmic system to detect shifts from normal to "abnormal" or failing states of network components. For example, if the traffic monitoring and the performance monitoring operations are performed at the origin versus the destination ends of a unidirectional network channel, failures at the channel/fiber level will be detected (see (Papantoni-Kazakos, 1992; Papantoni-Kazakos, Delic, Paterakis, & Liu, 1993). Generally, our approach can lead to a comprehensively designed and powerful performance-monitoring/failure-recognition system, where the accuracy of failure-decisions may be high. The overall system can be analyzed and evaluated, where the issues arising include: stability, and probabilities of correct versus false decisions.

Traffic and Performance Monitoring for Network Reconfigurations

The capacity of the wireless channels (signaling/medium access and transmission) is predetermined and limited. At the same time, the mobile user population is time-varying (due to mobility) and imposes a variety of constraints. It is thus important that powerful protocols for signaling/medium access and transmission be deployed, whose operations are insensitive to the user population and which also induce high channel utilization with simultaneous satisfaction of the constraints imposed by the users. Some of their operational characteristics depend (for throughput maximization), however, on the intensities of the user traffics, on the values of the constraints for accessing delays and blocking probabilities, and on the distributions of message lengths generated by the users. Based on relatively accurate projections of mobile user populations, the characteristics of the latter protocols may be designed to provide high performance (throughput and delays) for a range of user populations and traffic intensities and specifications. The protocols can then also effectively accommodate users who move across areas controlled by different base-stations, when hand-off techniques are superimposed. In addition, the performance of the designed protocols for signaling/medium access and transmission (throughput, delays) can be predicted for every given set of user characteristics; conversely, specific quantitative performance of these protocols can lead to conclusions about the characteristics of the acting wireless populations; such are the protocols in (Burrell, Papantoni-Kazakos, 1996; Burrell, Makrakis & Papantoni-Kazakos, 1998) and the medium access protocol in (Papantoni-Kazakos, P., Likhanov, N., & Tsybakov, B. S. (1995). This suggests that the deployment of an Automated-traffic and performance-Monitoring System (AMS) may facilitate network reconfigurations. We specifically propose that:

- The AMS be deployed at the base stations. The AMS may dynamically compute expected delays, blocking probabilities, and throughputs induced by the deployed protocols for signaling/medium access and transmission (for each of the heterogeneous traffic classes), and may continuously compare the found numbers against those predicted by the performance analysis of the deployed protocols. As a result of this comparison, the AMS can estimate characteristics of the mobile user populations (traffic intensities and specifications for all traffic classes). Using these estimates, in conjunction with pre-computed performance characteristics of the deployed protocols for signaling/medium access and transmission, the AMS may then implement appropriate changes in network architectures and protocols (whenever judged as necessary) and may notify the users accordingly.

The effective design of the AMS implies thorough quantitative studies of the deployed signaling/medium access and transmission protocols as well as of the monitoring algorithms in Section 4, for various characteristics of the heterogeneous traffics. The results of such studies can be maintained in memory and can be used by the AMS for the reconfiguration of network architectures and the adaptation of signaling/medium access and transmission protocols.

DISTRIBUTED MONITORING SUB-NETWORK AND ALGORITHMIC PERFORMANCE CHARACTERISTICS

The traffic and network performance monitoring operations are performed by a monitoring sub-network whose nodes are generally located in key nodes of the backbone network and execute distributed functions. Each sub-network node monitors a subset of network elements (nodes, channels, etc.). The performance monitoring characteristics of the monitoring algorithms, as executed by the distributed sub-network, affect the overall system performance and the induced tradeoffs. Below, we discuss such effects for traffic versus network performance monitoring.

Traffic Monitoring

Traffic monitoring may be used to dictate dynamic capacity allocations to the various multimedia heterogeneous traffics at the transmission stage, and to also facilitate the failure recognition and network reconfiguration processes (see above). The implementation of dynamic capacity allocation may be facilitated by frame-structures, where the capacity per frame allocated to each traffic category is a direct function of the corresponding acting traffic process decided upon by the Traffic Monitoring Algorithm (TMA) (Burrell & Papantoni-Kazakos, 1998).

When the combinations of traffic monitoring, dynamic capacity allocation, and either Time Domain or Code Division Multiple Access or hybrid transmission policies are considered, rejections of traffic messages are caused either by violations of possible imposed admission delay constraints or by decisions of the TMA that reduce capacity allocations to levels causing interruptions of messages in transmission, (see Burrell & Papantoni-Kazakos, 1996; Burrell, Makrakis & Papantoni-Kazakos, 1998]. For the TMA/Time Domain Multiple Access combinations, capacity waste results from the allocation of excess capacity by the TMA and due to transmission power-ups and synchronization, (see Burrell & Papantoni-Kazakos, 1996). For the TMA/Code Division Multiple Access combination, the encoding for the spreading is also contributing to the capacity waste via a bandwidth expansion factor, while an additional contribution to wasted capacity is due to the single common power-up and synchronization loss per frame, (see Burrell & Papantoni-Kazakos, 1996). At the same time, the contribution of power-up and synchronization loss for the Time Domain Access policy equals the average number of all messages in transmission per frame times the fraction of a slot required for a single power-up and synchronization loss.

We note that keeping the size of packets fixed (in number of bytes) and maintaining fixed frame sizes in terms of time length, the number of time slots per frame increases as the speed of the transmission channels increases. Channel speed should thus be expected to be an important factor in the selection between the TMA/Time Domain Multiple Access and the TMA/Code Division Multiple Access policies; for lower channel speeds, fewer messages will be concurrently in transmission per channel frame, and thus less power-up and synchronization losses will be induced by the Time Domain policy. Similarly, shorter message lengths will also reduce power-up and synchronization losses. In short, the Time Domain Multiple Access policy outperforms the TMA/Code Division Multiple Access policy when the speed of the transmission links is relatively low and the lengths of the transmitted messages are relatively short, (see Burrell & Papantoni-Kazakos, 1996).

The rejection rates of traffic messages and the wasted capacity rates induced by the traffic monitoring and dynamic capacity allocation combination are involved in a tradeoff that may be partially controlled by the selection of the thresholds in the monitoring algorithmic systems in Section 4 [Burrell, 1994; Burrell & Papantoni-Kazakos, 1996; Burrell, Makrakis & Papantoni-Kazakos, 1998).

The distributed sub-network nodes monitor local traffics and are fully capable of independent decisions about local traffic changes and subsequent local dynamically adapted capacity allocations. For global system optimality, however, to apply globally optimal capacity allocations and possible system topological reconfigurations, information about the overall system traffic is needed. Then, information exchange among traffic monitoring network nodes becomes a necessary attribute and induces a computational load versus bandwidth for information exchange tradeoff.

Network Performance Monitoring

As discussed earlier in this section, coupled with traffic monitoring, network performance monitoring may be used for failure recognition and for subsequent pertinent topological reconfigurations, and involves the continuous monitoring of the delays (D), rejection rates per traffic message (MRR), and wasted capacity rates (WCR) performance metrics (per traffic class). The activated monitoring algorithmic systems for the D, MRR, and WCR metrics are controlled by the corresponding traffic monitoring algorithms: per traffic class, the specific D, MRR, and WCR monitoring algorithms are associated with the stochastic process that the corresponding TMA has decided as being the one describing the acting traffic characteristics. Thus, the performances of the monitoring systems for the D, MRR, and WCR metrics are very sensitive to the accuracy of the decisions induced by the TMA. For given network topology, it is very important that the effects of the TMA performance on the performances of the monitoring systems for the D, MRR, and WCR metrics and the factors involved be thoroughly and quantitatively studied, for various signaling/medium access and transmission deployed multiple access protocols. Factors that influence strongly the specifics of these coupled performances (between TMAs and monitoring systems for the D, MRR, and WCR metrics) include the adopted set of stochastic processes that models the traffics and their variations (i.e., the Kullback-Leibler numbers between them, as in Section 4) and all the algorithmic thresholds (of all the monitoring algorithms involved).

The distributed nodes of the monitoring sub-network monitor local D, MRR, and WCR performance metrics using TMA decisions which are frequently performed by other monitoring nodes in other localities. Thus, the accurate and timely communication of information among the distributed sub-network nodes is a crucial issue here and a vital factor in the overall system performance. The importance of this issue is further amplified when global failure and topological reconfiguration decisions need to be made. The tradeoff between computational load and bandwidth for information exchange rises again, where the specific localities of the monitoring nodes affect this tradeoff and also impact the overall system performance.

MINIMAL SIZE SUB-NETWORK

To this point, we have discussed the nature of the network metrics monitored, the monitoring algorithms, and some performance characteristics inherent in the monitoring algorithmic systems, when they operate either interactively (as network performance monitoring does with traffic monitoring) or non-interactively. In this section, we focus on the issue of distributiveness for the sub-network that implements the monitoring: the minimal set of monitoring nodes needed for network "visibility", their localities, the induced information exchange versus computational loads tradeoffs and sub-network mobility and structure, as functions of dynamic network topologies.

Minimal Size of Monitoring Sub-Network for Given Fixed Network Topology

The performance of the mobile information network, as perceived by the users, is measured by the "success" of message transmission attempts, where "success" means satisfaction of all the imposed QOS as well as good delay characteristics, and where "failure" is synonymous to rejection. Thus, from the point of view of the network users, the identification of a transmission attempt as successful or non-successful is based on the overall origin-to-destination performance, where origins and destinations are local base stations. We note that local base stations are where traffics are both generated and disseminated. We also note that through measurements at the local base stations, in conjunction with the complete operational characterization of the deployed signaling/medium access, transmission, and routing protocols, as well as the deployed dynamic capacity allocation techniques, the global network D, MRR, and WCR performance metrics can be quantified. We finally note that the mobile network includes additional internal processing nodes, not included in the set of local base stations.

As can be easily concluded from the above discussion, data measurements taken solely at the local base stations suffice to identify and monitor overall network traffic rates and network performance metrics. The open question at this point is associated with the concept of failure identification for network components. In particular, the questions to be addressed are: Can end-to-end (local base station-to-local base station) data alone be used to effectively locate faulty network lines *anywhere in the network?* If yes, how; and if not, what kind of additional information is necessary and from where in the network should it be collected? The answers to these questions may provide the cardinality of the minimal set of monitoring sub-network nodes and their localities. As an illustration, Figure 4 shows a simple network with two ends A and B and hierarchical routing through the central processing nodes T_1, T_2, T_3.

To explore the above questions, a mathematical maximum likelihood statistical approach may be applied to a fixed network topology model: *a network with fixed nodes and connectivity, with point-to-point loads, and with fixed routing probabilistic structure* (Papantoni-Kazakos, Delic, Paterakis. & Liu, 1993). This approach allows sufficient conditions for the identifiability (estimation) of a fixed set of per link failure probabilities to be developed. These conditions depend only on the routing probabilities for the point-to-point traffic, and indicate that, while link failure probabilities for wireless networks cannot in general be completely determined from end-to-end observations, ambiguities can be resolved by the addition of observations on a minimal number of selected links from central processing nodes. Because of the dynamically changing nature of loads and routing in wireless networks, the minimal observation result may be of use only if associated with dynamic network reconfigurations and sub-network mobility.

The maximum likelihood approach also indicates the appropriate extension of the core algorithm in Section 4, when applied to detect shifts in per link call (communication attempt) failure probabilities for a large-scale wireless network. The extension uses the basic simplified assumption that the network routing structure is known and remains unchanged (Papantoni-Kazakos, Delic, Paterakis.

Figure 4. A simple hierarchical network

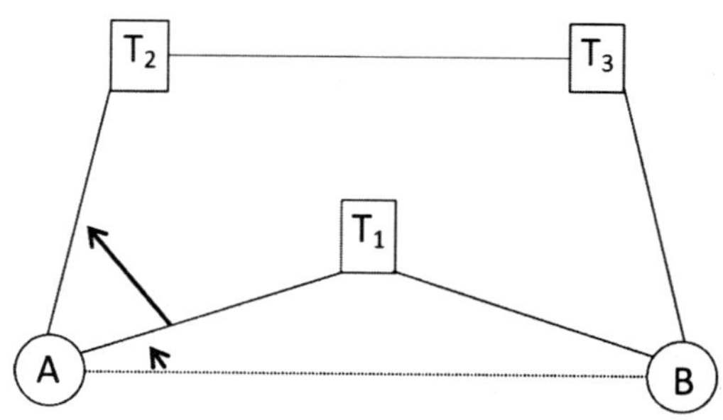

& Liu, 1993). This assumption may reflect average load network conditions (no large load fluctuations present), and may be closer to realistic when limited network portions are considered.

A Sample of the Maximum Likelihood Approach

Here, we give a sample of the maximum likelihood approach. Consider a given portion of the whole network, involving a number of local base stations that are connected with each other through a number of links and tandems. We use the term *call* from now on for communication request. Denote:

(kl): ordered end-to end communication, i.e., call originating at end k and addressing end l.

i; $1 \leq i \leq M$: link index, where M is the overall number of links in the network portion considered.

r_{kl} : the relative load associated with pair (kl) over the network portion considered.

Alternatively, probability that a random communication attempt made somewhere in the network portion is a (kl) attempt. Then, $\Sigma_{kl} r_{kl}=1$, where the summation is over all communicating network end pairs.

$q_{i,(kl)}$: probability that a (kl) call uses the link indexed by i. This is a routing probability.

v_i: failure rate of the link indexed by i. This is the probability that a call going through the link indexed by i fails.

p_i: the probability that a call attempt made somewhere in the network portion considered fails due to the link indexed by i.

p_o: the probability that one random call generated somewhere in the network does not fail.

$f_{(kl)}(x)$: the probability that a random call attempt is generated on the network, it is a (kl) attempt, and an outcome x is observed. When this outcome is a failure or success, and these two concepts are disjointly defined, then

$$x = \begin{cases} 1, & \text{if attempt fails} \\ 0, & \text{if attempt succeeds.} \end{cases}$$

We will assume that both the relative loads and the routing probabilities remain unchanged and they are well-known.

Under these assumptions, each end-to-end pair (kl) in the network portion considered generates a constraint fraction r_{kl} representing the relative call load generated from (kl) the way an outside observer sees it. The outside observer sees, in addition, the outcome (communication success or failure) of every communication attempt in the network, while the individual users see only the outcomes of their own attempts.

The outside observer evaluates the overall performance of the network portion considered through the appropriate processing of the observed dispositions of end-to-end call attempts; the observations may be made either by the assumed outside observer, or they may be reported by the individual users.

Let us now make the following important assumption: A call failure is caused by just one link and the call continues being routed (or flowing) after a failure. This assumption excludes the possibility of a call being actually stopped at the link where the failure occurs.

Under our assumption, the contribution of link i to communication failures in the network is represented by the number p_i, i.e., p_i represents the probability that link i fails a random call on the network. Obviously, we have then:

$$\sum_{i=0}^{M} p_i = 1$$

We will show now that the probabilities p_i can also represent the point-to-point performance of the network, i.e., performance as seen by the network users.

Using binary classification of the successful and unsuccessful call attempts, we obviously have:

$$\underset{(kl)}{f(1)} = \sum_{i=1}^{M} p_i \bullet P_r\{kl) \text{ attempt/random attempt, fails at link } i\}$$
$$= \sum_{i=1}^{M} p_i \frac{r_{kl} \bullet q_{i},_{(kl)}}{\sum_{m\rho} r_{m\rho} q_{i},_{(m\rho)}} \tag{7}$$

where in $\Sigma_{m\rho} r_{m\rho} q_{i},_{(m\rho)}$, the summation is overall the communicating $(m\rho)$ pairs in the network portion considered.

Generalizing (7) we easily see that:

$$\underset{(kl)}{f(x)} = r_{kl} \left[\sum_{i=1}^{M} p_i \frac{q_{i}\text{'}_{(kl)}}{\sum_{m\rho} r_{m\rho} q_{i}\text{'}_{(m\rho)}} \right]^{x} \bullet \left[1 - \sum_{i=1}^{M} p_i \frac{q_{i}\text{'}_{(kl)}}{\sum_{m\rho} r_{m\rho} q_{i}\text{'}_{(m\rho)}} \right]^{1-x} \tag{8}$$

From expression (8) or (7), one observes that the influence of link i to the point-to-point performance between nodes k and l is represented by the expression:

$$v_i q_{i}\text{'}_{(kl)} = p_i \frac{q_{i}\text{'}_{(kl)}}{\sum_{m\rho} r_{m\rho} q_{i}\text{'}_{(m\rho)}} \tag{9}$$

Summing over all the links gives the total point-to-point failure rate for pair kl.

Also, it is clear from (9) that there is a direct relationship between the p_i and the corresponding link failure rate v_i.

Let us now consider that the outside observer has collected a fixed number of observations for the network portion considered, and he is given the pair index (kl) for each of them and the outcome of each attempt (success or failure). Then, an ML estimation algorithm to estimate the p_i's assuming the r_{kl}'s, $q_{i,(kl)}$'s known, requires the maximum likelihood function:

$$f(\overline{p}) = \sum_{kl} \sum_{j=1}^{N_{kl}} \left[x_{j,kl} \log \left(\sum_{i=1}^{M} p_i \frac{q_{i,(kl)}}{\sum_{m\rho} r_{m\rho} q_{i,(m\rho)}} \right) + (1 - x_{j,kl}) \log \left(1 - \sum_{i=1}^{M} p_i \frac{q_{i,(kl)}}{\sum_{m\rho} r_{m\rho} q_{i,(m\rho)}} \right) \right] + \sum_{kl} \sum_{j=1}^{N_{kl}} \log r_{kl}$$

The ML optimal $\overline{p}$ value is found when the gradient of $f(\overline{p})$ is set equal to zero, where the identifiability of $\overline{p}$ is determined via the second gradient matrix of $f(\overline{p})$. In particular, $\overline{p}$ is ML identifiable if and only if the latter matrix is strictly negative definite. Alternatively, as it turns out [53], the maximum set of identifiable links is determined by the maximum set of linearly independent routing vectors $\left[q_{i,((kl)_1)}, \ldots, q_{i,((kl)_m)}, \ldots \right]$. The latter set is generally *not unique* and determines the links that are "visible" via the end-to-end measurements, where the remaining links should be monitored via direct (end-to-end per link) observations.

Minimal Size of Monitoring Sub-network — Tradeoffs

As suggested from the approach presented above, the localities of the minimal (for complete network "visibility") set of monitoring nodes include all the local base stations, plus some central processing nodes, where the set of the latter is generally not unique. The final selection of the central processing nodes used by the monitoring sub-network is controlled by tradeoffs and possible constraints:

- Some central processing nodes may be limited. That is, it may be that some monitoring nodes cannot function to their full potential at certain locations.
- The location of some central processing nodes may be more beneficial to the computational load versus bandwidth for information exchange tradeoff than others.

The above constraints and tradeoffs need to be fully explored before the final localities of the monitoring nodes are selected to comprise the **optimal minimal – size monitoring sub-network**. Given a network topology and its limitations, this must be pursued comprehensively and rigorously. In this pursuit, it is necessary that, for each selection of localities for the monitoring nodes:

- The rate of the necessary communication between monitoring nodes be quantified for maintaining sufficiently updated information about the state of the network (traffic rates, performance indices, failures, etc.), as required by the traffic and performance monitoring algorithms deployed. This rate depends on the traffic models selected (sets of stochastic processes that model various traffic states), in conjunction with the performance characteristics of the core algorithm in Section 4.

Sub-Network Mobility as Function of Varying Network Topologies

As we stated earlier in this section, a fixed network topology implies fixed set of nodes (local base stations and central processing stations), fixed connectivity, and fixed probabilistic routing structure. For fixed network topologies, we presented a mathematical methodology for the selection of the minimal set of monitoring nodes and their localities, and we discussed the induced tradeoffs. The issue we focus on now is mobility of the monitoring nodes and their localities as functions of varying network topologies. We note that changes in network topologies may occur due to: (a) solely changed probabilistic routing structure to accommodate either changed traffic loads or temporarily failing (sub-functioning) links or nodes; (b) reconfiguration of the mobile network (set of local base stations and central processing nodes and their connectivity) accompanied by an appropriately adjusted probabilistic routing structure.

Caused by any of the factors stated above, a changed network topology will require a reconfiguration of the optimal set of monitoring nodes and their localities as dictated by the ML methodology presented earlier in this section and the subsequent evaluation of the induced tradeoffs across equivalent minimal – size monitoring sub-networks. The new optimal minimal sets of monitoring nodes and their localities, as compared to those before the network topology changed, represents the outcome of sub-network mobility as function of changed network topology. Given a network topology, a number of interesting issues arise here:

- How much change in the optimal minimal set of monitoring nodes is caused by a sole change in the probabilistic routing structure, and what is then the resulting change in processing effort per monitoring node and in the information interchange among monitoring nodes.
- What is the effect of a single link failure on the optimal minimal sets of monitoring nodes and on the resulting processing loads and information exchanges. Generally, the answer dependents on the location of the link and the traffic load it carries.
- What are the effects of delays or errors in the decisions performed by the traffic and network performance monitoring algorithms on the motions of the monitoring nodes and what are the subsequent effects on the overall network performance.

LEARNING TECHNIQUES FOR ADAPTIVE MONITORING

As we have repeatedly stated, all the monitoring techniques performed by the distributed monitoring sub-network are based on the core algorithm in Section 4. The operational parameters of the latter algorithm consist of the log likelihood updating steps (that are functions of the observed data) and the set $\{\delta_i\}$ of decision thresholds. The analytical forms of the updating steps (as functions of the observed data) are determined by the set of stochastic processes which model the variations in the statistical characteristics of the metric modeled (e.g., traffic, delays, etc.). The set $\{\delta_i\}$ of thresholds are also selected based on the latter set of processes, in conjunction with the desired performance tradeoffs (probabilities of correct versus incorrect decisions). As can be shown, via the theory of statistical qualitative robustness, the log likelihood updating steps can be modified in a precise fashion to provide a "robust" algorithm [3], whose performance is relatively insensitive to variations in the models of the stochastic processes used. This result leaves the set $\{\delta_i\}$ of thresholds as the only set of parameters that strongly affect the performance of the core algorithm in Section 4, when variations in the stochastic processes describing the environment occur. This conclusion gives rise to the following question:

- Can the thresholds be "learned" via interaction with the environment, when the environment is dynamic and the models describing it are time-varying.

An affirmative answer to this question may be very significant for the design of effective monitoring sub-networks, since the mobile environment is highly dynamic to the point where precise traffic characterization may be impossible. This means that the selected stochastic models used in the design of the monitoring operations may be then inadequate for the accurate selection of the thresholds $\{\delta_i\}$.

Fortunately, there is a lot of experience about supervised learning. Effective learning techniques are sequential "stochastic approximation" algorithms (Zhang, Hafez, & Falconer, 1994). Those that are most effective are designed based on a performance criterion which is pertinent to the objective that the "learned" parameters serve (Papantoni-Kazakos, 1979, & Papantoni-Kazakos, 1994). For example, in the case of interest here, the objective the "learned" thresholds serve is detection of changes in stochastic models, and the pertinent performance criterion is the Kullback-Leibler relative information measure that we first saw in Section 4. Thus, supervised learning techniques for the set of thresholds $\{\delta_i\}$ in Section 4 may be devised, being based on the Kullback-Leibler performance criterion. Such techniques may converge to the correctly optimal threshold values with probability one, where such values are determined by pre-selected levels of error and correct decision probabilities. A learning algorithm in this class can be found in (Chandler, Hulburt, & McTiffin, 1991), for the detection of change between two processes.

SUGGESTIONS FOR FUTURE RESEARCH

In this chapter, we have laid out an approach towards the design of a dynamically re-configurable monitoring sub-network, whose function is to detect traffic and performance changes in a mobile heterogeneous network and to subsequently decide upon and implement network architectural and operational re-configurations. We have proposed a specific algorithm for the detection of changes and have identified the appropriate metrics to be monitored. For the actual design and deployment of a monitoring sub-network, a number of open research problems remain, however. Specifically, given a mobile heterogeneous network, there is need to:

- Characterize the traffic characteristics, to subsequently design the specific traffic monitoring algorithm, as in Section 4. The latter algorithm needs to be analyzed then, in terms of its non-asymptotic performance metrics, as stated in Section 4.

- Qualify and quantify the performance metrics discussed in Section 5 and to subsequently design and analyze the specific performance monitoring algorithms induced by these metrics, in conjunction with the core algorithm in Section 4.
- Analyze the architecture of the given network topology, to identify the nodes which will be parts of a minimum-size performance monitoring sub-network, utilizing the approach in Section 6. Also analyze the mobility characteristics of the given network, to identify the architectural dynamics of the minimum-size sub-network.
- Develop and analyze supervised learning techniques, for the dynamic, on-line, adaptation of pertinent algorithmic parameters, as discussed in Section 7, and with regard to the deployed traffic/performance monitoring algorithms.

SUMMARY

We presented a specific approach towards the design of a mobile and distributed sub-network whose function is the traffic and network performance monitoring of mobile networks. We proposed the adoption of a statistically sound core algorithm for the performance of the monitoring operations and discussed its performance characteristics and tradeoffs when implemented by a distributed sub-network. We also presented a mathematical approach for the selection of an "optimal" minimal set of monitoring nodes and their localities, and discussed mobility and time-varying node-localities as functions of changing network topologies. We finally presented the issue of "supervised learning" for the threshold parameters of the monitoring algorithms, and presented the gist of our approach towards the design of "learning" algorithms. Our approach is comprehensive and necessitates the integration of traffic and network management for failure identification and reconfiguration of network topologies. Such a comprehensive approach is a necessity for truly effective management of the information traffics carried by mobile heterogeneous networks.

REFERENCES

Acampora, A.S., & Naghshineh, M. (1994). Control and Quality-of-Service Provisioning in High-Speed Micro-Cellular Networks. *IEEE Personal Communications*, (2), 36-42.

Acampora, A.S. & Naghshineh, M. (1994). An Architecture and Methodology for Mobile-Executed Cell Hand-off in Wireless ATM Networks. *IEEE JSAC, 12*.

Bansal, P. K., & Papantoni-Kazakos, P. (1986). An Algorithm for Detecting a Change in a Stochastic Process. *IEEE Transactions on Information Theory*, *IT-32*, 227–235. doi:10.1109/TIT.1986.1057160

Bar-Noy, A., & Kessler, I. (1993). Tracking Mobile Users in Wireless Networks. *Proceedings - IEEE INFOCOM, 93*, 1232–1239.

Bar-Noy, A., & Kessler, I. (1994). Mobile Users: To Update or not to Update? *Proceedings - IEEE INFOCOM, 94*, 570–576.

Basagni, S., Chlamtac, I., Syrotiuk, V. R., & Woodward, B. A. (1998). A Distance Routing Effect Algorithm for Mobilty (DREAM). In *Fourth Annual ACM/IEEE International Conference on Mobile Computing and Networking*, (pp. 76-84).

Berruto, E., Eynard, C., Fiorina, E., & Napolitano, A. (1993). Issues in Protocol Evolution for Personal Telecommunications. In *Proceedings IEEE GLOBECOM '93*, (pp. 555-559).

Brady, P. T. (1965). A Technique for Investigating On-Off Patterns of Speech. *The Bell System Technical Journal*, 1–22.

Brady, P. T. (1968). A Statistical Analysis of On-Off Patterns in 16 Conversations. *The Bell System Technical Journal*, 73–91.

Burrell, A. T. (1994). Traffic Management in Broadband Integrated Services Digital Networks. unpublished doctoral dissertation, University of Virginia, Charlottesville, VA.

Burrell, A. T., Makrakis, D., & Papantoni-Kazakos, P. (1998). Traffic Monitoring for Capacity Allocation of Multimedia Traffic in ATM Broadband Networks. *IEEE Journal on High-Speed Networks*, *9*, 173–206.

Burrell, A. T., & Papantoni-Kazakos, P. (1996). Signaling, Transmission, and Dynamic Capacity Allocation Viewed in an Integrated Fashion. In *ITC Mini-Seminar Performance Modeling and Design of Wireless/PCS Networks*. Cambridge, MA: Wireless Networks in Hybrid Topologies.

Burrell, A. T., & Papantoni-Kazakos, P. (1998). Extended Sequential Algorithms for Detecting Changes in Acting Stochastic Processes. *IEEE Transactions on Systems, Man, and Cybernetics*, *28*(5), 703–710. doi:10.1109/3468.709621

Burrell, A. T., & Papantoni-Kazakos, P. (1999), On-Line Learning and Dynamic Capacity Allocation in the TrafficManagement of Integrated Services Networks. In European Transactions on Telecommunications, Special Issue on Architectures, Protocols, and Quality of Service for the Internet of the Future, 10(5), 202-214.

Burrell, A. T., Papantoni-Kazakos, P., & Stren, H. (1998). Dynamic Capacity Allocation and Hybrid Multiplexing Techniques For ATM Wireless Networks. *Journal on Wireless Networks*, *3*, 307–316.

Chandler, D. P., Hulburt, A. P., & McTiffin, M. J. M. J. (1991). An ATM-CDMA Air Interface for Mobile Personal Communications. In COST 231 TD (94).

Chlamtac, I. & Farago, A. (1994). Making Transmission Schedules Immune to Topology Changes in Multi-Hop Packet Radio Networks. *IEEE/ACM Transactions on Networking, 2* (1), 23-29.

Coviello, G. J., & Vena, G. P. (1975). Integration of Circuit/Packet Switching by a SENET (Slotted Envelope Network) Concept. In *Conference Rec. 1975 National Telecommunications Conference*, (pp. 42-12 -- 42-17).

Cox, D. C. (1992). Network Control for Wireless Communications Networks. *IEEE Communications Magazine*, 96–115. doi:10.1109/35.210361

Cox, D. C., Gifford, W. S., & Sherry, H. (1991). Low-Power Digital Radio as a Ubiquitous Subscriber Loop. *IEEE Communications Magazine*, 92–95. doi:10.1109/35.75532

De Prycker, M. (1993). *Asynchronous Transfer Mode—Solution for Broadband ISDN* (2nd ed.). New York: Ellis Horwood.

EIA/TIA. (1990). *Interim Standard IS-54*. Washington, D.C.: Cellular System Dual-Mode Mobile Station-Base Station Compatibility Standard.

EIA/TIA. (1991). *Cellular Radio Telecommunications Intersystem Operations*. Revision B, Technical Report IS-41, EIA/TIA.

Fischetti, M. (1993). The Cellular Phone Scare. [June.]. *IEEE Spectrum*, 43–47. doi:10.1109/6.214586

Gejji, R. (1992). Forward-Link-Power Control in CDMA Cellular Systems. In IEEE Transactions on Vehicular Technology (pp. 532 – 536).

Georgiadis, L., Merakos, L., & Papantoni-Kazakos, P. (1987). A Method for the Delay Analysis of Random Multiple Access Algorithms whose Delay Process is Regenerative. *IEEE Journal on Selected Areas in Communications*, *SAC-5*(6), 1051–1062. doi:10.1109/JSAC.1987.1146613

Gilhousen, K. S., Jacobs, I. M., Padovani, R., Viterbi, A. J., Weaver, L. A., & Wheatley, C. E. III. (1991). On the Capacity of a Cellular CDMA System. *IEEE Transactions on Vehicular Technology*, 303–312. doi:10.1109/25.289411

Goodman, D. J. (1991, June). Trends in Cellular and Cordless Communications. *IEEE Communications Magazine*, 31–40. doi:10.1109/35.79400

Goodman, D. J., Pollini, G. P., & Meier-Hellstern, K. S. (1992). Network Control for Wireless Communications Networks. *IEEE Communications Magazine*, 116–125. doi:10.1109/35.210362

Goodman, D. J., Valenzuela, R. A., Gayliard, K. T., & Ramamurthi, B. (1989). Packet Reservation Multiple Access for Local Wireless Communications. *IEEE Transactions on Communications*, *37*, 885–890. doi:10.1109/26.31190

Goodman, D. J., & Wei, S. X. (1991). Efficiency of Packet Reservation Multiple Access. *IEEE Transactions on Vehicular Technology*, *40*, 170–176. doi:10.1109/25.69985

Gruber, J. G. (1982). A Comparison of Measured and Calculated Temporal Patterns Relevant to Speech Activity Detection. *IEEE Transactions on Communications*, 728–738. doi:10.1109/TCOM.1982.1095514

Guo, N., & Morgera, S. D. (1993). The Grade-of-Service for Integrated Voice/Data Wireless DS-CDMA Networks. In *Proceedings IEEE ICC '93* (pp. 1104-1110).

IEEECommunications Magazine, 46(10). (2008, October).

(1987)... *IEEE Journal on Selected Areas in Communications*, *SAC-5*(5).

International Journal on Digital and Analog Cable Systems, 1*(4)*. *(*1988*)*.

Jain, R., Lin, Y. B., Lo, C., & Mohan, S. (1994). A Caching Strategy to Reduce Network Impact of PCS. *IEEE Journal on Selected Areas in Communications*, *12*(8), 1434–1444. doi:10.1109/49.329333

Jakes, W. C. Jr. (1974). *Microwave Mobile Communications*. New York: John Wiley and Sons.

Karn, P. (1990). MACA: A New Channel Access Method for Packet Radio. In *ARRL/CRRL Amateur Radio 9th Computer Networking Conference*.

Kummerle, K. (1974). Multiplexer Performance for Integrated Line- and Packet-Switched Traffic, *Proceedings of the ICCC*, Stockholm (pp. 508-515).

Lee, H. H., & Un, C. K. (1987). A Study of On-Off Characteristics of Conversational Speech. *IEEE Transactions on Communications*, 630–637.

Lee, W. C. Y. (1982). *Mobile Communications Engineering*. New York: McGraw-Hill.

Lee, W. C. Y. (1989). *Mobile Cellular Telecommunications Systems*. New York: McGraw-Hill.

Lee, W. C. Y. (1991). Overview of Cellular CDMA. In IEEE Transactions on Vehicular Technology, (pp. 291-302).

Lin, Y. B. (1994). Determining the User Locations for Personal Communications Services Networks. *IEEE Transactions on Vehicular Technology*, *43*(3), 466–473. doi:10.1109/25.312799

Liu, M., & Papantoni-Kazakos, P. (1992). A Random Access Algorithm for Data Networks Carrying High Priority Traffic. *IEEE Transactions on Communications*, *40*, 84–96. doi:10.1109/26.126710

Liu, M., & Papantoni-Kazakos, P. (1993). A Protocol for Cellular Radio Signaling Channels Carrying Data and High Priority Accessing Requests. *IEEE Transactions on Communications*, *41*, 570–582. doi:10.1109/26.223781

Madhow, U., Honig, M. L., & Steiglitz, K. (1994). Optimization of Wireless Resources for Personal Communications Mobility Tracking. *Proceedings - IEEE INFOCOM*, *94*, 577–584.

Mao, G. (2005, February). A Real-Time Loss Performance Monitoring Scheme. *Computer Communications*, *28*(2), 150–161. doi:10.1016/j.comcom.2004.06.007

Meier-Hellstern, K. S., Pollini, G. P., & Goodman, D. J. (1991). A Wireless Service for the IEEE 802.6 Metropolitan Area Network. In *Proceedings. IEEE GLOBECOM '91,* (pp. 1964-1968).

Mermelstein, P., Jalali, A., & Leib, H. (1993). Integrated Services on Wireless Multiple Access Networks. In IEEE ICC '93, (pp. 863-867).

Mohan, S., & Jain, R. (1994). Two User Location Strategies for Personal Communications Services. *IEEE Personal Communications*, *1*(1), 42–50.

Nanda, S., Goodman, D. J., & Timor, U. (1991). Performance of PRMA: A Packet Voice Protocol for Cellular Systems. *IEEE Transactions on Vehicular Technology*, *40*, 584–598. doi:10.1109/25.97513

Pados, D. A., & Papantoni-Kazakos, P. (1995). New Non-Least-Squares Neural Network Learning Algorithms for Hypothesis Testing. *IEEE Transactions on Neural Networks*, *6*(3), 596–609. doi:10.1109/72.377966

Pados, D. A., Papantoni-Kazakos, P., Kazakos, D., & Kogiantis, A. (1994). On-Line Threshold Learning for Neyman-Pearson Distributed Detection. *IEEE Transactions on Systems, Man, and Cybernetics*, *24*(10), 1519–1531. doi:10.1109/21.310534

Papantoni-Kazakos, P. (1979). Algorithms for Monitoring Changes in Quality of Communications Links. *IEEE Transactions on Communications*, *27*(4), 682–692. doi:10.1109/TCOM.1979.1094443

Papantoni-Kazakos, P. (1979). The Potential of End-to-End Observations in Trouble Localization and Quality Control of Network Links. *IEEE Transactions on Communications*, *27*(1), 16–30. doi:10.1109/TCOM.1979.1094254

Papantoni-Kazakos, P. (1992). Multiple Access Algorithms for a System with Mixed Traffic: High and Low Priority. *IEEE Transactions on Communications*, *40*, 541–555. doi:10.1109/26.135724

Papantoni-Kazakos, P. (1994). Accessing Protocols and Network Reconfiguration for Cellular-ISDN Systems. In. *Proceedings of IEEE ICC*, *94*, 1285–1296.

Papantoni-Kazakos, P., Delic, H., Paterakis, M., & Liu, M. (1993). Transmission Algorithms for a Multi-Channel Packet Radio System with Priority Users. *IJDACS*, *6*(4), 193–212.

Papantoni-Kazakos, P., Likhanov, N., & Tsybakov, B. S. (1995). A Protocol for Random Multiple Access of Packets with Mixed Priorities in Wireless Networks. *IEEE JSAC*, *13*(7), 1324–1331.

Paterakis, M., Georgiadis, L., & Papantoni-Kazakos, P. (1989). A Full Sensing Window Random-Access Algorithm for Messages with Strict Delay Constraints. *Algorithmica*, *4*(3), 313–329. doi:10.1007/BF01553894

Paterakis, M., & Papantoni-Kazakos, P. (1989). A Simple Window Random Access Algorithm with Advantageous Properties. *IEEE Transactions on Information Theory*, *35*, 1124–1130. doi:10.1109/18.42234

Prakash, R., Shivaratrai, N. G., & Singhal, M. (1995). Distributed Dynamic Channel Allocation For Mobile Computing. In *Proceedings of the Fourth Annual ACM Symposium on Principles on Distributed Computing*, (pp. 47-56).

Proakis, J. G. (1995). *Digital Communications* (3rd ed.). New York: McGraw-Hill.

Raychaudhuri, D. (1994). ATM Based Transport Architecture for Multi-services Wireless Personal Communications Networks. *Proceedings of the IEEE, 94*, 559–565.

Raychaudhuri, D., & Wilson, N. (1993). Multimedia Transport in Next-Generation Personal Communications Networks. *Proceedings of the IEEE, 93*, 858–862.

Ross, M. J., Gottschalck, J. H., & Harrington, E. A. (1980). An Architecture for a Flexible Integrated Voice/Data Switch. In *Conference. Rec. 1980 International Conference on Communications* (pp. 21.6-1-- 21.6-5).

Rozenbaum, Y., Papantoni-Kazakos, P., & Kazakos, D. (1995). Semidynamic and Dynamic Transmission Algorithms for Multiplexing Voice with Data. *Telecommunication Systems, 3*, 341–378. doi:10.1007/BF02110311

Schwartz, M. (1987). *Telecommunication Networks: Protocols, Modeling and Analysis*. Reading, MA: Addison-Wesley.

Steele, R. (1994). The Evolution of Personal Communications. *IEEE Personal Communications, 2*, 6–11. doi:10.1109/MPC.1994.298461

Stern, H. P., Mahmoud, S. A., & Wong, K. K. (1994). A Model for Generating On-Off Patterns in Conversational Speech, Including Short Silence Gaps and the Effects of Interaction between Parties. *IEEE Transactions on Vehicular Technology*, 1094–1100. doi:10.1109/25.330173

Tsybakov, B. S., & Mikhailov, V. A. (1979). Ergodicity of Slotted ALOHA System. *Probability. Peredachi Information, 15*, 73–87.

Wang, J. Z. (1993). A Fully Distributed Location Registration Strategy for Universal Personal Communication Systems. *IEEE Journal on Selected Areas in Communications, 11*(6), 850–860. doi:10.1109/49.232294

White, H. (1989). Some Asymptotic Results for Learning in Single Hidden-Layer Feedforward Network Models. *Journal of the American Statistical Association, 84*, 1003–1013. doi:10.2307/2290076

Winters, J. H. (1993). Signal Acquisition and Tracking with Adaptive Arrays in the Digital Mobile Radio System IS-54 with Flat Fading. *IEEE Transactions on Vehicular Technology, 42*(4), 377–380. doi:10.1109/25.260776

Woodruff, G., & Kositpaiboon, R. (1990). *Multimedia Traffic Management Principles for Guaranteed ATM Network Performance*. IEEE Journal on Selected Areas in Communications.

Zhang, C. G., Hafez, H. M., & Falconer, D. (1994). Traffic Handling Capacity of Broadband Indoor Network Using CDMA Multiple Access. *IEEE JSAC, 12*(12), 645–652.

APPENDIX

Recursions for the Poisson-Geometric Model

Let us define,

P_{ikj} (n, y): The probability that at the end of a channel frame the rate λ_i' is acting and the monitoring algorithm $\lambda_k \rightarrow \lambda_j$ is operating, while the value of the algorithm equals y and is operating for n frames without crossing its threshold.

Q_i (k): The probability that the interval during which the rate λ_i' is acting equals k slots.

$$Q_i(k) = (1-\rho_i)^{-1}\rho_i^{k-1} \; ; \quad k \geq 1$$

Then, in view of the algorithm steps in (1), Section 4, the following recursions are deduced, in a straight forward fashion, where the positive integer v_k denotes the common threshold of the monitoring algorithm, $\lambda_k \rightarrow \lambda_j$, $\forall\, k \neq j$.

$$\begin{aligned}
1 \leq \underset{n\geq 1}{y} \leq v_k \; ; \; \mathrm{P}_{ikj}(n,y) = & \sum_{m:\; 0\leq y-(-1)^{ime(k,j)}[s_{kj}m-t_{kj}]\leq v_k-1} [p_i^d e^{(-d\lambda_i')} \frac{(d\lambda_i')^m}{m!} * \\
& *\mathrm{p}_{ikj}(n-1, y-(-1)^{ime(k,j)}[s_{kj}m - dt_{kj}]) + \\
& + \frac{1}{\mathrm{n}-1}\sum_{p\neq i}(1-\rho_p^d)\, e^{(-d\lambda_i')}\frac{(d\lambda_i')^m}{m!}\mathrm{P}_{pkj}(n-1, y-(-1)^{ime(k,j)}[s_{kj}m - dt_{kj}])
\end{aligned}$$

$$\begin{aligned}
n \geq 1 \; ; \; \mathrm{p}_{ikj}(n,0) = & \sum_{0\leq w\leq v_k-1} [\, p_i^d \mathrm{P}_{ikj}(n-1,w) \sum_{m:\; w+(-1)^{ime(k,j)}[s_{kj}m-t_{kj}]\leq 0} e^{(-d\lambda_i')}\frac{(d\lambda_i')^m}{m!} + \\
& + \frac{1}{\mathrm{n}-1}\sum_{p\neq i}(1-\rho_p^d)\, \mathrm{P}_{pkj}(n-1,w) \sum_{m:\; w+(-1)^{ime(k,j)}[s_{kj}m-t_{kj}]\leq 0} e^{(-d\lambda_i')}\frac{(d\lambda_i')^m}{m!}\,]
\end{aligned}$$

If $P_{ikj}'(n,y)$ denotes the probability P_{ikj} (n, y), given that the acting rate λ_i' remains unchanged, then, the following recursions are easily deduced from the above expressions:

$$\underset{n\geq 1}{1\leq y\leq v_k} \;;\; \mathrm{P}'_{ikj}(n,y) = \sum_{m:\; 0\leq y-(-1)^{ime(k,j)}[s_{kj}m-t_{kj}]\leq v_k-1} e^{(-d\lambda_i')}\frac{(d\lambda_i')^m}{m!} *$$
$$*\mathrm{P}'_{ikj}(n-1, y-(-1)^{ime(k,j)}[s_{kj}m - d\,t_{kj}])$$

$$n\geq 1 \;;\; \mathrm{P}'_{ikj}(n,0) = \sum_{0\leq w\leq v_k-1} \mathrm{P}'_{ikj}(n-1,w) \sum_{m:\; w+(-1)^{ime(k,j)}[s_{kj}m-t_{kj}]\leq 0} e^{(-d\lambda_i')}\frac{(d\lambda_i')^m}{m!}$$

; with initial conditions $\mathrm{P}'_{ikj}(0,0)=1$.

Let $\mathrm{P}'_{ikj}(n)$ denote the probability that the $\lambda_k \rightarrow \lambda_j$ monitoring algorithm first crosses its threshold, v_k, in n frame steps after the beginning of its operation, given that the rate λ_i' is acting throughout. Then,

$$n\geq 1 \;;\; \mathrm{P}'_{ikj}(n) = \sum_{0\leq y\leq v_k-1} \mathrm{p}_{ikj}(n-1,y) \sum_{m:\; y+(-1)^{ime(k,j)}[s_{kj}m-\mathrm{d}t_{kj}]\geq v_k} e^{(-\mathrm{d}\lambda_i')}\frac{(\mathrm{d}\lambda_i')^m}{m!}$$

If $E\{N_{\{\lambda_k\rightarrow\lambda_j\}} / \lambda_i'\}$ denotes the expected stopping time of the $\lambda_k \rightarrow \lambda_j$ monitoring algorithm, given that the rate λ_i' is acting throughout, then,

$$E\{N_{\{\lambda_k\rightarrow\lambda_j\}} / \lambda_i'\} = \sum_{n\geq 1} nP'_{ikj}(n)$$

Chapter 12
Model Based Approach for QoS Constrained Communication and Data Integration among Multiple Agents

Manjunath Ramachandra
Philips - Bangalore, India

Vikas Jain
Philips - Bangalore, India

ABSTRACT

Meeting the agreed quality of service in a resource crunched data network is challenging. An intelligent element is required to carry out the activities involved. The inferences drawn with different rules need to be merged. Agents are useful for handling this responsibility in data networks and help in resource sharing. An agent is basically an entity that can be viewed as perceiving its environment through sensors and acting upon its environment through effectors. To handle the network traffic, the agents acquire the traffic status and provide the information on the availability of resources to the source of the traffic. Hence the study on agent communication has become important. Intelligent agents continuously perform the activities including perception of dynamic conditions in the environment, reasoning for interpretation of the perceptions, solve problems, draw inferences and determine actions.

INTRODUCTION

The Data getting exchanged among the distributed agents, that broker for computation or storage, often create problems up on integration with rest of the system, partly because it fails to meet the service quality constraints and partly because it fails to get updated at the right time.

Multiple agents are extremely used in applications involving distributed databases, smart user interfaces, world-wide web, mobile computing, distributed design and manufacturing, information gathering, decision support (using heterogeneous distributed data and knowledge sources), open systems, collaborative computing etc. In all these application, substantial data gets exchanged over the network resulting on the congestion. Agents driving

DOI: 10.4018/978-1-61520-791-6.ch012

these applications are to handle the utilization of the resources optimally and avoid the network getting in to congestion.

In this chapter the problem of quality based data exchange among the agents and data integration from multiple agents will be addressed. A probability of data loss or corruption will be associated with each agent and it changes dynamically with time as the data encounters any queue or dependency in the journey across the different agents. Specifically when the agents have to work on the shared resources, they need to fall in the queue. This resembles a distributed computing scenario.

At the destination, the agent will predict the trends in this feed back signal 'k' steps in advance and uses this information for controlling the size of the data originating from the source agent.

The shifted feedback information may be used to achieve some quality of service (QoS) deadlines such as the absolute delay guarantee, fraction of the data lost etc. Simulation results prove that the usage of shifted signals can reduce the data loss, resource requirement and improve the service quality in terms of overall successful operations in a given time.

The trend analysis will be done by an intelligent element. Although conventional neural networks can be used for this task, they suffer with two major drawbacks. Firstly, the training period is too large and it may not be possible to provide the requisite data. The second drawback is that of a large prediction error. In this work, a modified architecture called differentially fed artificial neural networks (DANN) has been made use. It overcomes both of these drawbacks. Here, a portion of the output is tapped, differentiated many times and used as the additional input. The new architecture comes with a wagon of interesting properties that are made use here.

BACKGROUND

The present day network traffic supporting the multimedia data with different QoS constraints have to be routed across the network in real time. Conventional techniques cannot catch up the fluctuations in the traffic making it necessary to use an intelligent element to memorize the changes. A comparison of different techniques used for providing the QoS is discussed in (Manjunath,R., & Shyam,V., 2008). Although a feedback based controller such as random early detection (RED) provides the congestion status information (Hollot, C., Misra, V., Towsley, D., & Gong, W, 2001) to the data source to alter the transmission rate subsequently, the technique is less adaptive for the fast changing network traffic. Hence, intelligent elements are required to predict the traffic in advance to provide sufficient time for the sources to act.

Neural networks exhibit massive parallelism making them ideal for real time application s. In any system making use of neural networks, when such an element is transferred to silicon the resources such as Buffer size, speed of decisions, area of the associated circuitry etc put stringent constraints making the algorithms of implementation competitive.

The traffic controller proposed here is based on the agents that implement a broker based model. The algorithm employs neural networks to compute desired transmission rate of the source in order to prevent congestion in the subnet. Obtained results prove that the neuro-computing approach is better than the conventional one. This is possible because of the unique learning and memorizing capabilities of the neural network based on the previous experiences.

AGENT BASED APPROACH FOR IMPLEMENTING QOS

Communication among homogeneous agents in narrow, precisely defined domains (e.g., distributed routing in communication networks) is relatively straightforward to be handled using appropriately defined protocols with specified syntax and semantics. Communication among heterogeneous agents involves collaborative problem solving and intelligent resource sharing and turns out to be challenging.

Multi-agent systems (MAS) are ones in which several computational objects (Nwana, 1996) called agents, interact with one another. The concept of 'agent' implies a problem solving entity that both perceives and acts upon the environment in which it is situated, applying its individual knowledge, skills, and other resources to accomplish high-level goals. Towards this end, agents thus integrate many of the algorithms and processes that have been independently developed in the field of artificial intelligence (Russell, S.,& Norvig, 1995) and more widely in computer science.

The built in intelligence of the agents stem up as a result of degree of freedom in how it interacts with other computational and human agents. The study of multi-agent systems involves the techniques and issues with this interaction.

Agents can communicate, cooperate, coordinate, and negotiate with each another, to enhance their individual knowledge and improve the performance of the overall system in which they are situated. Agents start collaborating (Sycara, K., Dekker, K., Pannu, A., Williamson, M., Zeng, D, 1996) to achieve the common goal with particular kinds of interactions among the agents. The agents with individual perspectives can together converge to systemic properties. The group of agents, each with expertise in a particular field needed by one another, can be deployed to collectively solve problems that are beyond their individual abilities. This collaboration among the agents can even be done on the fly, and include humans as well as heterogeneous computational agents (Demazeau, Y, 1998). MAS involve the knowledge from diverse areas (Ferber, J, 1999) such as physical, computational, natural, economical, social and life sciences.

Multi-agent systems were initially developed for system modeling (Bradshaw, J.M. (Ed), 1997) in natural, life, economical and social sciences, where in it is required to observe the individual behavior and to improve the communication capabilities (acquisition, sharing) with the other individuals.

Agents are increasingly used in the dynamic and resource constrained environments to perform a variety of tasks. Binding such agents is a tough task. The inter agent communications could lead to under or over utilization of the resources, as addressed in this chapter.

The MAS often faces the issue of scalability. However, because of the independent and modular nature of the implementation, it is possible to achieve the same unless there is conflict of interest in sharing the proprietary information, rights to use the information etc. However, some organizations find benefits in using the MAS to handle such information. If the agents are allowed to share the information, over a period of time, they form a system of experts, providing better adaptability for the organization in the changing business scenarios.

Multi agents are useful for fault tolerance. Agents share the task or responsibilities to achieve parallelism. In MAS, some of the agents that are free at a point of time share the load from the other agents providing the required redundancies. As a result, with the right choice of the routing for the control and data signals, it is possible to provide a reasonable degree of fault tolerance. However, sharing of load tend to compromise the privacy of the information in the organization as it requires the exchange of data and control signals. The priorities for performance, fault tolerance and privacy of the information are to be considered during the integration (Brenner, W., Zarnekow, R., & Hartmut, W, 1998) of the systems.

Multiple agents (Maes, P., 1997) are useful for time scheduling. When several options or solutions are available for real time problem, the one that optimizes the execution time will be the right solution. In this case, each agent has a local coordination module which interacts with its design-to-time scheduler. The coordination module develops commitments to other agents and the local scheduler validates whether all the current and proposed commitments can be met. In the case, they cannot be all met, the scheduler provides two type of information: alternative ways of partially satisfying the set of commitments and information about changes to the specifications of unsatisfied commitments that would make them to get satisfied. This information provides the basis for a negotiation process between scheduler and decision maker to find the best way to satisfy the decision makers requirements

BROKER BASED ARCHITECTURE FOR RESOURCE SHARING

The primary issue with the multiple agent system is the sharing of resources. A hierarchical organization of the processing as well as the command structure would bring in a kind of service based architecture for the multiple agent systems.

When the agents are of different types and heterogeneous nature, maintaining service quality is challenging. In such a scenario, in addition to the absolute quality performance figures, relative figures may be used. In (Manjunath, R., 2006) it has been explained how the information feed back can maintain the relative parameters consistent. The feedback in terms of data rate, loss rate, integration quality etc parameters seen by the end user of the information, may be provided to the source. This would enable the information sources to adjust the rate and quality of information transmission. The services get connected to these parameters either statically during the design of the service or dynamically when they get invoked.

A Broker based model shown in figures 1a and 1b goes well to handle this problem. The responsibility of providing appropriate data lies with the Broker. The service provider has to handle the delays, search the appropriate data with the quality constraints defined, integrate the same and finally render the required information to the end user in time.

The constraint is to meet these relative service parameters with minimal utilization of resources and minimum loss or rejection due to non conformance to these security parameters. It is interesting to observe the data gets dropped when the security constraints are not met at the broker. The broker may also drop them if the resources are full and no place to hold the data.

The effect of integration of the data is to average out the quality. While averaging, it so happens that the weighed average quality happens to be the quality parameter associated with one of the data sources. The quality distribution turns out to be Gaussian around this parameter. The mean value or the average parameter may be varied with the appropriate choice of the weights while fusing the data. The weighted average of different abstraction levels may be modeled as a swarm of ants (Abraham Ajith, Grosan Crina, Ramos Vitorino (Eds.), 2006). In a swarm of ants, the ants that move ahead of rest of the swarm in search of food leave behind the chemical footprints called pheromones. It provides important information and messages. It is then sensed and modified by the ants that follow. Thus the footprint will have the weighted history of pheromones from a number of ants.

It goes well with the common object broker architecture wherein the broker takes the responsibility of providing the best quality solution in a stipulated time. The broker himself contacts different sources of data or information that are transparent to the end user and generate the required response with agreed quality.

Figure 1.(a) Data flow in the broker model (b) command flow in the broker model

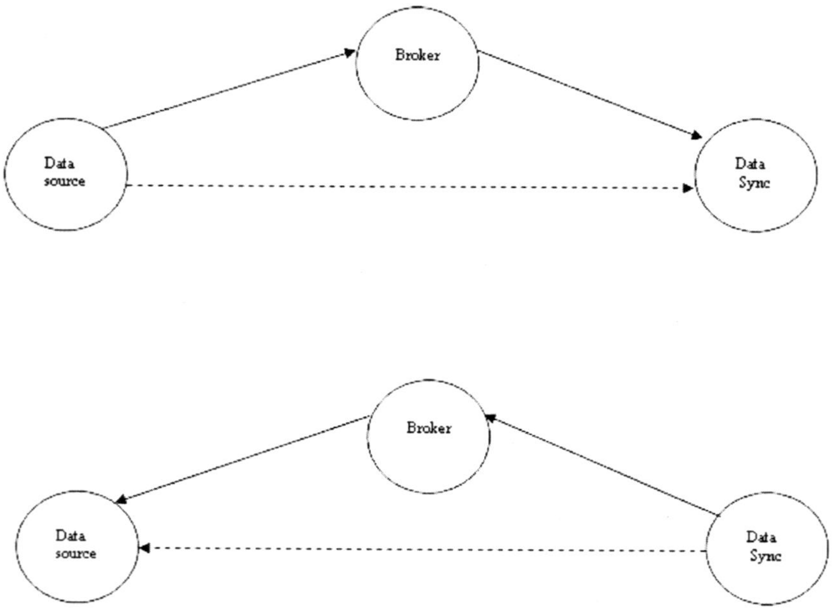

Taking the concept to the vector space where each data is represented as a point in the space, the different data representations may be thought of as the different components of the same resulting data. The integrated data is to be invariant in the representation. The components are not necessarily to be orthogonal, indicating the different representations of the data need not be totally different or distinct. The fused data would be of shortest distance from all the components. While resolving the conflicts that arise out of the different components, a knowledge based system may be used the broker that agrees to provide a time bound quality based solution would find this approach extremely useful. The multi resolution or hierarchical data bases may be implemented with the object oriented database concepts.

The broker model where by the intermediate agents apparently shield the actual source from the destination and often act as virtual sources down the line, may be taught of as an extreme case of the supply chain. In such a scenario, the service quality constraints are to be met by all the agents in between. The brokers take the responsibility of meeting the security constraints or parameters.

DIFFERENTIALLY FED NEURAL NETWORK BASED CONTROLLER

Here the constraint is to meet the relative service parameters with minimal utilization of resources and minimum loss or rejection due to non conformance to these security parameters. It is interesting to observe the data gets dropped when the security constraints are not met at the broker. The broker may also drop them if the resources are full and no place to hold the data.

DANN Architecture

The architecture is based on feed forward and feedback paths (Manjunath,R., & .Gurumurthy,K.S, 2003a). The feed forward path consists of the actual information or data or commodity flow departing from the source depending on the simulation application. It is data packets in a communica-

Figure 2. Differentially fed artificial neural network

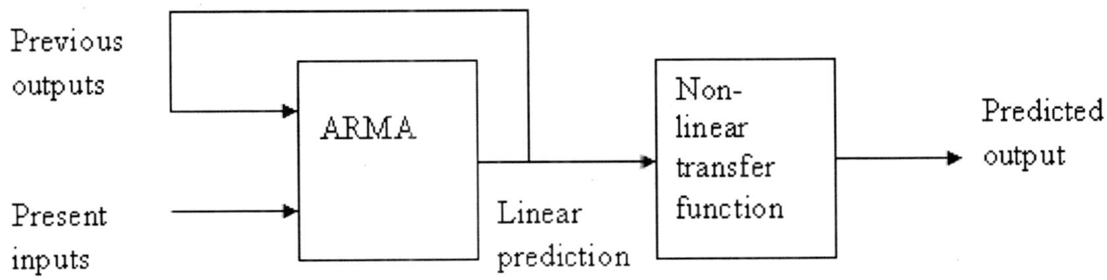

tion network. The feedback signal comprises of the position and status of the information at the destination that has departed from the source. The differentially fed neural network sits as a controller, as a part of the loop comprising of the source, the forward path, the destination and the feedback path. The architecture of a differentially fed neural network is shown in figure.2. The output y happens to be the weighted sum of the inputs as well as the differentials of the output.

The important properties(,R.,&.Gurumurthy,K.S, 2002) of this network that are useful to control the communication among agents are highlighted below:

- Output makes use of historical inputs
- For a given number of iterations, the square error is found to decrease with the order of differential feedback or work on a reduced set of training data
- For infinite feedback, the square error is zero
- The output with different orders of feed-back forms a manifold of hyper planes each of which is self similar to the other.
- The origin of self similarity is due to Long range dependency.
- The self similar outputs have varying degrees of abstraction each of which may be generated through the other by convolving with a Gaussian pulse

Since the differentially fed neural network is a part of the loop, its presence has profound effect on the data traffic in the loop. The DANNs make use of a large number of previous samples for decision making(,R., & .Gurumurthy,K.S, 2003). Decisions thrown out by such a system contributes to Long range dependency in the traffic.

One of the problems with the training of neural networks used in data mining is the over fitting of the data during training. It makes the network highly tuned to the data and useless as it loses the very purpose of decision making under noisy input conditions. The solution is to use a part of untrained data as test input. However it complicates the training procedure. Such a problem is not found in DANN (Manjunath,R., 2006) as the network is resistant for over fitting of the data. The commonly used clustering algorithms result in loss in the sense that a pert of the fine details would be lost while forming the clusters. DANN however retains all the details with different degrees of abstraction.

In essence, insertion of DANN in the traffic loop makes the entire network to behave as a differentially fed neural network, manifesting all its properties. The network here refers to the forward and feedback paths. Hence DANNs play a role more than replacing the conventional artificial neural networks (ANN) in traffic shaping. The traffic shaping involves maintaining the schedules, reduction in the delays and reduction in stranded times or reschedules while keeping up the agreed service parameters.

A multi bit closed loop feedback mechanism is proposed here, with the bits representing the cancellation probability of several connection requests, that also represent the congestion status of the network. The notification signal or feed back signal is time shifted to get better performance. This algorithm is called random early prediction (REP) (Manjunath,R., 2004).Feedback based control is in widespread use in systems that need precise adaptive control. Although there is feedback and an accurate model is not needed (only one that captures the 'dominant' behavior of the system), careful design of the controller is necessary. Otherwise it leads to instability.

Models of the communication among the agents are critical in providing high quality of service. A number of researchers have observed over the years that the traffic of communication does not obey Poisson distribution assumed in queuing analysis. The complexity of traffic in network is a result of integrating diverse ranges of members from different sources that significantly differ in their traffic patterns as well as their performance requirements over the same path.

Data Integration among Agents

In a multi agent scenario, fusion of the information from the different agents and removal of redundancies is tricky. Formulating the behavior and rules for each of the agents to achieve a desired common global behavior is an issue. The Bayesian networks capable of merging the rules may be used to get a common behavior. The agents are often distributed without a central server or program to control. The scenario represents a swarm and the techniques developed in swarm computing may be used in the inter agent communication. A differential feed back signal applied during the exchange of message or information can bring about a conscious global behavior from the individual behavior.

This global behavior is obtained by the weighted average of the individual behavior. It happens to be behavior of one of the elements of the group. The learning algorithms based on Genetic algorithm provide similar results.

The ability to fuse the service quality to the agent behavior is challenging. The feedback signals that get exchanged would provide a sophisticated platform for the same. Inter operability of the knowledge bases distributed across the globe in different regions is a major problem to be addressed. Semantic web provides the solution.

To handle the communication and queries in real time the agents are required to run sophisticated scheduling and learning algorithms. The scheduling and queue status may be coupled to the feedback signal that gets exchanged during communication. The feedback brings optimization for overall scheduling.

Handling the event queue and scheduling the events in an agent are tricky task. With differential feedback involving the agents, the event queue may be re organized in such a way that the overall QoS is met. Depending up on the QoS requirements, the position of an event (such as query) in the queue maps on to the probability of loss in the queue or to the probability of dropping the event. If the QoS parameter associated with the event is of higher priority, it would be positioned towards the head of the queue. The periodicity of evaluation may be fixed or once again event derived based on the arrival of the feedback signal.

For a given QoS, the queue position may be reflected on to the abstraction level of the information organization within a specified level of the knowledge hierarchy. Bayesian networks may be used for knowledge fusion. Bayesian networks map on to the knowledge base. If the conditional probability information is missing or uncertain, it may be predicted with the help of learning algorithms.

The Bayesian networks contain two parts-The deterministic part determined by the total probability and the time varying or dependent part dictated by the conditional probability. The conditional probability accounts for all uncertainties and dependencies in the know ledge supply chain including acquisition transfer etc. The fixed part of the knowledge is represented by zero feedback. The feedback provides built in intelligence as a result of previous history that account for powerful predictability. Hence, with differential feedback, it is possible to control or predict the missing part of the knowledge dependencies among the variables. With lapse of time i.e. when more previous history is available, the order of feedback increases and the resulting output is more & more abstract. Associated info is also less as it is almost predictable. Conditional probabilities represent the degree of dependence.

When the training set is small, the model parameters derived from it are generally less accurate because the noise associated with the data is also treated as the data. The noise gets cancelled out only when averaged over a large data set. It requires the model to work with a large data. No single model in practice, can work satisfactorily if the training data set is large. This is because it is very difficult to arrive at the consistent model parameters matching with the entire set of the data. An additional training set can always disagree with the model parameters derived from the training sets previously. However, a Gaussian model is overcomes this problem of over training (Karystinos,G., & Pados, D.,2000). A DANN based model, being Gaussian is resistant for over fitting.

In multiple agents the expertise is represented by a combination of declarative and procedural knowledge i.e., syntax and semantics. Therefore, each agent must operate independently to solve relevant sub problems and these individual solutions must be integrated into a globally consistent solution. This happens through a DANN by providing appropriate weightages to the individual solutions. An agent with only a local view of the search space cannot avoid producing sub problem solutions that conflict with other agents' solutions and cannot make intelligent decisions about managing conflicts that do occur.

The problem of local perspectives can be addressed by using learning techniques to enhance the global view at each agent. An agent embedded in a reusable-agent set is likely to propose solutions that conflict with the requirements of other agents. If the other agents can describe what is causing the conflicts, the proposing agent can begin to build a global perspective. This global perspective is typically not complete because not all conflicts can be readily described. However, any global information that can be readily shared will be useful in making local decisions. The global decision or perspective happens to be the scaled version of the individual agent decision or perspectives.

The search-oriented multi-agent systems often encounter the local perspective problem. This arises by constraining the information that gets distributed across the agent set but each individual agent perceives a search space bounded only by its local constraints rather than by the constraints of all agents in the system. This problem could be addressed if all expertise were represented in the form of explicit constraints or rules: the constraints could be collected and processed at one place to satisfy the constraints. A DANN can be used to merge the constraints and come out with an optimal constraint. Table I provides the simulation results of usage of DANN for merging the constraints for the communication among the agents.

Experimental Results

The simulation is carried out in Matlab software version 6. The functionalities of router, broker and the buffer of the data are all implemented within an agent. Four agents were considered to communicate simultaneously with four rules in the example. Each rule says who among the four connections are to be given the priority. Here, the agents 1 to 4 are assigned priority levels 1 to 4. If the data from agent with priority level 1 is contending with another agent with priority 4, the data from agent 4 is to be discarded to give

Table 1. Memory occupancy in different scheduling techniques

Method	Total cycles to clear all commands	Maximum memory utilization
ANN without differential feedback method	953	599
ANN with differential feedback method	927	423
ANN with self organization	936	447

space for the one from the agent 1. Likewise, a set or rules may be drafted down based on the contending priority levels. In the first experiment, as many estimators (neural networks) are used to learn the routing rules. In the second experiment, a single differentially fed neural network is used to learn the rules. In this case, the peak memory (resource) required to hold the results or growth of the buffer got reduced. The total time or cycles required to transfer all the packets considering the resource contention and retransmissions is also reduced.

It is clear from the table I that the differentially fed ANN can efficiently merge the ANNs reducing the resources as well as the time required to route the signals getting exchanged among the agents and provide a better quality of service for the communication.

Swarm of Agents

In a system making use of swarm computing, the basic unit of simulation is the swarm, a collection of agents executing a schedule of actions. Swarm supports hierarchical modeling approaches wherein agents can be composed of swarms of other agents in nested structures. Such a structure leads to abstraction of the commands.

The logical extension of distributed computing and memory paradigm blended with the Natural phenomenon of swarms gave birth to swarm computing. Here a group of computing elements or knowledge units each with a specific mission perform a common task and store its own contribution of the knowledge base and exchange the data over an adhoc network. There is no centralized server to control them. They communicate through the information left out by the others. The differential feedback may be explored for the effective utilization of this information for the communication among the members of the swarm. The model translates individual behavior to the collective behavior of the swarm. The entropy gets minimized with the differential feedback.

The ants use specific chemicals called pheromones for communication. Those insects that are ahead of rest of the swarm would leave some kind of footprints called pheromones for the detection and alteration by the others that follow them. The swarm members start changing these pheromones continuously. Each member while passing over the footprint of the other one will do that. It distorts it in its own way. What is left at the end will be having the previous history of all the foot prints i.e., a differential feedback or history.

The signal used for information exchange in a swarm comprises of two components, namely the Gaussian part and the bursty part. The Gaussian part of the signal corresponds to the aggregate of information over a period of time, whereas the bursty part models the information contribution by the swarm member. The Gaussian component imparts long range-dependence (LRD) to the signal, whereas the bursty component gives rise to spikiness. The investigation of random processes characterized by a wide range of timescales is becoming increasingly important in many experimental fields ranging from the investigation of earthquakes in earth science, to turbulence in fluids, or the price fluctuations in financial markets. In particular, many random processes exhibit a scale invariant structure. The self-similarity of the signal is reflected in the power law behavior of the power spectrum $S(f) = 1/f\alpha$, which lacks characteristic time scales. A collection of independent neurons require unsupervised learning.

In order to provide an inter-operable platform among agents in a multi-agent management environment, a minimal set of components and interfaces need to be specified. The important component is the message transport service that is used as an agent communication channel to route the messages among the agents. There are two kinds of routing-homogeneous and heterogeneous i.e. homogeneous agents are confined to within the platform. The heterogeneous agents reside on other platforms. The messages that get routed across these agents need to be queued and satisfy a certain degree of service quality. The techniques mentioned above will be useful here.

CONCLUSION

Agent based intelligent systems are extremely useful in on line and real time decision making systems. It calls for a powerful communication mechanism between the agents both within and across the platforms. The data routing mechanism requires built in intelligence. In this chapter a new class of neural networks called differentially fed artificial neural networks are introduced. With this, the signal exchange among the agents require minimal resources for a given service quality.

REFERENCES

Abraham, A., Grosan, C., & Ramos, V. (Eds.). (2006). *Swarm Intelligence in Data Mining Series: Studies in Computational Intelligence* (*Vol. 34*). Berlin: Springer-Verlag.

Bradshaw, J. M. (Ed.). (1997). *Software Agents*. Cambridge, MA: MIT Press.

Brenner, W., Zarnekow, R., & Hartmut, W. (1998). *Intelligent Software Agents*. Berlin: Springer.

Demazeau, Y. (1998). Preface. In *3rd International Conference on Multi-Agent Systems,* Paris, *ICMAS 98*.

Ferber, J. (1999). *Multi-Agent Systems*. New York: Addison-Wesley.

Hollot, C., Misra, V., Towsley, D., & Gong, W. (2001). *A Control Theoretic Analysis of RED*, INFOCOMM'01.

Karystinos, G., & Pados, D. (2000). On Overfitting, Generalization, and Randomly Expanded Training Sets. *IEEE Transactions on Neural Networks*, *11*(5), 1050–1057. doi:10.1109/72.870038

Maes, P. (1997). *Agents That Reduce Work and Information Overload. Software Agents*. Cambridge, MA: MIT Press.

Manjunath, R. (2006). *Compact architecture for the analysis and processing of subnet signals using differentiators as building blocks.* Unpublished doctoral dissertation, University of Bangalore, India

Manjunath, R. & Gurumurthy, K.S. (2002). *System design using differentially fed Artificial Neural networks*, TENCON'02.

Manjunath, R. & Gurumurthy, K.S. (2003). *Tensor domain analysis of differentially fed artificial neural networks, ITSim2003.*

Manjunath, R. & Gurumurthy, K.S. (2003a). Wavelet Representation of Differentially Fed ANN. *WSEAS Transactions On Circuits and systems*, Oct. 2003.

Manjunath, R. & Gurumurthy, K.S. (2004). *Maintaining Long-range dependency of traffic in a network*, CODEC'04.

Manjunath, R. & Shyam, V. (2008). *Improving Quality of Service through shifted prediction feedback*, CCNC'08.

Nwana, H. (1996). Software agents: an overview. *The Knowledge Engineering Review, 11*(3). doi:10.1017/S026988890000789X

Russell, S. & Norvig, (1995). *Artificial Intelligence: A Modern Approach.* New York: Prentice Hall.

Sycara, K., Dekker, K., Pannu, A., Williamson, M., & Zeng, D. (1996). Distributed Intelligent Agents. In IEEE Expert systems.

Chapter 13
Exploiting the Inter-Domain Hierarchy for the QoS Network Management

Marc-Antoine Weisser
SUPELEC, France

Joanna Tomasik
SUPELEC, France

Dominique Barth
PRiSM, The University of Versailles, France

ABSTRACT

The Internet is an interconnection of multiple networks called domains. Inter-domain routing is ensured by BGP which preserves each domain's independence and announces routes arbitrarily chosen by domains. BGP messages carry no information concerning quality parameters of announced routes. The authors' goal is to provide domains with information regarding the congestion state of other domains without any changes in BGP. A domain, which is aware of heavily congested domains, can choose a bypass instead of a route exhibiting possible problems with QoS satisfaction. They propose a mechanism which sends alert messages in order to notify domains about the congestion state of other domains. The major difficulty consists in avoiding flooding the Internet with signaling messages. The authors' solution limits the number of alerts by taking advantage of the hierarchical structure of the Internet set by P2C and P2P relationships. Their algorithm is distributed and heuristic because it is a solution to an NP-complete and inapproximable problem. They prove these properties by reducing the Steiner problem in directed acyclic graphs to our problem of alert diffusion. The simulations show that our mechanism significantly diminishes the number of unavailable domains and routes compared to those obtained with BGP routing and with a theoretical centralized mechanism.

DOI: 10.4018/978-1-61520-791-6.ch013

INTRODUCTION

The Internet is an interconnection of multiple networks called domains. We may see it as an inter-domain network. The transmission in the Internet may have to transit through several domains. The Internet connectivity is discovered by BGP (*Border Gateway Protocol*) (Rekhter, Watson, & Li, 1995) which is deployed in all the existing domains. This protocol was exclusively designed to transport information about possibilities of domain connections preserving at the same time the domain confidentiality and their independence, notably by letting domains choose connectivity information to be diffused on individual basis. It is well adapted to inter-domain routing because, despite of its possibly slow convergence and the complexity of routers, it is scalable.

The best-effort approach on both levels (IP, BGP) allows for the current Internet functioning thanks to over-dimensioning. Taking into consideration the growing number of Internet users and the development of different types of Internet applications, the introduction of QoS (*Quality of Service*) mechanisms is unavoidable. There are three ways to introduce the QoS into the inter-domain routing:

- replacing BGP by a new protocol,
- modifying BGP in order to adapt it to carry QoS information,
- deploying another protocol to transport QoS information, a protocol which works independently of BGP but collaborates with it.

As it is impossible to replace BGP incrementally by another protocol, the first of the possibilities listed above has to be rejected. The second approach seems to be more realistic, despite of the fact that incremental deployment is impossible. However, some attempts such as q-BGP (Boucadair, 2005) were proposed, which keeps routing tables for each class of service. This protocol also allows domains to have their own QoS criteria which are not necessarily adapted to being managed by normalized service definitions. Moreover, it does not take into account a current network state because a congestion detection mechanism is absent. In our opinion the most promising approach is the last one. In the next paragraph we discuss directions which have been taken in order to apply it in practice.

We consider two paradigms for the introduction of QoS into the Internet: flow-based and connectionless. The first one is based on an individual flow management. It requires the cooperation of network elements in order to set paths which satisfy required quality constraints and to allocate resources for individual flows. Propositions built on the flow-based paradigm are implemented on the intra-domain level (Braden, Zhang, Berson, Herzog, & Jamin, 1997). Generally, the flow-based paradigm is not adapted to the inter-domain level. The number of flows present on this level is too great to be managed individually. Moreover, domains are not interested in revealing information about their resources to other potentially competing domains. The flow-based paradigm should thus not be totally rejected as it is the only way to guarantee strict QoS requirements (Bless, 2004; Pan, Hahne, & Schulzrinne, 2000; Pelsser & Bonaventure, 2006). This paradigm may be applied to a small number of critical requests which need to satisfy strict QoS requirements. In practice, the number of strict QoS requests may be limited by assigning either a prohibitive price or an administrative restriction to them. For the other demands for QoS without strict guarantee, the second paradigm which is connectionless should be used.

The principle of the connectionless paradigm is represented by the rejection of flow management. Packets are divided into classes and the *priority traffic*, i.e. packets of the most privileged class, is, indeed, treated with priority. The connectionless paradigm is at the heart of the DiffServ architecture (Blake, Black, Carlson, Davies, Wang, & Weiss, 1998).

In (Weisser & Tomasik, 2006) we proposed an algorithm founded on the flow-based paradigm which finds multi-constraint paths in an inter-domain network. We then focused on the second approach which is connectionless (Weisser, Tomasik, & Barth, 2008). This chapter presents the complete theoretical study and simulation results we obtained to reach our goal which was to design a mechanism to find non-congested routes for priority traffic. It shows the influence of "non-standard" network characteristics as such the inter-domain hierarchy on the network performance and opens up new perspectives in the QoS network management.

PROPOSITION OF CONGESTION DETECTION

BGP is a protocol which constructs routing tables in an inter-domain network. We take as a hypothesis that a domain using BGP arbitrarily chooses one path from a set of possible paths, i.e. a domain uses the same BGP routing table for all its border routers (Feigenbaum, Papadimitriou, Sami, & Shenker, 2005). If a domain was aware of the congestion state of the other domains, it could choose a path which avoids the congested domains. Yet, such an approach is unrealistic because:

1. it would generate too many control messages,
2. domain operators would not want to give details of the configuration and resources of their domains.

We propose a mechanism which is external to BGP and which allows us to select paths avoiding congested domains. Our mechanism uses incomplete congestion state information to find bypasses which go around congested domains. Our mechanism copes with the two problems stated above.

Studies (Di Battista, Erlebach, Hall, Patrignani, Pizzonia, & Schank, 2007; Gao, 2001; Ge, Figueiredo, Jaiswal, & Gao, 2001; Subramanian, Agarwal, Rexford, & Katz, 2002) of BGP tables show a hierarchical structure of the inter-domain network. This hierarchy is induced by the different types of relationships assigned to links connecting two domains: *P2C (provider to customer)* and *P2P (peer to peer)*. Our mechanism uses this hierarchy to limit the number of control messages and solve the problem number 1.

A domain using our mechanism only needs to know about the congested domains which are found in its neighborhood. Moreover, a commercial contract defining relationships such as *P2C*, legitimates the exchange of the information concerning congestion. Providers have to warn their customers in order to allow them to change their routing and use networks of other providers. The warning obligation is legitimate because customers pay providers for a connectivity service. The problem number 2 stated above is solved because only a minimum of information is sent to a small number of domains.

BACKGROUND

Formerly examined approaches to introduce QoS into the inter-domain consist in either exchanging QoS characteristics between domains (Cristallo & Jacquenet, 2002) or guessing the QoS characteristics using probe messages (Xiao, Lui, Wang, & Nahrstedt, 2002). These approaches need a large amount of information which is difficult to collect and to use. Our approach proposes to use binary information regardless of whether a domain is congested or not. It is exchanged only by connected nodes.

A utilization of hierarchy in the context of QoS has already been dealt with in some papers

(Okumu, Mantar, Hwang, & Chapin, 2005; Subramanian, et al., 2005). The hierarchy described in (Okumu, Mantar, Hwang, & Chapin, 2005) is artificial and it has been constructed. Our proposition uses the existing hierarchy introduced by *P2P* and *P2C* relationships. We find a paper exploring this hierarchy in the routing context (Subramanian, et al., 2005). Its authors use it for a hybrid routing mechanism which works both with link-state vector and path vector.

To the best of our knowledge, the proposed utilization of alert message diffusion conditioned by the inter-domain hierarchy has never been studied. The present chapter demonstrates the interest of applying this hierarchy to congestion aware routing. We do not exclude that the knowledge of the hierarchy may be profitable in other aspects of inter-domain network management.

INTER-DOMAIN TOPOLOGY

An inter-domain network is composed of independent domains administrated by operators. Links connecting domains are characterized by different types of relationships. The relationships which depend on commercial contract signed by domain operators are:

- *P2C*, *provider-to-customer*, assigned to a link between a customer domain which buys a connectivity service from a provider domain, and
- *P2P*, *peer-to-peer*, assigned to a link existing between two domains which share connectivity.

The studies of BGP tables (Gao, 2001; Ge, Figueiredo, Jaiswal, & Gao, 2001; Subramanian, Agarwal, Rexford, & Katz, 2002) show that these types of relationships introduce a hierarchy imposing layers in the inter-domain network.

The core, *Tier-1*, is on the top of the hierarchy. It is a set of domains which are linked by *P2P* relationships. The domains of the core are not customers of any domain. Each domain of the core is connected to all (or almost all) other domains of the core. For this reason the core is close to a clique. Usually, the domains in the layer *Tier-i* are providers of domains in the layer *Tier-j* with $j > i$. The domains in the layer *Tier*-j are customers of domains in the *Tier-i*, $i < j$. The domains in the layer *Tier-i* and in *Tier-j* are linked together with *P2C* relationships. Domains in the same layer can be linked together with *P2P* or *P2C* relationships.

The average percentage of domains in each layer increases strictly (starting from the *Tier-1*). The average degree of a domain in a layer decreases strictly (starting from the *Tier-1*).

The inter-domain hierarchy has an impact on the current inter-domain routing because routes are established according to commercial relationships. According to the BGP operational principle which takes into account commercial agreements and financial compensation:

- a customer domain announces to its customers, peers, and providers the routes which it can establish,
- a provider domain announces its routes to its customers only,
- a peer announces available routes via its peers to its own customers only.

This principle implies that routes announced in the inter-domain network have a particular shape. They are made of downhill and uphill components connected by at most one *P2P* link. Speaking more precisely, a downhill component is a list of consecutive links labeled with a *P2C* relationship. An uphill component is a list of consecutive links labeled with a *C2P* relationship which is dual to a *P2C*. The uphill and downhill components are connected either by zero or by one *P2P* relationship. Such routes are called *valley-free* by Gao (Gao, 2001) and we adopt this term.

Figure 1 gives an example of *valley-free* routes. The possible *valley-free* routes from the domain *G*

Figure 1. Example of an inter-domain network: arcs indicate C2P relationships, undirected edges which are marked with dashed line indicate P2P relationships. The two solid paths are valley-free, the two pointed ones are not.

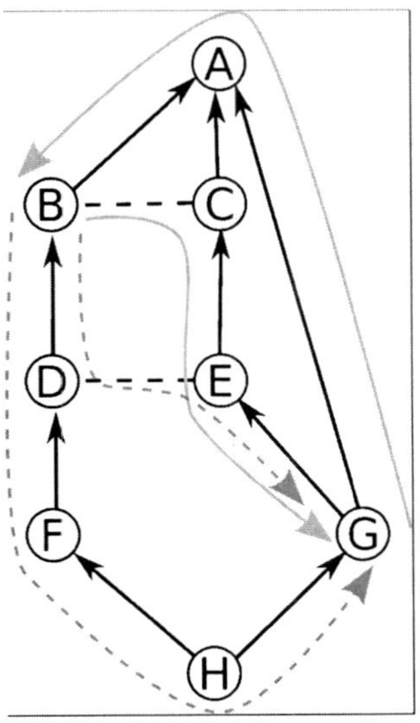

to the domain B are: (G, A, B), (G, E, C, A, B), and (G, E, C, B). The domain G has to pay for using any of these routes (either the provider A in the first case or the provider E in the two latter cases). As the reader may observe, the routes establishing connection from B to G, (B, A, G) and (B, C, E, G), are not symmetric to the ones mentioned above. The longer route is more advantageous for B because it does not have to pay to use it (B is a C peer). The shorter route is less advantageous for the domain B because it has to remunerate its provider A for transiting traffic.

Continuing the description of our example in Figure 1, we explain why routes which are not *valley-free* such as (B, D, E, G) and (B, D, F, H, G) do not exist in the Internet. The first route is never established because D does not transit for free the traffic of its provider B to its peer E (consequently, D does not announce the passage towards E to its provider B). The second route is never established because H is not interested in transiting the traffic sent by the domain F towards G and in paying for this transfer. For this raison H does not inform F about a connection to G.

These observations have helped us to detect possibly congested domains in the global network. We assumed that commercial relationships oblige providers to keep their customers informed about their current capacity of traffic transfer. This knowledge allows us to find routes with the best current quality to transit priority traffic. We say that a route is better than another when it is composed of fewer congested domains. We also take advantage of the inter-domain hierarchy to limit the number of control messages and the size of a sub-network in which they have to be diffused.

PROBLEM MODELING

We use a graph to model our problem. Let $G = (V,A,E)$ be a mixed graph (partially oriented as defined in (Raghavachari & Veerasamy, 1999) to which we refer later as *inter-domain graph*. A vertex $v \in V$ represents a domain in the inter-domain network. We enumerate the elements of V with natural numbers $1 \dots n$. An ordered pair $(p,c) \in A$ represents an existing *P2C* relationship between a provider p and its customer c. A pair $\{p_1,p_2\} \in E$ represents a *P2P* relationship between domains p_1 and p_2.

Relationships between domains are based on commercial contracts. A provider p, which sells connectivity to a customer c, cannot be a customer of c. We, therefore, consider that there is no cycle made of *P2C* relationships in an inter-domain network (Gao & Rexford, 2000) (Gao, Griffin, & Rexford, 2001). This means that (V,A) is a directed acyclic graph (DAG). The roots of this DAG are the vertices representing the domains of the core.

We define a capacity function $c\colon V \rightarrow \mathbb{R}^{>}$ (real positive). The value $c(v_i)$ represents an amount of traffic which can be transited by the domain v_i without overloading it.

Let $T: V^2 \rightarrow R^{\geq}$ (real non-negative) be a traffic matrix. Each value $T_{i,j}$ represents an amount of traffic which has to be sent from i to j. The traffic $T_{i,j}$ represents the internal traffic of the domain i.

Let $R: V^2 \rightarrow V$ be a routing matrix. Each value $R_{i,j}$ represents the next hop for a packet passing through the domain i which is to be sent to the domain j. We set $R_{i,i} = i$, for all $i \in \{1, \ldots, n\}$ for internal traffic. We say that a matrix R is *valley-free* if, and only if, all the routes which it represents are valley-free.

Given a network, a traffic matrix and a routing matrix, we say that a node is *perturbed* if the total amount of traffic transiting through it, emitted by it, and sending to it is greater than its capacity. A *perturbed path* is a path containing at least one perturbed node. Each $T_{i,j}$ is transmitted on a route induced by the routing. Traffic between i and j is perturbed if the route between i and j is perturbed. The *volume of a perturbed traffic* is the sum of traffic passing on perturbed paths.

Given a network and a traffic matrix, our problem is to find a valley-free routing matrix which minimizes

- the number of perturbed nodes (*network approach*);
- the volume of the traffic passing along perturbed paths (*traffic approach*).

This is an optimization problem with bi-criteria. We focus on the network approach only because we assume that minimizing the number of perturbed nodes may be a good heuristic approach to minimize the number of perturbed paths as well as the volume of perturbed traffic (see Results). Another reason for choosing the network approach criterion is implied by the operation mode of the proposed algorithm. As the reader will see in the section describing our method, the nodes which modify their state send alert messages. The minimization of the perturbed node number limits the number of sent messages.

Given a network and a traffic matrix, we refer to the above described problem as the *valley-free routing problem* (VFRP). The weight of its solution is the number of perturbed nodes.

REDUCTION TO THE STEINER PROBLEM

The definition of the *directed Steiner tree problem* (DSTP) is as follows: Given a DAG G, a root v, and a set of nodes S, find a directed tree of minimal weight containing each node in S. The weight of a solution is the number of nodes in the directed tree.

This problem is NP-complete (Hsu, Tsai, Wang, & Lee, 1996). We prove that VFRP is NP-complete and inapproximable. In an optimization problem, the aim is to minimize or maximize the value of a feasible solution considering a given objective function. Such an objective function could concern a benefit, the edge or vertex weight of a sub-graph, etc. The inapproximability of an optimization problem means that there is not a polynomial time algorithm which provides a solution whose value is bound with the optimal value of a solution by a constant ratio.

Theorem

Let $G = (V, A, E)$ be an inter-domain graph with a capacity function $c: V \rightarrow R^{>}$ and a traffic matrix $T: V^2 \rightarrow R^{\geq}$ associated. The problem of finding a valley-free routing which minimizes the number of perturbed nodes is NP-complete and inapproximable.

Proof

First, we observe that if we dispose of an instance of VFRP (consisted in an inter-domain graph, a capacity function, and a traffic matrix) and of a valley-free routing, we can compute in polynomial

Figure 2. Graph representing an instance I of DSTP (sink nodes are grey) and an instance I' of VFRP (all nodes but the root have a unitary capacity).

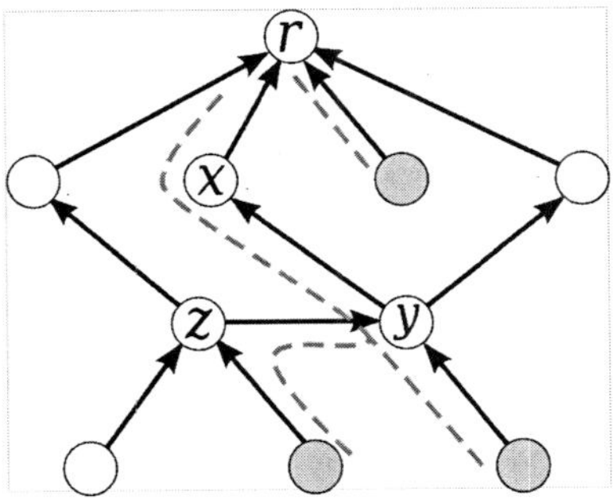

time how many nodes are perturbed. In other words, the certificate of VFRP is in the class P.

Second, we demonstrate that VFRP is NP-hard by reducing DSTP to VFRP. Let I be an instance of DSTP. Let $G = (V,A)$ be DAG rooted in r and S Í V a set of sink nodes. The solution of DSTP is a directed tree rooted in r which contains each node of S. Notice that a directed tree rooted in r and containing each node of S is made of valley-free routes from r to each node of S. Figure 2 presents a DAG $G = (V,A)$ with sink (grey) nodes. A minimal solution to DSTP is marked with dashed lines.

From I, we build an instance I' of VFRP. Let $G' = (V,A,E)$ be an inter-domain graph with $E = \emptyset$. Let $c(i) = 1$, for all $i \in V$¾$\{r\}$ and $c(r) = \infty$ be the capacity function. Let T be a traffic matrix

$$T_{i,j} = \begin{cases} 1+\varepsilon, i = r \wedge j \in S \\ 0, i \neq r \vee j \notin S \end{cases} \qquad (1)$$

Let us see now the graph in Figure 2 as an inter-domain graph $G' = (V,A,\emptyset)$ whose nodes have a unitary capacity (the root has an infinite capacity). According to the traffic matrix (Eq. (1)) non-zero traffic passes exclusively between the root r and sink nodes of S. We observe that the volume of traffic passing through nodes x, y, and z exceeds their capacity. For any path from r to s, $s \in S$, all nodes along the path but the root are perturbed. Therefore, the weight of a minimal solution to the instance I' of VFRP (the number of perturbed nodes) is the weight of a minimal solution of the instance I of DSTP minus one (the root is never perturbed).

We can reduce an instance of DSTP into an instance of VFRP in polynomial time. Thus, VFRP is NP-hard.

We remind the reader that, as we have seen before, the certificate of VFRP is in P. Consequently, VFRP is NP-complete.

In (Weisser & Tomasik, 2007) we prove that DSTP is inapproximable. VFRP is also inapproximable because the weight of the solution for the instances I minus one is equal to the weight of the instance I'. □

ALERT SENDING ALGORITHM

Our distributed algorithm is based upon the principle of sending alert messages which carry information about the domain congestion state. Each node informs its clients when it becomes perturbed in order to allow them to change their routing. Each node also keeps its neighbors informed when it returns to an operational state. To avoid taking the risk of flooding the entire network with alert messages, we aim to limit the range of their diffusion. We propose to take advantage of the inter-domain hierarchy to restrict the alert diffusion range.

We suppose that each node is provided with a BGP routing table and with a *priority table*. A priority table stores potentially congestion-free routes set aside for priority traffic. The priority table is the same as the BGP table if a node is not perturbed and neither are its neighbors (customers, peers, and providers). The BGP table is altered by classical BGP mechanisms only (Rekhter, Watson, & Li, 1995). The priority table is altered by our alerts and, occasionally, by changes in the BGP table.

Figure 3. The node x is red when either the traffic it has to transit is greater than its capacity or its provider and next hop a becomes red.

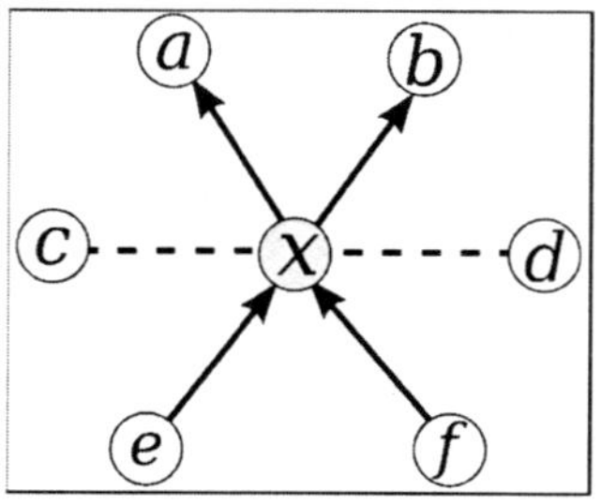

Each node contains a list of possible next hops towards every destination. These lists are constructed with routes announced by BGP. Their construction guarantees that all next hops satisfy the valley-free property of routes.

Each node can be in either of two distinct states: *green* or *red*. A node state is *red* (it is congested and/or is situated on a path containing congested nodes) if at least one of the two following conditions is satisfied:

- the amount of traffic transiting through the node, sending from it and sending to it, is greater than its capacity;
- at least one of its next hops which is a provider is in *red* state.

A node cannot become *red* because of its customer and peer congestion. Because of this fact, our algorithm avoids the spread of *red* nodes over the entire network when a single node becomes *red*. We use the hierarchy to limit the number of nodes in *red* state as well as the messages sent: a node which has a customer or a peer in *red* state as a next hop should not be in *red* state itself. The node which is not in *red* state is in *green* state. The *green* state is a domain stable state. The example is depicted in Figure 3. The domain *x* (grey) has two providers, *a* and *b*, two peers, *c* and *d*, and two customers, *e* and *f*. Let assume that *x* uses the domains *a*, *c*, and *e* as next hops. Other domains can be next hops for alternative paths. The node *x* is *red* when either the traffic it has to transit is greater than its capacity or its provider and next hop *a* becomes *red.*

Each node stores a table containing states of its neighbors. This table is updated by alert messages sent by the neighboring providers and customers when their state changes. A node changing its state sends messages to its customers and providers to inform them about its new state. The messages are sent up and down the hierarchy but the peers do not receive the message so that the spread of messages would remain limited. The alert message is composed of: an ID of the node (domain number), a new state, and a delay *d*. It enters into the scheduler of the node receiving the message where it is processed after the delay *d*. The received message replaces any older message which arrived from the same node and is present in the scheduler.

We introduce a notation in order to describe the behavior of a node processing an alert message. Let BR_i and PR_i be tables stored in the node *i*, containing the next hop for the BGP routing and the priority routing, respectively. The values contained in BR_i are computed by the classical BGP mechanism. The default values of PR_i are the same as those of BR_i.

Let LR_i be a table containing lists of the next hops which may be used to reach every destination. These lists are constructed using the routes announced by BGP. For a destination *j*, if there is a path from *i* to *j* via a customer of *i*, $LR_i[j]$ contains all next hops which are customers and which are announced by BGP. If a next hop is a peer, $LR_i[j]$ contains all the next hops announced by BGP which are peers. Otherwise, $LR_i[j]$ contains all next hops which are providers. These restrictions are useful to keep valley-free property preserved.

Let st_i be a table stored in the node *i* containing the known states of its neighbors. The default values in this table are *green*.

The following pseudocode details the behavior of a node *i* treating a message *m* received from the node *j*.

```
Input: message m = (j, color, delay) and
tables BR_i, PR_i, LR_i, st_i
Output:
1.  delete m from the scheduler
2.  st_i[j] › color
3.  if (color = red) then
4.    for all dest ∈ V do
5.      if (PR_i[dest] = j) then
6.        let S › {x ∈ LR_i[dest] | st_i[x] = green}
7.        if S = Ø then
8.          PR_i[dest] › BR_i[dest]
9.        else
10.         PR_i[dest] › choose_randomly_in(S)
11.       end if
12.     end if
13.   end for
14. else
15.   for all dest ∈ V do
16.     if (st_i[ PR_i[dest] ] = red) then
17.       if (j ∈ LR_i[dest]) then
18.         PR_i[dest] › j
19.       end if
20.     end if
21.     if (BR_i[dest] = j) then
22.       PR_i[dest] › j
23.     end if
24.   end for
25. end if
```

Steps 3-13 are executed when an incoming alert message arrives from a node *j* which is in *red* state. In this case, the node *i* selects destinations for which the node *j* is a designated next hop. The node *i* then looks for alternative next hops for the selected destinations. An alternative next hop is chosen according to a uniform distribution among domains stored in the set $LR_i[dest]$ and indicated as being in *green* state. If no node can be chosen, we use the default path stored in the BGP table in spite of its state. Obviously, a valley-free route does not include any cycle. Our mechanism keeps this route property preserved because the construction of the LR_i table permits us to replace a customer only by a customer, a peer only by a peer and a provider only by a provider.

Steps 14-24 are executed when the node *j* is in *green* state. In this situation, the node *i* replaces the nodes mentioned below by the node *j*

- the next hops whose state is *red* and which are leading to destinations for which *j* can be a next hop, or
- the next hops whose state is *green* towards all destinations for which *j* is a "natural" next hop according to BGP routing.

An objectionable phenomenon may emerge from exchanges of *green* and *red* alert messages. A customer *c* with two providers p_1 and p_2 can choose p_1 as a next hop for the destination *d* and perturb p_1. The perturbed node p_1 sends a *red* alert to *c* which changes its next hop to p_2. The provider p_1 is now *green* and the provider p_2 becomes *red*. The providers, p_1 and p_2, send a *green* and a *red* alert, respectively. The customer changes its next hop once again causing instability.

We avoid such instability by introducing a delay before the alert message is processed. Each alert message contains a field to store the delay *d* before the message processing. The messages are sent immediately but their processing is deferred. The delay is set according to a random distribution in order to avoid synchronization in the network. We use an exponential distribution whose mean is small for *red* alert and big for *green* alert.

The delay mechanism protecting the network against instability may unnecessarily introduce the *red* state into too many nodes. Therefore, the BGP table is used by default when no *green* next hop can be found and instability in the network leads our mechanism to work temporarily as BGP.

SIMULATIONS

We use simulation to evaluate the performance of our algorithm. Its performance will be compared to the performance of BGP and a theoretical centralized algorithm. The performance measures used to make comparisons are the numbers of perturbed nodes and paths, and the amount of perturbed traffic.

We expect that BGP will provide the worst results and we will use the results to obtain an upper bound for the number of perturbed elements. The next section will show that our algorithm always provides much better results than BGP.

The alert sending mechanism is distributed and operates in *on-line* mode, i.e. it processes each input in turn, without a detailed knowledge of future inputs (Atallah & Blanton, 1999). We define a centralized algorithm working in an *off-line* mode, i.e., it is given the entire sequence of inputs in advance.

We point out that such an algorithm, studied here for comparison purposes, cannot be considered as implementable in a network because of its complexity and the huge amount of data it has to process. We use it only to find a lower bound for the number of perturbed network elements.

Centralized Algorithm

Given an inter-domain graph G and a traffic matrix T, our goal is to find a routing matrix which minimizes the number of perturbed nodes in a network without consideration of the amount of traffic passing through perturbed nodes.

We consider that the minimum size for an inter-domain graph is 20 nodes (a nontrivial core, at least three layers, an increasing number of nodes in layers starting from the core, a number of paths between two nodes greater than one). This problem is NP-complete and inapproximable. We cannot use any exact algorithm to solve it because of the size of its instances. Thus, we have to use a heuristic algorithm.

Local modifications in the routing may have a global impact on the solution. Firstly, replacing a path by a new one may generate and remove perturbed nodes along both the new path and the old one. Secondly, changing a next hop may affect anything from one path to $n-1$ paths, where n is the number of nodes in the graph. For these reasons we propose a greedy heuristic algorithm i.e., which solves an optimization problem by finding locally optimal solutions (Atallah & Blanton, 1999) and which does not modify previous choices.

We observe that paths rising in the hierarchy are longer than the other paths. Moreover, they pass through nodes which may be used to satisfy many demands. These paths may cause the introduction of many perturbed nodes which degrade the network performance. For a traffic *demand* (s,d,t), where $t = T_{s,d}$, we define that a *preferred path* is a path which:

- minimizes the number of perturbed nodes;
- is preferably composed of nodes from lower layers.

To find such paths, we use an exhaustive route exploration. Such an exploration takes into account possible paths already introduced into the routing matrix. Exhaustive exploration runs in exponential time but we are not interested in the complexity of this algorithm. For most of the instances the complexity is polynomial. In practice, exploration time is quite short.

Our centralized algorithm is set out below. The steps 1-10 are the first phase of the algorithm during which we sort the demands in decreasing order of traffic amount and we satisfy as many demands as we can without perturbing any node.

The introduction of any demand which is not yet satisfied (steps 11-18), produces perturbed nodes. We search the worst demand and we satisfy it using a preferred path as long as unsatisfied demands persist. We define the *worst demand* as a demand:

- whose satisfaction using the preferred path introduces the maximum number of new perturbed nodes;
- whose amount of traffic is maximal.

Centralized Algorithm

```
Input: inter-domain graph G = (V,A,E) and list L of demands: (source, destination, traffic)
Output:
1.  let R be a routing matrix containing no path
2.  sort demands L in decreasing order of traffic
3.  for all q_i = (s_i,d_i,t_i) ∈ L do
4.     let p_i = find preferred path for q_i
5.     if (satisfying q_i using p_i does not perturb node) then
6.        add p_i to routing matrix R
7.        reduce capacity of node in p_i by t_i
8.        remove q_i of L
9.     end if
10. end for
11. while L ≠ Ø do
12.    let (s_j,d_j,t_j) := find the worst demand in L
13.    p_j := find best path for (s_j,d_j,t_j)
14.    add p_j to routing matrix R
15.    reduce capacity of node in p_j by t_j
16.    remove (s_j,d_j,t_j) of L
17. end while
18. return the routing matrix R
```

Simulation Plan

Our algorithm was tested for inter-domain topologies randomly generated with SHIIP, *SUPELEC Inter-domain Induction Program* (Weisser & Tomasik, 2007) which introduces the domain hierarchy into flat inter-domain topologies generated by BRITE (Medina, Lakhina, Matta, & Byers, 2001). The SHIIP software was written especially with the aim to validate our sending mechanism. Nevertheless, it may be useful for other purposes as well and for this reason it is available to the public on the Web. The chosen topologies have parameters (core size, layer size, node degree) close to the means of a series of topologies of a given size obtained with SHIIP. The results discussed in the next section were obtained for a network of 100 domains.

A traffic matrix $T: V^2 \rightarrow R^{\geq}$ is initially empty. At each step k the iterative matrix filling procedure determines a pair $(i^{(k)}, j^{(k)})$ where $i^{(k)}$ is uniformly chosen from the set V-$\{i^{(1)}, i^{(2)}, \ldots, i^{(k-1)}\}$ ($j^{(k)}$ is found in the same way in the set V-$\{j^{(1)}, j^{(2)}, \ldots, j^{(k-1)}\}$). Next, the procedure assigns a value $T(i^{(k)}, j^{(k)})$ indicating a traffic volume to be routed between two nodes $i^{(k)}$ and $j^{(k)}$. The volume of traffic $T(i^{(k)}, j^{(k)})$ is chosen according to a linearly scaled normal distribution. The diagonal element values $T(i^{(k)}, i^{(k)})$ represent a traffic to be carried inside the domain $i^{(k)}$. After $|V|^2$ iterations all matrix elements are examined and we consider the matrix as a full matrix. Starting from this point we vary the network load. We choose an (i,j) pair where both i and j are independently and uniformly distributed among the elements of V. We then set a new traffic value $T_{i,j}$ using the same normal distribution as before. In our simulation we use $(\alpha/|V|^2)$ Gauss(sqrt(5), 5) distribution limited to nonnegative values. The scaling factor α, $\alpha \geq 1$ allows us to study series of experiments with a growing traffic load. We do not specify a traffic unit, we speak of *Traffic Unit* (TU).

The choice of the time scale is not essential because we are interested in differences between the performances of our algorithm and two algorithms of reference expressed in terms of the number of perturbed nodes, paths, and the amount of perturbed traffic. We choose the exponential distribution with a mean equal to one time unit to determine a time passing between two consecutive traffic matrix changes.

We also choose the capacities in generated topologies to study networks which are not over-dimensioned. On the Internet, the largest domains with the largest capacities are at the top of the hierarchy. Domains with smaller capacities are at the bottom of the hierarchy. We suppose that the domains in the core are never perturbed. Thus, we choose to set the infinite capacity for all of them. We arbitrarily fix the capacity for domains in the *Tier-2* to 35 TU. For domains in the layers *Tier-3* and *Tier-4* we set capacities to 80% and 40% of the *Tier-2* capacity, respectively.

The first performance measure is obviously the number of perturbed nodes because it is also the optimization criterion for our algorithm. The second one is the number of perturbed paths and the third one is the amount of perturbed traffic. The second and the third are strongly influenced by the first one. These three measures are essential for the comparison of performance results of our distributed algorithm with the performance results of BGP and our theoretical centralized algorithm.

We are also interested in particular performance measures inherent to our distributed algorithm. We count the number of messages sent and the number of network state changes where a network state is a vector containing current congestion states of all network nodes.

RESULTS

In the first place we compare the number of perturbed nodes obtained for one simulation run with our distributed algorithm and BGP (Figure 4). The volume of transiting traffic is heavy enough (α=2.0) to saturate about 10% of nodes if the network uses BGP. Observe that the number of the perturbed nodes increases quickly and reaches eight nodes when the traffic matrix is filled up. The number of perturbed nodes oscillates around this value. Our algorithm considerably diminishes (about five times) the number of perturbed nodes. The initial heavy perturbation of six nodes is quickly reduced. Notice also that the shapes of these two diagrams are very similar.

Figure 4. The number of perturbed nodes for our algorithm (one simulation run, network of 100 nodes, heavy traffic α= 2.0).

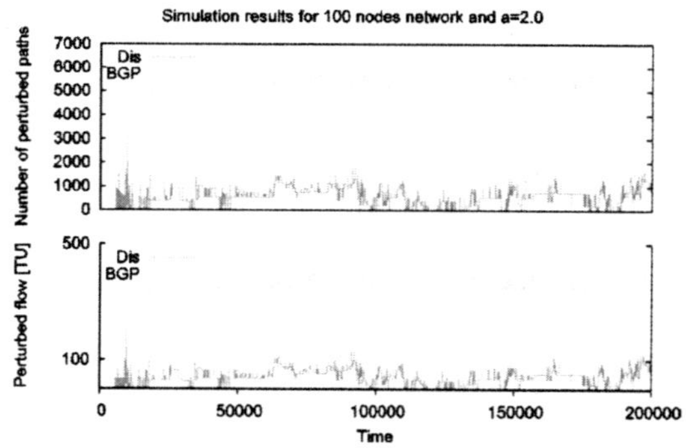

The number of alerts sent depends not only on the number of perturbed nodes but also on the layers in which these nodes are localized. The manifestation of four more perturbed nodes can cause the generation of the same number of alert messages as the manifestation of one perturbed node, but only if these nodes are situated far from the core.

Two other performance measures, the number of perturbed paths and the quantity of perturbed traffic, taken for the same network during the same simulation run, are depicted in Figure 5. As we expected in the section dedicated to problem modeling, the results for

Figure 5. Number of perturbed path and amount of perturbed traffic for our algorithm (one simulation run, network of 100 nodes, heavy traffic α=2.0).

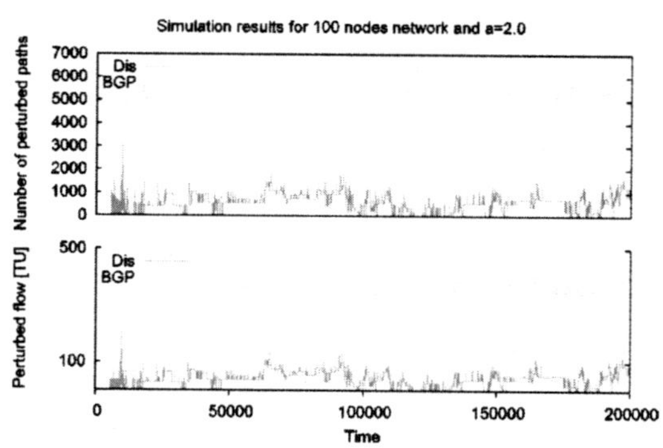

Figure 6. The number of perturbed nodes and paths averaged for a simulation run series, network of 100 nodes and heavy traffic α=2.0.

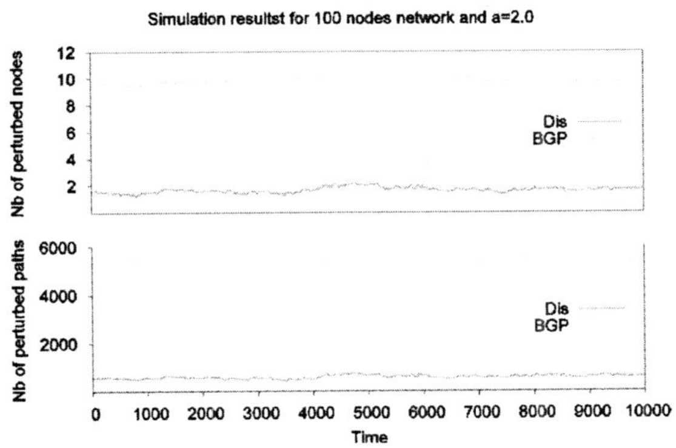

our algorithm are significantly better than for BGP although our method does not optimize them directly.

To verify the functioning of our method and that of BGP we performed a series of simulation runs for the same network and traffic load. The averages of the numbers of perturbed paths and nodes, presented in Figure 6, exhibit a strong tendency which appears in a simple simulation run; our algorithm works on average five times better than BGP for the given network.

The influence of the traffic load on the performance of our algorithm is presented in Figure

Figure 7. The number of perturbed nodes depending on the traffic load averaged for series of simulation runs for a 100 node network.

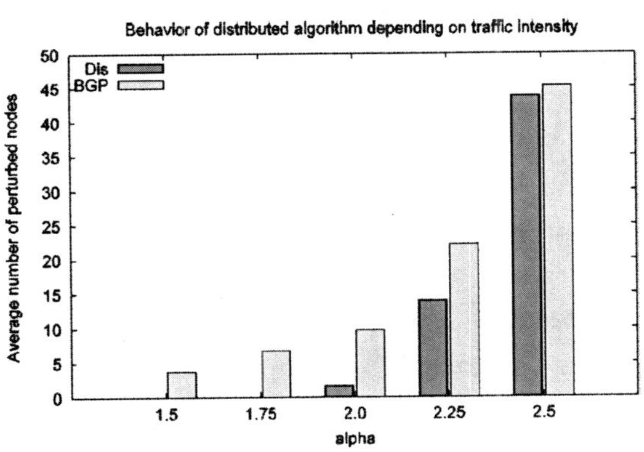

7. We used averaged series of simulation runs. Each series had a different load which varies from light load (α=1.5) to saturating load (α=2.5) with a step a equal to 0.25. In the same figure we show the results for the BGP performance. We observe that the saturating traffic α=2.5 is critical for the network because almost half of the network nodes are perturbed. In this case the performance of our algorithm approaches that of BGP.

The additional cost of our algorithm in relation to BGP is expressed in the number of transmitted alert messages. This number, for one simulation and for varying traffic loads, is plotted in an accumulative manner in Figure 8. For any traffic load the number of messages sent increases rapidly during the traffic matrix filling up period. Subsequently, the number of sent messages increases at a much slower rate. The increase in the number of sent messages is more significant for heavier traffic loads because more nodes become perturbed. As message transmission causes a change of node states, the number of network state changes depicted in Figure 9 follows the same pattern as that of alert messages.

The methodology applied to the comparison of our distributed algorithm and BGP cannot be used for a confrontation between the distributed and the centralized algorithms for two following

Figure 8. The cumulative number of sent messages for one simulation run depending on the traffic load for a network of 100 nodes.

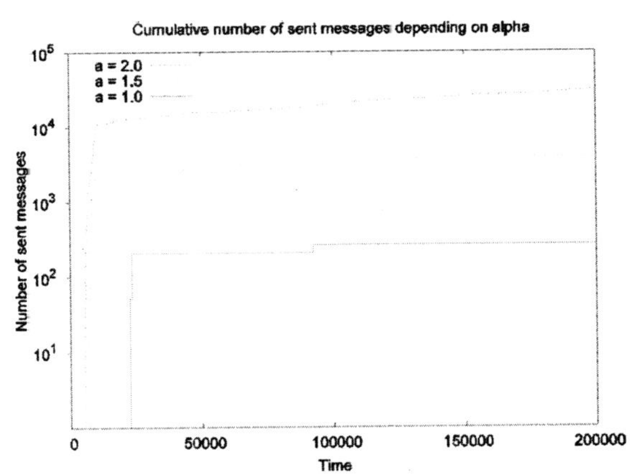

Figure 9. The cumulative number of state changes for one simulation run depending on the traffic load for a network of 100 nodes.

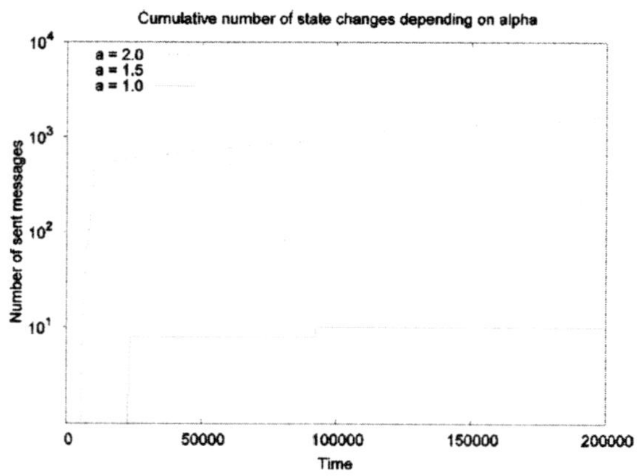

Figure 10. The number of perturbed nodes in a 100 node network averaged for series of initial instances with BGP, the centralized algorithm, and the distributed algorithm applied on routing obtained with BGP and our centralized algorithms together with a lower bound (heavy traffic, α= 2.0).

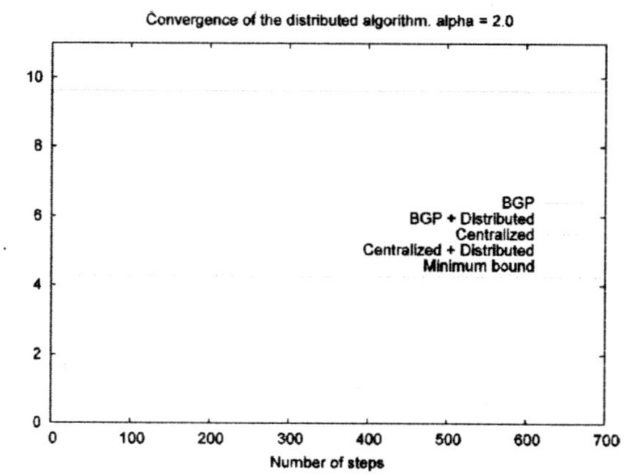

reasons. Firstly, computations performed by the theoretical centralized algorithm for each change in the traffic matrix are unacceptably time-consuming. The computations would make relevant simulation runs excessively long. Secondly, the variation of values of the elements of the traffic matrix one by one as described in the simulation plan could be seen as too advantageous for our distributed algorithm.

To evaluate our distributed algorithm, while retaining BGP as a practical reference, we start from an instant of the problem. It has been selected as a typical network state together with the traffic matrix from the simulation runs which have been discussed above. Starting from this point the traffic matrix is fixed and we activate our distributed alert mechanism with routing matrices produced with BGP and our centralized algorithm. We observe the rate with which it diminishes the number of perturbed nodes. We compare these results with the number of perturbed nodes when we use BGP and the centralized algorithm alone.

We compute a lower bound which is the number of nodes perturbed by traffic, whatever the routing matrix. For any routing matrix, a node i is perturbed if the sum of traffic sent by i and sent to i is greater than its capacity. We do not consider traffic transiting through it. This is a lower bound for our problem.

Figures 10 and 11 present results of our comparison averaged for series of initial instances with heavy traffic: α=2.0 and α=2.25, respectively. We observe that the distributed algorithm optimizes routing matrices produced with both BGP and our centralized algorithm.

For α=2.0 (Figure 10), the perturbation in the network is caused by the routing. A lower bound indicates that only 0.6% of nodes is perturbed, whatever the routing. This bound is reached by the combination of our centralized algorithm and the distributed one. This means that the bound is not only a lower bound but the optimum. With routing provided by BGP and our centralized algorithm, 9.6% and 4.3% of nodes are perturbed, respectively. This means that about 9.6-0.6 = 9.0% and 4.3-0.6 = 3.7% of nodes are perturbed only because of the transit traffic due to the BGP routing and the routing given by the centralized algorithm, respectively. The combination of BGP

Figure 11. The number of perturbed nodes in a 100 node network averaged for series of initial instances with BGP, the centralized algorithm, and the distributed algorithm applied on routing obtained with BGP and our centralized algorithms together with a lower bound (very heavy traffic, α = 2.25).

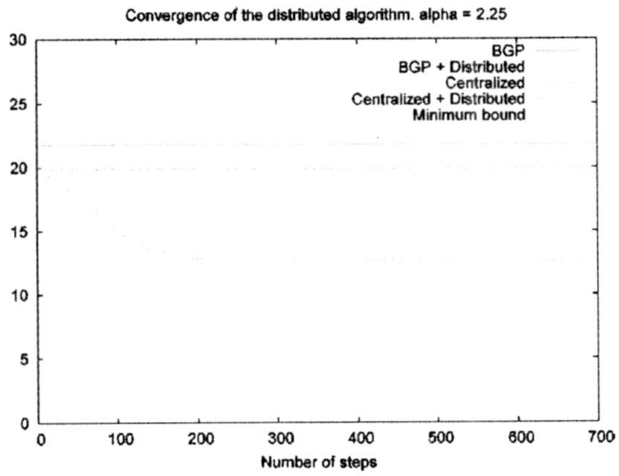

and our distributed algorithm is very good because the average percentage of perturbed nodes is stabilized around one percent. This is a better result than that provided by the centralized algorithm alone and only twice greater than the optimum.

For α = 2.25 (Figure 11), the perturbation in the network is substantial. There is 11.8 percent of nodes perturbed in the network, whatever the routing. BGP routing and our centralized algorithm provide results which are close (21.8% and 19.9%, respectively). Nonetheless, the combination of our centralized and distributed algorithm provides results which are much better than the combination of BGP and our distributed algorithm. The convergence is faster and the results are close to the minimum bound. The combination of BGP and our centralized algorithm is advantageous because it reduces by half the nodes whose perturbation is linked to the routing.

Figures 10 and 11 show that the distributed algorithm reduces efficiently the number of nodes perturbed only by transit traffic. Moreover, this number is close to the optimal number when the initial routing matrix is provided by the centralized algorithm. The centralized algorithm provides a solution which is a good initial solution for the distributed algorithm but it is not an available solution in practice.

SUMMARY AND FURTHER STUDIES

In this chapter we have proposed a BGP independent distributed mechanism in inter-domain networks to find non-congested routes which provides new possibilities missing from the state-of-art inter-domain traffic engineering. It sends out incomplete information concerning congestion state of domains by sending alert messages. The number of emitted alert messages and the range of their diffusion are limited by taking advantage of the hierarchy which is naturally established by the commercial relationships *P2C* and *P2P* existing between domains.

Because our distributed algorithm is heuristic, we performed exhaustive simulation experiments to evaluate the efficiency. On the one hand, we compared its performance with that of BGP and observed a considerable gain obtained when using our approach. On the other hand, we wanted to confront our mechanism with the one which always provides the precise results but cannot be implemented in a real network because of the computational effort it requires. For such comparison purposes we constructed a centralized off-line algorithm.

The obtained results are encouraging and we are convinced that the proposed distributed algorithm is worth further study.

First, we would like to verify the performance of our distributed algorithm for an inter-domain network model with the size and the hierarchy of the Internet. An open issue concerning the Internet hierarchy is notably the presence of *sibling to sibling* relationship which we have not investigated yet.

Second, we started our work from the hypothesis that information concerning congestion in the network allows an operator to route priority traffic on congestion-free paths. Notice that this is not a unique possibility to take advantage of the results of our distributed algorithm. An operator might prefer to place priority traffic on the best routes at his disposal despite their congestion state. In such a case, the operator redirects non-priority traffic on non-congested paths while saving the capacity of the best routes for privileged traffic. The operator decision may depend on route lengths and we would like to estimate them. The simulation studies presented in this chapter consider inter-domain networks with traffic entirely seen as priority traffic. In our algorithm, the introduction of two distinct classes of traffic requires two traffic matrices for each one of them.

Third, another issue which we see as a subject of further studies is the performance of our distributed algorithm in the case of its partial deployment in an inter-domain network. Our preliminary opinion is that it is naturally adapted to incremental deployment.

Finally, certain problems appear in our distributed algorithm. It would be interesting to see how to find delays before alert messages are processed depending on a given inter-domain network characteristic. We think that a more careful choice of their lengths may reduce momentary network state flickering.

REFERENCES

Atallah, M. J., & Blanton, M. (1999). *Algorithms and Theory of Computation Handbook*. Boca Raton, FL: CRC Press LLC.

Blake, S., Black, D., Carlson, M., Davies, E., Wang, Z., & Weiss, W. (1998). *An Architecture for Differentiated Service (RFC 2475).*

Bless, R. (2004). Towards Scalable Management of QoS-based End-to-End Services. In *Proc. of NOMS '04,* Seoul, Korea, (pp. 293-306).

Boucadair, M. (2005). *QoS-Enhanced Border Gateway Protocol. Technical report*. France Telecom.

Braden, R., Zhang, L., Berson, S., Herzog, S. & Jamin, S. (1997). *Resource ReSerVation Protocol (RSVP), RFC 2205.*

Cristallo, G., & Jacquenet, C. (2002). An Approach to Inter-domain Traffic Engineering. *Proc. of WTC '02,* Paris, France.

Di Battista, G., Erlebach, T., Hall, A., Patrignani, M., Pizzonia, M., & Schank, T. (2007). Computing the Types of the Relationships between Autonomous Systems. *Transactions on Networking, 15*(2), 267–280. doi:10.1109/TNET.2007.892878

Feigenbaum, J., Papadimitriou, C., Sami, R., & Shenker, S. (2005). A BGP-based mechanism for lowest-cost routing. *Distributed Computing, 18*(1), 61–72. doi:10.1007/s00446-005-0122-y

Gao, L. (2001). On inferring autonomous system relationships in the Internet. *Transactions on Networking, 9*(6), 733–745. doi:10.1109/90.974527

Gao, L., Griffin, T. G., & Rexford, J. (2001). Inherently safe backup routing with BGP. In *Proc. of INFOCOM'01*, Anchorage, AK, *1*, 547-556.

Gao, L., & Rexford, J. (2000). Stable Internet routing without global coordination. In *Proc. of SIGMETRICS'00* (pp. 307-317). Santa Clara, CA: ACM Press.

Ge, Z., Figueiredo, D. R., Jaiswal, S., & Gao, L. (2001). The hierarchical structure of the logical Internet graph. In *Proc. of SPIE-ITCOM'01, 4526,* (pp. 208-222).

Hsu, T., Tsai, K., Wang, D., & Lee, D. T. (1996). Steiner Problems on Directed Acyclic Graphs. In *Proc. of COCOON '96* (pp. 21-30). London: Springer-Verlag.

Medina, A., Lakhina, A., Matta, I., & Byers, J. (2001). BRITE: An Approach to Universal Topology Generation. In *Proc. of MASCOTS'01*, (pp. 346-354).

Okumu, I. T., Mantar, H. A., Hwang, J., & Chapin, S. J. (2005). Inter-domain QoS routing on DiffServ networks: a region-based approach. *Computer Communications*, *28*(2), 174–188. doi:10.1016/j.comcom.2004.08.018

Pan, P., Hahne, E., & Schulzrinne, H. (2000). BGRP: A Tree-Based Aggregation Protocol for Inter-domain Reservations. *Journal of Communications and Networks*, *2*(2), 157–167.

Pelsser, C., & Bonaventure, O. (2006). Path Selection Techniques to Establish Constrained Interdomain MPLS LSPs. In *Proc. of IFIP Networking,* Coimbra, Portugal.

Raghavachari, B., & Veerasamy, J. (1999). Approximation algorithms for mixed postman problem. *SIAM Journal on Discrete Mathematics*, *12*(4), 425–433. doi:10.1137/S0895480197331454

Rekhter, T., Li, T. & Hares, S. (2006). *RFC 4271 - A Border Gateway Protocol 4 (BGP-4).*

Subramanian, L., Agarwal, S., Rexford, J., & Katz, R. H. (2002). Characterizing the Internet Hierarchy from Multiple Vantage Points. In *Proc. of INFOCOM'02, 2*, (pp. 618-627), New York.

Subramanian, L., Caesar, M., Tien, C., Handley, M., Mao, M., Shenker, S., et al. (2005). HLP: a next generation inter-domain routing protocol. In *Proc. of SIGCOMM '05* (pp. 13-24). Philadelphia, PA: ACM Press.

Weisser, M.-A., & Tomasik, J. (2006). A distributed algorithm for inter-domain resources provisioning. In *Proc. of Second EuroNGI Conference*, (pp. 9-16), Valencia, Spain.

Weisser, M.-A., & Tomasik, J. (2007). Automatic induction of inter-domain hierarchy in randomly generated network topologies. In *Proc. of CNS'07* (pp. 77-84), Norfolk, VA. Retrieved from http://wwwsi.supelec.fr/~weisser/

Weisser, M.-A., & Tomasik, J. (2007). *Innapproximation proofs for directed Steiner tree and network problems. PRiSM Laboratory, University of Versailles Saint Quentin*. UVSQ.

Weisser, M.-A., Tomasik, J., & Barth, D. (2008). Congestion avoiding mechanism based on inter-domain hierarchy. IFIP Networking. (LNCS 4982, pp. 470-481). Singapore: Springer.

Xiao, L., Lui, K. S., Wang, J., & Nahrstedt, K. (2002). QoS extension to BGP. In *Proc. of ICNP '02*, (pp. 100-109), Paris, France.

Chapter 14
Scalable Intra and Inter Domain IPv6 QoS Management and Pricing Scheme

El-Bahlul Fgee
Dalhousie University, Canada

Shyamala Sivakumar
Saint Mary's University, Canada

William J. Phillips
Dalhousie University, Canada

William Robertson
Dalhousie University, Canada

ABSTRACT

Network multimedia applications constitute a large part of Internet traffic and guaranteed delivery of such traffic is a challenge because of their sensitivity to delay, packet loss and higher bandwidth requirement. The need for guaranteed traffic delivery is exacerbated by the increasing delay experienced by traffic propagating through more than one QoS domain. Hence, there is a need for a flexible and a scalable QoS manager that handles and manages the needs of traffic flows throughout multiple IPv6 domains. The IPv6 QoS manager, presented in this paper, uses a combination of the packets' flow ID and the source address (Domain Global Identifier (DGI)), to process and reserve resources inside an IPv6 domain. To ensure inter-domain QoS management, the QoS domain manager should also communicate with other QoS domains' managers to ensure that traffic flows are guaranteed delivery. In this scheme, the IPv6 QoS manager handles QoS requests by either processing them locally if the intended destination is located locally or forwards the request to the neighboring domain's QoS manager. End-to-end QoS is achieved with an integrated admission and management unit. The feasibility of the proposed QoS management scheme is illustrated for both intra- and inter-domain QoS management. The scalability of the QoS management scheme for inter-domain scenarios is illustrated with simulations for traffic flows propagating through two and three domains. Excellent average end-to-end delay results have been achieved when traffic flow propagates through more than one domain. Simulations show that

DOI: 10.4018/978-1-61520-791-6.ch014

packets belonging to non-conformant flows experience increased delay, and such packets are degraded to lower priority if they exceed their negotiated traffic flow rates. Many pricing schemes have been proposed for QoS-enabled networks. However, integrated pricing and admission control has not been studied in detail. A dynamic pricing model is integrated with the IPv6 QoS manager to study the effects of increasing traffic flows rates on the increased cost of delivering high priority traffic flows. The pricing agent assigns prices dynamically for each traffic flow accepted by the domain manager. Combining the pricing strategy with the QoS manager allows only higher priority traffic packets that are willing to pay more to be processed during congestion. This approach is flexible and scalable as end-to-end pricing is decoupled from packet forwarding and resource reservation decisions. Simulations show that additional revenue is generated as prices change dynamically according to the network congestion status.

INTRODUCTION

Quality of service (QoS) is defined as the ability of a network element (e.g. an application, host, router) to have some degree of assurance that its traffic and service requirements can be defined (Shaikh, McClellan, Singh, and Chakravarthy, 2002). In other words, QoS is the ability of a network provider to support a user application's requirements with regard to service categories through QoS parameters such as bandwidth, delay, jitter and traffic loss. These parameters are used to measure traffic flows at the end point to ensure that the users' requirements are meet. QoS goals can be achieved by measuring and improving characteristics such as transmission rate and error rate. In order to achieve good QoS results, it is necessary to differentiate between traffic flows according to their data contents. It is also necessary to find if there are enough network resources to handle QoS requests issued by non tolerant traffic flows. Therefore, each component in an IP network must be equipped with new logical QoS supporting facilities and functionalities including admission control, reservation policies, packet classification and traffic shaping (Stader, 2001). Providing some form of end-to-end service differentiation in the Internet has been an important research issue and creates various on-going challenges to support end-to-end QoS in the Internet.

Integrated Services and Differentiated Service mechanisms provide QoS to real-time applications (e.g., IP voice, video, IPTV) by treating different types of traffic flows differently. IntServ introduces end-to-end per flow reservation, such that each flow is guaranteed a certain bandwidth along its path from the source to the destination. However, this approach requires maintenance of individual flow states in the routers, and its signaling complexity grows with the number of users. The differentiated service (DiffServ) architecture (Blake, Black, Carlson, Davies, Wang, & Weiss, 1998) was proposed as a more scalable solution to the end-to-end QoS problem, compared to previous approaches such as integrated services (IntServ) architecture (White, 1997). Intra-domain reservation is easily handled by sending QoS requests to a bandwidth broker that allocates preferred services to users as requested. The BB handles domain reservations, and flows exceeding their committed rates are dropped. The DiffServ scheme is scalable, however the mapping of traffic flows to predefined service classes is time consuming and limit the flexibility in the types of service offered. Also, inter-domain QoS reservations present problems, for if a destination host is located in a different QoS domain, the user application requires QoS guaranteed delivery through all the domains the traffic flow traverses.

This chapter answers the question: Is it possible to provide end-to-end Quality of Service (QoS) in IP networks without compromising the scalability, flexibility and bandwidth efficiency of the current Internet infrastructure? The solution is to design a QoS method to meet the stated requirements, and to implement a QoS manager that administers controls and manages all the resources in the network domain. The proposed Ipv6 QoS scheme overcomes DiffServ's limited QoS handling capability, by allowing traffic flows to specify their required level of QoS without mapping them to predefined classes. First, the chapter presents arguments for why IPv6 provides better QoS management capabilities than IPv4. The chapter then provides the details of a suitable QoS method, and a QoS manager that can be deployed in IPv6 domains. In the QoS scheme presented core nodes simply forward and schedule traffic flows, and make no reservation decisions, while the complexity of QoS management is implemented at the edge nodes. In this paper, we demonstrate how the QoS manager handles both intra and inter- domain reservations using the IPv6 protocol. The QoS manager handles intra domain reservations by checking if there are enough resources and if the destination node is located in its domain. However, traffic flows are still aggregated to pre-defined classes and non-conformant traffic flows (traffic flows that violate their initial rates) are dropped. The scalability of the proposed QoS management scheme is demonstrated by extending the QoS management model so as to facilitate per-flow resource reservation across several network domains. Inter domain reservation is accomplished through exchanging QoS requests between co-operating QoS domains. Simulation results for intra and inter-domain QoS management demonstrate the feasibility of the QoS management scheme for IPv6 domains. Finally, we also present a pricing model that can be employed with in IPv6 networks by service providers to charge clients for end-to-end flow based QoS.

MOTIVATION FOR USING IPV6

The Internet protocol (IP) has undergone significant changes to support real-time applications. These applications require specific Quality of Service (QoS) guarantees. Internet Protocol version 4 (IPv4) provides best effort service and does not provide any guarantees as it has no provision for QoS at the network layer (Xiao & Ni, 1999). There are no mechanisms in IPv4 for policing or controlling unresponsive and high bandwidth flows that can cause congestion in the network. IPv4 best effort allows complexity to stay at the end hosts (sender and receiver applications control delivery) which scales well and allows the network to expand. As a result, all QoS management is left to the application. However, service degrades rapidly, and some applications cannot tolerate such a degradation of service caused, for example, by delay and jitter. Multimedia applications have very limited flow control options to stop them from causing congestion in the network. Consequently, QoS management for network multimedia applications over IPv4 is a significant and immediate challenge. To provide adequate service requires adding some "smarts" to the network to distinguish traffic with strict timing requirements from those that can tolerate delay, jitter and loss. This is what QoS protocols are designed to accomplish. QoS does not create bandwidth, but manages the bandwidth resource so that it may be used more effectively to meet the wide range of application requirements.

In the following subsections, some of the advantages to using IPv6 protocol are outlined. With a 32-bit address field, it is in principle possible to assign over 4 billion possible addresses. This number of addresses is not adequate as the two level structure of the IPv4 address space is wasteful of addresses. Also, growth of TCP/IP usage in new applications has resulted in a rapid growth in the demand for IPv4 addresses. To meet these needs, IPv6 which uses 128-bit addresses has been proposed. IPv4 is best employed for unicast addressing in which a single address bit pattern corresponds to a single host. Other forms of addressing are poorly supported, partly because no provision is made for certain addressing modes. For example, IPv6 includes the concept of an anycast address in which a packet is delivered to just one node in a set of nodes. The scalability of multicast routing is improved by adding a scope field to multicast address (Loukola & Skytta, 2003).

As more emerging multimedia applications become available over the Internet, core routers need to process and forward traffic at ever increasing data rates. Several aspects of IPv6 contribute to meeting such traffic flow performance requirements (Stallings, 1996). First, the number of fields in the IPv6 packet header is fewer than in IPv4. A number of IPv6 options are placed in separate optional header fields located between the IPv6 header and the transport layer header. The IPv6 header features simplify and speeds up the processing of IPv6 packets compared to IPv4 packets, since these optional headers are not examined by core routers. Secondly, the IPv6 packet header is fixed length whereas the IPv4 header is variable length again simplifying IPv6 packet processing. Thirdly, in contrast to IPv4, IPv6 enables labeling of packets belonging to a particular traffic flow when a sender requests special handling (Stallings, 1996). Hence, IPv6 makes it possible to associate packets with particular service classes, and afford preferential routing treatment on the basis of these classes. Therefore, IPv6 is better able to support real-time services and to specify priority levels to determine discard strategy in the event of congestion. Lastly, IPv4 provides no security capabilities other than an optional security label field. Although end-to-end security can be provided at the application level, there is little support for a standardized IP-level security service which any application can use. In addition, IPv6 provides a range of features that support authentication and privacy (Loukola & Skytta, 2003).

QoS can be provided in IPv6 with the use of "flow labels". Flow labels are used by the sender to request special handling of certain traffic flows, such as real-time applications. In addition to the flow label, IPv6 has an 8-bit traffic class (TC) field. The TC field is used to identify and distinguish IPv6 packets into classes with different priorities, enabling the provision of differentiated services (Loukola & Skytta, 2003). According to the IPv6 specification, the flow label can be used by the source to label packets (e.g., real-time traffic) that require special handling by intervening IPv6 routers. Packets belonging to the same flow are labeled with the same unique flow label value assigned to the flow by the source. A source can never label more than one flow with the same flow label at a given time (Loukola & Skytta, 2003; Rajahalme, Couta, Carpenter, & Deering, 2003). Employing the flow label for packet classification has several advantages. In IPv6 only traffic requiring special handling is labeled with a non-zero flow label. The great benefit for packet classification is that all information needed to classify packets is available within the IPv6 header. The flow label can facilitate implementation of QoS based flow routing mechanisms in which routers expedite processing packets with non-zero flow labels. In contrast, IPv4 intervening routers rely on the transport or application layer information for mapping packets to their reserved resources. This is known as the Layer Violation Problem and has some serious performance drawbacks with respect to packet classification.

QoS management in an IPv6 domain can use the flow label in conjunction with the source IP address, and this tuple is known as the domain global identifier (DGI) to uniquely identify flows. This allows efficient mapping of packets to flows to their flow specification policy as set out by the domain's QoS manager. Also, IPv6 overcomes the layer violation problem, as the flow label, source address tuple is used by routers to appropriately handle and forward packets. The DGI can now be employed by core routers in lookup procedures which reduces packet processing time resulting in smaller end-to-end delay of real time traffic. The use of the flow labels decreases the average processing load of the network routers since all packets from the same flow have identical headers. As a result, routers along the path of a flow need to process packets on a per flow basis rather than a per packet basis. Lastly, flow label usage facilitates end-to-end security mechanisms as IPv6 packet classification does not rely on higher layers. In contrast, IPv4 accesses higher layer information to distinguish between different flows, requiring intermediate routers to decrypt packets and encrypt the packet again before forwarding them to the next hop router. Repeated encryption and decryption of packets by core routers makes forwarding and processing more complicated and time consuming resulting in increasing end-to-end delay.

The priority field (Traffic Class) in the IPv6 header enables a source to identify the desired priority of its packets, relative to other packets from the same source. Values 0-7 are used to specify the priority of traffic for which the source is providing congestion control. Congestion controlled traffic refers to traffic for which the source "backs off" in response to congestion. IPv6 defines several categories of congestion-controlled traffic in order of decreasing priority. They include, Internet control traffic, interactive traffic, attended bulk transfer that is not delay sensitive (FTP and HTTP), unattended data transfer (e- mail) and best effort traffic. Values 8-15 are used to specify the priority of traffic that does not back off in response to congestion, e.g., real-time traffic. Non-congestion-controlled traffic is traffic for which a smooth data rate and a constant delivery delay are required. Examples include real time video and audio. Eight levels of priority are allocated for this type of traffic, from lowest priority (most willing to be discarded) to the highest priority 15 (least willing to be discarded). QoS management can employ these priority classes to implement queuing policies such as fair queuing or class-based queuing (Loukola & Skytta, 2003). The simulations presented later in this chapter make use of priority levels 15 and 12.

QOS APPROACHES IN LITERATURE

This section of the chapter discusses IntServ, DiffServ and MPLS, the three major QoS approaches, and how they have influenced the design of the proposed QoS manager.

Integrated Services

The philosophy behind IntServ is that routers must be able to reserve resources for individual flows to provide QoS guarantees to end users. IntServ QoS control framework supports two additional classes of service besides "best effort". They are guaranteed service (Shenker, Partridge, & Guerin, 1997) and controlled load service (Wroclawski, 1997). Guaranteed service provides quantitative and hard (deterministic) guarantees, e.g., lossless transmission and upper bound on end-to-end delay. Controlled load service is intended to support a broad class of applications that are highly sensitive to overload conditions. Both services must ensure that adequate bandwidth and packet processing resources are available to satisfy the level of service requested, and is accomplished through active admission control. Many research contributions have been made to define IntServ components needed to provide end-to-end QoS functionality, and to study their implementation issues. IntServ features include the use of a signaling protocol to set up and tear down reservations, e.g., resource Reservation Protocol (RSVP) (Braden, Zhang, Herzog, & Jamin, 1997), an application level interface (API) for applications to communicate QoS needs and, per-flow scheduling in the network (e.g., Weighted Fair Queuing (WFQ) or Class Based Queuing (CBQ)).

Unfortunately, IntServ faces the following major challenges that make deployment in intermediate core routers infeasible. The increase in per flow state maintenance at core routers is proportional to the number of flows, thus incurring huge storage and processing overhead at routers. Hence, IntServ does not scale well in the Internet core backbone. In the QoS management scheme proposed in this chapter, we overcome the issue of handling increasing numbers of flows by having edge routers communicate with a centralized QoS manager to reserve resources. The QoS manager handles intra domain reservations. A 20 bit flow label field, which is part of IPv6 header, is used to label packets belonging to a traffic flow for which the sender has requested special handling (Fgee, Kenney, Phillips, Robertson, & Sivakumar, 2004, 2005). Hence, core routers can classify packets based on IPv6 semantics allowing for efficient mapping of packets to their flows and hence to their flow specification policy. This labeling scheme has the advantages of IntServ in enabling traffic flows to individually specify their QoS requirements on a per flow basis. Core routers in the IPv6 domain merely process, forward, and schedule traffic flows based on the traffic class field in the header. In contrast, IPv4 routers rely on the transport protocol or application level information (socket port) to identify different flows of the same source.

Differentiated Services

DiffServ, on the other hand, aggregates multiple flows with similar traffic characteristics and performance into a few predefined classes. This approach requires that either end user applications, or ingress routers (interface where packets enter an administrative domain) mark the individual packets to indicate the service class. The QoS service class information is indicated in the Type of Service (ToS) field in the IPv4 packet header (Nicholas, Blake, Baker, & Black, 1998). The backbone routers provide per-hop differential treatments to different service classes as defined by the Per Hop Behaviors (PHBs) (Brim, Carpenter, & LeFaucheur, 2000). Individual flows are classified at the edge routers into one of the classes defined by the approach. Two service models have been proposed. These are assured service (Heinanen, Baker, & Weiss, 1999) and premium service (Jacobson, Nichols, & Poduri, 1999). Assured service is intended for customers that need reliable services from service providers. Premium service provides low delay and low jitter guarantees, and is suitable for Internet telephony, video conferencing and E-commerce applications.

The DiffServ approach has several advantages over IntServ. DiffServ is simpler than IntServ and does not require end-to-end signaling. DiffServ is more efficient at core routers, since classification and PHBs are based on a few bits rather than per-flow information. DiffServ requires minimum changes to the network infrastructure. Ingress routers mark packets while intermediate routers (core routers) can employ active queue management to provide service differentiation based on the packet headers. An advantage of Diffserv over IntServ is that DiffServ implements flow aggregation and is, therefore, highly scalable. Only a limited number of service classes are supported by ToS, and the amount of state information is proportional to the number of classes rather than number of flows. Hence, DiffServ suffers from limited QoS handling capability. The proposed Ipv6 QoS scheme overcomes DiffServ's limited QoS handling capability, by allowing traffic flows to specify their required level of QoS without mapping them to predefined classes. The 8-bit Traffic Class (TC) field in the IPv6 header is used to identify and discriminate traffic types. Like DiffServ which uses the Type of Service (ToS) field in the IPv4 packet header, the Traffic Class (TC) field indicates the level of QoS service required by an IPv6 traffic flow. In the IPv6 QoS scheme traffic class values are mapped to QoS flow specification policies set forth by the QoS domain manager. The core routers can now provide per-hop differential treatments to different flows by honoring the parameters implied by the traffic class field. Another disadvantage of DiffServ is that it does not ensure that adequate bandwidth and packet processing resources are available to satisfy the level of service requested and hence, cannot provide the same level of service provided for individual flows by IntServ. In the proposed QoS management scheme, we overcome the problem of ensuring adequate network resources for traffic flows by reserving these resources. The 20 bit flow label field in the IPv6 header is used in conjunction with the source address, known as the DGI, is used by the IPv6 QoS manager for reserving resources for a particular flow. The QoS manager guarantees resources and fair treatment before admitting the traffic flow.

MULTIPROTOCOL LABEL SWITCHING (MPLS)

In recent years, Multi-Protocol Label Switching (MPLS) has been proposed as a solution to overcome many of the performance and scaling problems that service providers are experiencing in their IP networks, and is the basis for more efficient traffic engineering methods. MPLS networks contain network nodes, called Label Switching Routers (LSRs), and network links connecting nodes (Rosen, Viswanathan, & Callon, 2001). MPLS organizes the network in domains. Edge LSRs define the boundaries of the domain and are the traffic demand ingress/egress nodes. Other nodes, named core LSRs, can exist on the network to provide communications between edge LSRs. The forwarding of IP packets from ingress to egress LSRs is done by means of routing paths, called Label Switched Paths (LSPs). In the ingress LSR, incoming IP packets are labeled based on their destination and required quality of service (QoS) and, depending on this classification, are forwarded through the appropriate LSP towards an egress LSR. MPLS enables source based routing, i.e. the forwarding path of a LSP from an ingress router to an egress router and is not constrained by the paths of other LSPs. In a similar fashion, the proposed IPv6 QoS scheme has core routers simply forwarding and scheduling traffic flows according to their traffic class. Domain edge routers forward resource reservation requests to a domain QoS manager that make reservation decisions. Hence, the complexity of QoS management is left to the edge nodes.

IPV6 QOS MANAGEMENT

The proposed IPv6 QoS management scheme has two subcomponents: the edge router and the QoS manager; and is shown in Figure 1. Edge routers handle QoS requests and communicate with the QoS manager. Traffic flows are classified based on the TC field so that each priority level is treated differently at routers. Thereby the class limitation is avoided and there is no need to map flows' packets to pre-defined classes, as in DiffServ. WFQ is used to separate the flows with separate queues assigned for each traffic flow as implied by its priority level. This scheme is unique in that the IPv6 network can be managed without invoking any other QoS signaling and admission protocols such as RSVP or MPLS.

When a node wants to send real time traffic, it sends a QoS request to the network edge router. Upon receiving requests from the sender, the edge router communicates with the QoS manager. The QoS manager sets up traffic handling policies for various TC values and communicates these policies as WFQ weights to all routers in its domain. The QoS manager uses the combination of the packet flow label and the source IPv6 address, together known as the **Domain Global Identifier (DGI),** for reserving resources and tracking traffic flows. The QoS manager approves or rejects the service requests, and the edge router forwards the QoS manager's responses to the sender as shown in Figure 1. When accepted, the source starts sending data packets to the edge router where packets are classified, scheduled and monitored.

Figure 1. IPv6 QoS management scheme

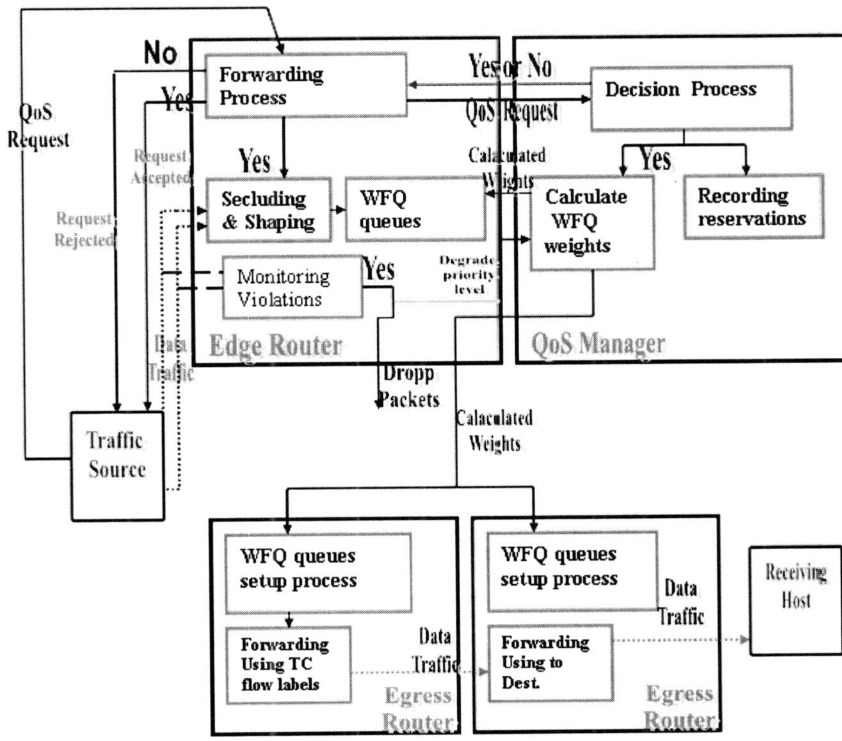

Packets are buffered, queued and handled based on their TC field value and on the policies set by the QoS manager. The edge router uses the leaky bucket algorithm to monitor and condition incoming traffic. The leaky bucket parameters for the accepted traffic are set up according to their traffic specifications. The WFQ weights are used by domain routers to buffer and queue the incoming packets according to the assured priority level implied by the TC field. When a flow violates its requested specification, its priority level is degraded or its packets are dropped. For degraded traffic, the edge router forwards a new priority level to the QoS manager who adjusts the WFQ weights. In case of transmission rate reduction in one of the accepted flows, the edge router sends the new rate to its QoS manager for freeing more resources resulting in dynamic adjustment of resources. The traffic class (TC) field is used for scheduling packets at the core routers' queues. The edge and core routers employ the DGI to make the next hop forwarding decision. The end-to-end delay is less as the time taken to find the next hop using DGI lookup is less than the longest prefix match procedure used typically by IPv4 routers resulting in a smaller processing time. In the following subsection, the QoS manager is described in detail.

IPv6 QoS Manager Model - Layout

The IPv6 QoS manager uses the DGI to uniquely identify traffic flows and make resource reservations for each flow. The IPv6 QoS manager that is used to control and manage network resources is shown in Figure 2. It consists of Request Processing Agent (RPA), Admission Control Agent (ACA), Management Reservation Agent (MRA), Traffic Control Data Box (TCDB) and WFQ Calculator Agent (WFQ-CA) (Fgee, 2005;

Figure 2. IPv6 QoS manager

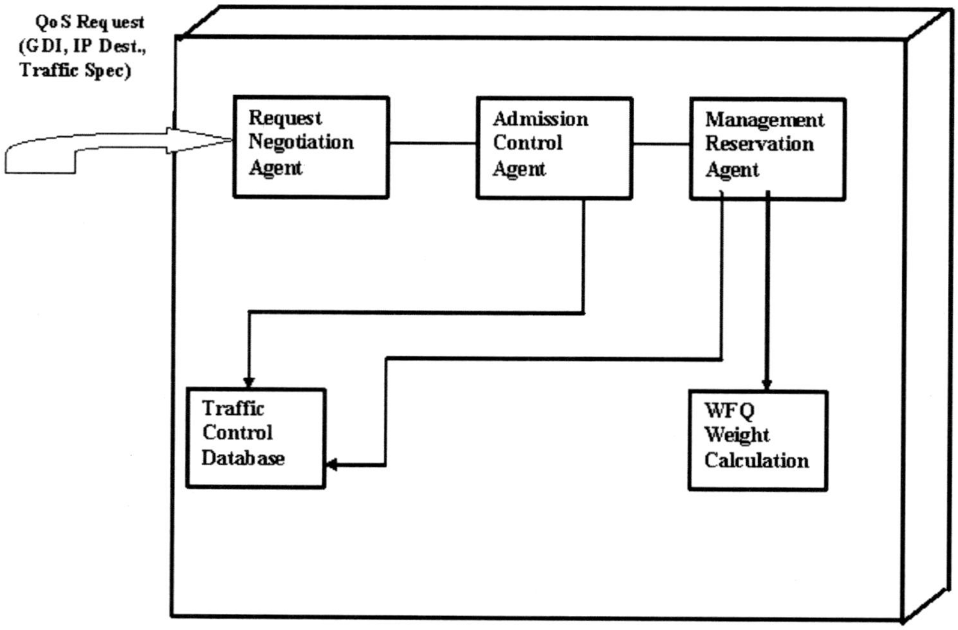

Fgee, Kenney, Phillips, Robertson, & Sivakumar, 2005). The RPA receives QoS requests from edge routers and forwards them to the decision block. The parameters used in each request are the DGI, destination address, and TC field value determines the peak rate, average rate, burst rate and delay. The ACA makes decisions on the received requests. If the destination is located in the manager's domain and there are enough resources, a positive response is sent to the source node applying for the request. For inter-domain QoS requests as is the case when the destination is located in a different domain, the service request is forwarded to the neighboring QoS manager. If sufficient resources are not available to meet the requested service anywhere along the path, the request is rejected. The MRA manages all reservations in the domain by recording all the accepted requests using the unique DGIs and their corresponding Tspec. It also sends the DGI of accepted traffic and their corresponding traffic classes to the WFQ-CA. Finally, this agent initiates policies, to handle traffic violations, to be implemented at the edge routers where traffic flows are monitored.

The TCDB records information, such as domain reservation, using the DGI and domain topology for tracing resources. WFQ-CA calculates the weights for all the accepted traffic flows and sends them to the edge routers that use them for classifying packets.

INTRA DOMAIN IPV6 QOS MANAGEMENT - SIMULATIONS

In this section we present simulation results to illustrate the feasibility of the proposed QoS management scheme. Network Simulator (NS) (The Network Simulator, 2004) was used in all simulations presented in this paper. The network topology for the intra domain case is shown in Figure 3. This IPv6 domain has ten nodes, three sending nodes (n6, n7, and n8), one receiving node (n9), two edge routers (n0, n1) and four core routers (n2, n3, n4, n5).

The simulations measure two QoS parameters: average end-to-end delay and packet loss rate when traffic of different priority levels traverses a

Figure 3. Intra-domain network topology

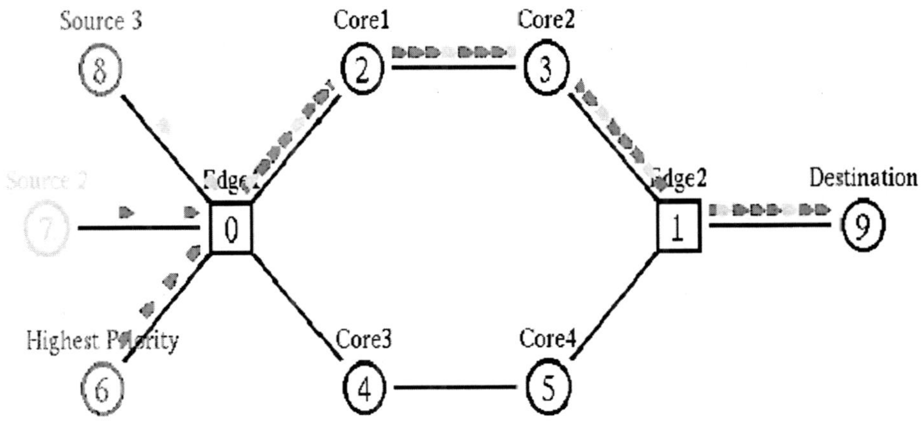

domain. Two scenarios are considered, first when traffic flows conform to their flow specification rates, and secondly when flows violate their slow specification rates. We measure the traffic degradation rate to confirm that traffic that violate their flow specification rates are degraded gracefully and then dropped. The sending nodes generate three traffic flows with different priority levels. The highest priority source generates constant bit rate (CBR) traffic at 0.5 Mbps rate and priority field set to 15 (highest level). Source 2 also generates CBR traffic but at 0.25 Mbps rate and priority level set to 12. Source 3 generates best effort traffic at a rate of 0.25 Mbps. The packets' size for all the flows is set to 500 bytes, the queues' buffers connecting edge 1 to core 2 and core 4 are set to 50 packets. The links throughput is set to 1 Mbps and the propagation delay is set to 1 mSec.

SIMULATION RESULTS ANALYSIS

Comparing IPv6 QoS Management with IntServ and DiffServ – Conformant Flows

Tables 1 and 2 compare the QoS parameters average delay, and packet loss rate for three traf-

Table 1. Delay and packet loss rate for conformant flows: IPv6 QoS management vs. IntServ, DiffServ, MPLS

			IPv6 QoS		**IntServ**		**DiffServ**		**MPLS with constraint routing**	
Traffic Source	Priority Level	Aver. Delay mSec	Traffic degrade rate	Packet Loss rate	Aver. Delay mSec	Packet Loss rate	Average Delay mSec	Packet Loss rate	Average Delay mSec	Packet Loss rate
Source 1-FID 100	15	13.71	0%	0%	15.85	0%	29.9	0%	31.75	0%
Source 2-FID 200	12	13.59	0%	0%	14.04	0%	26.88	0%	37.69	0%
Source 3-FID 300	Best Effort	18.35	0%	0%	17.87	0%	30.88	0%	29.39	0%

Table 2. Delay and packet loss rate for non-conformant flows: IPv6 QoS management vs. IntServ, Diff-Serv, MPLS

			IPv6 QoS		IntServ		DiffServ		MPLS with constraint routing	
Traffic Source	Priority Level	Aver. Delay mSec	Traffic degrade rate	Packet Loss rate	Average Delay mSec	Packet Loss rate	Average Delay mSec	Packet Loss rate	Average Delay mSec	Packet Loss rate
Source 1-FID 100	15	14.6	19.31%	0%	1604.9	0%	211.94	14.78%	209.62	22.93%
Source 2-FID 200	12	53.71	10.75%	8.6%	1692.3	0%	200.85	7.4%	205.64	9.24%
Source 3-FID 300	Best Ef-fort	102.4	0%	8.1%	136.97	24.17%	199.89	5.92%	208.46	18.66%

fic flows under conformant and non conformant conditions. Higher priority traffic flows with flow ID 100 and 200 experience lower end-to-end delay than the best effort traffic with flow ID 8, which experiences the highest delay.

Table 1 shows the average delay and packet loss rate for conformant traffic flows employing IPv6, IntServ, DiffServ, and MPLS with constraint routing. From Table 1, the following observations are made regarding the IPv6 QoS management scheme. Priority level 15 and 12 traffic flows have neither packets dropped nor degraded, as they conform to their rate policies. The end-to-end delay was 13.71 mSec for priority level 15 (flow ID 100) traffic. The delay was 13.59 mSec for priority level 12 traffic (flow ID 200), which is the smallest because this flow has a lower CBR compared to flow ID 100. Best effort has no packets dropped. The delay for best effort was 18.35mSec; the highest since packets belonging to this flow have the lowest WFQ weights. From Table 1, it is seen that the delay for priority traffic is the smallest for the proposed IPv6 scheme.

The network in Figure 3 was simulated for the IntServ case. All nodes involved in the simulation including source and destination nodes are set to become RSVP agents. All the links are set to be RSVP duplex links. Two sessions, A and B are set for FID 100 and FID 200 to set paths for both flows. Path messages are first exchanged for reservation purposes followed by data packets. The time set aside for messages exchange is 1 sec which is added to the end-to-end delay. From Table 1, for the IntServ case, it is seen that priority level 15 and 12 traffic experienced lower end-to-end delay of 15.85 mSec and 14.04 mSec respectively. All the packets belonging to these flows were delivered. Best effort traffic flow packets achieved average delay of 17.87msec higher than the other two sources since no resources were reserved for best effort traffic. In this scenario also no packets dropped.

The network in Figure 3 was simulated for the DiffServ scenario. An Active Resource Management (ARM) bandwidth broker that dynamically allocates resources has been used as a DiffServ bandwidth reservation manager. The token bucket is implemented at the edge routers for policing and monitoring traffic flows. All the nodes in the topology support DiffServ since core routers use DSCP for processing packets. Table 1 summarizes the results for the DiffServ case. Priority level 15 and 12 have achieved 29.90 msec and 26.88 msec end-to-end delay respectively. No packets belonging to these flows were dropped. Best effort flow experienced the maximum delay with an average delay of 30.88 msec.

The MPLS network simulator (MNS) patch was added to ns-2, and the constrained based routing using MPLS scenario was simulated. The same network topology setup used for the previous simulations is used here. However all the core nodes involved in the simulation become MPLS agents, different routing and labeling algorithms are supported. The links between nodes are set to duplex links and the MPLS domain queues are set to CBQ queue. At edge 1, packets are encapsulated and new MPLS labels are added to the IP packets. All traffic flows experience the highest end-to-end delay compared to the other schemes.

Comparing IPv6 QoS Management with IntServ and DiffServ – Non-Conformant Flows

Next, traffic flows are set to violate the bandwidth requested by a 30% increase shortly after start of simulation. The leaky bucket policies are set to degrade traffic flows from level 15 to level 12 and from level 12 to best effort when traffic flows do not meet their specifications. The network in Figure 3 was simulated for the IPv6, IntServ, DiffServ and MPLS. The results are presented in Table 2.

From Table 2, it is seen that for the IPv6 QoS management scheme, the highest priority traffic with Flow ID 15 has 19.31% of the total packets degraded to the next priority level 12. However, no packets are dropped. The delay was 14.60 msec, increased by approximately 1 msec as compared with the conformant case. Traffic flow with a lower priority level 12 has 10.75% of its total packets degraded to best effort. The delay increased by a factor of 4 to 53.71 msec. In addition, a packet loss rate of 8.62% was observed. The average packet loss rate for priority level 12 traffic in the IPv6 scheme is worse than that for IntServ, while DiffServ's packet loss rate is marginally better than that of the IPv6 scheme. The better performance of the IntServ and DiffServ schemes at priority level 12 may be attributed to the fact that 19.31% of the highest priority IPv6 traffic is accommodated at priority level 12 leading to congestion and traffic loss in the IPv6 scheme. IntServ's packet loss rate for non-conformant flows is 0% for high priority traffic even when such traffic do not confirm to their flow rate specifications. In the IntServ scheme, only best effort traffic packets are dropped when its rate is non conformant. For the IPv6 scheme, best effort traffic flow results in a very high delay of 102.44 msec and a higher packet loss rate of 8.09%. However, the packet loss rate in the IPv6 scheme at a priority level 12 is determined by the traffic degradation rate at priority level 15. Similarly, the packet loss rate for best effort traffic is determined by the traffic degradation rate at priority level 12 as some of the non-conformant higher priority traffic is accommodated at the next lower priority level. The MPLS with constraint routing experienced maximum delay for all three flows. Also, in the MPLS case the packet loss rate is the highest as non-conformant packets belonging to all three flows are dropped.

From Tables 1 and 2, it is seen that IPv6 QoS management scheme has achieved better average delay results for both conformant and non-conformant flow tests compared to IntServ, DiffServ and MPLS schemes. In addition non-conformant traffic flows that exceed their traffic flow specification rates are degraded to a lower priority level resulting in a larger delay and a higher packet loss rate.

Six Traffic Flows Simulation

The topology used in this simulation is the same as in Figure 3. Now six traffic sources generate traffic instead of the three traffic sources used previously. This simulation is performed to test how the proposed QoS management scheme handles additional traffic sources. Three priority levels are used, high, medium and low. The high priority has two flows, Source 1 with priority levels 15 and Source 2 with priority level 14. Medium priority traffic has two flows, Source 3 and Source 4 traffic flows with priority levels set to 12 and 11 respectively. The low priority traffic is

Table 3. End-to-end Delay and packet loss rate for 6 traffic sources scenario

Traffic Source	Priority level	Average end-to-end delay	Packet loss rate
Source 1	15 (highest priority)	13.58 ms	0%
Source 2	14	15.26 ms	0%
Source 3	12	15.15 ms	0%
Source 4	11	17.798 ms	0%
Source 5	9	21.08 ms	0%
Source 6	8	24.846	0%

simulated with two sources, Sources 5 and Source 6 traffic flows with priority levels set to 9 and 8 respectively. Table 3 shows the simulation results of the six sources scenario. From Table 3 it is seen that, the high and medium priority traffic flows achieved low end-to-end delay. The low priority traffic flows achieved higher delay than the other two levels as shown in Table 3. No packets have been dropped from all the six flows. The simulation results prove that the proposed QoS model scales well even if the number of traffic flows doubled. In summary, the proposed IPv6 QoS management model scales well when the number of traffic flows is increased, and simulation results show that the end-to-end delay experienced by for non-tolerant traffic flows with high priority is proportional to their priority level.

INTER DOMAIN IPV6 QOS MANAGEMENT (TWO AND THREE DOMAINS) SIMULATION RESULTS

In this section the scalability of the proposed approach is first demonstrated for two co-operating IPv6 domains. The feasibility of the approach is then demonstrated for three IPv6 domains.

Inter-Domain Simulations: Two Ipv6 QoS Domains

We first test whether the proposed QoS management scheme can handles resource reservation requests across more than one QoS domain. To achieve this we connect Destination 2 (node 16) to domain 2, while source 1, 2 and 3 (nodes 12, 13 and 14) are attached to Domain 1. Destination 1 and 3 (nodes 15 and 17) remain attached one to Domain 1 as shown in Figure 4. This topology allows testing the IPv6 model for inter domain reservations and measures how well the two QoS domains are co-operating to handle QoS requests.

- In this scenario, Source 1 to Destination 1 has the Highest Priority traffic (priority level 15) and Source 1 (node 12) sends a request for a CBR traffic flow at a rate of 0.5 Mbps. Destination 1 is located in Domain 1. Source 1 traffic packets have to traverse one domain to reach the destination.
- Source 2 to Destination 2 generates traffic with priority level 12. Source 2 (node 13) sends a request for CBR traffic flow at 0.25 Mbps CIR. Destination 2 is located in Domain 2. Source 2 traffic packets have to traverse across two domains to reach the destination. Source 2 packets have to traverse through two QoS domains and reservations are done in both Domain 1 and 2
- Source 3 (node 14) to Destination 3 is best effort traffic at 0.25Mbps. Sources 1, 2 and 3 are connected to Domain 1 through the Edge router 1.

All QoS requests to the Domain 1 QoS manager and all responses are forwarded by the

Figure 4. Two IPv6QoS domain topology

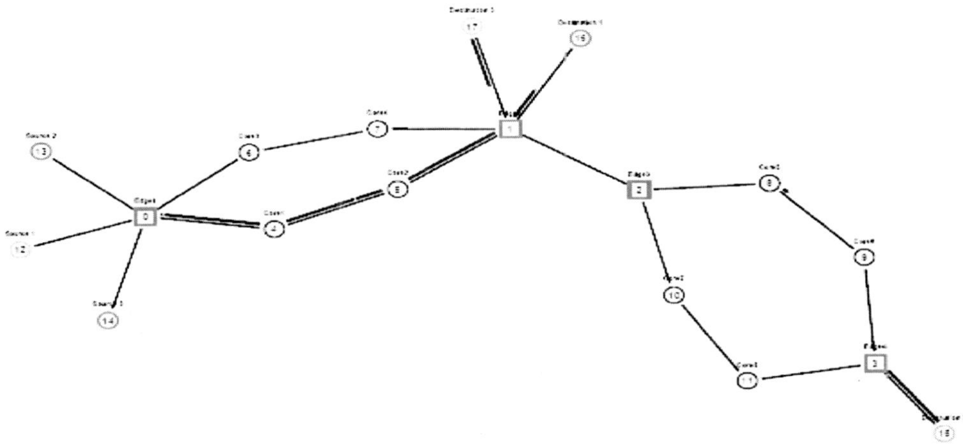

edge 1 router to the nodes that generated these requests. Similarly, all traffic passing through QoS Domain 2 pass through edge router 3. The Highest Priority source 1 requests are first processed locally inside Domain 1 to reserve resources in that domain. Next, Source 2's (priority level 12 traffic) request is handled by the Domain 1 QoS manager. It checks for resource availability in domain 1 and then forwards the QoS request to Domain 2 QoS manager as the Destination 2 (node 16) is located in Domain 2. The Domain 2 QoS manager checks if there are enough resources inside its domain to handle this QoS request. Source 3 (node 14) to Destination 3 (node17) is also processed locally by the Domain 1 manager. Token bucket is implemented at edge 1 router to monitor traffic flows and to apply Domain 1 QoS manager policies to non-conformant flows. During congestion, the Highest Priority packets are degraded to level 12, priority level 12 packets are degraded to best effort, and best effort packets may be dropped. The simulation setup procedure is the same as in the intra-domain section. QoS parameters average end-to-end delay and packet loss rate are measured.

Two Domain Results: Analysis

Table 4 summarizes the results obtained from simulating two IPv6 QoS domains. Delay and packet loss rate are measured for two scenarios, first during traffic conformance and next during traffic non conformance. To simulate network congestion traffic flows are set to violate the requested rate by a 30% increase. The delay and packet loss rates are recorded at the destinations. The following is the summary of simulation results:

- The end-to-end delay for the highest priority traffic with flow ID 100 was 14.21 ms. When Source 1 (highest priority) traffic is non-conformant, its packets are degraded to priority level-12. Under Source 1 traffic non-conformant conditions, the average delay experienced by Source 1 traffic increased to 14.94 ms.
- Under traffic conformant conditions, Source 2's average end-to-end delay was 24.22 ms as it had to traverse through two QoS domains. However, the delay experienced per domain by Source 2 traffic is 12.11 ms and is lower than the delay for Source 1 and Source 3 (best effort) traffic.

Table 4. Simulation results two IPv6 QoS domains

Traffic Source	Priority Level	Average Delay				Packet Loss rate	
		Conformant		Non conformant			
		End-to-end delay	Average Delay per domain traversed	End-to-end delay	Average Delay per domain traversed	Conformant	Non conformant
Source 1- FID 100	15	14.214 ms	14.214 ms	14.94 ms	14.94 ms	0%	0%
Source 2 - FID 200	12	24.22 ms	12.11 ms	25.66	12.83ms	0%	0%
Source 3- FID 300	Best Effort	18.39 ms	18.39ms	131.374	131.374	0%	20.866%

This may be accounted for by the fact that Source 2 has a lower CBR that Source 1 and a higher priority than Source 3. Under Source 2 traffic non-conformant conditions, its packets are degraded to best effort and may be dropped when congestion is encountered. Under Source 2 traffic non-conformant conditions, the average delay experienced by Source 2 packets increased to 25.66msec.

- Source 3 traffic is best effort traffic with no QoS guarantee for its flow when its traffic rate increases. Under Source 3 non conformant traffic conditions, Source 3 packets experienced an average delay of 131.37 msec and 20.86% of the best effort packets are dropped.
- Each time the Highest Priority traffic flow was non-conformant, the best effort traffic flow was delayed the most. For example, when both Source 1 and Source 2 traffic were non-conformant the delay experienced by the best effort traffic increased to 275ms and the delay of the level-12 traffic increased marginally to 25.8 ms.

INTER-DOMAIN SIMULATIONS: THREE IPV6 DOMAINS

In this simulation scenario, three IP QoS domains are tested and three destination nodes are attached to each one of the domains as shown in Figure 5. The purpose of this simulation scenario is to test the flexibility of the proposed QoS model. In this simulation scenario, source 1, 2 and 3 (nodes 12, 13 and 14) and destination 1 (node 21) is attached to Domain 1, destination 2 (node 22) is attached to Domain 2, and destination 3 (node 23) is attached to Domain 3 as shown in Figure 5. The objective of the simulation is to demonstrate that the delay experienced by priority flows is proportional to the number of domain traversed. The following is the setup of the traffic flows used in this simulation:

- Source 1 generates high priority traffic flow at an average rate of 0.5 Mbps. The priority level of this traffic flow is set to 15 the highest priority. Destination 3 is located in Domain 3. Source 1 traffic packets have to traverse all three domains to reach the destination and QoS reservation are done in all the three QoS domains.
- Source 2 generates a traffic flow at average rate of 0.25 Mbps. The priority level of this traffic is set to 12 corresponding to medium priority. The intended destination is Destination 2, located in Domain 2. Source 2 packets have to traverse through two QoS domains and reservations are done in both Domain 1 and 2.

Figure 5. Three IPv6 QoS domain topology

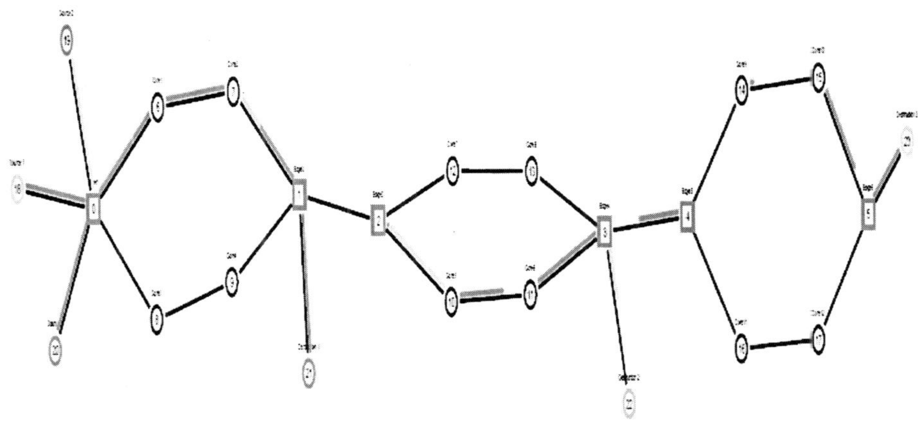

- Source 3 generates a best effort traffic flow at an average rate of 0.25 Mbps. Destination 1 is located in the same domain.

Three IPv6 Domains Simulation Result: Analysis

Table 5 summarizes the results obtained from simulating three IPv6 QoS domains. Delay and packet loss rate are measured for two scenarios, first during traffic conformance and next during Source 1 (highest priority) traffic non conformance. To simulate network congestion the traffic flow from Source 1 is set to violate the requested rate by a 30% increase and its impact on the delay and packet loss rates of level-12 and best effort traffic flows is studied. The following is the summary of simulation results:

- Source 1 (Flow ID 100) is assigned the highest priority level and traverses 3 QoS domains. These packets have achieved an average end-to-end delay of 35.14 ms as they traverse three domains under traffic conformant conditions. The delay per domain of 11.71 ms is better than that achieved by the other two flows. Under Source 1 non conformant conditions, no packets are dropped.
- Source 2 (Flow ID 200), medium priority packets, have also achieved low end-to-end delay of 25.66 msec as they traverse two QoS domains under traffic conformant conditions. The delay per domain of 12.83 ms is higher than that experienced by the highest priority traffic. However, the per-domain delay is better than that achieved by the best effort traffic. Also, no packets

Table 5. Three IPv6 QoS domains: end-to-end delay and packet loss rate

Traffic Source	Priority Level	Flow ID	End-to-end Delay	Average Delay per domain traversed	Average Packet Loss rate
Source 1	15	100	35.14 ms	11.71 ms	0%
Source 2	12	200	25.66 ms	12.83 ms	0%
Source 3	Best Effort	300	18.35 ms	18.35 ms	0%

are dropped. Under Source 1 traffic non-conformance conditions, the end-to-end delay for the level-12 traffic (Flow 200) increased by 11 msec to 36.7 msec, however no packets were lost.

- Flow ID 300, best effort packets, have achieved the highest delay of 18.35 msec as they traverse through one domain. Under Source 1 traffic nonconformance conditions, best effort packets are lost and the delay increased significantly to 137.5 msec.

In conclusion, the proposed QoS management model proves to be scalable as the delay experienced by priority flows is proportional to the number of domain traversed. Also, in the two-domain case, it was shown that when priority flows (level 15 and 12) do not conform to their flow specification rates they are degraded, and best effort traffic experiences maximum delay and higher packet loss rates in order to accommodate the non-conformant higher priority traffic flows. In the three three-domain case, it was shown that when Source 1 (highest priority traffic) did not conform to its flow specification rate, the traffic at priority level 12 was delayed considerably, and the best effort traffic experienced maximum delay in order to accommodate the non-conformant highest priority traffic.

IMPLEMENTING INTERNET BILLING IN THE IPV6 QOS MANAGER

Emerging integrated QoS capable networks provides a variety of services, such as telephony, video, interactive games, teleconferencing, and other Internet services. Upon accepting a user connection, the QoS system must be capable of negotiating QoS parameters and guaranteeing the agreed quality. This differentiation of traffic flows causes Internet elements to process traffic according to their data contents, and therefore, pricing becomes an important issue. Traditionally, users have not been charged for their use of networks resources, and have not generally been aware of the impact of their use on network performance. As a result, traditional Internet pricing schemes that institutionalize one rate for unlimited usage are unfair as they have no differentiation between traffic flows with different QoS requirements.

REVIEW OF THE INTERNET PRICING SCHEMES

Recently, pricing schemes for the Internet has been an active research area. In this section some of the known pricing approaches are reviewed.

Flat Pricing

Under a flat pricing scheme the user is charged a fixed amount per unit time, irrespective of usage (Falkner, Devetsikiotis, & Lambadaris,2000). This scheme has desirable advantages in that flat pricing is simple and convenient as no assumptions are made about the underlying deployed network, and no measurements are required for billing and accounting. The scheme assumes that there is relatively stable demand for resources, and makes no attempt to influence the individual traffic flows. For this reason the scheme is unsuitable for congestion control or traffic management. All users are charged the same even if some of them suffer packet loss due to other user's traffic consuming more resources.

Priority Pricing

Priority pricing requires users to indicate their traffic value by setting the priority field in the IP packet header (Falkner, Devetsikiotis, & Lambadaris,2000). In this scheme, measurements are required for billing and accounting to keep track of the priority level of each user transmitted packet. During periods of congestion, traffic is transmitted by priority level, and low priority traffic is either delayed or dropped. Priority pricing scheme, $P_{b1,b2}$ is defined by two flag bits, b1 priority flag and b2 non-drop flag. This results in four service classes including $P_{0,0}$ Base class (best-effort), $P_{1,0}$ non-drop and low priority class, $P_{0,1}$ drop and high priority class, $P_{1,1}$ non-drop and high priority (real time) class. The cost relation between these classes are $P_{1,1}$ cost = 3* $P_{0,0}$ cost, and $P_{1,0}$ cost = $P_{0,1}$ cost = 2* $P_{0,0}$ cost. Priority pricing raises the economy efficiency of the network since only low value packets are dropped. Under this scheme, the user selects one of the four classes to maximize overall satisfaction (QoS assurance). The network processes all the incoming packets by priority, maintaining different queues for each class. The packets are queued on an FIFO basis and transmitted by priority level.

Smart-Market Pricing

Smart-market pricing focuses on the issues of capacity expansion and costs imposed on customers. The latter includes connection cost and per packet cost that covers the incremental cost of sending a packet. Mason and Varian (Mackie-Masson, & Varian, 1994) introduced a usage charge during network congestion which is determined through an auction. The user inserts a bid price in each packet's header, communicating the user's willingness to pay for transmitting the packet. The network collects and sorts all the bids and sets a threshold value. All packets whose bid exceeds the threshold value are transmitted. The threshold valued is determined by the network's capacity and represents the marginal cost of congestion. Each transmitted packet is then charged this marginal cost. This scheme performs like a priority scheme in which traffic flows with low QoS demand are not guaranteed resources. Traffic packets are transmitted according to their relative priority and bid prices during congestion.

Edge Pricing

Edge pricing combines the approximation of congestion conditions such as time of day and expected path, where charge depends only on the source(s) and destination(s). Therefore, the resulting prices can be determined and charges are assessed locally at the access point. Prices are computed at the domain providers' edges where the users' packets enter the domain network rather than computing them in a distributed fashion along the entire path (Shenker, Clark, Estrin, & Herzog, 1996). Therefore, the focus is shifted to locally computed charges based on expected values of congestion and route. Such a pricing scheme is much simpler than the previous one, and facilitates receiver payments. Traffic management can be supported when this scheme is associated with ATM/RSVP. However, traffic measurements for billing and accounting may still be required.

Per-Packet Pricing Scheme

In this scheme each packet carries electronic money, which is used to pay routers in return for services (Elovici, Ben-Shimol, & Shabtai, 2003). Each packet header includes a user identity header which is used to identify the user by the billing system, accumulated charge field that includes the total amount of electronic money that the user is to be charged and is updated by routers based on pricing scheme, money field is used to set an upper limit to the total amount that can be charged by the network for servicing transmitted packets. Each router in the per-packet billing domain has a field that is used to accumulate the payments for its services. This field is incremented for each packet serviced when the packet arrives at the last hop. Information about the user is sent to a central billing data base. Users are charged according to the accumulated information for the packets they sent.

Figure 6. General pricing strategy

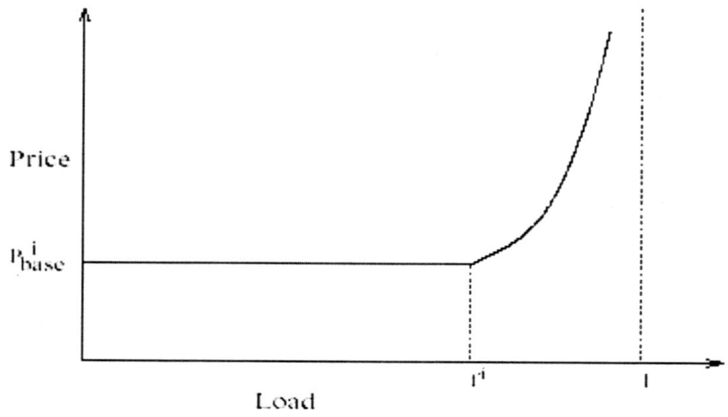

A DYNAMIC PRICING MODEL FOR IPV6 QOS DOMAINS

The proposed pricing model is based on the DiffServ end-to-end pricing scheme introduced in (Boudec, & Thiran, 2004). This model is based on the market model where the value for the base price P^i_{base} and fill factor f^i is set by the network provider for each traffic type. The fill factor is defined as the ratio of target capacity T_i to the maximum capacity C^i_{max} for a class of service *i*. The price is computed using (Li, Iraqi, & Boutaba, 2003; Li, Iraqi, & Boutaba, R., 2004)

$$P_i(t) = P_i(t-1) + \alpha_i(D_i - T_i) / T_i$$

Here $P_i(t)$ denotes the price for a class *i* at time *t* and D_i is the demand or current load for class *i* and α_i is the convergence rate factor that determines how the price converges to its maximum. Figure 6 illustrates the general pricing strategy. When the load for a particular service class is lower than its targeted capacity, the price is the base price P^i_{base} for that particular service class. As the load exceeds its target capacity and when the load is close to the maximum capacity, the price is increased rapidly i.e. we have a dynamic pricing scheme where the price is a function of current network conditions.

During demand increase the exponential pricing strategy is adopted:

$$P_i(t) = \left\{ \begin{array}{ll} P^i_{base} & if \quad D_i \le T_i \\ P^i_{base} e^{\alpha\, [\frac{D_i}{T_i} - 1]} & otherwise \end{array} \right\}$$

A price limit, P^i_{max}, can be set for each class service and this indicates the price when the demand reaches the maximum capacity. It is calculated using:

$$P^i_{max} = P^i_{base} e^{\alpha_i [\frac{D_i}{T_i} - 1]}$$

Therefore knowing, P^i_{base}, P^i_{max} and the fill factor f^i for a class service i gives the solution for the convergence factor α_i which determines how the price converges to the maximum.

$$\alpha_i = \log(\frac{P^i_{max}}{P^i_{base}}) * (\frac{f^i}{1-f^i})$$

The total revenue is the sum of all classes' prices.

Figure 7. IPv6 pricing model

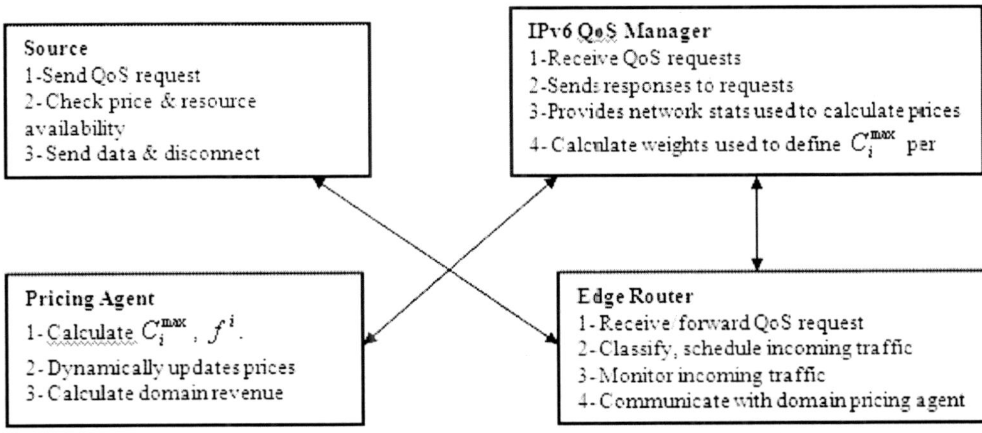

PRICING INTEGRATED QOS MANAGER

Figure 7 summarizes the functions performed by the various network entities in implementing the proposed pricing strategy. The source initiates the QoS request and waits for responses that include the acceptance messages and the associated prices. The edge router forwards requests and responses. It monitors all traffic packets entering the domain. The IPv6 QoS manager processes the QoS requests and then sends the network status for each accepted traffic flow to the pricing agent. The pricing agent calculates the price for each accepted traffic flow by first finding f^i using the information received from the domain QoS manager which includes the expected traffic rate (T_i) and the max allowed rate (C^i_{max}). The pricing agent attached to the edge router initiates the price according to the network status and the defined base price (P^i_{base}) for each traffic class accepted by the manager. All the prices then are sent to the customers that initiate requests. The customer accepts or rejects the price.

PRICING SIMULATION RESULTS

The robustness and behavior of the integrated pricing model in an IPv6 QoS capable network environment is studied using the ns-2 simulator. Figure 8 illustrates the network topology used. The topology consists of 4 core routers and 2 edge routers. Ingress router connects the source nodes and the egress router connects the destination nodes. The Ingress router acts as the pricing agent and handles QoS requests generated by the Source 1 and Source 2 nodes. The total capacity of each link is 1 Mpbs and propagation delay is 1 msec. The specification for the generated traffic flows are: Source 1 has a traffic rate of 500 Kbps with priority 15 and Flow ID-15. Source 2 has a traffic rate of 250 Kbps with priority 12 and flow ID 12. Source 3 has a traffic rate is 250 Kbps, is classified as Best effort type and flow ID- 8.

The base prices P^i_{base} for each class are set to \$0.16, \$0.09 and \$0.04 per unit time respectively starting with the flow with the highest priority. Our simulation was performed on three flows with FID-15 having the highest priority when the total link capacity reaches 50%, FID-12 has the 2rd highest priority when the total link capacity reaches 70% and FID-8 is classified as Best Effort for all link capacities.

Figure 8. Simulated pricing model network

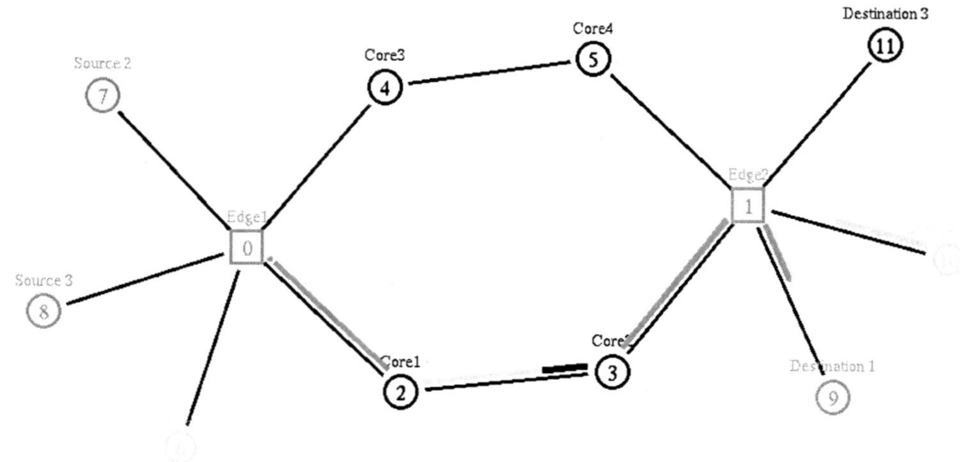

Two simulation scenarios have been tested for each traffic flow, one when the total link load is less than the percentage assigned for each flow and the second case when the non conformant traffic exceeds these assigned percentages. Figure 9 shows the change of the prices for traffic flow FID-15. From this figure it is seen that the prices change rapidly as the load increases which results in more revenue corresponding to the QoS assurance for this flow. It is seen that the changes in price for traffic flow with FID-12 does not change much since its percentage is set to 70% and the packets of this flow are not as critical as those of FID-15, thus resulting in a small revenue increase when compared with the first case. However, during congestion packets belonging to FID-12 are degraded to best effort as per the policies set by the QoS manager. Best Effort flow packets have no change in prices as the expected load is set to 100%; however, they are the first to be dropped during congestion.

Figure 9. Prices for the three traffic flows: highest priority-FID(15), high priority-FID(12) and best-effort-FID(8)

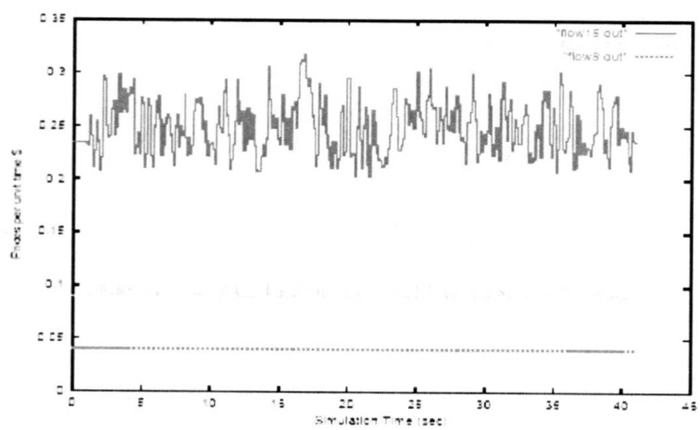

CONCLUSION

A scalable IPv6 QoS management model that guarantees network resources and achieves low end-to-end delay was proposed. The QoS management scheme has been designed to facilitate per flow resource reservation across IPv6 network domains. The key ideas that contribute to scalability and simplicity are: that QoS requests are sent to ingress- edge routers which communicate with their QoS domain manager; core routers merely forward, and schedule traffic flows. Core routers do not participate in resource reservation decisions. This scheme is simple and less complex than IntServ, as only the edge routers are involved in the admission, monitoring and reshaping procedures. The second key idea that contributes to faster forwarding and reservation is the use of DGI field in the IPv6 header to request, reserve and trace resources. Packets are processed faster as the core routers merely forward packets based on their DGI, especially when compared with IPv4 routing lookup that typically involves 5 fields. The third key idea that supports QoS sensitive traffic flow is the degrading of higher priority traffic flows to a lower priority during network congestion instead of tagging the packets as non-conformant. In this scheme, non conformant traffic packets are gracefully degraded and then if their priority is low, they may be dropped. The feasibility of the QoS management scheme is demonstrated with simulation in ns-2 for intra and inter-domain QoS management for conformant and non conformant traffic flows. Intra-domain QoS management, simulations show that the QoS model results in a lower end-to end delay than both DiffServ and IntServ the currently used models. Simulations for non conformant traffic show a slightly higher delay for higher priority packets but with no traffic loss. Simulations for inter-domain QoS management were done with two and three cooperating domains. In both inter-domain scenarios, the end-to-end delay for traffic applications that request QoS in more than one domain was found to be proportional to the delay across one domain. Even with the addition of more domains, the QoS performance of higher priority traffic did not degrade and packets arrived with a shorter end-to-end delay and zero loss. In both the conformant and non conformant traffic scenarios, the highest priority traffic flows recorded lower delay than best effort traffic. This indicates that the proposed model is scalable and works well in multiple domains. In summary, the IPv6 QoS management scheme has achieved low end-to-end and packet loss rates for both Intra and Inter domain QoS management. A dynamic pricing policy was integrated with the IPv6 QoS management scheme to control resources during various network loads. Simulations show that only customers willing to pay more during network congestion were allowed to transmit their traffic packets. Simulation results show higher profits and no higher priority packet loss thus proving that the proposed QoS manager can be used to the advantage of the service provider and customers who are prepared to pay higher costs.

ACKNOWLEDGMENT

The authors acknowledge the assistance of Jason D. Kenney for his assistance with the implementations in NS2. The authors also acknowledge that the excellent comments provided by the anonymous reviewers helped shape the writing of this chapter.

REFERENCES

Agrawal, R., Cruz, R., Okino, C., & Rajan, R., (1999, June). Performance Bounds for Flow Control Protocols. *IEEE/ACM Transaction on Networking, 7* (3).

Blake, S., Black, D., Carlson, M., Davies, E., Wang, Z., & Weiss, W. (1998). An Architecture for Differentiated Services. In Internet Engineering Task Force Request for Comment - IETF RFC 2475.

Boudec, J., & Thiran, P. (2004, May 10). Network Calculus: A Theory of Deterministic Queuing Systems for the Internet. In *LNCS 2050*. Berlin: Springer-Verlag.

Braden, R., Zhang, L., Herzog, S., & Jamin, S. (1997). Resource ReSerVation Protocol (RSVP)- Version 1 Functional Specification. In Internet Engineering Task Force Request for Comment – IETF RFC2205.

Brim, S., Carpenter, B., & LeFaucheur, F. (2000). Per Hop Behavior Identification Codes. In Internet Engineering Task Force Request for Comment – IETF RFC 2836.

Elovici, Y., Ben-Shimol, Y., & Shabtai, A. (2003). Per-Packet Pricing Scheme for IP Networks. In *10th International Conference on Telecommunications IEEE, 2*, 1494-1500.

Falkner, M., Devetsikiotis, M., & Lambadaris, I., (2000). An Overview of Pricing Concepts for Broadband IP Networks. *IEEE Communication Surveys,* (2), 2-13.

Fgee, E., Kenney, J., Phillips, W. I., Robertson, W., & Sivakumar, S. (2004, May 4-7). Implementing an IPv6 QoS management scheme using flow label & class of service fields. *IEEE CCECE 2004, Canadian Conference, 2*, 851 - 854.

Fgee, E. B. (2005). *Scalable QoS and QoS Management Models for IP Networks*. PhD Thesis, Dalhousie University, Halifax, Canada.

Fgee, E.-B., Kenney, J. D., Phillips, W. J., Robertson, W., & Sivakumar, S. (2005, May 18). Comparison of QoS Performance between IPv6 QoS Management Model and IntServ and DiffServ QoS Models. In *Proceedings of the 3rd Annual Communication Networks and Services Research Conference*, (pp. 287 - 292).

Firoiu, V., Boudec, J., Towsley, D., & Zhang, Z. (2002). Theories of Models for Internet Quality of Service. *Proceedings of the IEEE, 90*(9), 1565–1591. doi:10.1109/JPROC.2002.802002

Heinanen, J., Baker, F., & Weiss, W. (1999). Assured Forwarding PHB Group. In Internet Engineering Task Force Request for Comment – IETF RFC 2597.

Jacobson, V., Nichols, K., & Poduri, K. (1999). An Expedited Forwarding PHB. In Internet Engineering Task Force Request for Comment – IETF RFC 2598.

Li, T., Iraqi, Y., & Boutaba, R. (2003). Traffic-Based Pricing and Admission Control for Diff-Serv Networks. In *IFIP/IEEE 8th International Symposium on Integrated Network Management,* (pp. 73-86).

Li, T., Iraqi, Y., & Boutaba, R. (2004). Pricing and admission control for QoS-enabled Internet. In *Computer Networks*. New York: Elsevier.

Loukola, M. V., & Skytta, J. (2003). *New possibilities offered by IPv6*. Retrieved from http://www.hut.fi/~mloukola/pub7/p1.pdf

Mackie-Masson, J. K., & Varian, H. R. (1994, March). Pricing the Internet. In *International Conference of Telecommunication Systems Modelling,* Nashville, TN, (pp. 378-93). Retrieved from http://www.spp.umich.edu/papers/listing.html

Nicholas, K., Blake, S., Baker, F., & Black, D. (1998). (DS Field) in the IPv4 and IPv6 Headers. In *Internet Engineering Task Force Request for Comment – IETF RFC 2474*. Definition of the Differentiated Services Field.

NS-2 The Network Simulator ns-2. (n.d.). Retrieved Oct. 30, 2004 from http://www.isi.edu/nsnam/ns/

Rajahalme, J., Couta, A., Carpenter, A. & Deering, S. (2003). *IPv6 Flow label specification*. Retrieved March from draft-ietf-ipv6flow-label-0.1.txt

Rosen, E., Viswanathan, A., & Callon, R. (2001). (MPLS)Architecture. In *Internet Engineering Task Force Request for Comment – IETF RFC3031*. Multiprotocol Label Switching.

Shaikh, F. A., McClellan, S., Singh, M., & Chakravarthy, S. (2002). End-to-End Testing of IP QoS Mechanisms. *IEEE Computer Magazine*, *35*(5), 80–87.

Shenker, S., Clark, D., Estrin, D., & Herzog, S. (1996). Pricing in Computer Networks: Reshaping the Research Agenda. *ACM Computer Communication Review*, *26*(2), 19–43. doi:10.1145/231699.231703

Shenker, S., Partridge, C., & Guerin, R. (1997). Specification of Guaranteed Quality of Service. In Internet Engineering Task Force Request for Comment – RFC 2212.

Stader, R. (2001). *QoS Provisioning for IP Telephony Networks by Advanced bandwidth management*. Masters of Science Thesis, Hochschule Konstanz Technik, Wirtschaft und Gestaltung.

Stallings, W. (1996). IPv6: The New Internet Protocol. *IEEE Communications Magazine*, (July): 96–108. doi:10.1109/35.526895

White, P. P. (1997). RSVP and Integrated Services in the Internet: A Tutorial. *IEEE Communications Magazine*, 100–106. doi:10.1109/35.592102

Wroclawski, J. (1997). Specification of the Controlled-load Network Element Service. In Internet Engineering Task Force Request for Comment – IETF RFC 2211.

Xiao, V., Ni, L.M., (1999). Internet QoS: The Big Picture. *IEEE Network Magazine (*March/April), 8-18.

Chapter 15
Providing Quality of Service across Multiple Providers:
The Case of European Research and Academic Space

Christos Bouras
University of Patras, Greece

Apostolos Gkamas
University of Patras, Greece

Kostas Stamos
University of Patras, Greece

ABSTRACT

In this chapter, the authors present some of the latest developments related to the provisioning of Quality of Service (QoS) in today's networks and the associated network management structures that are or will be deployed to support them. They first give a brief overview of the most important Quality of Service proposals in the areas of Layer 2 (L2) and Layer 3 (L3) QoS provisioning in backbone networks, and they discuss the network management structures and brokers that have been proposed in order to implement these services. As a case study, they describe the pan-european research and academic network, which is supported centrally by GEANT and which encompasses multiple independent NRENs (National Research and Education Networks). In the last few years, GEANT has developed and deployed a number of production and pilot services meant for the delivery of quality network services to the end users across Europe.

INTRODUCTION

The GN2 European project GÉANT2 (2009) encompasses a range of research activities to advance both networking and user services in Europe. Central to this project, is the goal of providing high-quality services from one end user to another over multiple interconnected networks. The GÉANT2 (2009) network connects 34 countries via 30 national research and education networks (NRENs), using multiple 10Gbps wavelengths. GÉANT2 also connects to worldwide NRENs and the public Internet

DOI: 10.4018/978-1-61520-791-6.ch015

to ensure a global Gigabit-per-second connectivity for all users.

Quality of Service has been developed as a concept for several years and has reached maturity especially related to L3 implementations, although user demand and provider uptake has not always been as high as expected. The emergence of L2-based network architectures that try to avoid the high costs of high-end routing capabilities and take advantage of direct administration of optical circuits by organizations such as European NRENs, has led to the need for L2 QoS and Bandwidth on Demand services.

GEANT has deployed services in two main areas: The provisioning of L3 QoS based on DiffServ architecture, and the provisioning of Bandwidth on Demand (BoD) based on dynamic allocation of L2 circuits. The GN2 activity that has specified and is now prototyping a Bandwidth on Demand service intended to operate in a multi-domain environment using heterogeneous transmission technologies is called AutoBAHN, while the GN2 activity that has developed a L3 QoS provisioning framework is called AMPS. In addition GN2 has developed a monitoring system for the AutoBAHN service, which has proved in itself a complex and challenging task.

This chapter presents some of the latest developments related to the provisioning of Quality of Service (QoS) in today's networks and the associated network management structures that are or will be deployed to support them. The remaining of this chapter is structured as follows: The next section presents the international experience in the area of L2 and L3 QoS. Section 3 presents the efforts of GEANT in order to implement and deploy L2 and L3 QoS services. Section 4 presents the future trends in the area. Finally, Section 5 concludes this chapter.

BACKGROUND

QoS Architectures at Layer 3

IP networks are built around the idea of best effort networking, which makes no guarantees regarding the delivery, the speed and the accuracy of the transmitted data. While this model is suitable for a large number of applications and works well for almost all applications when the network load is low (and therefore there is no congestion), there are two main factors that combine to lead to the need for an additional capability of quality of service guarantees. One factor is that the amount of real-time and other multimedia data transmitted over the Internet increases, and this type of data have stricter service requirements. The other factor is that Internet usage in general is steadily increasing, and although the network infrastructure is often also updated, it is not always certain that network resources offering will be ahead of network usage demand. Several researchers for example, argue that there are signs that Internet demand is outstripping capacity (Nemertes, 2007). Furthermore, several providers are implementing usage caps to alleviate the problem.

The two main architectures that have been proposed for Quality of Service are IntServ and DiffServ. They follow different philosophy as they approach the topic of Quality of Service from different point of views.

The IntServ architecture tries to provide absolute guarantees via resource reservations across the paths that the traffic class follows. The main protocol that works with this architecture is the Reservation Protocol (RSVP). However, its operation is quite complicated and it also inserts significant network overhead. On the other hand, DiffServ architecture is more flexible and efficient as it tries to provide Quality of Service via a different approach. It classifies all the network traffic into classes and tries to treat each class differently, according to the level of QoS guarantees that each class needs. In the DiffServ architecture, 2 different types (per hop behaviours, Nichols, 2001) have been proposed, the expedited forwarding (Jacobson et al., 1999) and the assured forwarding (Heinanen et al., 1999), and their difference is on the packet forwarding behaviour. Expedited forwarding (EF) aims at providing QoS for the class by minimizing the jitter and is generally focused on providing stricter guarantees. This type tries to simulate the virtual leased lines and its policy profile should be very tight. Assured forwarding (AF) inserts at most 4 classes with at most 3 levels of dropping packets. Every time the traffic of each class exceeds the policy criteria then it is marked as lower level QoS class.

The operation of DiffServ architecture is based on several mechanisms such as packet classification, packet marking, metering, shaping and queue management. The classification is done via marking the DSCP (Differentiated Service CodePoint) field.

Although QoS provisioning mechanisms have been extensively tested and deployed in several networks, the biggest hurdle in wider application of the idea has been the fact that the Internet is fragmented in separate administrative sections (domains). Even if a domain implements some form of QoS provisioning and guarantees, there is no guarantee that traffic will receive the same treatment end to end, because there is no widespread availability and deployment of multi-domain automated provisioning systems. The research effort in GEANT2 has largely been devoted in changing this situation.

IP Premium Service

The IP Premium service has been defined in the framework of the SEQUIN project (Bouras et al., 2003) and aims at providing absolute bandwidth guarantees and minimum delay and jitter to a subset of the overall network traffic. Its main characteristic is that it follows the classic DiffServ architecture. It classifies the packets using the DSCP values for admitted and downgraded packets. The policing is performed at the edge of the network and high priority queuing is applied in the core and access routers at the outgoing interfaces.

QoS at Layer 2 and Bandwidth on Demand

In recent years, rapid technological developments combined with strong growth in demand for transmission capacity has encouraged network carriers to invest heavily in optical network infrastructure. The following paragraphs give an overview of the standardization efforts that have taken place in this area, and specifically the related technologies and standards proposed by the Internet Engineering Task Force (IETF), the International Telecommunication Union (ITU-T) and the Optical Internetworking Forum (OIF).

Generalised Multi Protocol Label Switching (GMPLS)

Generalised Multi Protocol Label Switching (GMPLS) is a technological framework proposed by the Internet Engineering Task Force (IETF) and targeted at enabling dynamic provisioning capabilities in optical networks. The approach followed by IETF has been to extend the well-known Multi Protocol Label Switching (MPLS) technological framework to encompass devices used for building optical networks.

According to the Generalised MPLS (GMPLS) framework RFC3945 (2004), the MPLS Traffic Engineering (TE) control plane is extended to include network elements such as Add-Drop Multiplexers (ADMs) and Optical Cross-Connects. The MPLS framework RFC3031 (2001) was designed for network elements capable of recognizing packet or cell boundaries. In contrast, the GMPLS framework has been proposed for network elements that can also recognise time-slots, lambdas or ranges of lambdas and fibres. More specifically, according to the GMPLS architecture the following interfaces are defined:

1. *Packet Switch Capable (PSC)* interfaces are able to recognise packet boundaries and forward data based on the content of a specific field in the packet header. Examples of this type of interface include router interfaces.
2. *Layer-2 Switch Capable (L2SC)* interfaces are able to recognise frame or cell boundaries and switch data based either on the value of the MAC header for Ethernet frames or on the value of the VPI/VCI pair for ATM cells. Examples of this type of interface include Ethernet and ATM switches interfaces.
3. *Time-Division Multiplex Capable (TDM)* interfaces switch data based on time-slots. An example of this type of interface is an SDH interface.
4. *Lambda Switch Capable (LSC)* interfaces switch data based on the wavelength on which incoming signal is modulated. These kinds of interfaces may also be able to switch contiguous groups of wavelengths (waveband switching). An example is the Optical Add Drop Multiplexer (OADM).
5. *Fibre-Switch Capable (FSC)* interfaces switch data based on the fibre or fibres that they are using. An example is the interface of a photonic cross connect.

Automatically Switched Optical Network (ASON)

To overcome the limitations of centralised manual provisioning, ITU-T Study Group 15 started, following a top down approach, the development of complete definition of the operation of an Automatically Switched Transport Network G.807 (2001). Automatically Switched Optical Network (ASON) G.8080 (2001) is not a protocol or collection of protocols. It is a framework that defines the components in an optical control plane and the interactions between these components. An Automatically Switched Optical Network is an optical transport network that is capable of dynamically adding and removing connections. This capability is accomplished by using a control plane that performs the call and connection control functions in real time.

ASON can be thought of as an improved optical transport network (OTN) that adds sufficient intelligence to the optical nodes to permit dynamic provisioning that can respond to changing traffic patterns. ASON is an architecture that defines the components of an optical control plane and the interactions between those components. In itself, it does not define any protocols. A key principle of ASON is to explicitly build a framework that supports legacy network equipment.

The ASON architecture is based on the assumption that a network's design and segmentation is dictated by the operator's decisions and criteria (e.g. geography, administration, technology). Network subdivisions are defined in ASON as 'routing areas'. Recommendation G.8080 defines a routing area as a set of subnetworks. A routing area contains smaller routing areas interconnected by Subnetwork Termination Point Pool (SNPP) links. Routing uses a hierarchical structure based on a decomposition of the network into a subnetwork hierarchy. Each subnetwork has its own dynamic connection control, which knows its own topology but does not know the topology of other subnetworks belonging to either the same hierarchical level or different levels.

Optical Internetworking Forum (OIF)

The Optical Internetworking Forum (OIF) has as its main objective to foster the development of a low-cost and scalable internet using optical technologies. In order to achieve this, OIF brings together the architectures and requirements defined by ITU-T as well as the protocols defined by IETF into a complete working solution. OIF has defined two interfaces:

- User to Network Interface (UNI): The UNI 1.0 recommendation was defined by OIF in December 2001, the current release was published in February 2004. The OIF UNI 1.0 enables clients to establish optical connections dynamically using signalling procedures compatible with GMPLS signalling. The UNI 2.0 specification finalized in 2008. It extends UNI 1.0 by adding various functionalities such as the separation of call and connection control and non disruptive connection modification.
- External Network to Network Interface (E-NNI): The purpose of E-NNI is to support deployment of an optical control plane in a heterogeneous environment. The support for such technically heterogeneous networks is achieved by introducing the concept of control domains. Signalling and routing information exchange between those domains is performed over the E-NNI. Thus the OIF specifies the E-NNI to be a interface for signalling messages, attributes and flows for the creation of transport connections across multiple heterogeneous domains.

Other Research Approaches

Several other research networks have dealt with similar issues and devised their own approaches. For example, the DRAGON project (Leung et al., 2006) has also conducted research and developed technologies to enable dynamic provisioning of network resources on an interdomain basis across heterogeneous network technologies. The OSCARS/BRUW project (Guok, 2005) focuses on L3 MPLS QoS and adopts SNMP queries to the routers for monitoring LSP teardown and usage. The UCLP community project and the related Argia commercial product enable users to control and manage network elements for the purposes of establishing End-to-End (E2E) lightpaths (Wu et al., 2003, Argia Web site, 2007). The MUPBED project attempts to integrate and validate, in the context of user-driven large-scale testbeds, ASON/GMPLS technology and network solutions (Cavazzoni, 2007). MUPBED takes into account that for an optical network operated according to OTN, specific fields of the frame are reserved to user's monitoring of a connection. VIOLA (VIOLA Web site, 2007) is another related project for the development and test of software tools for the user-driven dynamical provision of bandwidth but does not focus on the development of tools for the monitoring of the provisioned resources. VIOLA is focused instead on the area of network technology and application development as part of a testbed environment.

IETF has worked on the concept of Path Computation Element (PCE) which aims to separate routing decisions from the packet forwarding procedures (RFC4655, 2006). GEANT2 approach has been similar to the one proposed by IETF, in that path finding decisions are taken at an overlay control layer. Because of the multi-domain requirements of GEANT2, it has placed greater focus on the abstraction and limited information exchange, and less focus on optimal path selection mechanisms.

THE CASE OF EUROPEAN RESEARCH AND ACADEMIC SPACE

Description of GEANT2 Activities

Within the GN2 project, a number of service activities (SAs) and joint research activities (JRAs) are being pursued. Service activities represent more mature services that are considered to be ready for production deployment, while research activities lead to pilot deployments of services. Since the issue of Quality of Service in layer 3 had been researched and numerous experimental deployments had taken place, it was decided that such a service should be available in a mature level within GEANT. It has also been understood that in the research and academic environment, there are applications and research fields (such as radioastronomy, high-energy physics and general Grid applications) with strict demands for the provisioning of guaranteed and dedicated capacity. For this reason, the GN2 project has also developed the AutoBAHN (Bandwidth on Demand – BoD) Joint Research Activity 3.

The main purpose of the relevant GEANT2 activities was to design, implement and deploy systems for the interoperation of provisioning mechanisms between different domains, so that traffic from one end of Europe could reach another end at a potentially different country with a network managed by a different entity, while at the same time receiving guaranteed service (in the case of Layer 3 QoS provisioning) or even a dedicated circuit (in the case of Bandwidth on Demand service). Several research and academic networks across Europe had already developed their own solutions for their inner network, however these solutions were not interoperable and could therefore only guarantee service until the boundary of the specific domain. The GEANT2 design of these services has therefore gone to great length in order to make sure that the deployed systems are modular enough so that pre-existing solutions can "plug-in" and interoperate in an international context. Although this design choice adds some complexity to the system, a monolithic solution would be unacceptable as few, if any, network domains would agree to give up on their installed and tested provisioning systems for a completely new solution. Furthermore, GEANT2 research activities have designed the provisioning systems in such a way that as little information as possible is shared between domains, since separate network management entities are not willing to freely share detailed information about their inner network.

Since both the AMPS and AutoBAHN systems faced the above requirements, they have taken a similar approach in general system design and interoperability, as will be seen in more detail in the following paragraphs.

GN2 L3 QoS Service (AMPS)

AMPS (ADS, 2006) implements the recommendations of the SEQUIN (Bouras et al., 2003) project for providing premium IP service across multiple, independent networks. The purpose of AMPS is to regulate the maximum allowed amount of prioritised IP traffic in a given domain, thus ensuring that approved traffic continues to receive a top-quality service (low delay, low packet loss) in the event of network congestion. It does this by evaluating each new request for Premium IP (PIP) against existing, approved PIP requests and the total available network resources, and then only approving those new requests which will not adversely affect any existing reservations. AMPS also includes a communication module which enables it work with neighbouring peers in order to establish a PIP service that crosses multiple domains.

AMPS has been developed for IP-based domains, and is based on the assumption that they are either over-provisioned, or use the DiffServ architecture. Currently, AMPS does not always directly configure the network devices (routers), although several AMPS deployments, such as the one in the Greek NREN GRNET do support automatic router configuration.

The overall AMPS architecture is shown in Figure 1. Communication between the 4 subsystems takes place through web services so that they can be easily upgraded or switched with equivalent modules developed independently (Bouras et al., 2007).

AMPS, similarly to the AutoBAHN system described later, take the approach of developing reference implementations for all their subsystems, but with maximum modularity so that they can be replaced by modules already existing in an organization and so that they can easily be upgraded to support more technologies.

Figure 1 displays 3 AMPS instances in 3 neighbouring domains, with the middle one enlarged so that its subsystems and their interactions are

Figure 1. AMPS architecture

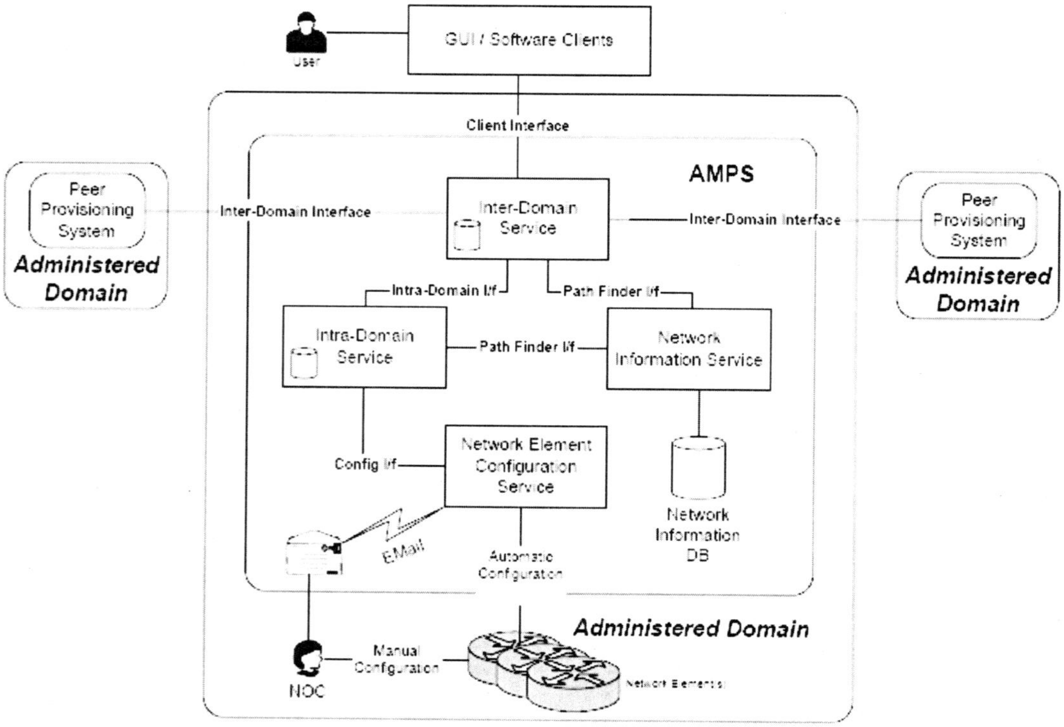

visible. A user is also displayed as an example connecting to the middle AMPS instance.

Inter-Domain Subsystem

The Inter-Domain subsystem is the core of the AMPS multi-domain functionality, and the module that is expected to be deployed in most, if not all, deployments of the AMPS system. It is responsible for receiving messages from and sending messages to external systems as well as handling transactions. These external systems may be either an end-client or the AMPS system in an adjacent domain. Through the Inter-Domain subsystem a reservation request is relayed from one end of the path to the other end and the reservation decision is negotiated before being announced to the end user. AMPS implements a chain communication model, where an AMPS Inter-Domain system cannot directly communicate with another Inter-Domain system in a domain to which it is not directly connected, but such messages can be relayed to the distant Inter-Domain system via intermediate Inter-Domain systems.

Intra-Domain Subsystem

The Intra-Domain subsystem is responsible for its own domain and it keeps a record of all approved PIP reservations that pass though its domain. Requests for new reservations are passed to it by the Inter-Domain subsystem. The reservation includes basic parameters such as the ID of the user submitting the reservation, source and destination end-point, required capacity, start and stop time. The Intra-Domain subsystem will first check that the request is valid according to several sanity and policy tests (for example, whether the capacity and time period requested are within the rights of the user). This is done by querying its Policy Module. If a request is within policy limits then the Intra-Domain subsystem requests the intra-domain path from the cNIS database. The reservation database is then checked to see if that path has sufficient spare PIP capacity for the requested period. If so, the reservation database is updated with the new information and the Inter-Domain subsystem is informed of a successful reservation.

Reservation Status and Transaction Manager

Since a reservation requests might have to traverse multiple remote domains, and since resources might not be automatically allocated in all domains, AMPS has to implement a method of gradual updates to the end user regarding a submitted reservation's status. Therefore, when the Inter-Domain subsystem receives a request for a new PIP reservation it immediately responds to the client with a service id and status as "pending". The domain where a request is submitted is called the home domain. The Inter-Domain subsystem of the home domain then, acting as a transaction manager, starts a new transaction. It then contacts cNIS using the pathfinder interface to check which is the next domain (if any) and what is the current domain's egress interface and next domain's ingress interface. It then sends the reservation request to the Intra-Domain subsystem. Once the Intra-Domain subsystem reports that reservation request is successful then the request is forwarded to the Provisioning System of the next domain along the path. Assuming that the reservation is successful in the next domain this chain process continues until the last domain along the path is reached. Once the request is successful in the last domain; a message indicating that the request is successful is relayed back to the originating domain. This end-to-end chaining process completes the transaction and the status is updated as "accepted". If any domain in the path rejects the request, a message indicating the request is unsuccessful is relayed back to the originating domain. The transaction manager is then responsible to send a rollback message to all domains along the path where a reservation may have been made to cancel the reservation. Once all domains have rolled back their reservation the transaction manager is notified. This completes the transaction and the request status is changed to 'rejected', with a reason given for rejection. The transaction manager will keep sending the rollback until it receives the acknowledgement (or will notify some human administrator). If any service along the path does not respond, a timeout mechanism will be triggered on the transaction manager and a rollback process will be started automatically. Once all domains have rolled back their reservations the transaction manager is notified. This completes the transaction and status is changed to "rejected", and a reason given for rejection.

The client can periodically query the status of the request. Once the transaction is complete the status will be updated from "pending" to "accepted" or "rejected". If the reservation is submitted to a domain but it starts in another (in other words, if the home domain is different from the source domain), the request will be forwarded to the source domain. Even though the reservation starts in the source domain, the home domain will act as the transaction manager. In all other respects AMPS behaves as described above.

cNIS Database

The Network Information Service subsystem uses the Network Information database to calculate what route a given flow will take across the network. The database must therefore have a record of all the links in the network, it must know each link's metric, and it must be informed (by a client, using the NIS's PathFinder interface) the start and end points of the flow. The NIS will then return to the client (using the same PathFinder interface), the link by link path that the specified flow will follow.

The cNIS database started from the AMPS activity but its use has been generalized in the

GN2 project, and can therefore store information about layers 1, 2, and 3 and is also used by the AutoBAHN service described below.

GN2 BoD Service (AutoBAHN)

Similarly to AMPS, the architecture of AutoBAHN system which implements the GN2 BoD service has been designed to meet the fundamental requirement for operation in a multi-domain, multi-technology environment. The BoD service was defined so that it could provide end-to-end, multi-domain, point-to-point symmetric (in terms of bandwidth capacity and path selection) guarantees. Point-to-multipoint services may be realized as a set of point-to-point ones. Furthermore, a BoD service instance may be requested in advance, and a reservation is expected to last from days to years. A minimum time period is required between the request and the actual provisioning of the service, which is due to the level of automation in the resource allocation process. The provisioned paths can be either unprotected, partially or fully protected. All services with full protection require the set-up of two completely separate paths from source to destination, including the physical layer, so as to survive failures even in the case of events such as fibre cuts.

The GN2 BoD system is composed of the modules presented in Figure 2. Its architecture is modularized in order for individual modules to be easily upgraded or replaced, and the communication between these modules is heavily based on web services interfaces.

Inter-Domain Manager (IDM)

The IDM module, similarly to the AMPS Inter-Domain subsystem is the key component of the AutoBAHN system. As the only ingress point to the system, it is responsible for receiving BoD service requests directly from a user or application, or indirectly by another domain and is then responsible for the admission and instantiation of these requests. The IDM functionality is also independent of the underlying individual per-domain implementations and can apply to both automated and manual per-domain BoD provisioning.

When service end points are in different domains, the IDMs involved will cooperate on a peer-to-peer basis to create the requested end-to-end path. Each domain can independently choose the policies and technologies for the BoD service. The peering model also allows scaling to a large number of domains and eases the synchronization constraints of the implementation.

Upon receiving a reservation request, the IDM module uses the Inter-domain pathfinder to contact the next domain and establish an end-to-end path. In order to commit to the reservation request, IDMs use a chain model, similar to the one used by RSVP (Resource ReSerVation Protocol).

The IDM relies on the local DM to implement the service requested in the form of a provisioned circuit. The DM deals, through the Technology Proxy, with the physical details of the particular network domains and the different technologies used to implement the BoD circuit. For more details refer to DJ3.3.1 (2008) and FSIDM (2007).

If needed, the IDM module also communicates with the AAI service, in order to authenticate the AutoBAHN user and the associated privileges for the BoD service, always applying the local domain rules and policies.

Domain Manager (DM)

The Domain Manager (DM) module is responsible for instantiating the reservations within the single domain where it has been deployed. It has detailed knowledge of the topology of its domain and participates in the inter-domain pathfinding process by examining the feasibility of providing an end-to-end path within its local domain. For the actual, technology-specific configuration to take place, the DM contacts the Technology Proxy module.

Figure 2. AutoBAHN system modules

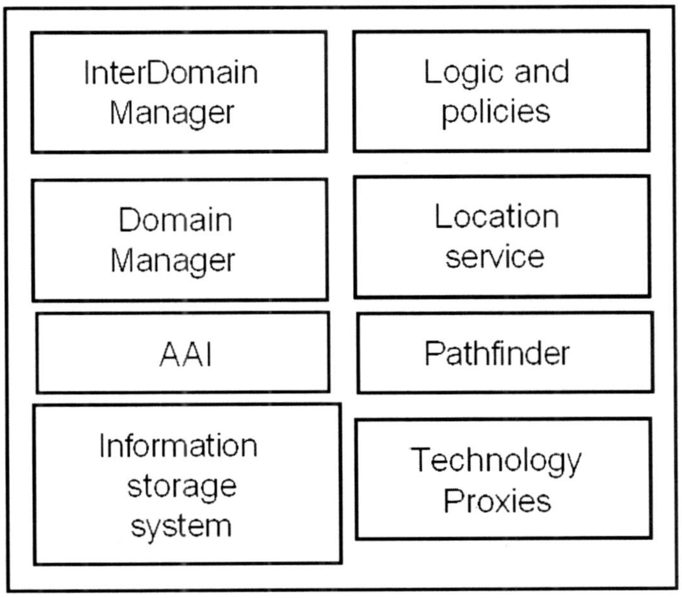

Technology Proxy (and Resource Modelling) Module

The Technology Proxy module performs the translation of requests received by the DM (in abstract network language) into vendor- or equipment-specific configurations. It is the AutoBAHN module that is expected to be more frequently upgraded and replaced for various deployments depending on the existing low-level technologies in each domain. The proxy module may configure the network via an existing Network Management System (NMS) or act as a GMPLS agent; consequently it does not act directly upon the network, but relies on an intermediate control layer.

Other Modules

The *Policy module* contains all the rules and policies which are available for use by other modules when inspecting and elaborating on a request. The rules are collected in a single module for easy maintenance, modification and to enforce coherence.

The *Pathfinder* module contains the algorithms and the logic to search for a path that satisfies each BoD reservation request according to specific sets of constraints, algorithms and policies. The module actually consists of two independent blocks, one for inter-domain pathfinding and one for intra-domain pathfinding, which are respectively incorporated in the IDM and DM modules.

The *Information Storage System* and the *Location Service* function mainly offer support to the other modules. The Information Storage System is responsible for providing storage, archival and database functionalities for data explicitly relevant to the BoD system, while the Location Service locates the addresses of all type of services and modules.

The Inter-Domain Pathfinder

The inter-domain Pathfinder module is responsible for producing a list of paths that satisfy the reservation requests. It receives a set of parameters from each reservation request, takes into account the local policies and the information received by other IDMs and computes a list of candidate end-to-end paths over which the request can potentially be implemented.

While in a standard routing protocol, signaling, topology discovery and update, routing policies and route computation are tightly coupled, in the BoD architecture, these functionalities are decoupled and placed in different modules.

- Inter-domain topology signaling is placed in the IDM.
- Inter-domain topology discovery and update is performed at the IDM, which receives updates from all other IDMs and creates an abstracted inter-domain topology.
- The routing algorithms operate on the abstracted topology produced by the Pathfinder.
- Policies are applied both in the IDM and in the Pathfinder. Various set of policies exist, such as signaling policies (filtering) and request handling policies (which includes user access policies) in the IDM and path computation policies (algorithm parameter values) in the Pathfinder.

The Pathfinder module, located in the source domain, computes the complete path from the source domain to the destination domain. Then, the source domain IDM contacts the next domain in the path, which in its turn contacts the next one using the announced path (or using its own routing computation in case of a mismatch) in a chained model.

The source domain's view of the abstracted inter-domain BoD topology is built from the announcements from other IDMs. For each specific request, the Pathfinder routing algorithm uses the abstracted topology to return a list of feasible paths based on the parameters of the reservation request. In order to return multiple paths, k-shortest path algorithms (Shier (1979), Eppstein (1994)) are used.

Since the Pathfinder uses a chained model, it is preferable to have the source domain compute the path and announce it to the subsequent domains. Even if all domains may re-compute the same end-to-end path, announcement of the path is useful in order to reduce load and ensure consistency. In case the chained reservation process fails at some point, the source domain will use a different path (either from the set already computed by the Pathfinder or by calling the Pathfinder module again) and start again.

The Pathfinder implementation is based on the OSPF protocol to distribute information about the links and build the database necessary for path computation. In order to carry Traffic Engineering information using OSPF, the Pathfinder module will use Opaque LSAs of type 9, 10, 11 according to RFC 2370 (Coltum, 1998).

Reservations

A service request is submitted at the source domain (Home Domain) and is examined using a chain communication model, so that each domain is only in contact with its direct neighbour. When a reservation request is submitted, the Home Domain performs a local validation procedure and executes inter-domain pathfinding in order to identify a list of feasible paths. If it has sufficient resources available to perform the reservation, it propagates the request forward to the next domain of the selected inter-domain reservation path. Attached to the propagated request are the reservation constraints, which are subsequently propagated all the way to the last domain on the reservation path. A reverse propagation of the status of the request then takes place, so that domains are informed whether the request was accepted by the subsequent domains or not.

Implementing a Brokering and Monitoring Service

An integral part of the AutoBAHN service is the monitoring of the provisioned end-to-end connections. This section describes in more detail the architectural design and decisions taken in order to implement this module of the system (Bouras et al., 2008).

The basic concepts for the End to End (E2E) Monitoring were:

- *Intradomain link:* Intradomain link is a link between two nodes (routers or switches) that both belong to the same domain.
- *irtual link:* Virtual link is the conceptual link which connects two border nodes (routers or switches) that both belong to the same domain. A virtual link is the result of the conjunction of many Intradomain links. Virtual links are the kind of information that a domain presents to the outside world about its internal state: it does not propagate detailed information about its internal links; instead it provides aggregated information about Edge to Edge connections represented by Virtual links.
- *Interdomain link:* Interdomain link is a link between two border nodes (routers or switches) of two different domains. Interdomain links are typically monitored by both domains they connect to, but the case where only one domain monitors an interdomain link can also be handled.
- *E2E (End to End) link:* E2E link is the conceptual link which connects two end points from different domains. An E2E link is the result of the conjunction of many Interdomain and Virtual links.

Figure 3. Information flow for the monitoring module

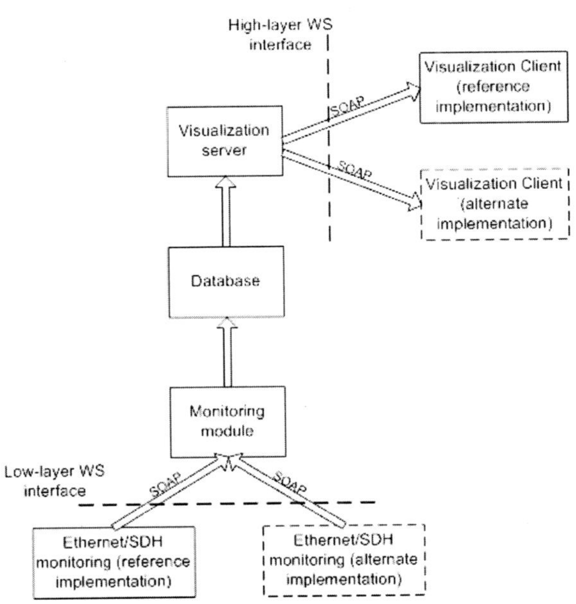

Each domain provides information about the links it monitors (these links can be either Virtual links or Interdomain links). The E2E Monitoring system computes the overall status of an E2E link by aggregating the status information from the involved domains.

The overall architecture of the E2E monitoring system consists of the following modules:

- *Low-level reference implementation:* This module can be a secure scripting server, if the underlying network is based on Ethernet technology, or it can be a technology proxy to the NMS (Network Management System) if the underlying network is based on SDH. It is responsible for the low-level, technology specific communication with the network devices of the domain in order to check the status of the physical links.
- *DM monitoring module:* The monitoring module of the DM is responsible for monitoring the status of both Virtual and Interdomain links and provide this information to the Visualisation server via the Database.
- *Database:* The database functions as an intermediary level between the DM monitoring module and the visualization server. It stores persistent information that can be asynchronously retrieved by the upper layers, thereby insulating low-level functions from user requests.
- *Visualisation server:* The visualisation

server collects monitoring information from the DMs (through the corresponding monitoring module) of the domains involved in the E2E monitored link and presents monitoring information to the user/administrator through a graphical interface.

As displayed in Figure 3. the modular architecture in combination with the usage of standards such as SOAP for the implementation of the interfaces allows modules to be easily and transparently changed or upgraded, allowing the full or partial deployment of the monitoring system in various NREN environments.

During the monitoring of an end-to-end Bandwidth on Demand circuit over Ethernet Infrastructure the following steps take place:

The IDMs and DMs of the involved domains cooperate, as described in the relevant section above, in order to establish an end-to-end Bandwidth on Demand circuit over the existing infrastructure. The results of this establishment will be an end-to-end circuit in the abstracted topology of the involved domains. This end-to-end Bandwidth on Demand circuit or E2E link for shortness is the input for the E2E monitoring system which is responsible to monitor the status of the E2E link. The E2E monitoring system extracts from the abstracted topology the domains and the corresponding interdomain and virtual links which comprise the E2E link. In repeated time intervals the E2E monitoring system polls the DM monitoring modules of the involved domains and aggregates all the status information. Each DM monitoring module reports aggregate status about the links that it monitors to the E2E monitoring system. In order for the DM monitoring module to check the status of an interdomain link or an intradomain link, it has to communicate (via web services) with the low-level technology specific implementation. For example, a reference implementation has been

Figure 4. AutoBahn GUI

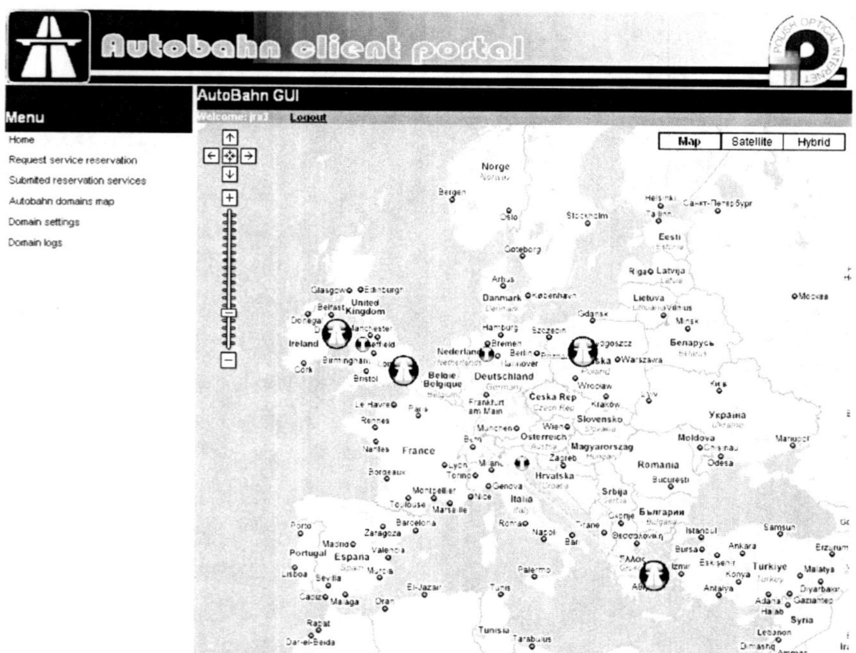

developed for Ethernet, where communication is done using a Secure Scripting Server. This communication for security reasons in based on SSH. The Secure Scripting Server communicates with the corresponding routers / switches in order to check the status of the physical link that corresponds to an intradomain or interdomain link. An interdomain link can be monitored by either one of the domains connected by this interdomain link or by both connected domains. In the latter case the E2E monitoring system is responsible for combining the monitoring information from both involved domains into a unified status for the link. The E2E monitoring system computes the overall status of an E2E link by aggregating the status information of the involved domains and presents the overall status of an E2E link through the visualization server. The communication between the visualization server and the DM monitoring system is also based on web services.

The E2E monitoring system in its current version provides information for two monitoring parameters: The Operational State, which is derived from the operational state of the involved physical devices, and the Administrative State, which reflects the management processes performed by the domains.

Figure 5. Demonstration topology

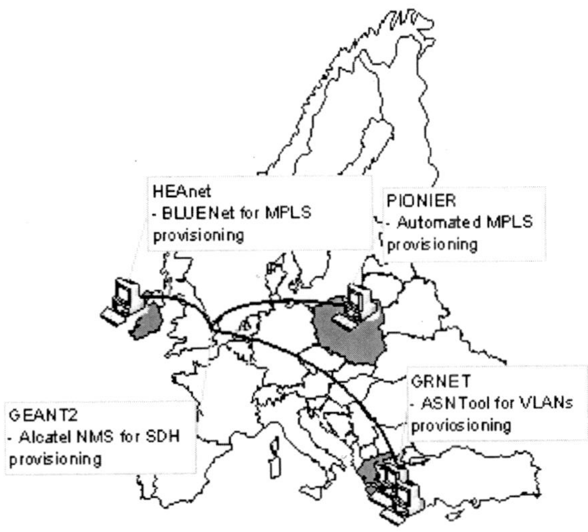

Demonstrations

The AutoBahn team has made various demonstrations of the AutoBahn BoD service during the last years. During the GEANT2 Workshop in January 2008 the following demonstration took place: Multiple parallel connections between end points were supported by data plane, while domains' resource management was fully automated and performed without administrator attention. The following figures show the AutoBahn GUI and topology of the demonstration.

In addition in November 2007, AutoBAHN was presented at the SuperComputing'07 event, where the European test environment was interconnected with a similar research environment in the USA. Four European domains were involved and collaborated with the USA system. The following figure shows the topology of the demonstration and some performance graphs.

FUTURE RESEARCH DIRECTIONS

GEANT and the European NREN community intend to continue working on and expand the described services in the future, and in particular in the context of the upcoming research projects.

One of the most emerging issues in the area of L2 QoS is the standardization and interoperability of services like the AutoBAHN service of GEANT. This will allow the simplification of the deployment of the end to end L2 BoD services and will reduce the cost of such service deployment both in terms of equipment cost and map power cost. Standardization and interoperability issues will have to be studied in two directions:

Figure 6. Demonstration topology

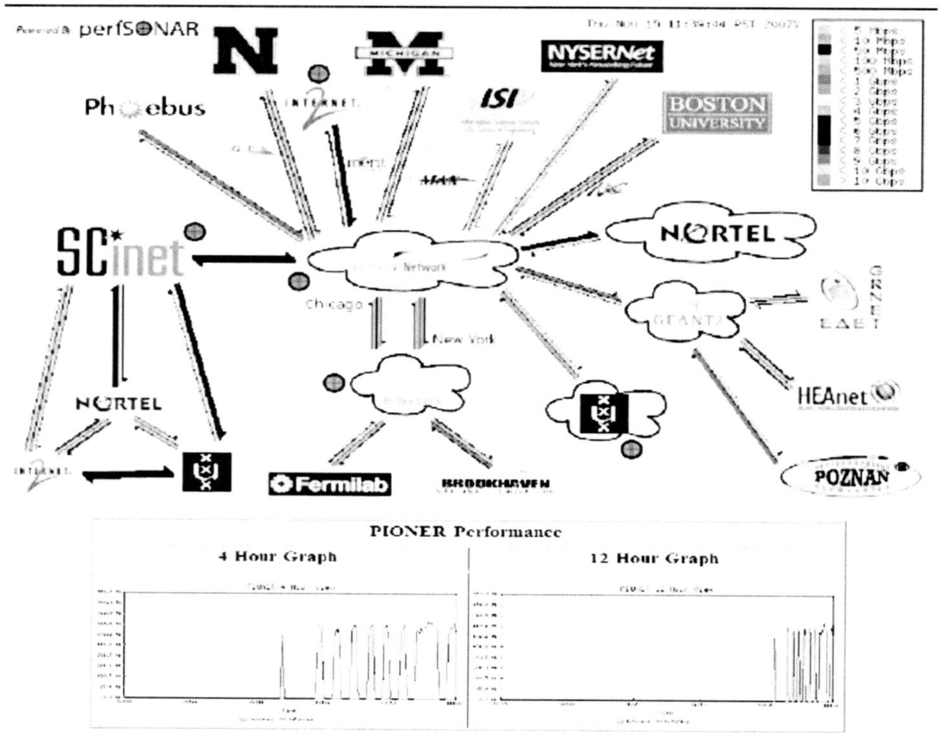

- Standardization and interoperability in the interface between similar L2 QoS services: In this direction protocols must be standardized for the communication of IDM entities of various L2 QoS services.
- Standardization and interoperability in the interface between the service and the domains participating to the L2 QoS cloud. In this direction protocols must be standardized for the communication of DM entities and the technology proxy of a participating domain to the L2 QoS cloud.

The current experience suggests the standardization of the above interfaces to be based on XML. This will allow the easy implementation of the relative protocols and will increase the interoperability among different implementation platforms.

Furthermore, GEANT intends to further investigate L3 QoS provisioning as a production-level service and streamline the reservation procedure so that the users can more seamlessly take advantage of dynamic network resource allocation.

CONCLUSION

Designing and implementing the services for Quality of Service at layer 3 and Bandwidth on Demand in such a large scale for GEANT has proven to be a complex and challenging task. At the completion of the GEANT project, both services were operating at a functional level, with multiple deployments across European NRENs. For the AutoBAHN system, the network abstraction and a network description language, technology stitching and inter-domain pathfinding were the most significant areas where research and development effort was required. The AMPS system spawned the creation of a generalized persistency layer in the form of cNIS database and was successful in interoperating with several pre-existing single domain tools, which it incorporated in a multiple federation domain setting. Furthermore, the introduction of a complex monitoring solution across multiple heterogeneous domains was achieved by modularizing the system using several levels of abstraction and by isolating compartments of the overall task.

It is important to note that in each case, a domain can adopt the parts of the AMPS or AutoBAHN and the accompanying monitoring module system that it sees fit, and it can put in place its own custom components in the remaining places by obeying to the standardized provided interfaces.

Current development and deployment has focused on specific popular technologies such as IP, ethernet and SDH. However the design concepts are absolutely valid for a heterogeneous technology environment, and the design has been general enough to accommodate heterogeneous technology environments from the start.

REFERENCES

ADS. (2006). GEANT2, deliverable GN2-04-153v4 "AMPS – Design Specification."

Bouras, C., Campanella, M., Przybylski, M., & Sevasti, A. (2003, February). QoS and SLA aspects across multiple management domains: the SEQUIN approach. *Future Generation Computer Systems archive, 19*(2), 313 – 326.

Bouras, C., Gkamas, A., & Stamos, K. (2008). Monitoring End to End Bandwidth on Demand Circuits over Ethernet Infrastructure. In *Seventh International Network Conference – INC 2008,* Plymouth, UK, 8 - 10 July 2008.

Bouras, C., Haniotakis, V., Primpas, D., Stamos, K., & Varvitsiotis, A. (2007). AMPS - ANStool: Interoperability of automated tools for the provisioning of QoS services. *TERENA Networking Conference 2007,* Lyngby, Denmark, 21 - 24 May 2007.

Campanella, M., Krzywania, R., Reijs, V., Sevasti, A., Stamos, K., Tziouvaras, C., & Wilson, D. (2006). Bandwidth on Demand Services for European Research and Education Networks. In *1st IEEE International Workshop on Bandwidth on Demand,* 27 Nov 2006, San Francisco.

Cavazzoni, C. (2007). MUPBED Overview and Architecture. In *TERENA Networking Conference 2007,* Copenhagen, Denmark.

Coltum, R. (1998 July). The OSPF Opaque LSA Option. *RFC 2370.*

DJ3.2.2.3. (2007). *Third review of Bandwidth on Demand related technologies (DJ3.2.2.3).*

DJ3.3.1. (2008). Definition of Bandwidth on Demand Framework and General Architecture (DJ3.3.1).

Eppstein, D. (1994). *Finding the k shortest paths. In 35th* (pp. 154–165). Santa Fe: IEEE Symp. Foundations of Comp. Science.

FSIDM. (2007). *Functional Specification of GÉANT2 Inter-domain Manager (IDM).* Prototype.

G.807. (2001 July). ITU-T Rec. G.807/Y.1302. *Requirements for Automatic Transport Networks (ASTN).*

G.8080 (2001). ITU-T Rec. G.8080/Y.1304. In *Architecture for the Automatically Switched Optical Networks, November 2001 and Amendment 1, March2003.*

GÉANT2. (2009). *GÉANT2: The pan-European R&E network.* Retrieved from http://www.geant2.net/

Heinanen, J., Baker, F., Weiss, W. & Wroclawski, J. (June 1999). *Assured Forwarding PHB Group, RFC 2597.*

Inocybe technologies Inc. (n.d.). *Argia product.* Retrieved from http://www.inocybe.ca/

Jacobson, V., Nichols, K. & Poduri, K. (1999 June). *An Expedited Forwarding PHB, RFC 2598.*

Lehman, T. (2006). InterDomain Peering and Provisioning via GMPLS and Web Services. In 6th Global Lambda Workshop, Tokyo, Sep. 1-13, 2006.

Nichols, K. & Carpenter, B. (2001 April). *Definition of Differentiated Services Per Domain Behaviors and Rules for their Specification, RFC 3086.*

RFC3031 & Rosen, E., et al (2001, January). *IETF RFC 3031, Multiprotocol Label Switching Architecture.*

RFC3945 & Mannie, E., (2004 October). IETF RFC 3945. *Generalised Multi-Protocol Label Switching (GMPLS) Architecture.*

RFC4655, Farrel, A., & Vasseur, J.-P. (2006 August). A Path Computation Element (PCE)-Based Architecture. *IETF RFC 4655.*

Shier, D. (1979). On algorithms for finding the k shortest paths in a network. *Networks, 9*(3), 195–214. doi:10.1002/net.3230090303

The Internet Singularity, Delayed: Why Limits in Internet Capacity Will Stifle Innovation on the Web. (2007, November). Mokena, IL: Nemertes Research. Leung, F., Flidr, J., Tracy, C., Yang, X., Lehman, T., Jabbari, B., Riley, D. & Sobieski, J. (2006). The DRAGON Project and Application Specific Topologies. In *Broadnets 2006,* San Jose, CA. Guok, C. (2005). ESnet On-Demand Secure Circuits and Advance Reservation System (OSCARS). In *Internet2 Joint Techs Workshop,* Salt Lake City, Utah, February 15, 2005.

VIOLA project - Vertically Integrated Optical Testbed for Large Applications in DFN. (n.d.). Retrieved from http://www.viola-testbed.de/

Wu, J., Campbell, S., Savoie, J. M., Zhang, H., Bochmann, G. v., & St.Arnaud, B. (2003, Sept. 7-11). User-managed end-to-end lightpath provisioning over CA*net 4. In *Proceedings of the National Fiber Optic Engineers Conference (NFOEC)*, Orlando, FL, (pp. 275-282).

Chapter 16
QoS Guaranteed Based Network Management Policies in the Integration of Wired and Wireless Architecture of a Healthcare Network

Pattarasinee Bhattarakosol
Chulalongkorn University, Thailand

Watcharaporn Tanchotsrinon
Chulalongkorn University, Thailand

ABSTRACT

Every community in the world expects to have a high value of life. Therefore, budgets are pooling to the local healthcare unit to increase healthcare and medical services to their citizen. One common implementation in the healthcare system is a healthcare network, where all necessary information are transferred to safe patients' lives. Various developments in medical equipments integrate communication circuit to enhance ability to transmit data direct from patients to medical staffs so that their lives can be safe in time. Since the implementation of wireless network is widely spread, this paper proposes the integration of the wireless network and wired network to serve a healthcare system under a management policy. The results have shown that the proposed architecture with policy has a better quality of services than another alternative solution using QoS standard metrics. Thus, the paper ensures that a qualified healthcare network can be achieved under the condition that the suitable architecture must be implemented and the right management policies are also applied.

INTRODUCTION IN HEALTHCARE NETWORK

People life is very important. Therefore, a healthcare system must be properly installed for every commune. The components in the system are patients, medical staffs, hardware and software for medical equipments; these components must be cooperated in the suitable time line to save a person's life. Additionally, one important factor that must be granted to doctors and nurses for saving patients

DOI: 10.4018/978-1-61520-791-6.ch016

is their information, especially medical treatment information and current symptoms.

There are various methods to store and send patients' information and medical treatment, including some medical services over a healthcare network (HN). However, this HN must be guaranteed with quality of services in many aspects. However, services of an HN must relate to various persons (Raman, Jagannathan & Reddy,1997), such as medical staffs, health insurance companies, government sections, clinics and other hospitals. Therefore, the network management model to enhance QoS of an HN must ensure that the security of the HN is maintained as necessary.

Although the security issue is a sensitive point in the healthcare system, the performance of the HN is also vital, since patients' lives are always depended on their health information, these information must be delivered to the medical doctor in the right time, right person without a long delay. Therefore, performance of the HN has to be well managed. Even though the HN might be installed based on high quality architecture, having unsuitable policy may not increase performance of the HN as expected. Thus, the success of QoS of an HN can be obtained from the suitable architecture and the management policy.

In this chapter, before the QoS of a HN are mentioned, the requirements of an HN will be described in the following section following by types of data over the HN. After that the requirement for QoS of the HN is illustrated where performance issue is discussed. Moreover, a case study from a Thai hospital with two alternative solutions is elaborated and discussed. The last section will be the conclusion.

REQUIREMENTS IN HN

Saving lives is very important and very sensitive processes; it must consist of various factors, including information and time. Generally, information of patients in the legacy system of the healthcare unit was manually transferred. Moreover, some patients might get sick or feel uncomfortable according to sudden physical abnormality. Thus, under these conditions, the patients' lives might not be able to be protected or taking care off because of lacking of necessary information in the required time interval. Therefore, functions of the healthcare system can be classified in three aspects: patients, medical staffs, and administration.

The functions of a healthcare system in the patients' aspect refer to the patient's monitoring system. Since some patients need special care or special tracking from medical staffs according to their illness, such as heart disease, diabetic, etc. The monitoring system needs to be installed for individual patient; so, whenever they are in bad condition alone, especially the elderly person, the monitoring system can directly report to the medical staff to save their lives in the proper time, or patients can inform their medical unit for help.

In the aspects of the medical staffs, functions of the healthcare system are the medical services that have to provide to patients. It is the truth that people expect high quality of medical services from all medical staffs when needed. The medical services include emergency lives saving, health consulting, illness treatment, laboratory test and diagnosis, etc. Although every government gives a high priority in granting budgets to the healthcare system, most rural areas always lack of critical medical services from their local healthcare units. Therefore, implementing an efficient HN supports these critical medical services for long distance requests. For examples, patients can send their questions via mobile system consulting their doctors for first aid treatment to prevent serious consequences of any physical or mental problems. In some countries, a telemedicine system was implemented to serve people in the rural area from serious injuries; operations can be performed by a local doctor guiding by specialist from the medical school or other central hospital.

According to the administration's aspects, functions of the healthcare system must depend on information that flows around the system to support all lives' saving processes. Considering the situation that medical staffs meet patients when they admit to the healthcare unit. The most important document to be obtained before the curing starts is the patient's sickness profile. Since each patient will have different physical treatment condition, the doctor must know these medical records before starting their treatment; otherwise, patients might be in danger situation for unsuitable treatments. Since computers are implemented in the healthcare organization for decades, some healthcare organizations have implemented the Electronic Health Records (EHR) and Electronic Medical Records (EMR) retrieval system of patients. This system supports fast data retrieval for doctors and the expected result is that patients' lives can be highly secure in the doctor's hands. However, although the EHR and EMR have been implemented for healthcare units and links between departments as an effective HN, the problem of the network delay based on improper network management can cause critical damage to human's lives as same as the non-network environment. Thus, the implemented HN must have good network design architecture as same as management policy.

By conclusion, every high quality of services of HN must support three main functions: patient's monitoring, medical services, and EHR and EMR retrieval functions. Considering each functions, the requirements related to each main functions are different although they share some part of information to serve patients as needed. Therefore, before setting the QoS of HN system, the requirements of each main function must be separately clarified.

For the patient's monitoring system in HN, the requirements of this system is to send message to the medical staff whenever patients are in the bad condition and needs help. Therefore, the system must be able to correctly locate the patient, and send the request for help with location to the medical center in time. In some situation, the information about the current state of patient's sickness must be the additional message that must be sent to the medical center. Thus, the size of all information that must be sent from the monitoring device might be large comparing with the general GPS system or SMS from a mobile phone. Besides, these messages must not be lost. So, the QoS of this system is considered based on the lost of these messages, including with the reliability of the HN system.

In the situation of medical services from HN, the important data could be the information of patients' sickness, symptom, and results from labs' diagnostic. Thus, these information must be sent to patients in any suitable time line without any lost. So, the reliability and availability of the HN must be guaranteed. Since the information of the medical services are very important to lives, the integrity of information must be assured. Moreover, the information must be sent to the right person, not only for security but also, mainly, for the safety of each patient. If the medical advices or lab diagnostic was sent to the wrong person, doctors or patients, these can affect to the medical treatment which finally affect to the people's lives. Thus, all information must be able to indicate the sender; otherwise, the lives of people cannot be fully protected by law. So, the characteristics of information security must be fully applied to this medical services information as a significant requirement of the installed HN.

Considering the EHR and EMR retrieval system that serves medical staffs while taking care of patients, this system needs a high speed transfer data between data storage and a clinical unit. The clinical unit can be either remote or local area. Therefore, the transfer speed should be adjusted according to types of transferred data.

According to the above paragraphs, the requirements of HN depend on applications that must be served. Some applications require high performance, while some applications require information security. Furthermore, the reliability and availability are two features that cannot be overlooked because life can be in a danger situation in every second.

TYPES OF DATA OVER HN

Since there are three main functions of a healthcare unit as mentioned above, there are various types of data are sending over the communication channel. These data may be transferred among patients' equipments to medical staffs, or among healthcare staffs, or between a medical device and a healthcare staff. The types of transferred data are based on the processing functions.

Consider data that are generated under the patients' monitoring system. These data can be text, voice, audio file, or video streaming. These data are usually sent from patients, or devices attached to patients, to medical staffs for life supports. So, these data can be generated in different situations by different equipments and methods. Most data that are generated by the medical devices are in the text mode, such as heart beat rate, blood pressure, and sugar level, etc. However, some data are in the graphic mode, such as the measurement from the EKG device that attached to unconscious patients. In some situation, patients can make a call to the HN centre for help; such data is classified as voice or an audio file for an automatic calling system. On the other hand, patients may send sms (short message service) asking for life saving when he or she does not have any alternatives. In a modern patient monitoring system, a video streaming system to capture movements of patients is installed. Thus, all movements of patients will be sent as a video streaming via the connection channel to the monitoring room of the medical staffs; this method can ensure that patients will be in a good care when needed.

As similar to the patients' monitoring system, the data of the medical services can be in every format: text, voice, audio file, images, or video streaming. The difference between the patients' monitoring system and the medical services is that data generated by this system is much longer and larger than the patients' monitoring system. Some examples of data in the medical services are data generated under the Telemedical service system. Most data under this system is classified as the video streaming because the online communication is performed for medical treatment and consulting for patients in the rural areas. Moreover, doctors may send the medical instructions to their patients via email or provide an online counselling room for their patients via a web site. Thus, these medical service data is in the text stream. However, in some automatic response system, patients may receive an automatic voice mail for any fundamental information for healthcare services. So, this replied information is classified as voice or audio files. Additionally, some patients might need to have a lab test or x-ray before taking any treats, the results from these tests are usually presented in the form of images.

After receiving all services from medical staffs, these medical treatment records must be stored for references. Thus, the data generated for the EHR and EMR basically is obtained from the medical service system, and some data are obtained from the monitoring system as a patients' symptom. Therefore, data stored in the EHR and EMR are in the same format of the data exists in the medical service system.

Referring to data for all system mentioned above, there are various types of data are flowed in the HN, text, image, digital photography, audio, video and multimedia files. Each type required different capacities and reliability since some of them are in different categories. Therefore, the HN must set the QoS to quarantine the transferring data will be achieved as needed.

QUALITY OF SERVICES ISSUES IN HN

Generally, the quality of services of a network can be measured under different conditions and variables; many metrics are applied to measure the QoS of the network, such as performance, reliability, availability, delay, sometimes the quality of presentation is included. Therefore, many factors must be involved in the network implementation in order to obtain and maintain their QoS. These factors are listed below.

- the use of communication media: wire, or wireless
- the design and implementation of network architecture
- the implementation and development of equipment and communication devices
- the implementation of network management policy

Since an HN is a kind of specific network, consequently, the HN that can be claimed to have QoS must be implemented under the consideration of the factors mentioned above. However, the data and applications of medical services system are very vital. Therefore, these elements must be delivered to the suitable place, people, and time, with guarantee of correctness, and integrity of data is maintained. This delivery is mainly relied on the efficiency of the available HN. Thus, the QoS factors for the HN must be seriously considered. In another word, all medical tasks, objects or resources have to be well managed and manipulated. Consequently, tremendous researches have proposes methods to obtain and maintain QoS. Some of these researches are summarised below.

As the fact that there are various types of data flowed in an HN system, these data are separately stored based on the system generators and usages. Each type of data generators or devices usually generates different data formats and sizes, then stored in various patterns because there is no standard to be enforced among those devices. As a consequence, these data required different bandwidths while transferring to the destination (Lage & Martins & Oliveira, 2004; Philip & Istepanian, 2007).

In a qualified HN system, QoS of the HN can be described in various aspects: reliability, availability, and performance. The reliability of the HN is based on the quality of the connection over the entire system: wired or wireless. Each type of connections provides different quality of services. Moreover, the reliability, availability, and performance can be measured using different values, such as mean time between failures (MTBF), mean time between critical failures (MTBCF), number of packet loss, average network delay, capacity or throughput, and jitter. Therefore, each HN can be trusted when various factors are considered to prevent the failure of the entire or partial network.

Based on variety of applications over the HN, data are classified in different classes. So, diversities of communication methods are applied. Presently, there are tremendous methods to help human communication, such as CSCW (computer supported cooperative work) as mentioned in (Ray & Weerakkody, 1999), e-mail, SMS, MMS, mobile applications (Philip & Istepanian, 2007), and teleconference (Lage & Martins & Oliveira, 2004). Each communication methods required dissimilar media to transfer data. However, most communication methods are moving from wired to wireless communication according that it is easy to be installed, changed location, managed, and most of all, cost effective. Furthermore, many mobile companies realize the significant of their customers' lives; then, they have installed life support software as a part of mobile applications for patients or elderly in order to increase the quality of life and to make sure that they can get help anytime-anywhere when needed.

Although the applications over an HN are grouped in various classes, QoS of a network cannot be claimed unless the network architecture is designed properly. Thus, the second factor is the network architecture. As a result of the study of (Lage & Martins & Oliveira, 2004; Philip & Istepanian, 2007), the delay over a network is related to the network architecture. If the network designer chooses the right topology and suitable architecture for the healthcare organization, the delay over the entire network will be small (Tanchotsrinon & Bhattarakosol, 2008). Therefore, whenever a large volume of data is transferred over the improper designed network, a long delay of packets occurs.

Nevertheless, only a good designed HN may not have a short delay time. Then, the suitable network management policy is applied to be the last factors that affects to the QoS; otherwise the unbalanced traffic will occur in the communication channel. As result, a long packet delay cannot be avoided. Moreover, from the research of (Hiranpongsin & Bhattarakosol, 2009), the growth of traffic flow can be controlled by selecting a suitable management policy along with appropriate architectures. According to this research, most packets will be filtered and sent to the destinations without broadcasting to the Internet or the main traffic flow. Thus, numbers of packets flow out to the Internet or the main line will be small comparing with the architecture that has no filtering algorithm. As a consequence, the delay of every packet will be reduced.

In real lives, there are factors affect to QoS of an HN system. Moreover, there are other factors that have not been point out in details, such as the collaborative methods between services granted from different organizations toward a patient, or human's role in the HN system (Tentori & Favela, 2008). Generally, most of QoS problems are focused in two areas which are performance, and security of the HN. However, since the data and devices in the HN might be shared according to the integration of the existing HNs around the world, the additional problem is the standardization of data format that are sent through the communication lines using various medical applications. In this paper, only the performance issue will be considered as a main point of QoS for HN services. Therefore, the following subsection will describes some related researches that also focus in the performance of the HN.

PERFORMANCE ISSUES IN HN

Performance of a network is an important part of QoS that users always concern in every moment of their usages, especially the performance of the HN system because it relates to live and dead of people. In the legacy system, the network of an HN was implemented based on the cabling system. Thus, services were limited according to the cable. Once the wireless technology has been introduced and widely developed, it becomes a practical tool for the HN that brings tremendous advantages to the healthcare system. The high benefit of combination among wireless and wired architecture appears to be a flexible solution for every healthcare unit, as mentioned in (Goldberg & Wickramasinghe, 2003). This combination required a new management policy in order to have a secure data transfer under low cost of investment and maintenance. However, QoS of the HN is maintained. Various researches have shown that mobile/wireless solutions for healthcare can achieve four critical goals of improvement of patient care, reducing transaction costs, increasing healthcare quality, and enhancing teaching and research (Goldberg & Wickramasinghe, 2003; Seshadri, Liotta, Gopal, & Liotta, 2001).

As similar to the wireless technology, the improvement of the mobile system and equipment bring high advantage for all functions of HN mentioned above. Pavlovski, et al. (2004) presented a proven reference architecture for a secure enterprise mobile healthcare solution for hospital physicians and nurses. The solution furnishes access to several medical information systems whilst supporting a capability to roam within and outside the hospital environment.

This was obtained by seamless roaming between the 802.11 and GSM/CDMA mobile networks. Furthermore, a monitoring tool named MRTG was proposed as an infrastructure for recording environmental and biological variables, in order to achieve a remote, reliable, secure and efficient real-time access to this data which may be displayed on a PDA (Lubrin & Lawrence & Navarro, 2005). Moreover, Lim & Singh (2005) had proposed a network architecture using eye blinking as a passing parameter to communicate with the medical staffs for helping especially for paralyzed persons. Therefore, there lives are much secure and in a good care as needed.

Moreover, Varshney (2006) proposed ad hoc networks that can be formed among patients' devices for improving transmission of emergency messages. This technique puts forward several design enhancements to improve the quality and coverage of patient monitoring. With this recommended architecture, the message can be sent through the HN with low delays and high reliability. In addition, performing multicast or broadcast-based routing scheme also maintains a low delay as needed.

According to the improvement of the wireless network and cellular communication, Yau & Chung (2007) mentioned that the integrating of the wireless network and cellular network help expanding the coverage range and enhance the mobility of the system. The mobile healthcare applications have eased the mobile users to merge cellular phone with the wireless enabled devices for entitling in flexi and portable healthcare solution at any places. This helps empowering communication between doctors and patients as patients' health condition can be reported to their doctors any time when needed. Besides in the year 2008, a wearable ECG monitoring system for ubiquitous healthcare that offers a powerful new way in keeping track of a patient's heart status and predict impending events was proposed (Yang et al., 2008). The post-layout simulation results show that the smart electronic electrode with ultra low power consumption is quite feasible for a hand-held PHA which uses a battery as energy source. During the monitoring period, vital signs of patients could fluctuate significantly and/or match certain undesirable patterns and, therefore, "alerts" or emergency messages must be delivered to healthcare professionals. Moreover, the gap between body sensor networks (BSN) and Wireless Sensor Network (WSN) was solved by implementing a three-tier structure to enhance the patient's monitoring system (Pan & Wu, 2008).

In order to improve the efficiency of the EHR and EMR retrieval system, (Lee et.al.,2007) proposed a query supported healthcare system that is capable of obtaining physiological data from sensor attached to patient's body and transfers it wirelessly to a remote base-station in an ad-hoc network, following IEEE802.15.4 standard (Zigbee) for wireless communication. The additional benefit of this system is that it supports the energy consumption problem because it enables nodes to transfer data only when desired and sleep for the rest of the time. As the fact that the monitoring system must co-operate with the EHR and EMR when the monitored patient falls into a critical condition, the information from these systems must be transferred to the medical staffs in the proper time. Thus, Lee, Lee & Chung (2008) introduced and implemented a query processor of broadcasting type and flooding type for reliability query transmits to destination node. This proposed solution has shown that the flooding type query processor has better performance than broadcasting type query for the query losses and reliability from terminal PC to destination node. In the same year, Mateo, Salvo, & Lee (2008) have proposed a balanced clustering method that controls the load balance of the communication channel to reduce the delay over the network. Thus, the critical injury of life and dead is decrease. This method performs the balancing of the agents' distribution within a base station network. It considered the minimum load variation of the network by deploying agents from the loaded base station to other least loaded base station. The algorithm considers the QoS by employing the nearest neighbor deployments. The mobile agent distribution is based on a threshold value to optimize the load distribution. Simulation evaluation shows that the proposed balanced clustering is efficient in distribution of loads and considers the QoS from clients by minimizing the communication hops in deploying the mobile agents.

In order to obtain QoS for the HN system, the proper policy must be set up. The suitable policy enhances the performance of the entire system, such as enhancing QoS, authorization, and reliable transmission. While there are several of services to be granted from a HN, many groups of users, and applications have to be managed and classified based on their behavior and services (Schmutzler et.al.,2008). Thus, interconnections between medical staffs and patients are perfectly maintained. Consequently, patients will be placed in a good caring system under their serious conditions. Similar to Schmutzler et.al. (2008), the research of Zhu Y., et.al. (2008) proposed a policy-driven management system on the biosensor. Therefore, the dynamic loading can be performed without shutting down nodes and the fine-grained access control is possible through authorization policies on biosensors. The results have shown that the policy system is viable and can accelerate application development of biosensor networks for healthcare.

According to the development of the mobile technology, mobiles become useful and efficient tools in the HN, called m-Health. Various researches and solutions of using mobiles have been proposed to support all HN functions mentioned previously. The benefits of m-health have been presented in the year 2005 by Istepanian (2005) although there was no standard communication rule has been announced. Additionally, in the year 2006, (Cho et.al, 2006) had presented a mobile healthcare system prototype based on surrogate host system using Proxy-based security control. The experimental results showed that the developed system could be utilized to provide patients with real-time heart disease diagnosis based on Grid computing in a secure and convenient manner.

Referring to all researches above, the development of QoS in the HN is mainly focussed in the creaing abilities of devices and communination mechanism, including network management policy as same as network QoS factors mentioned previously. These progresses lead to the situation that a high QoS HN can be obtained under the high investment cost. Umfortunately, it cannot be applied or implemented in poor countries such as Thailand. Therefore, in the next section, a case study of a Thai hospital was studied to find an altertanative network for the healthcare department under the conditions of low investment cost and maintenance with guaranteed QoS.

A CASE STUDY FROM A THAI HOSPITAL

The case study was performed at a Thai hospital that is composed of 14 buildings, which are Outpatient2, Administration, Ear Nose Throat, Medical Supply, Medicine, Emergency, Outpatient1, Radiology, Nuclear Medicine, X-ray, Operating, Cobalt, Cancer, and Lab, as shown in Figure 1. Currently, these buildings are connected via a wired network. However, the information usage over the current network is rapidly growth. Therefore, the management level of the hospital would like to upgrade the current network under a large amount of investment. However, since the wireless technology is widely used and implemented with low cost, the solution proposed for this hospital, another wireless solution with a management policy is proposed as an alternative model for this hospital. Therefore, all necessary comparisons in QoS metrics between common upgrade solution and the proposed solution must be performed; the following section describes the models that are considered in this paper.

The Current Network (CN)

Referring to Figure 1, the current system has only one server (node 1), which is in the Outpatient2 building. Moreover, the core network is Asynchronous Transfer Mode (ATM), while all LANs in each building are implemented as Fast Ethernet.

The First Alternative Network (FAN)

The FAN solution is the solution that proposed by the management level of the hospital. All components of this FAN are mainly similar to the CN, except that wired technologies, which are ATM in the core network as well as Fast Ethernet in the accessed network, are changed to the Gigabit Ethernet in order to support the increased requirements of users. Therefore, the Gigabit Ethernet is installed of both the core and the accessed network of this upgrade network. Furthermore, this model is also added a second link, which is 10Gigabit Ethernet, between two core switches to lighten the traffic load connected to the server.

PROBLEM STATEMENTS

From the fact that the growth of network usage in the hospital is continuously increase, the congestion and delay problems cannot be avoided in the system. Additionally, hospital services are sometimes significantly in vital so that these

Figure 1. The CN of the healthcare system

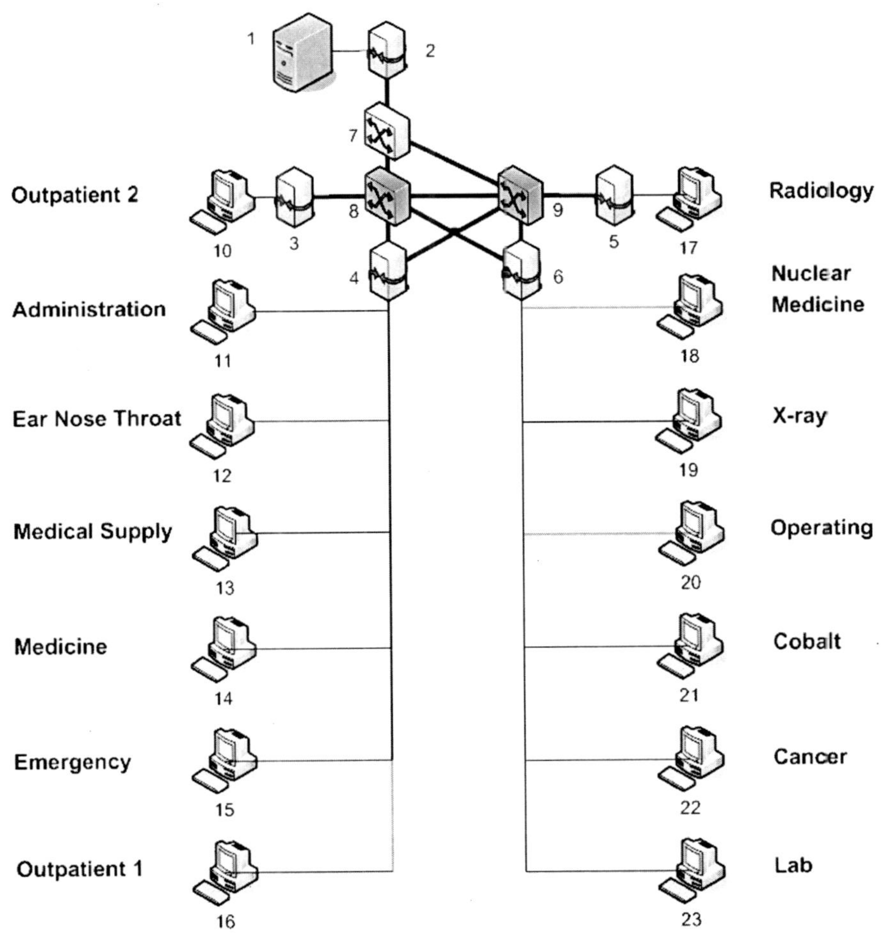

Figure 2. The first alternative network (FAN) of the healthcare system

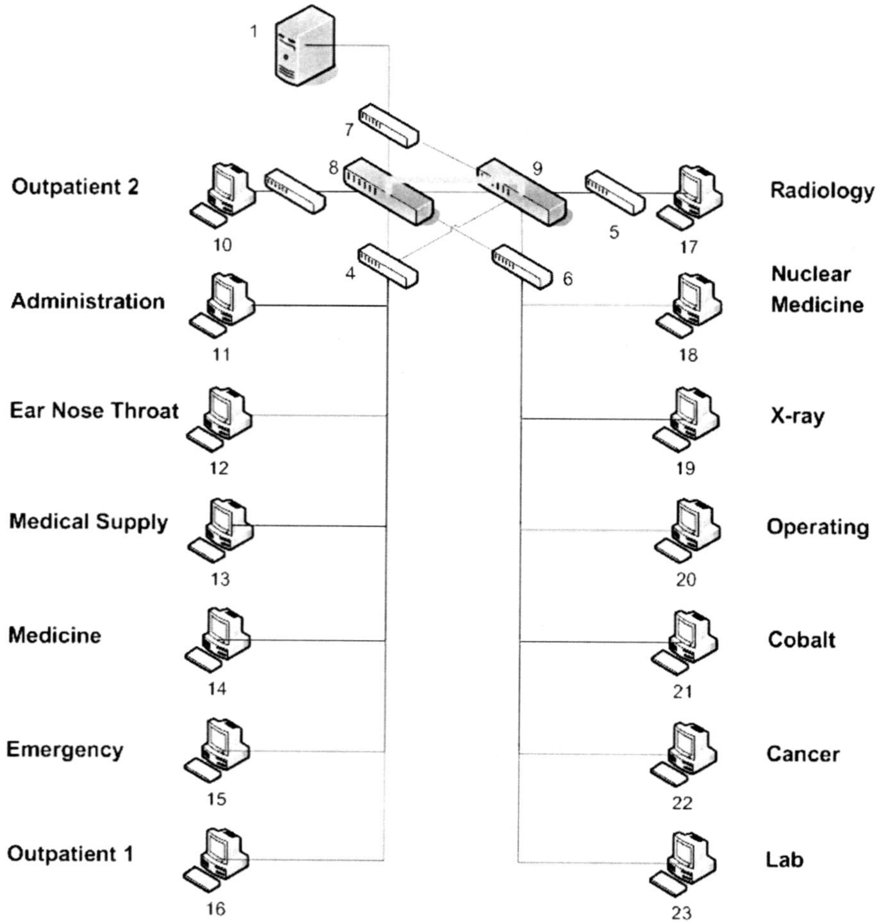

problems can be a serious one in some emergency cases. The general solution that the network administrator chooses to apply is to create new high-performance network system, or upgrade an existing network with high capacity equipments. In doing so, the cabling system must be expanded. Although this basic solution can enhance the network performance while obtaining a reliable authentication and authorization of their information, it will cost a large amount of money and implementation time. Besides, the old network system must be terminated and replaced by the new one iteratively.

Since the healthcare system consists of various types of data, including critical data that causes life and dead of patients. Therefore, the transferring system can be counted as the delay sensitive system. In addition, the transferring system must be reliable. Consequently, this research emphasizes on improvement the healthcare system, that originally implemented with the cabling system, with a wireless system for cost saving. Under this new architecture, the network must also be well-managed with a good policy; otherwise, all sensitive data will be affected by bad management and cause vital damage to patients' lives. Accordingly, this situation requires an improvement of a core network by installing a wireless network with a suitable network management policy in the healthcare system.

Then, the objective of this paper is to propose suitable network management policies that are efficient to manage the overlapping among wired and wireless networks under low cost of investment and maintenance, as well as maintaining scalability for the organization. The expected outcome of this proposed architecture is the HN with guaranteed QoS.

PROPOSED SOLUTION

In this paper, a wireless network implemented on top of the existing wired network is proposed as an alternative solution for hospital management level. This architecture is not only determined from the viewpoint of cost, but also emphasized on reducing the delay time in critical information of patients' lives within the system. Thus, the QoS of the HN can be achieved.

The second alternative network (SAN) is performed by installing a wireless technology, Wi-Fi, over the original wired network, as shown in Figure 3. The detail of SAN is presented in Figure 4. Moreover, the network management policies for both of the wired and wireless networks are also applied to this model in order to enhance the performance of transmission the significant applications through this network.

In this architecture, the original CN was unchanged except that every building is installed a wireless network (IEEE 802.11g-Wi-Fi), including with suitable network management policies of both wired and wireless for improving the performance in transmitting the significant applications.

Details of this alternative network are described as follow.

- **Wired**: It is similar to the CN, except that cables are added between servers and a Wi-Fi switch, between Wi-Fi switches, and between a Wi-Fi switch and access points due to installation of the wireless technology.
- **Wi-Fi**: all wireless devices will

Figrue 3. 3D-view of SAN in the healthcare system

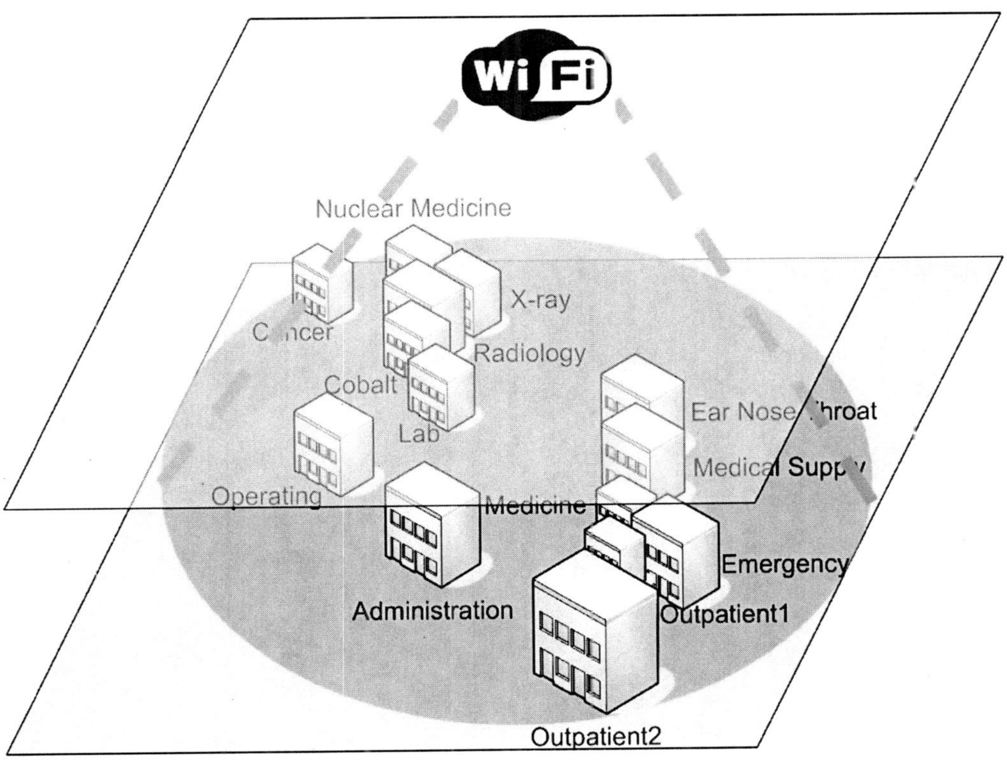

communicate with a server (node 1) via access points for obtaining information used in the hospital, or even Internet services. Thus, an access point is installed in each building (node 24-37).

Due to consideration of appropriate locations in the real situation, there are 2 Wi-Fi switches. The first one is located in the Outpatient2 building (near the server), while the second is located in the Operating building. In this experiment, there are 3 types of applications from wireless devices. So, all wireless devices are grouped into 3 categories: devices from doctors who would like patients' information for helping them diagnosis (Node 38-51), devices from doctors who access the Internet (Node 52-65), and devices from patients surfing over the Internet (Node 66-79).

Management Policies

Although the SAN is installed to mitigate a congestion problem occurred in the CN, it is required to manage applications that run within in the system in order to enhance performance and maintain QoS of this network. Therefore, suitable network management policies of both wired and wireless for this network are determined as follow.

Wired Policy

The wired policy was set up by considering an important of routine work in each building. Thus, the highest priority is set for buildings that provide medical treatments which are occasionally significant in vital or some tasks may be affect even in a short delay time of an incoming message. Then, the middle priority is set for buildings that involve in various kinds of applications, or their information are, sometimes, need to be transmit-

Figure 4. The details of SAN in the healthcare system

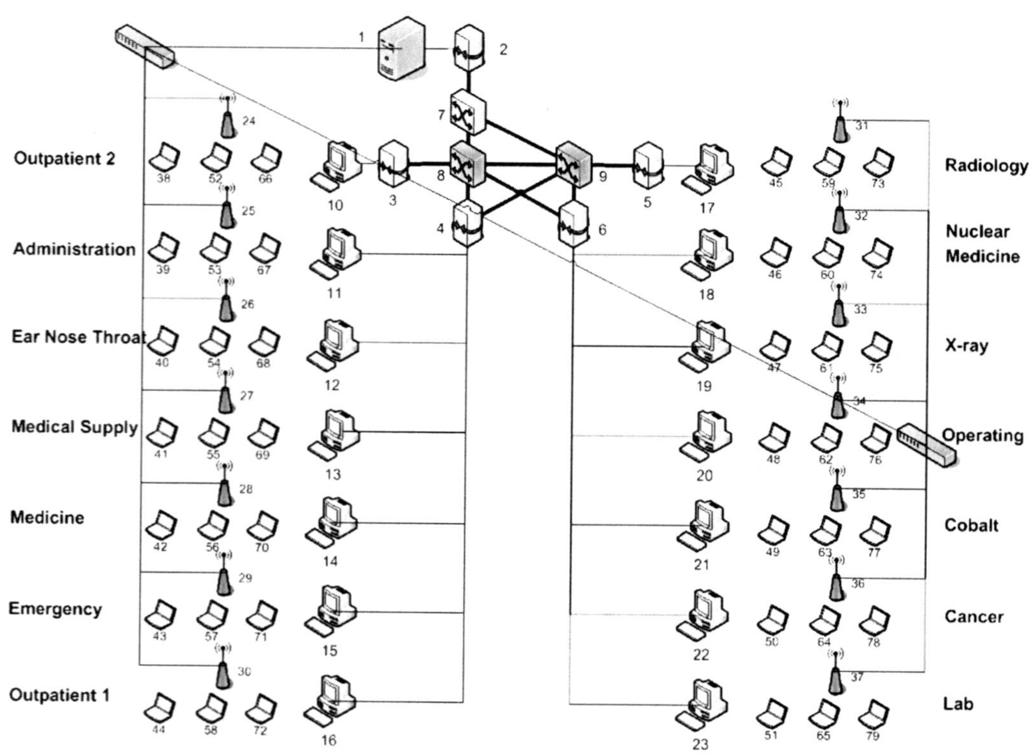

Table 1. Wired policy for SAN

Priority	Building
Highest	Outpatient2, Administration, Ear Nose Throat, Emergency, Outpatient1, and Operating
Middle	Radiology, Nuclear Medicine, X-ray, Cobalt, Cancer, and Lab
Lowest	Medical Supply, and Medicine

ted to doctors as requested. Lastly, setting up the lowest priority is for buildings that require only routine data, or a long delay is acceptable. As a result, the wired policy for the SAN is illustrated in Table 1.

Wireless Policy

In the wireless network setting up the policy is differed from the wired network; it is because transmitted applications from the wired are the only task served for the needs of the hospital. In contrast, applications from the wireless network can be transmitted from doctors who request information to support their diagnosis, or transmitted from the patients surf the Internet during their waiting time. Moreover, if this wireless policy was set up by considering only the important of each department, according to the wired, the applications for significant information from the lower priority departments can be blocked by the Internet applications from the higher priority departments. So, the wireless policy was determined based on the objectives and user types. Besides, all priority levels of applications from the wireless are under the lowest priority level of the wired policy due to avoidance of the full stack in the queue.

Referring to 3 types of applications mentioned previously, the wireless policy for the SAN is illustrated in Table 2.

Simulation Model

In this section, the simulation models of the CN, the FAN, and the SAN are elaborated. In this experiment, the analysis of the throughput loss rate in each building is divided into 3 main conditions. First is the condition that the real load is less than the maximum load that a line can support, or where the ratios stand at 1:2 and 3:4. Second is the condition that the real load is equal to the maximum, or where the ratio stands at 1:1. The last is the condition that the real load is greater than the maximum, or where the ratio stands at 5:4.

Due to differences of wired technologies in these 3 models, simulations are performed under the same conditions. For that reason, the loads, which are offered to the CN and the SAN, are 50, 75, 100, and 125 Mbps, based on the maximum load of Fast Ethernet in their access networks. In addition, real loads for the FAN are 500, 750, 1000 and 1250 Mbps, since the wired technology in this model is Gigabit Ethernet. Hence, the performance of these 3 network models will be evaluated reasonably.

Table 2. Wireless policy for SAN

Priority	Type of Wi-Fi application
Highest	Patient information for doctors
Middle	Internet services for doctors
Lowest	Internet services for patients

CN Model

For the simulation model of this network, IP Queue type is First In First Out (FIFO), the number of priorities are eight, and scheduler type of this queue is the strict priority. Furthermore, the service transfer type is the Constant Bit Rate (CBR), the MAC frame size is 1024 bytes, and the simulation time is 40 min. Also, these configurations are used in the simulations of the FAN, and the SAN with policies.

The simulation is performed based on the real CN model as mentioned previously.

- ATM: a core network with the link bandwidth is 155 Mbps.
- Fast Ethernet: LAN in each building connects to the ATM with the nominal rate of 100 Mbps, full duplex mode.

FAN Model

The simulation of the FAN is the Gigabit Ethernet (IEEE 802.3), full duplex mode of both the core and the accessed network. Additionally, the 10Gigabit Ethernet line is added as the second link between two core switches.

SAN Model

The simulation of this architecture will compose of 2 parts:

Wired: A core network is ATM with 155 Mbps data rate, and buildings' LANs are Fast Ethernet in the full duplex mode, as mentioned previously. Due to installation of Wi-Fi, there is a link of a Gigabit Ethernet between a server and the Wi-Fi switch as same as links among Wi-Fi switches in the same network. Additionally, the links existed between the Wi-Fi switches and access points are the Fast Ethernet.

Wi-Fi: IEEE 802.11g with 54 Mbps data rate is installed as the wireless network for each building. Although the data rate of this technology can be reach up to 54 Mbps, in theory, its typical throughput is about 20 Mbps. Thus, for 14 buildings, the overall wireless throughput is approximately 280 Mbps. So, some applications of patient information, which all have the data rate 20 Mbps, are split from wired and transmitted via Wi-Fi instead. To illustrate this point, 20 Mbps. of data rate is split from the entire system that has the real loads as 50, 75, 100 and 125 Mbps, and then the wired network will transmit at 30, 55, 80, and 105 Mbps, respectively. After transmitting patient information with the data rate of 20 Mbps. via Wi-Fi, it remains 260 Mbps. under the bandwidth of this wireless network. Therefore, this rest bandwidth is provided for Internet access of doctors and patients in each building. As a result, the wireless applications can be separated into 3 flow types: patient information for doctors with data rate 20 Mbps, the Internet access for doctors with data rate 130 Mbps, and the Internet access for patients with data rate 130 Mbps.

Simulation Results

In this section, the results from the simulation process will be reported. The network performance metric is measured in various collecting parameters, such as utilization, throughputs, and delay of both FAN and SAN. The performance of all testing models will be measured under 3 situations related to the maximum capability of the entire network; this value is called as maximum load. The simulation is performed by setting the value of network usage which is called as the real load against the maximum load in three conditions.

The first situation is simulated under the condition that the real load is less than the maximum load. Thus, the ratios of the real load served for the main task in the hospital to the maximum load are set to be 1:2 and 3:4. The second situation for this simulation is considered when the maximum load is equal to the real load. Finally, the last condition to be simulated is the situation where the maximum load is less than the entire hospital real load; the ratio of the real load served for the main task in the hospital to the maximum load stands at 5:4.

Based on the above conditions, all simulations results are elaborated as follows.

Channel Utilization

In simulation method, the system will be stable after the channel utilization has reached to its maximum value, and then performance parameters, such as throughput, delay, and jitter, are constants. Since the channel utilization depends on the simulation time, the investigation of the channel utilization at various times is required in order to detect the minimum simulation time that the channel utilization has reached to its maximum. Therefore, the channel utilization of the CN is investigated by varying times. From Figure 5, the result has shown that the channel utilization will increase sharply at the beginning and then rise moderately. Until the simulation time is 40 minutes, the channel utilization begins to change slightly which value is 6.869 * 10^{-3}. Thus, it can be specified that 40 minutes is the first point that the channel utilization begins to reach to its maximum. Accordingly, all architectures, which include CN, FAN, and SAN, will be simulated at 40 minutes.

Overall Throughput

According to Figure 6, there is no throughput loss rates from the CN and the FAN because the real load is less than the maximum load, while the throughput from the SAN is slightly lost according to Wi-Fi communication. The throughput loss rates of the CN and the FAN are much higher than the SAN when the real load is grater or equal to the maximum load of the entire system. This is because this SAN model is well-managed in transmiting applications through the policies in addition to considering of resource allocation by installation of the wireless network.

Figure 5. Channel utilization of the CN

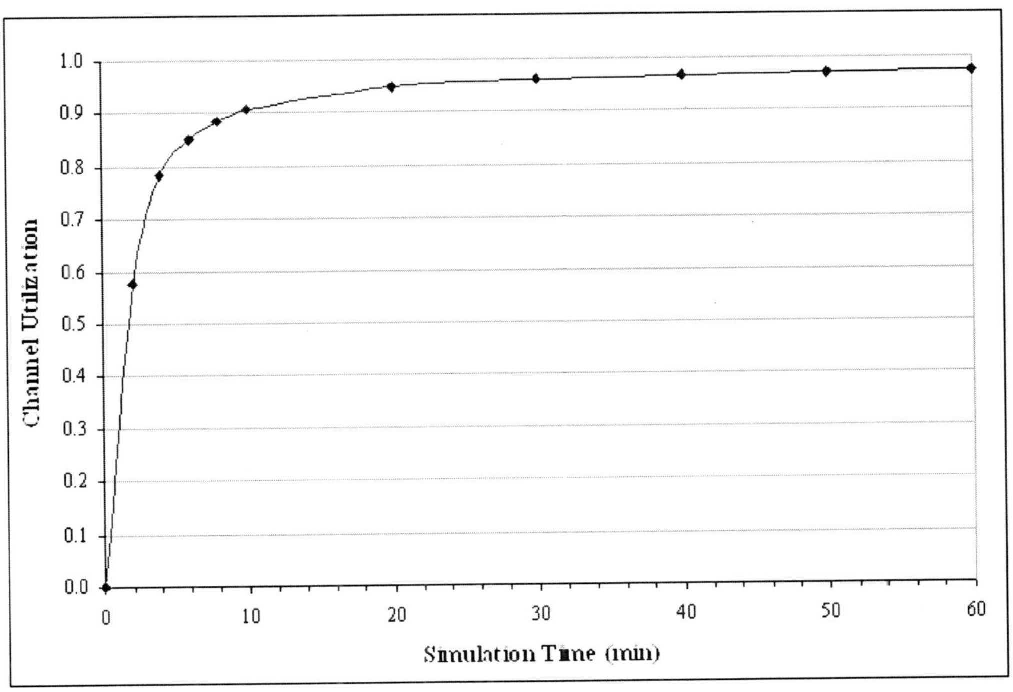

Figure 6. The overall throughput loss rate of the Healthcare System where the ratios of the real loads to the maximum load stand at 1:2, 3:4, 1:1 and 5:4.

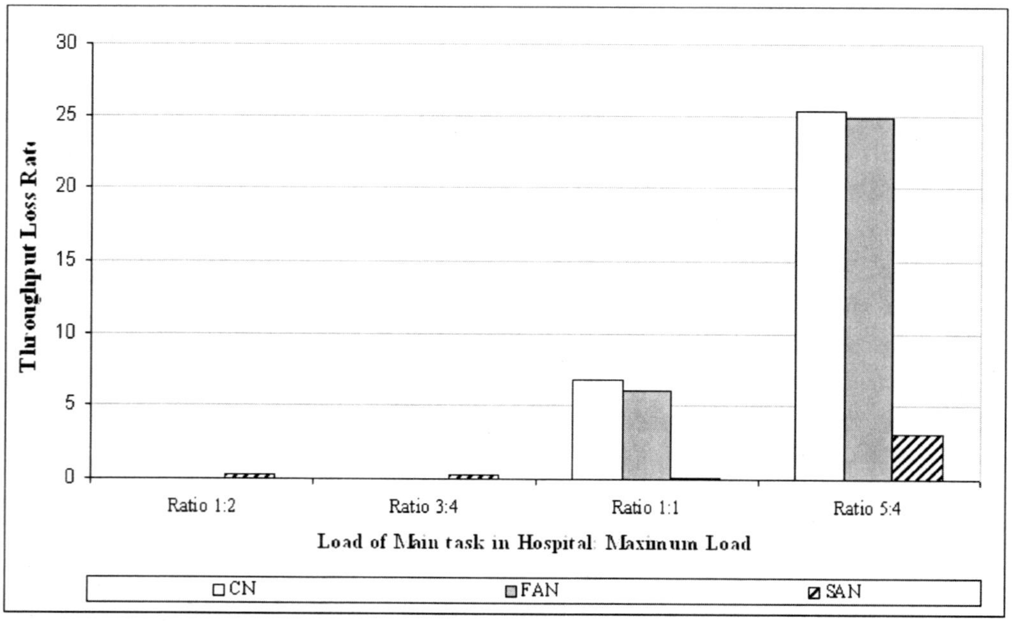

Building Throughput

Although the SAN can achieve the minimum throughput loss rate of the overall system, it is not explicitly illustrated the impact of the wired policy to this model. Hence, it is required to determine the throughput loss rate occurred in each building so that the building throughput loss rate will be analyzed in 3 main conditions as mentioned above.

Condition 1: The real load is less than the maximum load.

Based on Figure 7 and Figure 8, there is no throughput loss rate in each building of the FAN, while this value is slightly lost in the CN and the SAN. However, the throughput loss rates from each building in the CN and the SAN are randomly lost, since their loss rates are not consistent with the implemented policies: FIFO for the CN, and the prioritization of the wired policy for the SAN.

Condition 2: The real load is equal to the maximum load.

Figure 9 has shown that there are a great number of the throughput loss rates in the lab building of both the CN and the FAN due to FIFO of the queue types and no management policy. This can imply that when the load reaches to the maximum value of the line, transmitted applications for the lab building are blocked by the former ones. In contrast, there is no throughput loss in every building of the SAN model due to appropriate management of the transmitted application through the proposed policy as well as considering of resource allocation by installing a wireless network to relieve the congestion problem. For this condition, the result has shown that applying the suitable network management policies to the SAN model can efficiently prevent the loss of throughput in every building of the hospital, which applications must be routed within the healthcare system, and these transmitted applications are occasionally significant in patients' life.

Condition 3: The real load is more than the maximum load.

According to the results presented in Figure 10, there are a great number of throughput loss

Figure 7. The average loss rate of the Healthcare System in each building where the ratio of real loads to the maximum load stands at 1:2.

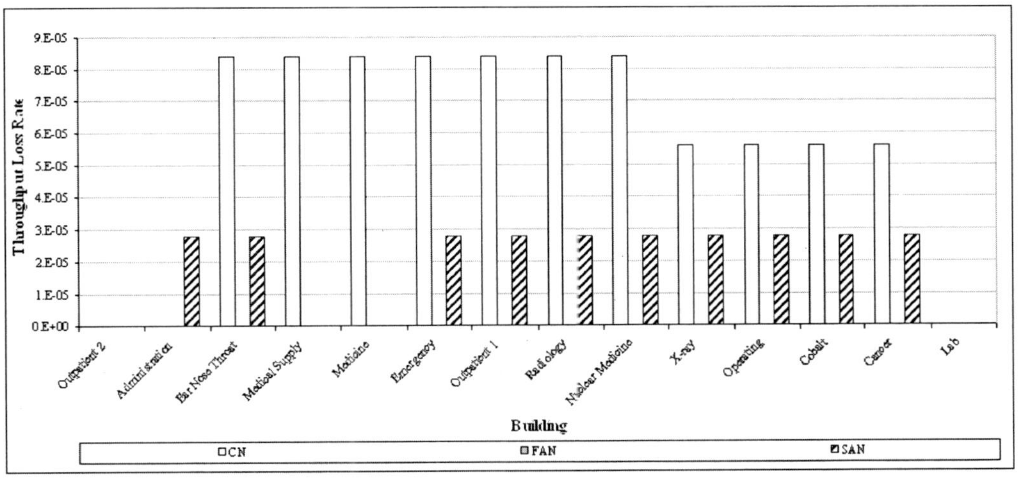

rates in the last four buildings of both the CN and the FAN, while it is lost in the lowest priority buildings of the SAN. In the CN and the FAN, due to FIFO of the queue types without a policy, the throughput is extremely lost in the operating building, cobalt building, cancer building, and lab building, which the loss of throughput must be avoided according that mission critical may be needed. For instance, the routine work of the operating building involves in surgery; therefore, a small loss of some transmitted applications can cause in a patient's life, while the information from cobalt building, cancer building, and lab building are necessary for doctors to help

Figure 8. The average loss rate of the Healthcare System in each building where the ratio of real loads to the maximum load stands at 3:4.

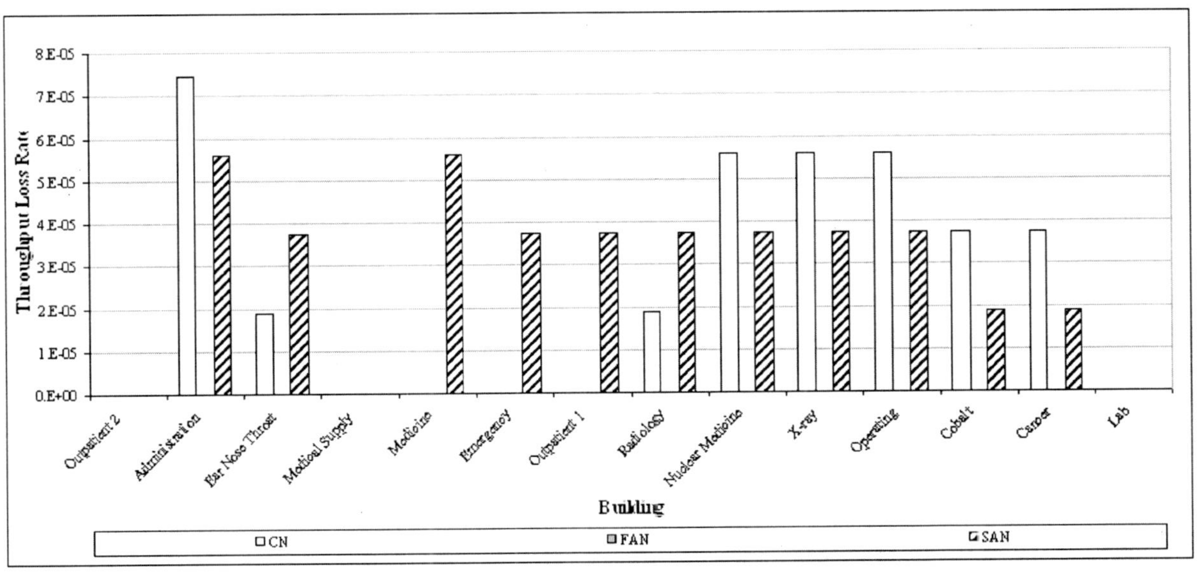

Figure 9. The average loss rate of the Healthcare System in each building where the ratio of real loads to the maximum load stands at 1:1.

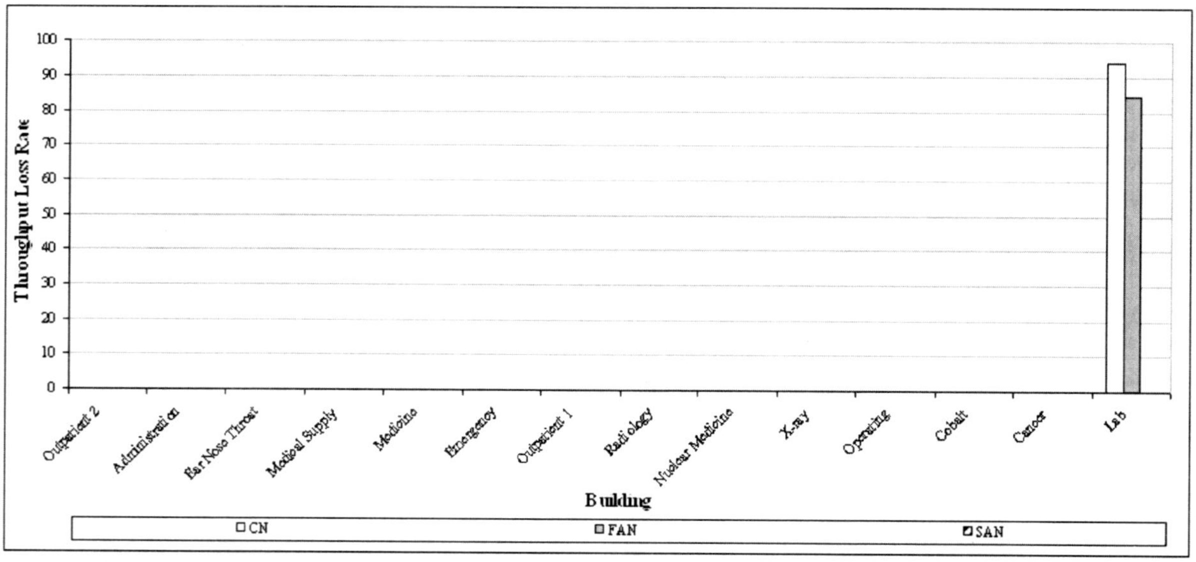

them diagnosis; unfortunately, the throughput is totally lost in these 3 buildings. In contrast, the insignificant loss of throughput is occurred in the medical supply building and the medicine building of SAN model due to prioritization of the wired policy. Consequently, it can be noticed that although it is in the congestion situation, the loss of throughput in the SAN is not only less than others, but it also occurred in the buildings that their routine work doesn't involve in any critical operations.

Wired Delay

Since the delay time of an incoming message is vital in the healthcare system, the delay time of transmitted applications is also analyzed in this experiment. Likewise, the analysis of wired delay will be divided into 3 main conditions as same as the throughput values.

Condition 1: The real load is less than the maximum load.

Figure 11 and Figure 12 show that the delay per throughput of every building in the SAN model is higher than the delay of the CN and the FAN models. According to the management policy of the SAN, the results shows that the values of the delay of the SAN model is low in the highest priority buildings, moderate in the middle priority buildings, and high in the lowest priority buildings. Thus, applying the wired policy to SAN model under this condition may not help reducing the delay as expected.

Condition 2: Real load is equal to the maximum load.

Figure 13 has shown that only the delay per throughput from the CN is very high for every building until the delays of the FAN and SAN models cannot be seen since they are both in the low values and no rapid change in every building.

Condition 3: The real load is more than the maximum load.

According to Figure 14, most buildings in the SAN model has very low delay, except the both lowest priority buildings: medicine and medical supply. Thus, patients' lives can be taking care off as needed. Unlike the SAN model, delay values in the CN and the FAN models are high in the three

Figure 10. The average loss rate of the Healthcare System in each building where the ratio of real loads to the maximum load stands at 5:4.

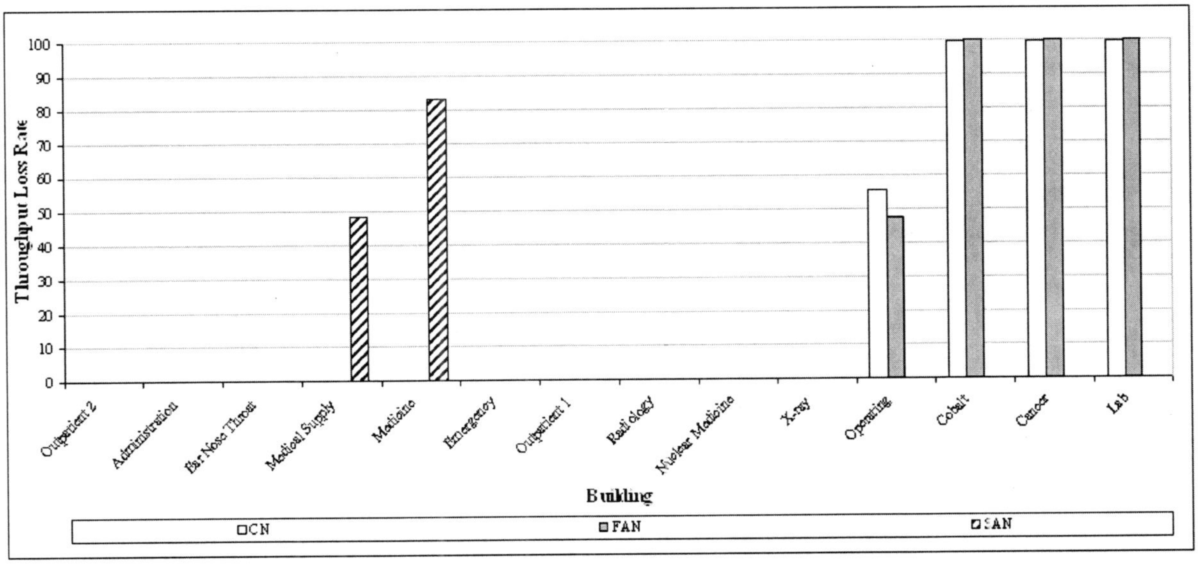

important buildings: Lab, Cancer, and Cobalt. This is the significant effect of the FIFO of the queue types. Thus, the patients' lives can be in danger under the stress of network condition.

Wi-Fi Throughput and Delay

Based on the SAN wireless policies, the simulation result has shown in Figure 15 that there is no throughput loss in the flow of patient information

Figure 11. The average delay per throughput of the Healthcare System in each building where the ratio of real loads to the maximum load stands at 1:2

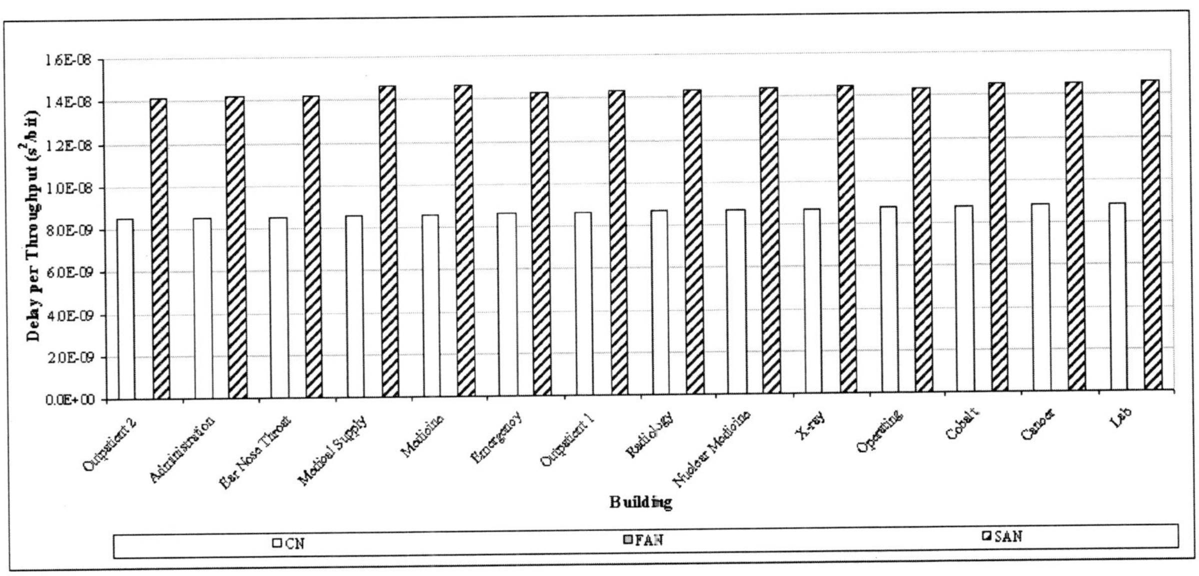

Figure 12. The average delay per throughput of the Healthcare System in each building where the ratio of real loads to the maximum load stands at 3:4

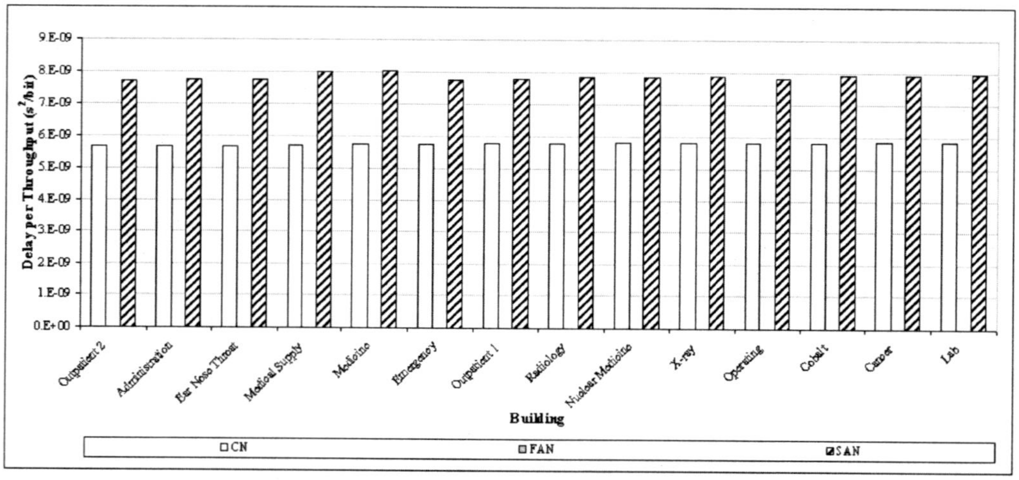

for doctors, which is the highest priority flow in the wireless policy. Likewise, there are a few losses in the flow of the Internet services for doctors, which is the middle priority flow. Consequently, it can be noticed that applying this wireless policy can efficiently support a transmission of significant applications via Wi-Fi, without loss. Even though the throughput loss rate is increased in the flow of Internet services for patients, this value is low. So, patients can fluently surf the Internet or even access e-services while they are waiting for diagnosis.

Figure 16 shows that the delay per throughput of the flow of patient information for doctors and the flow of the Internet for doctors is very low. Consequently, the efficient transmission of significant applications via Wi-Fi can be obtained by this SAN model. Although the delay per throughput from the flow of the Internet for patients has increased, it is very low

Figure 13. The average delay per throughput of the Healthcare System in each building where the ratio of real loads to the maximum load stands at 1:1

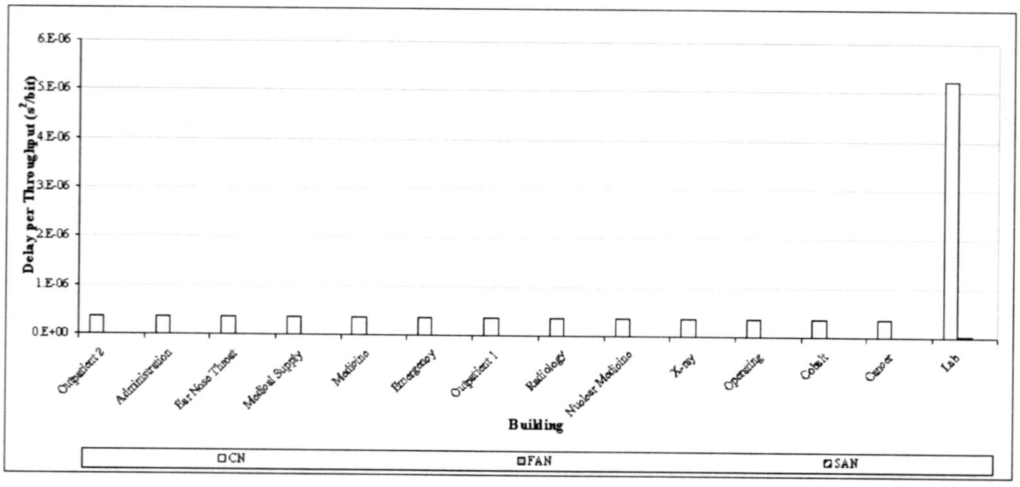

Figure 14. The average delay per throughput of the Healthcare System in each building where the ratio of real loads to the maximum load stands at 5:4

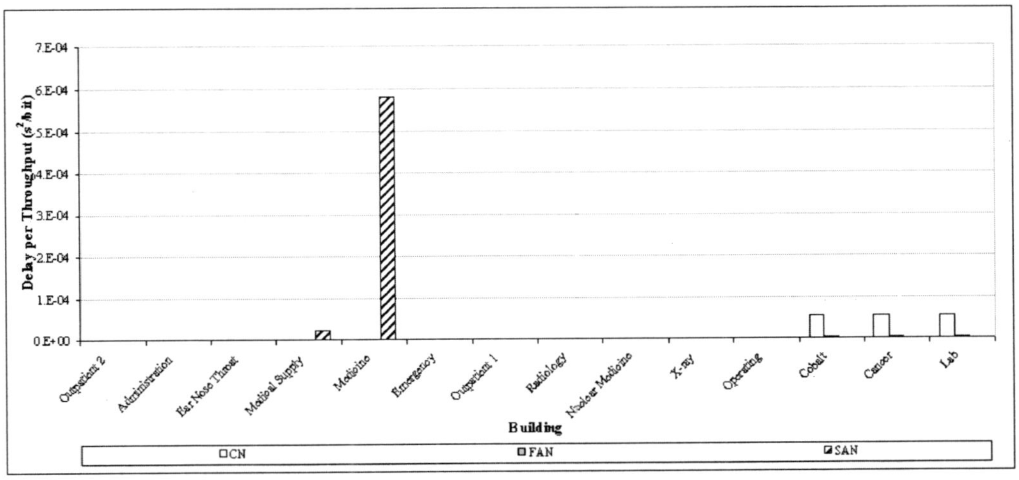

so that patients can surf the Internet, access e-services, or even access multimedia web sites efficiently.

DISCUSSION

The healthcare network, HN, is an important network because it must deal with human's life. Basically, there are three types of services of the HN: patient monitoring, medical services, and EHR and EMR retrieval system. Therefore, all services have to be guaranteed that medical staffs or responsible persons will receive all they need correctly in the proper time, and place so patients' lives can be saved. Thus, various researches proposed terrific solutions which are software, algorithms and communication methods, and medical with communication devices. However, these solutions need a large change in the real situ-

Figure 15. The average loss rate of each wireless flow type in the SAN when the real loads of Patient Information for doctors, the Internet for doctors, and the Internet for patients are 20 Mbps, 130 Mbps, and 130 Mbps, respectively.

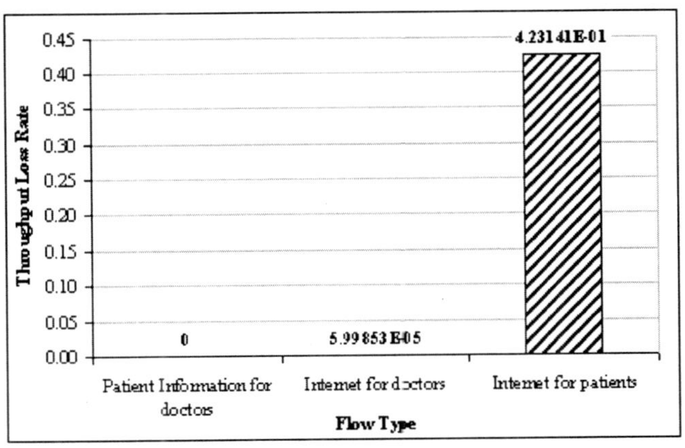

Figure 16. The average delay per throughput of each wireless flow type in SAN when the real loads of Patient Information for doctors, the Internet for doctors, and the Internet for patients are 20 Mbps, 130 Mbps, and 130 Mbps, respectively

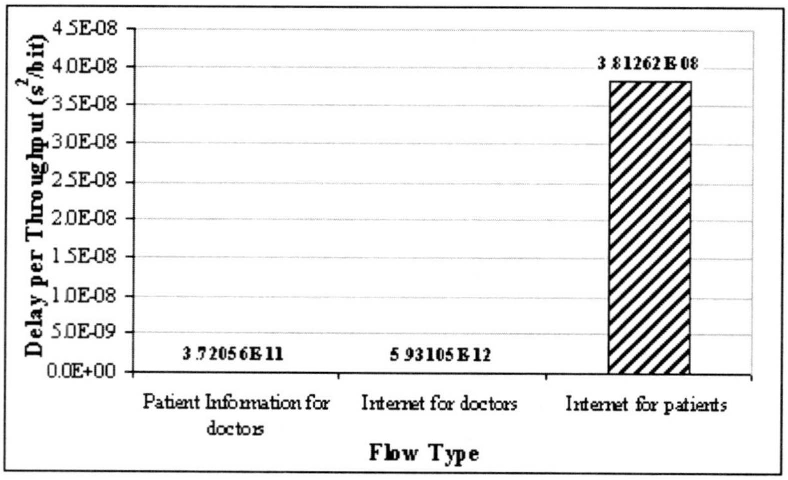

ation, and some solutions need a high investment cost which might not be suitable for a poor country like Thailand. Therefore, this paper has proposed a simple method that provides a simple, low cost of investment and maintenance. Moreover, the proof for QoS of the proposed architecture and management policies has been demonstrated that it can serve needs of any healthcare systems.

The difference between the solution proposed in this paper and other researches is the method to obtain QoS for the HN because the proposed solution uses all available technologies and management technique to reach the QoS requirements while others must re-implement new mechanism or new devices into the existing system. Consequently, the simplicity of implementing and maintaining this qualified HN system also arise and becomes a benefit to the implemented organization in the long term.

CONCLUSION

Although the original objective of network development was to support business process, this technology has been adjusted to the healthcare system in order to improve all services provided to human being. Various technologies and techniques have been developed and implemented to enhance medical activities so that people can be saved in an unpredictable world. Healthcare network was installed to support all significant functions of healthcare system: patient's monitoring, medical services, and EHR and EMR retrieval functions. These healthcare functions are implemented either in wired or wireless network devices, running over wired or wireless environment. However, the quality of healthcare services based on these functions must be guaranteed.

In order to claim that an HN is guaranteed its QoS, the performance measurement of data delivered to right persons, right time must be performed since data is the vital object related to life and dead. Therefore, the performance indicators are the data loss rate, and the packet delay time. However, values of these indicators are related to many factors, especially the network architecture, network management policies.

This paper has shown that choosing the right network architecture by implementing a wireless network with suitable management policies can maintain all medical data deliveries especially when the network is in the congestion situation much better than the original architecture, CN, and another alternative solution, FAN. Moreover, when comparing to the other two architectures, the proposed solution, SAN, is a cost effective, easy to be installed, and supports scalability in the future time.

Even though the result of this experiment has pointed out that setting the management policy is an effective method to obtain QoS but the management policy for traffic controlling has been setup as a static policy. Therefore, in a real implementation, a dynamic policy for traffic load balancing between wired and wireless should be applied; then, the expected outcome for packet loss rate and other measurement metrics should be better than these results.

Another significant outcome of this paper is that it confirms the idea of right implementation and right management method can bring quality of services to the network no matter how traffic has grown. In the other words, QoS can be achieved only using suitable network architecture with qualified management policy.

FURTHER INTERESTING PROBLEMS

This paper has considered the situation of an HN that runs for only one healthcare environment. However, in the real world, patients might have to transfer between healthcare systems in an unavoidable case. Thus, their EHR and EMR must be transferred between healthcare systems so that medical treatment can be correctly performed. Unfortunately, these data are not completely transferred according to unpractical medical's documents or files. Moreover, these data have not been transferred through the Internet because of data security and integrity problems, including that there is no private link between healthcare systems. Thus, many researches problem are opened and waiting to be solved such as,

1. How can the Internet be used to transfer data between healthcare systems?
2. Should new transmission protocol be implemented in the application layer to serve needs of HN over the Internet?
3. As a consequence of the installation of WiMAX, a MAN technology, should this technology bring a big change for data transfer among healthcare systems?

REFERENCES

Cho, H. S., Lee, B. H., Kim, M. K., Lee, S. Y., & Youn, C. H. (2006). A Secure Mobile Healthcare System based on Surrogate Host. *The Sixth IEEE International Conference on Computer and Information Technology*. (pp. 153-157).

Goldberg, S., & Wickramasinghe, N. (2003). 21ST Century Healthcare - The Wireless Panacea. *The 36th Annual Hawaii International Conference on System Sciences*, (pp.163b). Manoa, HI: University of Hawaii.

Hiranpongsin, S., & Bhattarakosol, P. (2009). Intelligent Cache Farming Architecture with the Recommender System. *International Journal of Engineering Science and Technology*, *4*(2), 206–219.

Istepanian, R. S. H. (2005). Wireless Security for Personalized and Mobile Healthcare Services. In *The 29th Annual International Computer Software and Applications Conference*. (Vol. 1, pp.86).

Lage, A. L., Martins, J. S. B , & Oliveira, J. C. (2004). A quality of service framework for telemedicine applications. In *Conference on WebMedia and LA-Web*, (pp. 18 – 20).

Lee, S. C., Lee, Y. D., & Chung, W. Y. (2008). Design and Implementation of Reliable Query Process for Indoor Environmental and Healthcare Monitoring System. In *The Third International Conference on Convergence and Hybrid Information Technology,* (pp. 398 – 402). Busan, Republic of Korea: IEEE Computer Society.

Lee, Y. D., Lee, D. S., Walia, G., Alasaarela, E., & Chung, W. Y. (2007). Design and Evaluation of Query Supported Healthcare Information System Using Wireless Sensor Ad-hoc Network. *The International Conference on Convergence Information Technology,* (pp. 997-1002). Bangladesh: United International University.

Lim, H., & Singh, V. K. (2005). Design of Healthcare System for Disabled Person Using Eye Blinking. In *The Fourth Annual ACIS International Conference on Computer and Information Science,* (pp. 551-555). Jeuu Island, South Korea: IEEE Computer Society.

Lubrin, E., Lawrence, E., & Navarro, K. F. (2005). Wireless Remote Healthcare Monitoring with Motes. In *The International Conference on Mobile Business (ICMB'05)*, (pp.235-241). Sydney, Australia: IEEE Computer Society.

Mateo, R. M., Salvo, M. A., & Lee, J. (2008). Balanced Clustering using Mobile Agents for the Ubiquitous Healthcare Systems. In *The Third International Conference on Convergence and Hybrid Information Technology*. (pp.686-691). Busan, Korea: IEEE Computer Society.

Pan, J., Li, S., & Wu, Z. (2008). Towards a Novel In-community Healthcare Monitoring System over Wireless Sensor Networks. In *The International Conference on Internet Computing in Science and Engineering*. (pp.160-165). Harbin, China: IEEE Computer Society.

Pavlovski, C., Kim, H., & Wood, D. (2004).Ubiquitous Mobility in Clinical Healthcare. In *IDEAS Workshop on Medical Information Systems: The Digital Hospital*. (pp.147-153). Beijing, China: IEEE Computer Society.

Philip, N., & Istepanian, R. S. H. (2007). Medical Quality of Service for Wireless Ultrasound Streaming in Robotic Tele-Ultrasonography System. In *The IEEE International Conference on Networking, Sensing and Control,* (pp. 245 – 250). London: IEEE Computer Society.

Raman, R. S., Jagannathan, V., & Reddy, R. (1997). Security Collaboration Technology for Healthcare Enterprises. In Sixth IEEE Workshops on Enabling Technologies: Infrastructure for Collaborative Enterprises. (pp. 263-268). Cambridge, UK: IEEE Computer Society.

Ray, P., & Weerakkody, G. (1999). Quality of Service Management in Healthcare Organizations: A Case Study. In *The 12th IEEE Symposium on Computer-Based Medical Systems*, (pp. 80 – 85). Stamford, CT: IEEE Computer Society.

Schmutzler, J., Foley, C., Michaelis, S., van der Meer, S., & Wietfeld, C. (2008). Dynamic group management as an enhancement to emergency healthcare using policies. In e-health Networking, Applications and Services (HealthCom 2008). Biopolis, Singapore: IEEE computer Society.

Seshadri, K., Liotta, L., Gopal, R., & Liotta, T. (2001). A Wireless Internet Application for Healthcare. In *The 14th IEEE Symposium on Computer-Based Medical Systems,* (pp.109-114). Bethesda, MD: IEEE Computer Society.

Tanchotsrinon, W., & Bhattarakosol, P. (2008). Enhancing Services in Healthcare System using Overlapping Network Models. In *The 7th International Conference on e-Business*, (pp.128 – 134). Bangkok: Rangsit University Press.

Tentori, M., & Favela, J. (2008). Activity-Aware Computing for Healthcare. *IEEE Pervasive Computing / IEEE Computer Society [and] IEEE Communications Society*, 7(2), 51–57. doi:10.1109/MPRV.2008.24

Varshney, U. (2006).Transmission of Emergency Messages in Wireless Patient Monitoring: Routing and Performance Evaluation. In *The 39th Annual Hawaii International Conference on System Sciences,* (pp.91a). Manoa, HI: University of Hawaii.

Yang, G., Cao, Y., Chen, J., Tenhunen, H., & Zheng, L. R. (2008). An Active-Cable Connected ECG Monitoring System for Ubiquitous Healthcare. In *The Third International Conference on Convergence and Hybrid Information Technology*, (pp. 392-397). Busan, Korea: IEEE Computer Society.

Yau, C. L., & Chung, W. Y. (2007). IEEE 802.15.4 Wireless Mobile Application for Healthcare System. In *The 2007 International Conference on Convergence Information Technology*, (pp.1433-1438). Gyeongju, Korea: IEEE Computer Society.

Zhu, Y., Keoh, S. L., Sloman, M., Lupu, E., Dulay, N., & Pryce, N. (2008). An Efficient Policy System for Body Sensor Networks. In *14th IEEE International Conference on Parallel and Distributed Systems*. (pp. 383, 390). Melbourne, Australia: IEEE Computer Society.

Chapter 17
QoS Signaling Security in Mobile Ad Hoc Networks

Ohm Sornil
National Institute of Development Administration, Thailand

ABSTRACT

A quality of service (QoS) signaling system is necessary for QoS provision in a mobile ad hoc network (MANET). A QoS signaling system in MANETs is vulnerable to various types of attacks, ranging from fabrication and modification of messages to denial of services, which can cause failures of QoS provisions. Security is thus a critical issue for a signaling system. However, distinctive characteristics of MANETs make security mechanisms effective in conventional networks inapplicable in this environment. This chapter describes issues and challenges, and examines mechanisms specifically designed to provide security for QoS signaling systems in MANETs.

INTRODUCTION

A Mobile Ad Hoc Network (MANET) is a network of mobile nodes such as laptops and PDAs, connected via a wireless medium with no fixed infrastructure, e.g., wireless access point or router. This type of wireless network has become increasingly popular due to several advantages, including infrastructure-lessness, dynamical self-organization, self-adaptation, self-healing, robustness, and scalability (Marwaha et al., 2008). MANETs are suitable for a variety of applications (Reinisch et al.,2007 ; Toh, 2007), such as public safety, military, intelligent transportation, metropolitan area networks, building automation, as well as providing wireless network coverage to remote and inaccessible areas. Quality of service (QoS) is a set of bounds, such as latency, jitter, throughput, and packet loss to be maintained by the network for a particular data flow (Crawley et al., 1998). With the emergence of real-time applications such as Voice over Internet Protocol (VoIP) and video streaming, e.g., Video on Demand (VoD), strict QoS supports are required.

To provide QoS in a MANET, a signaling protocol is required to search for routes with sufficient resources for the desired QoS, to reserve and release

DOI: 10.4018/978-1-61520-791-6.ch017

resources, to set up, tear down, and renegotiate flows in the networks. Various types of attacks on a signaling protocol are possible such as signaling message fabrication, interception of QoS requests, modifications of QoS parameters, etc. Security is thus a critical aspect for the signaling system. Security properties that should be supported for QoS signaling systems in MANETs include confidentiality, availability, authenticity, integrity, and non-repudiation. Confidentiality requires the secrecy of the communication to be protected. Availability requires that services are available to an authorized entity. Authenticity ensures that an entity is who it claims to be. Integrity ensures that a message transmitted is not maliciously altered, and non-repudiation ensures that a node transmitting a message cannot deny the transmission.

Characteristics of MANETs, such as absence of fixed infrastructure, rapid topology change, high node mobility, and limited node capability, impose difficulties on security protection. Current approaches proposed for intrusion detection and security prevention on QoS signaling in wired networks (such as SDS/CD (Wu et al., 1999) and RSVP-SQOS (Talwar et al., 2001)) cannot be applied to MANETs, and new security techniques are necessary. Cryptographic mechanisms by themselves can only address a subset of security problems that exist with current QoS signaling. While attacks on routing generally focus on disrupting network connectivity, attacks on QoS signaling can affect routes established by secure routing protocols (Lu & Pooch, 2005). Without proper protection from security mechanisms, attacks on a QoS signaling system could result in QoS routing malfunction, interference of resource reservation, or even failure of QoS provision.

This chapter describes issues and challenges, and examines the state of the art in QoS signaling security in MANETs. The rest of the chapter is organized as follows. Section 2 discusses security issues in QoS signaling systems. Section 3 describes and analyzes two prominent security mechanisms specifically designed to protect QoS signaling systems. Section 4 provides concluding remarks.

VULNERABILITIES AND ATTACKS ON QOS SIGNALING SYSTEMS IN MANETS

QoS Signaling Systems in MANETs

A signaling protocol is required to propagate QoS reservation messages and establish appropriate QoS reservations. Two main QoS provisioning models in the Internet have been developed by IETF: Integrated Services (IntServ) (Braden et al., 1994) and Differentiated Services (Blake et al., 2009). The stateful IntServ, which maintains per-flow reservation state at QoS network entities, has a greater level of accuracy at a finer level of granularity. The stateless DiffServ does not maintain per-flow reservation state at QoS network entities and only relies on coarse classification and differential treatment of traffic. The two models are also adopted to provisioning QoS in MANETs. A number of QoS signaling protocols have been proposed for MANETs, for example, INSIGNIA, QoS AODV, SWAN, etc. (Chen & Nahrstedt, 1998)

In-Band Signaling System for Supporting QoS in MANET (INSIGNIA) (Lee et al., 200) employs the option part of every IP packet to carry the signaling control. It is a per-flow based protocol (the IntServ approach) where the state of each flow is managed individually over a session in response to topology and end-to-end QoS condition changes. INSIGNIA uses a soft-state method to maintain its state information. Bandwidth is allocated to a particular flow if the QoS resource requirements of that flow can be satisfied. Otherwise, if the required resources are not available, the flow will be downgraded to a best-effort service. To be able to respond quickly to topology changes and varying end-to-end QoS conditions, INSIGNIA uses QoS reports to inform the source node of the status of its real-time flows. The destination node actively monitors the received flows and calculates QoS statistics, such as loss rate, delay, and throughput. The reports are sent back to the source node periodically. The source node then takes appropriate steps in order to adapt to the changing network conditions.

QoS Signaling System for Ad hoc On-demand Distance Vector (QoS AODV) (Perkins & Belding-Royer, 2001) also employs the IntServ approach. The original AODV is extended by adding new fields, including bandwidth and delay parameters, on the Route Request (RREQ) and Route Reply (RREP) messages, that must be met by nodes forwarding an RREQ from the source or an RREP from the destination during the route discovery phase. If an intermediate node is unable to keep the QoS promises made to the source of the flow, it will send an ICMP QOS_LOST message back to the source.

Service Differentiation in Stateless Wireless Ad hoc networks (SWAN) (Ahn et al., 2002) uses the DiffServ approach and offers a stateless QoS model for MANETs. It does not require intermediate nodes to maintain per-flow reservation states. To check whether the required bandwidth is available on a path, a probe message with the bandwidth requirement is sent to the destination on a previously established route. Upon receiving the packet, an intermediate node compares the required value with the available bandwidth on its outgoing routes, and overwrites the requested bandwidth if the available bandwidth is smaller. Once the destination receives the packet, it sends a reply packet back to the source node. The source node decides whether or not to establish a real-time flow based on the rate indicated in the packet. Resources are not explicitly reserved for each flow.

Vulnerabilities of QoS Signaling Systems in MANETs

An attacker can exploit a vulnerability of a QoS signaling protocol to launch an attack on a system. Main vulnerabilities of QoS signaling systems in MANETs are as follows (Lu & Pooch, 2005; Zouridaki et al., 2005):

1. *Open Network Topology*: In a MANET, the address and the identity of a node are independent of the node's location. The open topology and overlaps in radio transmissions and reception ranges make it easier for attackers to overhear QoS requests and control messages, and to actively interfere with such messages. In addition, the link between two nodes is shared among network nodes in the range, and available bandwidth can be perceived differently by different nodes. This leaves the signaling protocol vulnerable to attacks on confidentiality, authenticity, integrity, and availability.
2. *Homogenous Nodes in QoS Provision*: All nodes in a MANET have homogenous roles in QoS provisioning. A node can serve as a core node at one time and as an edge node at another time.
3. *Node Mobility*: In a fixed and wired network, the IP address of a host is considered to be its identity and indicative of its location in the network topology. In a MANET setting, it is difficult to trace and verify the legitimacy of QoS requests due to mobility of nodes. Mobility can cause link capacity to change. Moreover, the promised QoS can be broken when the communication capacity between two nodes dramatically changes.
4. *Intermittent Connectivity*: Due to intermittent connectivity, control messages may be lost, or protocol timing dependencies may be modulated. Such effects are difficult to distinguish from real attacks.

5. *Limited Node Capabilities*: Typical nodes in a MANET have stringent resource constraints, such as limited energy, memory, and CPU cycles. Any processing must be very efficient, and information stored must be managed efficiently in each node.

Attacks on QoS Signaling Systems in MANETs

In this section, common attacks on QoS signaling in MANET environments are discussed (Lu & Pooch, 2005; Zouridaki et al., 2005) which include signaling message fabrication, interception of QoS requests, malicious modifications of QoS parameters, over reservation of resources, reporting false state information, flooding denial of service, and replay attacks. Most attacks apply to both reservation-based and reservation-less QoS signaling protocols with an exception of over reservation of resources which applies only to reservation-based protocols. We assume that a secure routing protocol is available in the system to determine a route between the source and the destination nodes while reliable and resistant to malicious attacks.

1. *Signaling Message Fabrication*: An attacker can exploit a signaling protocol by fabricating a message with a legitimate entity's identity to reserve resources for its own traffics, to make resources unavailable to other nodes, or to release resources in order to disrupt QoS services which would degrade the network performance. This kind of attack is possible since a protocol neither authenticates the sender nor verifies usage of reservation, and detecting QoS is quite difficult for devices in MANETs due to limited node capability.
2. *Interception of QoS Requests*: An attacker can intercept or drop reservation messages so that the QoS reservation and the channel setup will be failed or tremendously delayed. This attack can prohibit the QoS resources from being available to the victim.
3. *Malicious Modifications of QoS Parameters*: An attacker can modify QoS parameters without authorization. In addition, an attacker can act as an intermediate node and increase delay or jitter of a traffic to an unacceptable level causing the degradation or re-initialization of QoS for a particular service; or decrease the values of the requested resources in an RREQ message. This can result in a reservation of incorrect amount resources which disrupt the quality of the service provided to the flow.
4. *Over Reservation of Resources*: A greedy node can reserve bandwidth more than what it actually needs in order to ensure that its traffic will be supported in the near future or to perform a denial of service attack. For a protocol with refreshment, a node can send data packets in the specified refresh-time interval to keep reservation refreshed. This causes underutilization of the resources, and legitimate sessions may be denied services.
5. *Reporting False State Information*: An attacker may falsely report state information in order to disrupt the service, for example, a node falsely reports available bandwidth on an outgoing link. The source node then transmits at a rate not matching the actual bandwidth available on the path which can cause congestion.
6. *Flooding Denial of Service Attacks*: An attacker can act as a source node and flood the network with data traffic that consumes all the available bandwidth. This causes legitimate sessions to be denied service. The attack is possible since a protocol does not verify resource usage, does not identify the source, and does not take measures against flooding.
7. *Replay Attacks*: Since a wireless channel is a broadcast medium, each mobile node

can hear the transmission of every node in its transmission range. Attackers can duplicate or modify signaling information and forward the modified messages to the next hop. Resources are wasted, and legitimate flows are denied service. A replay attack can happen to protocols that allow exchange of unauthenticated information and do not protect the integrity of signaling information. These protocols cannot distinguish a replay from an authentic one.

SECURITY MECHANISMS FOR QOS SIGNALING SYSTEMS IN MANETS

Though security is important to a QoS signaling system, there is little work proposed on this aspect in MANET environments. In this section, two prominent mechanisms specifically devised to provide security for QoS signaling in MANETs are discussed and analyzed.

Security Mechanism for QoS Signaling Systems in MANETs by Lu and Pooch

Lu and Pooch (Lu & Pooch, 2005) proposed a security mechanism for MANET QoS signaling systems which provides authentication and detects intrusions on QoS parameters in the absence of adjacent colluding nodes. The mechanism consists of 3 major components working together: (1) a hop-by-hop authentication protocol, (2) an end-to-end authentication protocol, and (3) neighboring node cooperation.

1. *A Hop-by-Hop Authentication Protocol*: As discussed above, an attacker can tamper QoS signaling messages with falsified data to steal or deplete resources used or reserved by other nodes. These attacks can result in degraded performance of the network, interference of resource reservation, unauthorized uses of resources, or even failure of QoS provision. To thwart these attacks, a light-weight hop-by-hop authentication protocol ensures that the sender of a message is an authentic and legitimate node. The protocol utilizes one-way hash chains to create authentication keys. A one-way hash function H maps an input of any length into a fixed length bit string. To generate a key chain of length $n+1$ in a one-way hash chain authentication, the first key is randomly picked by a transmitting node, and the chain of keys is generated by repeatedly applying the one-way function to the result of the previous iteration.

To use a hash chain in the protocol, the keys are used and distributed in reverse order of the generated keys, starting from h_n which is calculated from the entire key sequence. The validity of a key h_i can be verified from h_j $(0 \le j < i \le n)$ by applying function H for *i-j* times since $h_i = H^{i-j}(h_j)$.

When a node (say node A) wants to send a message, it computes a message authentication code (MAC) on the message using the current key h_i and unicasts the message to the receiving node (say node B), or multicasts (or broadcasts) the message to the receivers in the following format: $A \to B(or\ *) : M, MAC(M, h_i^A)$ where M is the message to be sent, and h_i^A is the current key used by node A. To prevent the man-in-the-middle attack, the key is broadcasted in a KEYUPDATE message: $A \to * : A, h_i^A$ after a time delay interval, and the receiver can verify the key using the previously released key h_{i+1}^A. The broadcasted key enables the receiver to verify MAC of the message. The time delay is determined by the sender and announced in data packets that are protected with the key. Before knowing the key, messages cannot be verified and thus stored in cache at the receiving node until the key is disclosed.

A MAC is generated at each intermediate node with its currently used hash chain key, and the RREQ message is relayed to its adjacent downstream node. After the key is disclosed, the downstream node will use the disclosed key to verify authenticity and integrity of the parameters. In case that the authentication fails, the node will raise an intrusion alarm to its downstream node on the path as well as all the other neighbors. This mechanism can prevent spoofing of signaling messages and protect legitimate messages from man-in-the-middle attacks.

2. *An End-to-End Authentication Protocol*: The second component in this QoS signaling security system is an end-to-end (source to destination) authentication protocol. The QoS parameter part of the route request (RREQ) message is digitally signed by the source node's private key, and that part in the route reply (RREP) message is signed by the destination node.

Each intermediate node on a path can voluntarily verify the digital signature to assure that QoS parameters have not been maliciously altered during the transmission. After the RREQ reaches the destination node, the destination checks integrity of the QoS parameters via MAC verification. If the parameters have been altered during transmission, the destination node will raise an alarm. Otherwise, it generates an RREP message, hashes the QoS parameters, and sends it back to the source of the request. The source will verify the authenticity and integrity of the QoS parameters upon receiving the RRep packet from the destination.

3. *Neighboring Node Cooperation*: Neighboring nodes play significant roles in detecting distributions of false QoS state information while providing integrity and authenticity of signaling messages.

A misbehavior by a node can be detected by neighboring nodes through a watchdog scheme. This scheme requires that each intermediate node on the route sends a signaling message to all of its neighbors so that its upstream nodes can listen to the broadcasted message and verify whether its neighbors are maliciously distributing false QoS status. This mechanism can be applied to various QoS parameters, e.g., maximum permissible delay, maximum permissible jitter, minimum available bandwidth, etc.

Under a circumstance that a node experiences a significant change that keeps it from reserving the promised service, it will send an ICMP QoS_LOST message. Keeping track of nodes sending QoS_LOST messages helps detect malicious attacks. To prevent a malicious node from acting normal during the QoS signaling but failing to keep the promise intentionally, the destination node and volunteer intermediate nodes monitor a flow against the promised QoS level and periodically report to other nodes including the source of the flow for detection.

Even though the watchdog scheme is implemented, there are some instances that the attacker's neighbors are not able to overhear the fallacious information. For example, a malicious node (say node B) intentionally sends false QoS status to the downstream node C when node A's radio channel is busy in order to cause a signal conflict at A, thus A will not be able to overhear the fallacious information. Later B sends the correct information to node A while taking advantage of signal conflicts at node C so that node C would not be able to detect that node B sends different values. In this case, node A will fail to detect the fallacious QoS information distributed.

In this case, neighbors of an intermediate node on a path are needed in the detection since some of them are likely to hear from two broadcasted signaling messages and able to detect the misbehavior. To implement this scheme, a non-repudiation mechanism using two MACs, created from two consecutive keys, are used to produce

Figure 1. Neighboring node cooperation

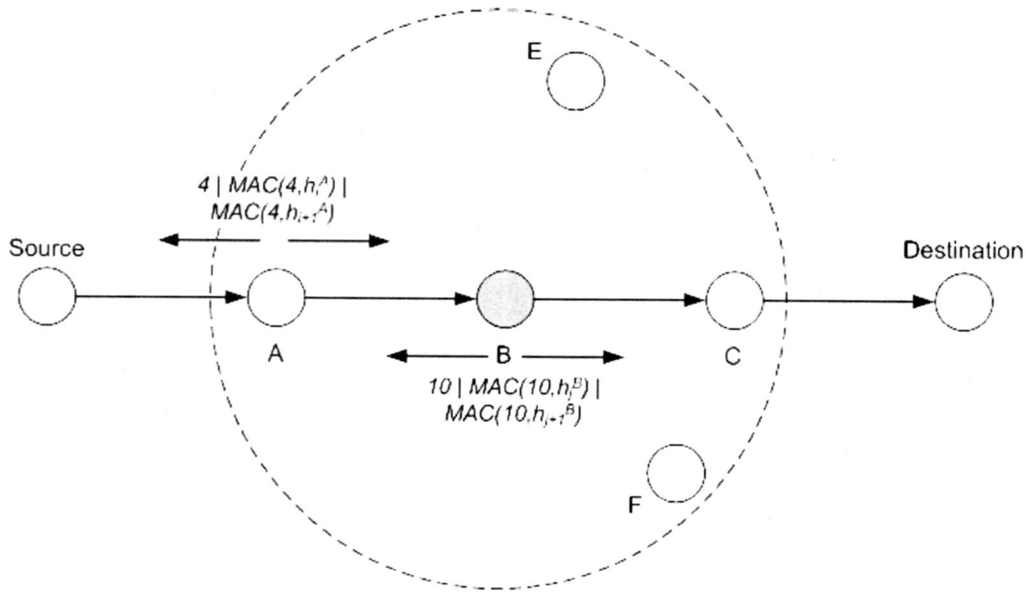

evidences of attacks while the attacker cannot deny its action.

Two MACs are calculated for QoS parameters: one generated using the key that will be disclosed the next h_i^A, the other generated with the key h_{i-1}^A that will be disclosed a short while after h_i^A. For example, as shown in Figure 1, node A sends the maximum permissible jitter parameter of 4 ms generated with key h_i^A. Disclosure of h_i^A provides timely authentication for the signaling message, and the delayed disclosure of h_{i-1}^A provides non-repudiation for the attacker's action.

If node B sends a signaling message with a different value of the maximum permissible jitter parameter to nodes A and C. This behavior will be noticed by node E and/or F. They will raise an intrusion alarm with the two messages. The only way for B to deny this action is to release the second key h_{i-1}^B and proves that the second MAC of the message is not generated with h_{i-1}^B which is easily authenticated by applying H to h_i^B.

Denial-of-Service Resistant Quality-of-Service Signaling Scheme (DRQoS)

Denial-of-Service Resistant QoS Signaling Scheme (DRQoS) (Hejmo et al., 2005) is a distributed, stateful QoS signaling protocol, designed to be resistant to a large class of DoS attacks. Each node (say node B) maintains a state for the aggregate stream from node A to node C, where A and C are one-hop neighbors of B. An entry (A, C) in B's state table records: (1) the assigned transmission rate R_{AC}, (2) a counter of bits arrived during the current measurement window X_{AC}, and (3) a measured rate $\widehat{R}_{AC}$ from the previous measurement window.

DRQoS consists of two phrases: bandwidth probing phase and data transmission phase. The first phase employs two control messages: Bandwidth Probe Request (BPRep) and Bandwidth Probe Reply (BPRep). The BPReq contains IP addresses of source and destination, message type, flow ID, and requested data rate (stored in the bottleneck bandwidth field, BB).

Initially, the source node sends a BPReq message to the destination. Upon receiving the message, an intermediate node along the path compares the available bandwidth on its outgoing link to C (ABW_C) with the value in the BB field of the BPReq packet. If $BB > ABW_C$, the node replaces the BB field with ABW_C and forwards the message to node C. When BPReq reaches the destination node, it creates a BPRep message, copies the value in BB field onto BPRep, and sends the message back to the source node on the reverse path.

Upon receiving a BPRep on the reverse path, an intermediate node compares ABW_C and the BB field value in the BPRep packet, replaces the BB field with the smaller value, adds the BB value to the assigned rate R_{AC} in the state table, and forwards the BPRep upward. Once the BPRep reaches the source node, the source establishes a real-time flow based on the value of the requested data rate (BB field) in the BPRep packet.

1. *DRQoS Distributed Rate Control Mechanism*:The process above is utilized by a rate control mechanism. DRQoS includes a distributed rate control mechanism which performs two main functions: (1) traffic policing and (2) rate monitoring and adjustment.

Traffic policing is performed at each node to ensure that a traffic passing through it does not exceed the assigned rate R_{AC} recorded in the state table. The rate of a traffic is measured; and if the measured rate $\widehat{R}_{AC}$ is lower than the assigned rate by a large margin, R_{AC} is decreased by a factor (γ). The actual rate that is used to police a traffic stream is $R'_{AC} = \gamma \cdot R_{AC}$ where $0 < \gamma < 1$ is a reduction factor, defined by: $\gamma = \min(Capacity_C / \sum_i R_{iC})$ where $Capacity_c$ is the estimated outgoing link capacity to node C. The reduced rate ensures that the sum of the policed rate over all in-hop link *i*'s toward node C does not exceed the estimated link capacity. Packets of a traffic that violate the assigned rate would either be dropped immediately, marked as low priority, or delayed.

Estimation of $Capacity_c$ depends on the type of MAC layer used in the network. DRQoS applies the approach proposed in (Kazantzidis & Gerla, 2002) for estimating it for the IEEE 802.11 MAC layer. An intermediate node uses the available bandwidth ABW_C to determine the value that should be recorded in the BB field of a BPRep packet passing through it, where $ABW_C = \max\{0, (Capacity_C - \sum_i R_{iC})\}$.

The rate monitoring function measures the traffic rate of a given stream over a time interval *T*. A counter X_{AC} is incremented by the size of each message. After the time period of *T* elapses, the measured rate $\widehat{R}_{AC}$ is computed as: $\widehat{R}_{AC} = X_{AC} / T$. To adjust the transmission rate, if the measured rate $\widehat{R}_{AC}$ is less than the assigned rate R_{AC} by more than $p\%$. The assigned rate R_{AC} will be decreased by a factor $(1 - \alpha \cdot p)$, where $0 < \alpha < 1$ is a user-supplied parameter. If the assigned traffic rate for a stream is decreased below a certain threshold, the stream is removed from the state table (treated as inactive).

Analysis of the QoS Signaling Security Mechanisms

The mechanism proposed by Lu and Pooch focuses on the first five types of attacks which include: signaling message fabrication, interception of QoS requests, malicious modifications of QoS parameters, intentional reporting of false state information, and replay attacks. To protect against fabricated signaling messages, QoS parameters are signed by the source's or the destination's private key, and every node can voluntarily check for the authenticity of the sender. An interception of QoS requests can be detected by the coopera-

Figure 2. The response to an over-reservation attack by DRQoS

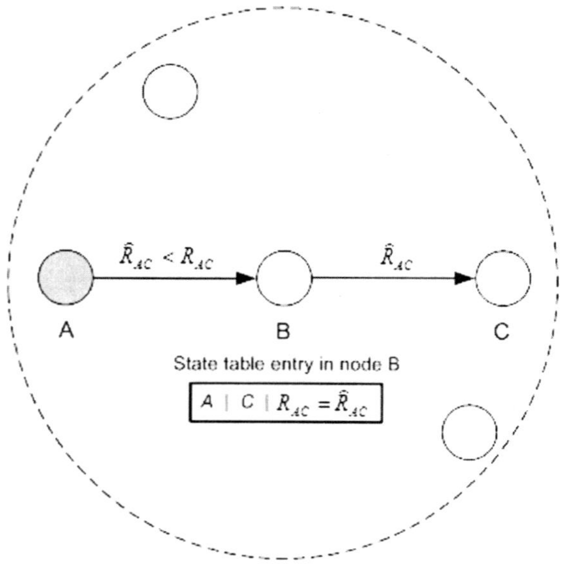

Figure 3. The response to a flooding attack by DRQoS

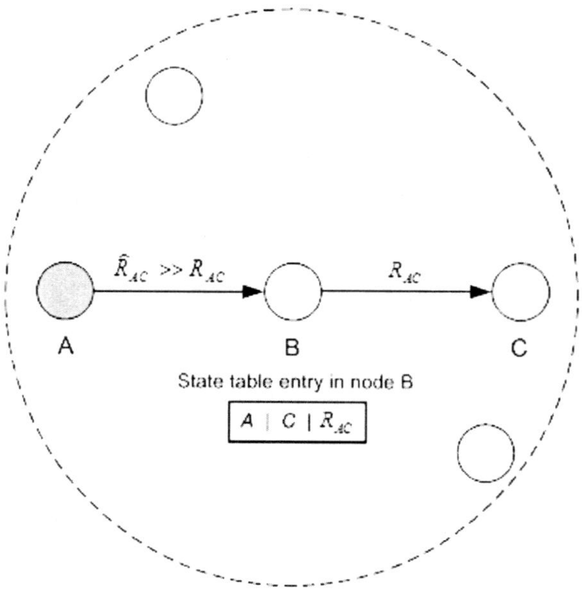

tion of neighboring nodes as well as that of their neighbors. A drop of QoS message from a node can be overheard by the upstream node which can analyze whether the drop has malicious intentions. Malicious modifications of QoS parameters are handled by the lightweight hop-by-hop authentication protocol with delayed key disclosure providing authentication and integrity of the parameters in signaling messages. The delayed key disclosure guarantees that a malicious node is not able to forge MACs with an already released key, and the identity of a legitimate node cannot be spoofed by an attacker. A replay attack can be prevented by the hash chain scheme together with the delayed key disclosure scheme. Finally, the intentional reporting of false state information can be identified by adjacent downstream nodes which can detect both the attack as well as the malicious node on the path. The two-MAC scheme provides evidences for non-repudiation while allowing timely message authentication.

DRQoS is specifically designed to protect the QoS signaling system against denial of service attacks, e.g., over reservation of resources and flooding. Over-reservation attacks can be detected from the mismatch between the rate measured periodically and the assigned rate in the state table. The assigned rate which is much larger than the measured rate is thus reduced until matching with the actual rate, freeing wasted bandwidth on the outgoing link of the detecting node. For example, in Figure 2 the attacking node A transmits at a rate far below the assigned rate R_{AC}, node B measures $\hat{R}_{AC}$, detects this mismatch, and reduces the assigned rate R_{AC} until it matches the actual rate of transmission. A flooding attack where an attacker transmits at a rate faster than the assigned rate is handled by the traffic policing. For example, in Figure 3 node B which is downstream from the attacker A maintains a state table entry for the stream from A and polices the outgoing traffic at the assigned rate. The violating traffic is dropped, insulating other nodes downstream from B from the flooding attack by node A.

CONCLUSION

A signaling protocol is necessary for QoS provision in a MANET. A QoS signaling system in this type of environment is susceptible to a variety of attacks, including signaling message fabrication, interception of QoS requests, malicious modifications of QoS parameters, over reservation of resources, etc. Security is thus critical for the signaling system. However, the distinctive characteristics of MANETs impose difficulties for security protection causing conventional security measures inapplicable, and new security mechanisms are required. Two prominent mechanisms specifically designed to provide security for QoS signaling in MANETs are examined in this chapter. We can see that with the complexities of the environments and attacks, each mechanism (even with sophisticated components working together) is effective only for some classes of attacks. Satisfying all security requirements for QoS signaling in MANETs is a challenging task. A complete solution to secure QoS signaling security in MANETs should incorporate: intelligent traffic management, light-weight intrusion detection scheme, and efficient cryptographic primitives (Zouridaki et al., 2005). With the current state-of-the-art, this aspect remains largely open for research.

REFERENCES

Ahn, G.-S., Campbell, A. T., Veres, A., & Sun, L. H. (2002). Supporting Service Differentiation for Real-Time and Best-Effort Traffic in Stateless Wireless Ad Hoc Networks (SWAN). *IEEE Transactions on Mobile Computing*, *1*, 192–207. doi:10.1109/TMC.2002.1081755

Blake, S., Black, D., Carlson, M., Davies, E., Wang, Z., & Weiss, W. (n.d.). *IETF RFC: 2475, An Architecture for Differentiated Service*. Retrieved August 9, 2009 from http://www.ietf.org/rfc/rfc2475.txt

Braden, R., Clark, D., & Shenker, S. (1994). *IETF RFC: 1633, Integrated Services in the Internet Architecture: an Overview*. Retrieved August 9, 2009 from http://www.ietf.org/rfc/rfc1633.txt

Chen, S., & Nahrstedt, K. (1998). Distributed Quality-of-Service Routing in the Ad-Hoc Networks. *IEEE Journal on Special Areas in Communications*, *17*(8), 1488–1505. doi:10.1109/49.780354

Crawley, E., Nair, R., Rajagopalan, B., & Sandick, H. (1998). *IETF RFC: 2386, A Framework for QoS-Based Routing in the Internet*. Retrieved August 9, 2009 from http://www.ietf.org/rfc/rfc2386.txt

Hejmo, M., Mark, B. L., Zouridaki, C., & Thomas, R. K. (2005). A denial-of-service resistant quality-of-service signaling protocol for mobile ad hoc networks. In *Proceedings of the Second Conference on Quality of Service in Heterogeneous Wired. Wireless Networks, 2005*, 9–32.

Kazantzidis, M., & Gerla, M. (2002). End-to-end versus explicit feedback measurement in 802.11 networks. In *Proceedings of the 7th IEEE International Symposium on Computers and Communications (ISCC)* (pp.429–434).

Lee, B., Ahn, G.S., Zhang, X., & Campbell, A.T. (2000). INSIGNIA: an IPbased quality of service framework for mobile ad hoc networks. *Journal of Parallel and Distributed Computing, Special issue on Wireless and Mobile Computations and Communications, 60*, 374–406.

Lu, B., & Pooch, U. W. (2005). Security in QoS signaling systems for mobile ad hoc networks. In *Proceedings of IEEE International Conference on Wireless And Mobile Computing, Networking. Communications*, *3*, 213–220.

Marwaha, S., Indulska, J., & Portmann, M. (2008). Challenges and Recent Advances in QoS Provisioning, Signaling, Routing and MAC protocols for MANETs. In. *Proceedings of Telecommunication Networks and Applications Conference, 2008*, 97–102.

Perkins, C. E., & Belding-Royer, E. M. (2001). Quality of Service for Ad Hoc On-Demand Distance Vector Routing. *Internet Draft*. Retrieved August 9, 2009, from http://tools.ietf.org

Reinisch, C., Kastner, W., Neugschwandtner, G., & Granzer, W. (2007). Wireless Technologies in Home and Building Automation. In *Proceedings of the 5th IEEE International Conference on Industrial Informatics, 1,* 93-98.

Talwar, V., Nath, S. K., & Nahrstedt, K. (2001). RSVP-SQoS: A Secure RSVP Protocol. In *Proceedings of International Conference on Multimedia and Exposition* (pp.579-582).

Toh, C.-K. (2007). Future Application Scenarios for MANET-Based Intelligent Transportation Systems. In *Proceedings of Future Generation Communication and Networking (FGCN 2007),* (Vol.2, pp. 414-417).

Wu, T., Wu, S. F., Fu, Z., Huang, H., & Gong, F. (1999). Securing QoS: Threats to RSVP Messages and Their Countermeasures. In *Proceedings of the Seventh International Workshop on Quality of Service* (pp. 62-64).

Zouridaki, C., Hejmo, M., Mark, B. L., Thomas, R. K., & Gaj, K. (2005). Analysis of Attacks and Defense Mechanisms for QoS Signaling Protocols in MANETs. In Proceedings of Wireless Information Systems (WIS) Workshop, 2005, (pp.61–70).

Compilation of References

Abbott, L. (1955). *Quality and Competition: An Essay in Economie Theory*. New York: Columbia University Press.

Abd El-kader, S., Eissa, H. & Baraka, H. (2001). A New Proposed No-Loss\No-Delay Effective Network Resources Consumer Meter. The Egyptian Computer Journal. Institute of Statistical Studies and Research, 29(1), 34–44.

Abd El-kader. S. (2003). A New Scalable Quality Guaranteed Model For The Real-Time Multimedia Communications Across the Internet. Ph.D thesis, Faculty of Engineering, Cairo University, Cairo, Egypt.

Abd El-kader. S., Eissa, H. & Baraka, H. (2002). Real-time Voice Quality Guarantee on the IP Based Networks. In The 8th IEEE International Conference On Communication Systems, (pp. 510-514).

Abraham, A., Grosan, C., & Ramos, V. (Eds.). (2006). *Swarm Intelligence in Data Mining Series: Studies in Computational Intelligence* (*Vol. 34*). Berlin: Springer-Verlag.

Acampora, A.S. & Naghshineh, M. (1994). An Architecture and Methodology for Mobile-Executed Cell Hand-off in Wireless ATM Networks. *IEEE JSAC, 12*.

Acampora, A.S., & Naghshineh, M. (1994). Control and Quality-of-Service Provisioning in High-Speed Micro-Cellular Networks. *IEEE Personal Communications*, (2), 36-42.

Adami, D., Callegari, C., Giordano, S., Mustacchio, F., Pagano, M., & Vitucci, F. (2005). Signalling protocols in diffserv-aware MPLS networks: design and implementation of RSVP-TE network simulator. *IEEE Global Telecommunications Conference (GLOBECOM '05)*, 792-796.

Addie, R. G., Zukerman, M., & Neame, T. (1995). Fractal traffic: measurements, modelling and performance evaluation. In *Proceedings of the Fourteenth Annual Joint Conference of the IEEE Computer and Communication Societies Infocom '95, 3,* (pp. 977-984).

Adner, R. (2002). When are technologies disruptive? A demand-based view of the emergence of competition. *Strategic Management Journal, 23*, 667–668. doi:10.1002/smj.246

ADS. (2006). GEANT2, deliverable GN2-04-153v4 "AMPS – Design Specification."

Agrawal, R., Cruz, R., Okino, C., & Rajan, R., (1999, June). Performance Bounds for Flow Control Protocols. *IEEE/ACM Transaction on Networking, 7* (3).

Ahmed, T., Asgari, A., Mehaoua, A., Borcoci, E., Berti-Equille, L., & Georgios, K. (2006). End-to-end quality of service provisioning through an integrated management system for multimedia content delivery. *Computer Communications, 30*(3), 638–651. doi:10.1016/j.comcom.2006.10.009

Ahn, G.-S., Campbell, A. T., Veres, A., & Sun, L. H. (2002). Supporting Service Differentiation for Real-Time and Best-Effort Traffic in Stateless Wireless Ad Hoc Networks (SWAN). *IEEE Transactions on Mobile Computing, 1*, 192–207. doi:10.1109/TMC.2002.1081755

Ahn, G.S., Campbell, A.T., Lee, S.B., & Zhang, X. (1999). INSIGNIA. IETF MANET WG Internet Draft: draft-ietf-manet-insignia-01.

Ahn, J. S., Hong, S. W., & Heidemann, J. (2005). An Adaptive FEC Code Control Algorithm for Mobile Wireless Sensor Networks. *Journal of Communication and Networks*, *7*(4), 1–10.

Akan, O.B., & Akyildiz, I.F. (2005). Event-to-sink reliable transport in wireless sensor networks. *IEEE/ACM Transactions on Networking, 13*(5), 1003-1016.

Akkaya, K., & Younis, M. (2003). An energy-aware QoS routing protocol for wireless sensor networks. In *Proceedings of the 23rd International Conference on Distributed Computing Systems Workshops*, (pp. 710–715).

Akyildiz, I. F., Su, W., Sankarasubramaniam, Y., & Cayirci, E. (2002). Wireless Sensor Networks: A Survey. *Elsevier Computer Networks*, *38*(4), 393–422. doi:10.1016/S1389-1286(01)00302-4

Akyildiz, I., Su, W., Sankarasubramaniam, Y., & Cayirci, E. (2002). A Survey on Sensor Networks. *Computer Networks*, *38*(4), 393–422. doi:10.1016/S1389-1286(01)00302-4

Alena, R. L., & Lee, C. (2005). Adaptive bio-inspired wireless network routing for planetary surface exploration. IEEE Aerospace Conference (pp.1438 – 1443).

Ali, A. A., & Fisal, N. (2008). A real-time routing protocol with load distribution in wireless sensor networks. *Computer Communications*, *31*(14), 3190–3203. doi:10.1016/j.comcom.2008.04.030

Anand, M., Cronin, E., Sherr, M., Blaze, M., Ives, Z., & Lee, I. (2006). Sensor Network Security: More Interesting Than You Think. In *Proc. of 1st USENIX Workshop on Hot Topics in Security.*

Anderson, E. W., & Sullivan, M. W. (1993). The Antecedents and Consequences of Customer Satisfaction for Firms. *Marketing Science*, *12*(2), 125–143. doi:10.1287/mksc.12.2.125

Andersson, J. (2002). *Addressing VoIP speech quality with non-intrusive measurements.* Retrieved January 02, 2005 from http://www.techonline.com/community/tech_group/comm/tech_paper/21663

Andersson, L., Doolan, P., Feldman, N., Fredette, A., & Thomas, B. (2001). *LDP Specification, RFC 3036.*

Andersson, L., Minei, I. & Thomas, B. (2007, October). *LDP Specification.* RFC 5036. IETF.

Apostolopoulos, G., Guerin, R., Kamat, S., & Tripathi, S. (1999). Improving QoS routing performance under inaccurate link state information. In *16th International Teletraffic Congress* (ITC. 16).

Apostolopoulos, G., Kama, S., Williams, D., Guerin, R., Orda, A. & Przygienda, T. (1999, August). *QoS Routing Mechanisms and OSPF Extensions.* RFC 2676. IETF.

Aslam, F., Uzmi, Z. A., & Farrel, A. (2007). Interdomain Path Computation: Challenges and Solutions for Label Switched Networks. *IEEE Communications Magazine*, *45*(10), 94–101. doi:10.1109/MCOM.2007.4342830

Aspirot, L., Belzarena, P., Bermolen, P., Ferragut, A., Perera, G., & Simon, M. (2005). Quality of service parameters and link operating point estimation based on effective bandwidths. *Performance Evaluation*, *59*(2-3), 103–120. doi:10.1016/j.peva.2004.07.006

Atallah, M. J., & Blanton, M. (1999). *Algorithms and Theory of Computation Handbook.* Boca Raton, FL: CRC Press LLC.

Aukia, P., Kodialam, M., Koppol, P., Lakshman, T., Sarin, H., & Suter, B. (2000). Rates: a server for MPLS traffic engineering. *IEEE Network*, *14*, 34–41. doi:10.1109/65.826370

Avallone, S., Kuipers, F., Ventre, G., & Mieghem, P. V. (2006). Dynamic Routing in QoSaware Traffic Engineered Networks. In *EUNICE 2005: Networks and applications towards a ubiquitously connected world* (pp. 45–58). Boston: Springer. doi:10.1007/0-387-31170-X_4

Awduche, D. (1999). MPLS and traffic engineering in IP networks. *IEEE Communications Magazine*, *37*, 42–47. doi:10.1109/35.809383

Awduche, D., Berger, L., Gan, D., Li, T., Srinivasan, V., & Swallow, G.. (2001). *RSVP-TE: Extensions to RSVP for LSP Tunnels, RFC 3209, updated by RFCs 3936, 4420.*

Awduche, D., Chiu, A., Elwalid, A., Widjaja, I. & Xiao, X. (2002, May). *Overview and Principles of Internet traffic Engineering.* RFC 3272. IETF.

Awduche, D., Malcolm, J., Agogbua, J., O'Dell, M. & McManus, J. (1999, September). *Requirements for traffic Engineering Over MPLS.* RFC 2702. IETF.

Bacco, G. D., Melodia, T., & Cuomo, F. (2004). A MAC protocol for Delay-Bounded applications in Wireless Sensor Networks. In *Proc of Third Annual Mediterranean Ad Hoc Networking Workshop (Med-Hoc-Net 2004),* (pp. 208-220).

Badis, H., & Agha, K. A. (2004). QOLSR multi-path routing for mobile ad hoc networks based on multiple metrics: bandwidth and delay. IEEE Vehicular Technology Conference, (Vol. 4, pp. 2181-2184).

Badis, H., & Agha, K. A. (2006). CEQMM: a complete and efficient quality of service model for MANETs. ACM Intlernational workshop on Performance Evaluation of wireless ad hoc, sensor & ubiquitous networks (pp. 25–32).

Bagula, A., Botha, M., & Krzesinki, A. (2004). The least interference optimization algorithm. In. *Proceedings of the IEEE International Conference on Communications, 2,* 1232–1236.

Bansal, P. K., & Papantoni-Kazakos, P. (1986). An Algorithm for Detecting a Change in a Stochastic Process. *IEEE Transactions on Information Theory, IT-32,* 227–235. doi:10.1109/TIT.1986.1057160

Barakovic, J., Bajric, H., & Husic, A. (2007). QoS Design Issues and Traffic Engineering in Next Generation IP/ MPLS Network. In *proceedings of the 9th International Conference on Telecommunications (ConTel 2007),* (pp. 203-210).

Bar-Noy, A., & Kessler, I. (1993). Tracking Mobile Users in Wireless Networks. *Proceedings - IEEE INFOCOM, 93,* 1232–1239.

Bar-Noy, A., & Kessler, I. (1994). Mobile Users: To Update or not to Update? *Proceedings - IEEE INFOCOM, 94,* 570–576.

Basagni, S., Chlamtac, I., Syrotiuk, V. R., & Woodward, B. A. (1998). A Distance Routing Effect Algorithm for Mobilty (DREAM). In *Fourth Annual ACM / IEEE International Conference on Mobile Computing and Networking,* (pp. 76-84).

Beker, S., Puech, N., & Friderikos, V. (2004). A Tabu Search Heuristic for the Offline MPLS Reduced Complexity Layout Design Problem. In *Networking* (p. 514525). Berlin, Germany: Springer.

Benmohamed, L., Liang, C., Naber, E. & Terzis, A. (2006). *QoS Enhancements to BGP in Support of Multiple Classes of Service.* draftliangbgpqos00.txt, work in progress, IETF.

Bernet, Y., Ford, P., Yavatkar, R., Baker, F., Zhang, L., Speer, M., Braden, R., Davie, B., Wroclawski, J., & Felstaine, E., (2000). *A Framework for Integrated Services Operation over Diffserv Networks, RFC 2998.*

Berruto, E., Eynard, C., Fiorina, E., & Napolitano, A. (1993). Issues in Protocol Evolution for Personal Telecommunications. In *Proceedings IEEE GLOBECOM '93,* (pp. 555-559).

Bertrand, G., Lahoud, S., Molnar, M., & Texier, G. (2008). *InterDomain Path Computation with Multiple Constraints* (Tech. Rep. No. 1902). IRISA Campus de Beaulieu 35042 Rennes Cedex: IRISA. Retrieved from http://hal.inria.fr

Bertrand, G., Lahoud, S., Texier, G., & Molnár, M. (2009). Computation of Multi-Constrained Paths in Multi-Domain MPLS-TE Networks. In *NGI 2009: Fifth EuroNGI Conference on Next Generation Internet Networks* (to appear). Piscataway, NJ: IEEE Computer Society.

Bianchi, G. R., Vieira, F. H. T., & Ling, L. L. (2004). A novel network traffic predictor based on multifractal traffic characteristic. In *Proceedings of the IEEE Global Telecommunications Conference, 2004. GLOBECOM'04, 2,* (pp. 680-684).

Black, D., Brim, S., Carpenter, B., & Le Faucheur, F. (2001). Per Hop Behavior Identification Codes. RFC 3140.

Blake, S., Black, D., Carlson, M., Davies, E., Wang, Z. & Weiss, W. (1998, December). *An Architecture for Differentiated Service.* RFC 2475. IETF.

Bless, R. (2004). Towards Scalable Management of QoS-based End-to-End Services. In *Proc. of NOMS '04,* Seoul, Korea, (pp. 293-306).

Boucadair, M. (2005). *QoS-Enhanced Border Gateway Protocol. Technical report.* France Telecom.

Bouch, A., & Sasse, M. A. (1999). *It ain't what you charge, it's the way that you do it: a user perspective of network QoS and pricing.* Proceedings of the Sixth IFIP/IEEE International Symposium on Distributed Management for the Networked Millennium, Boston.

Bouch, A., & Sasse, M. A. (1999). *Network Quality of Service – An Integrated Perspective.* Paper presented at the 4th International distributed conference (IDC'99), Madrid, Spain.

Bouch, A., Kuchinsky, A., & Bhatti, N. (2000). *Quality is in the eye of the beholder: meeting users' requirements for Internet quality.* Paper presented at the Proceedings of the SIGCHI conference on Human factors in computing systems The Hague, The Netherlands

Bouch, A., Sasse, M. A., & DeMeer, H. (2000). *Of packets and people: a user-centered approach to quality of service.* Paper presented at the Eight International Workshop on Quality of Service, Pittsburgh, PA, USA.

Boudec, J., & Thiran, P. (2004, May 10). Network Calculus: A Theory of Deterministic Queuing Systems for the Internet. In *LNCS 2050.* Berlin: Springer-Verlag.

Bouras, C., Campanella, M., Przybylski, M., & Sevasti, A. (2003, February). QoS and SLA aspects across multiple management domains: the SEQUIN approach. *Future Generation Computer Systems archive, 19*(2), 313 – 326.

Bouras, C., Gkamas, A., & Stamos, K. (2008). Monitoring End to End Bandwidth on Demand Circuits over Ethernet Infrastructure. In *Seventh International Network Conference – INC 2008,* Plymouth, UK, 8 - 10 July 2008.

Bouras, C., Haniotakis, V., Primpas, D., Stamos, K., & Varvitsiotis, A. (2007). AMPS - ANStool: Interoperability of automated tools for the provisioning of QoS services. *TERENA Networking Conference 2007,* Lyngby, Denmark, 21 - 24 May 2007.

Boutaba, R., & Xiao, J. (2002). Network management: state of the art. In Communication systems: The state of the art IFIP world computer congress (pp. 127-146). Deventer, Netherlands: Kluwer, B.V.

Bower, J. (1970). Planing within the firm. *The American Economic Review, 60*(2), 186–194.

Bower, J. L. (1970). *Managing the resource allocation process.* Homewood, IL: Richard D. Irwin, Inc.

Bower, J. L., & Christensen, C. M. (1995, January-February). Diusruptive technologies: Catching the wave. *Harvard Business Review,* 43–53.

Braden, R. (Ed.). (1997). Resource ReSerVation Protocol (RSVP) - Version 1 Functional Specification. IETF RFC 2205.

Braden, R., Clark, D. & Shenker, S. (1994, June). *Integrated Services in the Internet architecture: an Overview.* RFC 1633. IETF.

Bradshaw, J. M. (Ed.). (1997). *Software Agents.* Cambridge, MA: MIT Press.

Brady, P. T. (1965). A Technique for Investigating On-Off Patterns of Speech. *The Bell System Technical Journal,* 1–22.

Brady, P. T. (1968). A Statistical Analysis of On-Off Patterns in 16 Conversations. *The Bell System Technical Journal,* 73–91.

Brenner, W., Zarnekow, R., & Hartmut, W. (1998). *Intelligent Software Agents.* Berlin: Springer.

Brim, S., Carpenter, B., & LeFaucheur, F. (2000). Per Hop Behavior Identification Codes. In Internet Engineering Task Force Request for Comment – IETF RFC 2836.

Britt, R. (2000, 5.12). *Ip-telephony*. Paper presented at the FCC Industry Meeting.

Bross, J. F. M., & Meinel, C. (2008), Can VoIP Live up to the QoS Standards of Traditional Wireline Telephony? *AICT, Fourth Advanced International Conference on Telecommunications,* (pp.126-132).

Bruckner, D., Sallans, B., & Russ, G. (2007). Hidden Markov Models for Traffic Observation. In *5th IEEE International Conference on Industrial Informatics,* (pp. 23-27).

Bucklew, J. (1990). *Large deviation techniques in decision, simulation, and estimation.* New York: John Wiley & Sons.

BuddeComm. (2007). *June 2007 Global NGN IP VoIP – Analyses Statistics and Forecasts.* BuddeComm.

Burgelman, R. (1983). A model of the interaction of strategic behaviour, corporate context, and the concept of strategy. *Academy of Management Review, 3*(1), 61–69. doi:10.2307/257168

Burgelman, R. (1983). A process model of internal corporate venturing in teh diversified major firm. *Administrative Science Quarterly, 28*(2), 223–244. doi:10.2307/2392619

Burrell, A. T. (1994). Traffic Management in Broadband Integrated Services Digital Networks. unpublished doctoral dissertation, University of Virginia, Charlottesville, VA.

Burrell, A. T., & Papantoni-Kazakos, P. (1996). Signaling, Transmission, and Dynamic Capacity Allocation Viewed in an Integrated Fashion. In *ITC Mini-Seminar Performance Modeling and Design of Wireless/PCS Networks.* Cambridge, MA: Wireless Networks in Hybrid Topologies.

Burrell, A. T., & Papantoni-Kazakos, P. (1998). Extended Sequential Algorithms for Detecting Changes in Acting Stochastic Processes. *IEEE Transactions on Systems, Man, and Cybernetics, 28*(5), 703–710. doi:10.1109/3468.709621

Burrell, A. T., & Papantoni-Kazakos, P. (1999), On-Line Learning and Dynamic Capacity Allocation in the TrafficManagement of Integrated Services Networks. In European Transactions on Telecommunications, Special Issue on Architectures, Protocols, and Quality of Service for the Internet of the Future, 10(5), 202-214.

Burrell, A. T., Makrakis, D., & Papantoni-Kazakos, P. (1998). Traffic Monitoring for Capacity Allocation of Multimedia Traffic in ATM Broadband Networks. *IEEE Journal on High-Speed Networks, 9,* 173–206.

Burrell, A. T., Papantoni-Kazakos, P., & Stren, H. (1998). Dynamic Capacity Allocation and Hybrid Multiplexing Techniques For ATM Wireless Networks. *Journal on Wireless Networks, 3,* 307–316.

Busch, C., Ismail, M. M., Sivrikaya, F., & Yener, B. (2004). Contention-Free MAC Protocols for Wireless Sensor Networks", *In Proc. Of 18th International Conference on Distributed Computing, DISC'04, Amsterdam,* (pp. 245-259).

Calafate, C. T., Manzoni, P., & Malumbres, M. P. (2006). A Novel QoS Framework for Medium-Sized MANETs Supporting Multipath Routing Protocols. In 11th IEEE Symposium on Computers and Communications (pp. 213- 219).

Campanella, M., Krzywania, R., Reijs, V., Sevasti, A., Stamos, K., Tziouvaras, C., & Wilson, D. (2006). Bandwidth on Demand Services for European Research and Education Networks. In *1st IEEE International Workshop on Bandwidth on Demand,* 27 Nov 2006, San Francisco.

Capone, A., Fratta, L., & Martignon, F. (2003). Virtual Flow Deviation: Dynamic Routing of Bandwidth Guaranteed Connections. In *QoSIP 2003: Proceedings of the second international workshop on quality of service in multiservice IP networks* (pp. 592-605). London: SpringerVerlag.

Carlson, E., Karl, H., Wolisz, A., & Prehofer, C. (2006). Distributed allocation of time-slots for real-time traffic in a wireless multi-hop network. *IEEE JSAC, 24*(11), 2018–2027.

Carroll, G. R. (1985). Concentration and specialization: Dynamics of niche width in populations of organizations. *American Journal of Sociology, 90*, 1262–1283. doi:10.1086/228210

Cavazzoni, C. (2007). MUPBED Overview and Architecture. In *TERENA Networking Conference 2007*, Copenhagen, Denmark.

Chandler, D. P., Hulburt, A. P., & McTiffin, M. J. M. J. (1991). An ATM-CDMA Air Interface for Mobile Personal Communications. In COST 231 TD (94).

Chandrasekaran, G. (2001). Performance Evaluation of Scheduling Mechanisms for Broadband Networks. Chennai, India: Master of Science, Anna University.

Chandy, R. K., & Tellis, G. J. (1998, November). Organizing for radical product innovation: The overlooked role of willingness to cannibalize. *JMR, Journal of Marketing Research, 35*, 474–487. doi:10.2307/3152166

Chang, C. S. (1994). Stability, Queue Length and Delay of Deterministic and Stochastic Queueing Networks. *IEEE Transactions on Automatic Control, 39*(5), 913–931. doi:10.1109/9.284868

Chang, C. S., & Thomas, J. A. (1995). Effective bandwidth in high-speed digital networks. *IEEE Journal on Selected Areas in Communications, 13*(6), 1091–1100. doi:10.1109/49.400664

Chaudet, C., & Lassous, I. G. (2002). BRuIT: Bandwidth Reservation under InTerferences influence. Paper presented at the European Wireless, Florence, Italy.

Chaudet, C., & Lassous, I. G. (2005). Evaluation of the BRuIT protocol. IEEE 61st Vehicular Technology Conference, (Vol. 4, pp. 2493 – 2497).

Chen, C.-L. (2006). *The signaling protocol for intserv operation over diffserv model.* Tech Rep. No. 2002 ICS, Feng Chia University, Taiwan.

Chen, D., & Varshney, P. (2004). QoS Support in Wireless Sensor Networks: A Survey. In *Proceedings of the International Conference on Wireless Networks (ICWN 2004)*, Las Vegas, NV, (pp. 227-233).

Chen, J.-L., Chen, M.-C., & Chian, Y.-R. (2007). QoS management in heterogeneous home networks. *Computer Networks, 51*(12), 3368–3379. doi:10.1016/j.comnet.2007.01.032

Chen, S. & Nahrstedt, K. (1998-2). An overview of quality-of-service routing for the next generation high-speed networks: Problems and solutions. *IEEE Network, Nov/Dec, 12*(6), 64-79.

Chen, S., & Nahrstedt, K. (1998). Distributed Quality-of-Service Routing in the Ad-Hoc Networks. *IEEE Journal on Special Areas in Communications, 17*(8), 1488–1505. doi:10.1109/49.780354

Chen, S., & Nahrstedt, K. (1998). On finding multi-constrained paths. *IEEE International Conference on Communications*, (vol. 2, pp. 874-879).

Chen, S., & Nahrstedt, K. (1999). Distributed quality of service routing in ad hoc networks. *IEEE Journal on Selected Areas in Communications, 17*(8), 1488–1505. doi:10.1109/49.780354

Chesbrough, H. W. (2003). Environmental influences upon firm ebtry into new sub-markets: Evidence from the worldwqide hard disk drive industry conditionally. *Research Policy, 32*, 659–678. doi:10.1016/S0048-7333(02)00033-1

Chipara, O., He, Z., Xing, G., Chen, Q., Wang, X., Lu, C., et al. (2006). Real-time Power-Aware Routing in Sensor Networks. In *Proc. 14th IEEE International Workshop on Quality of Service (IWQoS 2006)*, (pp. 83-92).

Chiu, J.-F., Huang, Z.-P., Lo, C.-W., Hwang, W.-S., & Shieh, C.-K. (2003). Supporting end-to-end QoS in DiffServ/MPLS networks. In *10th International Conference on Telecommunications (ICT 2003), 1*, (pp. 261-266).

Chlamtac, I. & Farago, A. (1994). Making Transmission Schedules Immune to Topology Changes in Multi-Hop Packet Radio Networks. *IEEE/ACM Transactions on Networking, 2* (1), 23-29.

Cho, H. S., Lee, B. H., Kim, M. K., Lee, S. Y., & Youn, C. H. (2006). A Secure Mobile Healthcare System based on Surrogate Host. *The Sixth IEEE International*

Conference on Computer and Information Technology. (pp. 153-157).

Christensen, C. M. (1993). The rigid disk drive industry: A history of commercial and technological turbulence. *Business History Review*, (67): 531–588. doi:10.2307/3116804

Christensen, C. M. (1997). *The innovator's dilemma: When new technologies cause great firms to fail.* Boston: Harvard Business School Press.

Christensen, C. M. (2002). The rules of innovation. *Technology Review*, *105*, 32–38.

Christensen, C. M., & Bower, J. (1996). Customer power, strategic investment, and the failure of leading firms. *Strategic Management Journal*, *17*, 197–218. doi:10.1002/(SICI)1097-0266(199603)17:3<197::AID-SMJ804>3.0.CO;2-U

Christensen, C. M., & Rosenbloom, R. S. (1994). Technological discontinuities, organizational capabilities, and strategic commitments. *Industrial and Corporate Change*, (3): 655–685.

Christensen, C. M., & Rosenbloom, R. S. (1995). Explaining the attacker's advantage: The technological paradigms, organizational dynamics, and the value network. *Research Policy*, *24*, 233–257. doi:10.1016/0048-7333(93)00764-K

Christiansen, M., Jeffay, K., Ott, D. & Smith, F.D. (2001 June).Tuning RED for Web Traffic. *IEEE/ACM Transactions on Networking.*

Chui, C. K. (1992). *An introduction to wavelets.* San Diego, CA: Academic Press Professional, Inc.

Cisco. (1997). *Configuring OSPF.* Documentation at http://www.cisco.com/en/US/docs/ios/ 12_0/np1/configuration/guide/1cospf.pdf

Claypool, M., & Tanner, J. (1999). The Effects of Jitter on the Perceptual Quality of Video. In *Proc. ACM Multimedia*, (pp. 115-118).

Cohen, A. J. (1984). Technological change as historical process: The case of the U.S. Pulp and paper industry, 1915-1940. *The Journal of Economic History*, *44*(3), 775–799. doi:10.1017/S0022050700032368

Coltum, R. (1998 July). The OSPF Opaque LSA Option. *RFC 2370.*

Conner, W., Heidemann, J., Krishnamurthy, L., Wang, X., & Yarvis, M. (2004). Workplace applications of sensor networks. In Bulusu, N., & Jha, S. (Eds.), *Wireless Sensor Networks: A Systems Perspective.* Boston: Artech House.

Conti, M., Giordano, S., Maselli, G., & Turi, G. (2003). MobileMAN: Mobile Metropolitan Ad Hoc Networks. Berlin: Springer. *Lecture Notes in Computer Science*, *2775*, 169–174.

Cooper, A., & Schendel, D. (1976, Feb.). Strategic responses to technological threats. *Business Horizons*, *19*, 61–69. doi:10.1016/0007-6813(76)90024-0

Courcoubetis, C., & Weber, R. (1996). Buffer overflow asymptotics for a buffer handling many traffic sources. *Journal of Applied Probability*, *33*, 886–903. doi:10.2307/3215366

Courcoubetis, C., Siris, V. A., & Stamoulis, G. D. (1999). Application of the many sources asymptotic and effective bandwidths to traffic engineering. *Telecommunication Systems*, *12*, 167–191. doi:10.1023/A:1019194628625

Coviello, G. J., & Vena, G. P. (1975). Integration of Circuit/Packet Switching by a SENET (Slotted Envelope Network) Concept. In *Conference Rec. 1975 National Telecommunications Conference*, (pp. 42-12 -- 42-17).

Cox, D. C. (1992). Network Control for Wireless Communications Networks. *IEEE Communications Magazine*, 96–115. doi:10.1109/35.210361

Cox, D. C., Gifford, W. S., & Sherry, H. (1991). Low-Power Digital Radio as a Ubiquitous Subscriber Loop. *IEEE Communications Magazine*, 92–95. doi:10.1109/35.75532

Crawley, E., Nair, R., Rajagopalan, B., & Sandick, H. (1998). *A framework for QoS- based routing in the internet. In Internet Engineering Task Force Request for*

Comment – IETF RFC2386. Retrieved from http://www.ietf.org/rfc/rfc2386.txt

Cristallo, G., & Jacquenet, C. (2002). An Approach to Inter-domain Traffic Engineering. *Proc. of WTC '02*, Paris, France.

Crosby, P. B. (1979). *Quality is Free: The Art of Making Quality Certain*. New York: New American Library.

Crovella, M. E., & Bestavros, A. (1997). Self-similarity in World Wide Web traffic: evidence and possiblecauses. *IEEE/ACM Transactions on networking, 5*(6), 835-846.

Crowcroft, J., Hand, S., Mortier, R., Roscoe, T., & Warfield, A. (2003). *QoS's downfall: at the bottom, or not at all!* Paper presented at the Conference ACM SIGCOMM workshop on Revisiting IP QoS: What have we learned, why do we care? Karlsruhe, Germany.

Dale, B. G., & Cooper, C. L. (1994). Introducing TQM. *Management Decision, 32*(1), 20–26. doi:10.1108/00251749410050660

Dam, T. V., & Langendoen, K. (2003). An Adaptive Energy-Efficient MAC Protocol for Wireless Sensor Networks. In *Proc. of ACM Conference on Embedded Networked Sensor System, Los Angeles, CA*.

De Neve, H., & Van Mieghem, P. (2000). Tamcra: A tunable accuracy multiple constraints routing algorithm. *Computer Communications, 23*, 667–679. doi:10.1016/S0140-3664(99)00225-X

De Prycker, M. (1993). *Asynchronous Transfer Mode—Solution for Broadband ISDN* (2nd ed.). New York: Ellis Horwood.

De, S., Das, S. K., Wu, H., & Qiao, C. (2002). Trigger-based distributed QoS routing in mobile ad hoc networks. *ACM SIGMOBILE Mobile Computing and Communications Review, 6*(3), 22–35. doi:10.1145/581291.581298

Dehbi, Y., & Mikou, N. (2008). Priority Assignment for Multimedia Packets Scheduling in MANET. IEEE International Conference on Signal Image Technology and Internet Based Systems (pp. 32-37).

Delgado, G. D., Frias, V. C., & Igartua, M. A. (2006). Video-streaming Transmission with QoS over Cross-Layered Ad hoc Networks. International Conference on Software in Telecommunications and Computer Networks, SoftCOM, (pp.102 – 106).

Demazeau, Y. (1998). Preface. In *3rd International Conference on Multi-Agent Systems*, Paris, *ICMAS 98*.

Demirkol, I., Ersoy, C. & Alagoz, F. (2006). MAC Protocols for Wireless Sensor Networks: A Survey. *IEEE Comm. Magzine*, 115-121.

Deng, J., & Haas, Z. (1998). Dual Busy Tone Multiple Access (DBTMA), A New Medium Access Control for Packet Radio Networks. IEEE International Conference on Universal Personal Communications, (Vol. 2, pp. 973-977).

Deshpande, A., Guestrin, C., Madden, S., Hellerstein, J., & Hong, W. (2004). Model-Driven Data Acquisition in Sensor Networks. In *Proc. of the 13th international conference on Very large data bases*, Canada.

Dewar, R. D., & Dutton, J. E. (1986). The adoption of radical and incremental innovations: An empirical analysis. *Management Science, 32*(11), 1422–1433. doi:10.1287/mnsc.32.11.1422

Di Battista, G., Erlebach, T., Hall, A., Patrignani, M., Pizzonia, M., & Schank, T. (2007). Computing the Types of the Relationships between Autonomous Systems. *Transactions on Networking, 15*(2), 267–280. doi:10.1109/TNET.2007.892878

DJ3.2.2.3. (2007). *Third review of Bandwidth on Demand related technologies (DJ3.2.2.3)*.

DJ3.3.1. (2008). Definition of Bandwidth on Demand Framework and General Architecture (DJ3.3.1).

Doshi, B. T., Eggenschwiler, D., Rao, A., Samadi, B., Wang, Y. T., & Wolfson, J. (2003). Voip network architectures and qos strategy. *Bell Labs Technical Journal, 7*(4), 41–59. doi:10.1002/bltj.10033

Dosi, G. (1982). Technological paradigms and technological trajectories. *Research Policy, 11*, 147–162. doi:10.1016/0048-7333(82)90016-6

Douville, R., Le Roux, J. L., Rougier, J. L., & Secci, S. (2008, June). A Service Plane over the PCE Architecture for Automatic Multidomain ConnectionOriented Services. *IEEE Communications Magazine*, *46*(6), 94–101. doi:10.1109/MCOM.2008.4539472

DTAG. (2004). *Vendor market report - insights into the telecommunication and information technology equipment and software markets (internal paper)*. Deutsche Telekom AG - Zentralbereich Technologie und Plattformen.

Du, J., Liu, H., & Chen, P. (2007). OMR: An Opportunistic Multi-Path Reliable Routing Protocol in Wireless Sensor Networks. In *Proc. of International Conference on Parallel Processing Workshops*.

Duffield, N. G., & O'Connell, N. (1995). Large deviations and overflow probabilities for the general single-server queue, with applications. *Mathematical Proceedings of the Cambridge Philosophical Society*, *118*, 363–374. doi:10.1017/S0305004100073709

Dulman, S., Nieberg, T., Wu, J., & Havinga, P. (2003). Trade-off between Traffic Overhead and Reliability in Multipath Routing for Wireless Sensor Networks. In *Proc. of WCNC Workshop*, New Orleans, LA.

Durham, D., Boyle, J., Cohen, R., Herzog, S., Rajan, R., & Sastry, A. (2000). *The COPS (Common Open Policy Service) Protocol, RFC 2748*.

Dutton, J., & Thomas, A. (1985). Relating technological change and learnign by doing. *Research on Technological innovation. Management and Policy*, *2*, 187–224.

EIA/TIA. (1990). *Interim Standard IS-54*. Washington, D.C.: Cellular System Dual-Mode Mobile Station-Base Station Compatibility Standard.

EIA/TIA. (1991). *Cellular Radio Telecommunications Intersystem Operations*. Revision B, Technical Report IS-41, EIA/TIA.

El-Gendy, M. A., & Shin, K. G. (2003). Evolution of the Internet QoS and Support for Soft Real-time Applications. *Proceedings of the IEEE*, *91*(7). doi:10.1109/JPROC.2003.814615

El-Haddadeh, R., Taylor, G. A., & Watts, S. J. (2004). Towards scalable end-to-end QoS provision for VoIP applications. Telecommunications Quality of Services: The Business of Success, (pp.132-135).

El-Haddadeh, R., Watts, S. J., & Taylor, G. A. (2006). Charging QoS Inter-Domain Networks: IntServ over DiffServ. In *IEEE Global Telecommunications Conference, (GLOBECOM '06)*, (pp. 1-5).

Elovici, Y., Ben-Shimol, Y., & Shabtai, A. (2003). Per-Packet Pricing Scheme for IP Networks. In *10th International Conference on Telecommunications IEEE, 2*, 1494-1500.

Elwalid, A. & Mitra, D. (1993). Effective bandwidth of general Markovian traffic sources and admission control of high speed networks. *IEEE/ACM Transactions on networking, 1*(3), 329-343.

Eppstein, D. (1994). *Finding the k shortest paths. In 35th* (pp. 154–165). Santa Fe: IEEE Symp. Foundations of Comp. Science.

Erbas, S. C., & Erbas, C. (2003, Aug.Sep.). A Multiobjective Offline Routing Model for MPLS Networks. In J. Charzinski, R. Lehnert, & P. TranGia (Eds.), Providing quality of service in heterogeneous environments, 5, proceedings of the 18th international teletraffic congress. Amsterdam, Netherlands: Elsevier B.V.

Ergen, S. C., & Varaiya, P. (2006). PEDAMACS: Power Efficient and Delay Aware Medium Access Protocol for Sensor Networks. *IEEE Transactions on Mobile Computing*, *5*(7), 920–930. doi:10.1109/TMC.2006.100

Erramilli, A., Narayan, O., & Willinger, W. (1996). Experimental queueing analysis with long-range dependent packet traffic. *IEEE/ACM Transactions on Networking, 4*(2). 209-223.

Erramilli, A., Narayan, O., Neidhardt, A., Saniee, I., & Qnetworx, M. (2000). Performance impacts of multi-scaling in wide area TCP/IP traffic. In *Proceedings of the Nineteenth Annual Joint Conference of the IEEE Computer and Communications Societies (INFOCOM 2000), 1*, (pp. 352-359).

ETSI. (1994). ETR 003: Network Aspects (NA); General aspects of Quality of Service (QoS) and Network Performance (NP).

ETSI. (2001). *Telecommunications and internet protocol harmonization over networks (tiphon) release 3; end-to-end quality of service in tiphon systems; part 2: Definition of speech quality of service (qos) classes.* ETSI.

ETSI. (2003). TR 102 276: User's Quality of Service Criteria for Internet Access in Europe.

ETSI. (2005). EG 202 057: Speech Processing, Transmission and Quality Aspects (STQ); User related QoS parameter definitions and measurements.

ETSI. (2007). EG 202 009-1: Quality of telecom services; Part 1: Methodology for identification of parameters relevant to the users.

ETSI. (2007). EG 202 009-2: Quality of telecom services; Part 2: User related parameters on a service specific basis.

Falkner, M., Devetsikiotis, M., & Lambadaris, I., (2000). An Overview of Pricing Concepts for Broadband IP Networks. *IEEE Communication Surveys,* (2), 2-13.

Fang, Y., & McDonald, B. (2004). Dynamic codeword routing (DCR): a cross-layer approach for performance enhancement of general multi-hop wireless routing. In *Proc. of IEEE SECON'04,* (pp. 255-263).

Farrel, A., Vasseur, J.P. & Ash, J. (2006, August*). A Path Computation Element (PCE)Based Architecture.* RFC 4655. IETF.

Farrel, A., Vasseur, J.P. & Ayyangar, A. (2006, November). *A Framework for InterDomain Multiprotocol Label Switching traffic Engineering.* RFC 4726. IETF.

Feigenbaum, J., Papadimitriou, C., Sami, R., & Shenker, S. (2005). A BGP-based mechanism for lowest-cost routing. *Distributed Computing, 18*(1), 61–72. doi:10.1007/s00446-005-0122-y

Feldmann, A., Gilbert, A. A., & Willinger, W. (1998). Data networks as cascades: investigating the multifractal nature of Internet WAN traffic. In *Proceedings of the ACM SIGCOMM '98 conference on Applications, technologies, architectures, and protocols for computer communication,* (pp. 42-55).

Feldmann, A., Gilbert, A. C., Willinger, W., & Kurtz, T. G. (1998). The changing nature of network traffic: Scaling phenomena. *ACM SIGCOMM Computer Communication Review, 28*(2), 5–29. doi:10.1145/279345.279346

Felemban, E., Lee, C., & Ekici, E. (2006). MMSPEED: multipath Multi-SPEED protocol for QoS guarantee of reliability and Timeliness in wireless sensor networks. *IEEE Transactions on Mobile Computing, 5*(6), 738–754. doi:10.1109/TMC.2006.79

Feng, W-C., Kapadia, A. & Thulasidasan, S. (n.d.). GREEN: proactive queue management over a best-effort network. *IEEE GLOBECOM,* (pp 1774 - 1778).

Ferber, J. (1999). *Multi-Agent Systems.* New York: Addison-Wesley.

Fgee, E. B. (2005). *Scalable QoS and QoS Management Models for IP Networks.* PhD Thesis, Dalhousie University, Halifax, Canada.

Fgee, E., Kenney, J., Phillips, W. I., Robertson, W., & Sivakumar, S. (2004, May 4-7). Implementing an IPv6 QoS management scheme using flow label & class of service fields. *IEEE CCECE 2004, Canadian Conference, 2,* 851 - 854.

Fgee, E.-B., Kenney, J. D., Phillips, W. J., Robertson, W., & Sivakumar, S. (2005, May 18). Comparison of QoS Performance between IPv6 QoS Management Model and IntServ and DiffServ QoS Models. In *Proceedings of the 3rd Annual Communication Networks and Services Research Conference,* (pp. 287 - 292).

Figueiredo, G., da Fonseca, N., & Monteiro, J. (2006). A minimum interference routing algorithm with reduced computational complexity. *Computer Networks: The International Journal of Computer and Telecommunications Networking, 50*(11), 1710–1732.

Firoiu, V., Boudec, J., Towsley, D., & Zhang, Z. (2002). Theories of Models for Internet Quality of Service. *Proceedings of the IEEE, 90*(9), 1565–1591. doi:10.1109/JPROC.2002.802002

Fischetti, M. (1993). The Cellular Phone Scare. [June.]. *IEEE Spectrum*, 43–47. doi:10.1109/6.214586

Fitzek, F. H. P., & Reisslein, M. (2001). MPEG-4 and H. 263 video traces for network performance evaluation. *Network, IEEE, 15*(6), 40–54. doi:10.1109/65.967596

Flegkas, P., Trimintzios, P., Pavlou, G., Andrikopoulos, I., & Cavalcanti, C. F. (2001). On Policy Based Extensible Hierarchical Network Management in QoSEnabled IP Networks. In *Policy '01: Proceedings ofthe international workshop on policies for distributed systems and networks* (pp. 230-246). London: SpringerVerlag.

Floyd, S. & Jacobson, V. (1993). Random Early Detection gateways for Congestion Avoidance. *IEEE/ACM Transactions on Networking, 1*(4), 397-413.

Floyd, S. (2003). *High Speed TCP for Large Congestion Windows*, RFC 3649.

Fonte, A., Curado, M., & Monteiro, E. (2008, December). Interdomai quality of service routing: setting the grounds for the way ahead. *Annales des Télécommunications, 63*(1), 683–695. doi:10.1007/s12243-008-0065-y

Fonte, A., Monteiro, E., & Yannuzzi, M. MasipBruin, X. & DomingoPascual, J. (2005). A Framework for Cooperative InterDomain QoS Routing. In EUNICE (pp. 91104). Secaucus, NJ: SpringerVerlag, Inc.

Fortz, B., & Thorup, M. (2004). Increasing Internet Capacity Using Local Search. *Computational Optimization and Applications, 29*(1), 13–48. doi:10.1023/B:COAP.0000039487.35027.02

Foster, R. N. (1986). *Innovation: The attacker's advantage*. New York: Summit Books.

FSIDM. (2007). *Functional Specification of GÉANT2 Inter-domain Manager (IDM)*. Prototype.

Fu, X., Wang, J., Zhou, W., & Song, J. (2006, Nov.). EndtoEnd QoS Architecture and Interdomain QoS Model across Multiple Domains. In *International Conference on Communication Technology. (ICCT)* (p. 14). New York: IEEE Communications Society.

Fu, Z., Yang, Y., Lee, T. S., & Park, M. S. (2006). Adapted Listening in Wireless Sensor Network MAC Protocol. In *Proc. of 3rd International Conference, UIC 2006, Wuhan, China*, (pp. 546-555).

Fullmer, C. L., & Garcia-Luna-Aceves, J. J. (1995). Floor Acquisition Multiple Access (FAMA) for Packet-Radio Networks. Conference on Applications, Technologies, Architectures, and Protocols for Computer Communication (SIGCOMM), (pp.262-273).

G.807. (2001 July). ITU-T Rec. G.807/Y.1302. *Requirements for Automatic Transport Networks (ASTN).*

G.8080 (2001). ITU-T Rec. G.8080/Y.1304. In *Architecture for the Automatically Switched Optical Networks, November 2001 and Amendment 1, March2003.*

Galluccio, L., Leonardi, A., Morabito, G., & Palazzo, S. (2007). A MAC/Routing cross-layer approach to geographic forwarding in wireless sensor networks. *Ad Hoc Networks, 5*(6), 872–884. doi:10.1016/j.adhoc.2007.02.004

Gao, J., & Rubin, I. (1999). Multifractal analysis and modeling of long-range-dependent traffic. *Proceedings of the IEEE International Conference on Communications, 1999, (ICC '99). 1,* 382-386.

Gao, J., & Rubin, I. (2000). Superposition of multiplicative multifractal traffic streams. In *Proceedings of the IEEE International Conference on Communications, 2000 (ICC 2000), 2,* (pp. 816-820).

Gao, L. (2001). On inferring autonomous system relationships in the Internet. *Transactions on Networking, 9*(6), 733–745. doi:10.1109/90.974527

Gao, L., & Rexford, J. (2000). Stable Internet routing without global coordination. In *Proc. ofSIGMETRICS'00* (pp. 307-317). Santa Clara, CA: ACM Press.

Gao, L., Griffin, T. G., & Rexford, J. (2001). Inherently safe backup routing with BGP. In *Proc. ofINFOCOM'01*, Anchorage, AK, *1*, 547-556.

Gardner, M. T., Frost, V. S., & Petr, D. W. (2003). *Using optimization to achieve efficient quality of service in voice over IP networks.* Retrieved January 03, 2009 from http://www.ittc.ku.edu/publications/documents/Gardner2003_ipc31-Todd-Gardner-VoIP-Optimization.pdf

Garrett, M. W., & Willinger, W. (1994). Analysis, modeling and generation of self-similar VBR video traffic. *Computer Communication Review, ACM SIGCOMM, 24*(4), 269–280. doi:10.1145/190809.190339

Gavalas, D., Greenwood, D., Ghanbari, M., & O'Mahony, M. (2002). Hierarchical network management: a scalable and dynamic mobile agentbased approach. *Computer Networks, 38*(6), 693–711. doi:10.1016/S1389-1286(01)00277-8

Ge, Z., Figueiredo, D. R., Jaiswal, S., & Gao, L. (2001). The hierarchical structure of the logical Internet graph. In *Proc. of SPIE-ITCOM'01, 4526*, (pp. 208-222).

GÉANT2. (2009). *GÉANT2: The pan-European R&E network*. Retrieved from http://www.geant2.net/

Gejji, R. (1992). Forward-Link-Power Control in CDMA Cellular Systems. In IEEE Transactions on Vehicular Technology (pp. 532 – 536).

Georgiadis, L., Merakos, L., & Papantoni-Kazakos, P. (1987). A Method for the Delay Analysis of Random Multiple Access Algorithms whose Delay Process is Regenerative. *IEEE Journal on Selected Areas in Communications, SAC-5*(6), 1051–1062. doi:10.1109/JSAC.1987.1146613

Gibbens, R. J., & Hunt, P. J. (1991). Effective bandwidths for the multi-type UAS channel. *Queueing Systems, 9*(1-2), 17–28. doi:10.1007/BF01158790

Gilbert, C. G., & Bower, J. (2002). Disruptive change - when trying harder is part of the problem. *Harvard Business Review*, 94–101.

Gilhousen, K. S., Jacobs, I. M., Padovani, R., Viterbi, A. J., Weaver, L. A., & Wheatley, C. E. III. (1991). On the Capacity of a Cellular CDMA System. *IEEE Transactions on Vehicular Technology*, 303–312. doi:10.1109/25.289411

Goldberg, S., & Wickramasinghe, N. (2003). 21ST Century Healthcare - The Wireless Panacea. *The 36th Annual Hawaii International Conference on System Sciences*, (pp.163b). Manoa, HI: University of Hawaii.

Goodman, D. J. (1991, June). Trends in Cellular and Cordless Communications. *IEEE Communications Magazine*, 31–40. doi:10.1109/35.79400

Goodman, D. J., & Wei, S. X. (1991). Efficiency of Packet Reservation Multiple Access. *IEEE Transactions on Vehicular Technology, 40*, 170–176. doi:10.1109/25.69985

Goodman, D. J., Pollini, G. P., & Meier-Hellstern, K. S. (1992). Network Control for Wireless Communications Networks. *IEEE Communications Magazine*, 116–125. doi:10.1109/35.210362

Goodman, D. J., Valenzuela, R. A., Gayliard, K. T., & Ramamurthi, B. (1989). Packet Reservation Multiple Access for Local Wireless Communications. *IEEE Transactions on Communications, 37*, 885–890. doi:10.1109/26.31190

Goodridge, W., Robertson, W., Phillips, W. J., & Sivakumar, S. (2004). *Multiple metric QoS in differentiated services networks using preference functions measurement concepts. Lecture Notes in Computer Science* (pp. 390–399). Berlin: Springer Verlag.

Goodridge, W., Robertson, W., Phillips, W. J., & Sivakumar, S. (2004). Over-constraint QoS routing in large networks. In. *Proceedings of the London Communications Symposium, 2*, 61–64.

Goodridge, W., Robertson, W., Phillips, W. J., & Sivakumar, S. (2005). Traffic driven multiple constraint-optimization for QoS routing. *International Journal of Internet Protocol Technology, 1*, 1–11. doi:10.1504/IJIPT.2005.007555

Gozdecki, J., Jajszczyk, A., & Stankiewicz, R. (2003). Quality of service terminology in IP networks. *IEEE Communications Magazine, 41*(3), 153–159. doi:10.1109/MCOM.2003.1186560

Griffin, D., Spencer, J., Griem, J., Boucadair, M., Morand, P., & Howarth, M. (2007, Feb.). Interdomain routing through QoSclass planes [QualityofServiceBased Routing Algorithms for Heterogeneous Networks]. *IEEE Communications Magazine, 45*(2), 8895.

Grossglauser, M., & Bolot, J. C. (1999). On the relevance

of long-range dependence in network traffic. *IEEE/ACM Transactions on Networking, 7*(5), 629-640.

Gruber, J. G. (1982). A Comparison of Measured and Calculated Temporal Patterns Relevant to Speech Activity Detection. *IEEE Transactions on Communications*, 728–738. doi:10.1109/TCOM.1982.1095514

Guerin, R. & Orda, A. (1999). QoS-based routing in networks with inaccurate information: Theory and algorithms. *IEEE/ACM Transactions on Networking, 7*(6), 350-364.

Guerin, R. A., Orda, A., & Williams, D. (1997, November). QoS routing mechanisms and OSPF extensions. In *IEEE Global Telecommunications Conference (GLOBECOM)* (Vol. 3, pp. 1903-1908). Piscataway, NJ: IEEE Computer Society.

Guérin, R., Ahmadi, H., & Naghshineh, M. (1991). Equivalent capacity and its application to bandwidth allocation in high-speed networks. *IEEE Journal on Selected Areas in Communications, 9*(7), 968–981. doi:10.1109/49.103545

Gungor, V. C., & Akan, O. B. (2007). Delay aware reliable transport in wireless sensor networks. *International Journal of Communication Systems, 20*(10), 1155–1177. doi:10.1002/dac.869

Guo, N., & Morgera, S. D. (1993). The Grade-of-Service for Integrated Voice/Data Wireless DS-CDMA Networks. In *Proceedings IEEE ICC '93* (pp. 1104-1110).

Guok, C. (2005). ESnet On-Demand Secure Circuits and Advance Reservation System (OSCARS). In *Internet2 Joint Techs Workshop*, Salt Lake City, Utah, February 15, 2005.

Hardy, W. C. (2001). *QoS: Measurement and Evaluation of Telecommunications Quality of Service*. Chichester, UK: John Wiley & Sons, Inc.

Harry, M. J., & Schroeder, R. R. (2000). *Six Sigma: The Breakthrough Management Strategy Revolutionizing the World's Top Corporations*. New York: Doubleday.

Hayes, M. H. (1996). *Statistical digital signal processing and modeling*. New York: John Wiley & Sons, Inc.

He, T., Stankovic, J., Lu, C., & Abdelzaher, T. (2003). SPEED: A stateless protocol for real-time communication in sensor networks. In *Proceedings of 23rd International Conference on Distributed Computing Systems*, (pp. 46–55).

He, W., Liu, X., Nguyen, H., Nahrstedt, K., & Abdelzaher, T. (2007). PDA: Privacy-preserving Data Aggregation in Wireless Sensor Networks. In *Proc. of IEEE INFOCOM'07.*

Hein, M., Reisner, M., & Voß, A. (2002). *Voice over IP: Sprach-daten-konvergenz richtig nutzen*. Berlin: Franzis Verlag GmbH.

Heinanen, J., Baker, F., Weiss, W. & Wroclawski, J. (June 1999). *Assured Forwarding PHB Group, RFC 2597.*

Heinzelman, W. (2000). *Application specific protocol architectures for wireless networks*. PhD Thesis, MIT, Cambridge, MA.

Hejmo, M., Mark, B. L., Zouridaki, C., & Thomas, R. K. (2005). A denial-of-service resistant quality-of-service signaling protocol for mobile ad hoc networks. In *Proceedings of the Second Conference on Quality of Service in Heterogeneous Wired. Wireless Networks, 2005*, 9–32.

Henderson, R. M. (1993). Underinvestment and incompetence as responses to radical innovation: Evidence from the photolithographic alignment equipment industry. *The Rand Journal of Economics, 24*(2), 248–270. doi:10.2307/2555761

Henderson, R. M., & Clark, K. B. (1990). Architectural innovation: The reconfiguration of existing systems abd the failure of established firms. *Administrative Science Quarterly, 35*, 9–30. doi:10.2307/2393549

Heyman, D. P. & Lakshman, T. V. (1996). What are the implications of long-range dependence for VBR-video traffic engineering? *IEEE/ACM Transactions on Networking (TON), 4*(3), 301-317.

Hiranpongsin, S., & Bhattarakosol, P. (2009). Intelligent

Cache Farming Architecture with the Recommender System. *International Journal of Engineering Science and Technology*, *4*(2), 206–219.

Hollot, C., Misra, V., Towsley, D., & Gong, W. (2001). *A Control Theoretic Analysis of RED*, INFOCOMM'01.

Hollot, C., Misra, V., Towsley, D., & Gong, W. (2002). Analysis and design of controllers for AQM routers supporting TCP flows. *IEEE Transactions on Automatic Control*, *47*(6). doi:10.1109/TAC.2002.1008360

Houck, D. J., & Yang, W. (2004). *Voicer over internet protocol - voice quality of service.* White Paper, Lucent Technologies - Bell Labs Innovators, Murray Hill, NJ.

Hsu, T., Tsai, K., Wang, D., & Lee, D. T. (1996). Steiner Problems on Directed Acyclic Graphs. In *Proc. of COCOON '96* (pp. 21-30). London: Springer-Verlag.

Hu, N., Li, L. E., Mao, Z. M., Steenkiste, P., & Wang, J. (2004). Locating internet bottlenecks: algorithms, measurements, and implications. *SIGCOMM Computer Communication Review*, *34*(4), 41–54. doi:10.1145/1030194.1015474

Hu, N., Zou, P., Zhu, P., & Liu, X. (2008). Cooperative Management Framework for interdomain Routing System. In *ATC '08: Proceedings of the 5th international conference on autonomic and trusted computing* (pp. 567-576). Berlin: SpringerVerlag.

Hu, Y., Hu, N., & Jia, X. (2006). Energy Efficient Real-Time Data Aggregation in Wireless Sensor Networks. In *Proc. of ACM IWCMC'06.*

Hu, Y., Xue, Y., Li, B., Xie, J., & Yang, H. (2005). A congestion control protocol for wireless sensor networks. *Journal of Information and Computational Science*, *2*(1), 41–50.

Hu, Y., Yu, F., & Deng, P. (2007). A Novel Data Query Method for Wireless Sensor Networks. In *Proc. of International Conference on Wireless Communications, Networking and Mobile Computing.*

Huang C., Tseng Y. & Wu, H. (2008). Distributed Protocols for Ensuring Both Coverage and Connectivity of a Wireless Sensor Network. *ACM Transactions on Sensor Networks, 3*(1).

Huang, C., & Tseng, Y. (2005). The Coverage Problem in a Wireless Sensor Network. [MONET]. *ACM Mobile Networks and Applications*, *10*(4), 519–528. doi:10.1007/s11036-005-1564-y

Huang, J. (2005). eTOM and ITIL: Should you be bi-lingual as an IT Outsourcing Service Provider? *BPTrends.*

Huang, X., & Fang, Y. (2008). Multiconstrained QoS multipath routing in wireless sensor networks. *Wireless Networks*, *14*(4), 465–478. doi:10.1007/s11276-006-0731-9

Hui-Lan, L., & Faynberg, I. (2003). An architectural framework for support of quality of service in packet networks. *IEEE Communications Magazine*, *41*, 98–105. doi:10.1109/MCOM.2003.1204754

Huston, G. (2000). Next Steps for the IP QoS Architecture. RFC 2990.

IEEE 802.11 Standard. (1999). Wireless LAN MAC and PHY specifications.

IEEE 802.11e Draft 3.1. (2002). Wireless LAN Medium Access Control (MAC) and Physical Layer (PHY) Specifications: Medium Access Control (MAC) Enhancements for Quality of Service (QoS).

IETF-IPPM. (1994). *RFC 1633: Integrated Services in the Internet Architecture: an Overview.*

IETF-IPPM. (1998). *RFC 2330: Framework for IP Performance Metrics.*

IETF-IPPM. (1998). *RFC 2475: An Architecture for Differentiated Services.*

IETF-IPPM. (2001). *RFC 3031: Multiprotocol Label Switching Architecture.*

Inocybe technologies Inc. (n.d.). *Argia product.* Retrieved from http://www.inocybe.ca/

Intanagonwiwat, C., Govindan, R., & Estrin, D. (2000). Directed diffusion: A scalable and robust communication paradigm for sensor networks. In *Proceedings of the 6th Annual ACM/IEEE International Conference on Mobile Computing and Networking (MobiCom'00)*, Boston, (pp. 56-67).

Ishibashi, K. (2007). Maintaining Quality of Service Based on ITIL-Based IT Service Management. *Fujitsu Scientific and Technical Journal*, *43*(3), 334–344.

Ishikawa, K. (1985). *What is total quality control? The japanese way*. Englewood Cliffs, NJ: Prentice Hall.

ISO 2005. (2005). *ISO 9000:2005. Quality management systems - Fundamentals and vocabulary.*

ISO 8402. (1986). *ISO 8402:1996. Quality management and quality assurance - Vocabulary.*

ISO/IEC 13236. (1998). *ISO/IEC 13236: Information technology -- Quality of service: Framework.*

Istepanian, R. S. H. (2005). Wireless Security for Personalized and Mobile Healthcare Services. In *The 29th Annual International Computer Software and Applications Conference*, (Vol. 1, pp.86).

ITU-T. (1988). *ITU-T recommendation g.711: Pulse code modulation (pcm) of voice frequencies*. ITU.

ITU-T. (1994). [Terms and definitions related to quality of service and network performance including dependability.]. *E (Norwalk, Conn.)*, 800.

ITU-T. (1996). ITU-T recommendation p.800: Methods for objective and subjective assessment of quality:ITU.

ITU-T. (1996). P.800: Methods for subjective determination of transmission quality.

ITU-T. (1999). *ITU-T recommendation g.109: Definition of categories of speech transmission quality*. ITU.

ITU-T. (2001). *G.1000: Communications quality of service: A framework and definitions.*

ITU-T. (2001). *G.1010: End-user multimedia QoS categories.*

ITU-T. (2001). *ITU-T recommendation g.113: Transmission impairments due to speech processing*. Telecommunications and Standardization Sector of the ITU.

ITU-T. (2001). ITU-T recommendation p.862: Methods for objective and subjective assessment of quality: ITU.

ITU-T. (2002). [*Framework of a service level agreement.*]. *E (Norwalk, Conn.)*, 860.

ITU-T. (2003). *ITU-T recommondation g.107: Definition of categories of speech transmission quality*. Telecommunications and Standardization Sector of the ITU.

ITU-T. (2005). G.1030: Estimating end-to-end performance in IP networks for data applications.

ITU-T. (2006). [Framework for achieving end-to-end IP performance objectives.]. *Y (Dayton, Ohio)*, 1542.

ITU-T. (2007). [Framework and methodologies for the determination and application of QoS parameters.]. *E (Norwalk, Conn.)*, 802.

ITU-T. (2007). [Internet protocol data communication service – IP packet transfer and availability performance parameters: ITU-T.]. *Y (Dayton, Ohio)*, 1540.

ITU-T. (2007). [Measurements in IP networks for inter-domain performance assessment.]. *Y (Dayton, Ohio)*, 1543.

ITU-T. (2007). *G.1070: Opinion model for video-telephony applications: ITU-T.*

ITU-T. (2008). J.247: Objective perceptual multimedia video quality measurement in the presence of a full reference: ITU-T.

ITU-T. (2008a). [Definitions of terms related to Quality of Service.]. *E (Norwalk, Conn.)*, 800.

ITU-T. (2008b). *G.1081: Performance monitoring points for IPTV: ITU-T.*

Iwata, A., & Fujita, N. (2000). A hierarchical multilayer QoS routing system with dynamic SLA management. *IEEE Journal on Selected Areas in Communications*, *18*(12), 2603–2616. doi:10.1109/49.898740

Jacobson, V., Nichols, K., & Poduri, K. (1999). An Expedited Forwarding PHB. In Internet Engineering Task Force Request for Comment – IETF RFC 2598.

Jaffe, J. (1984). Algorithms for finding paths with multi constraints. *Networks*, 95–116. doi:10.1002/net.3230140109

Jain, R. (2004). Quality of experience. *Multimedia, IEEE*, *11*(1), 96–95. doi:10.1109/MMUL.2004.1261114

Jain, R., Lin, Y. B., Lo, C., & Mohan, S. (1994). A Caching Strategy to Reduce Network Impact of PCS. *IEEE Journal on Selected Areas in Communications*, *12*(8), 1434–1444. doi:10.1109/49.329333

Jakes, W. C. Jr. (1974). *Microwave Mobile Communications*. New York: John Wiley and Sons.

Jamoussi, B., Andersson, L., Callon, R., Dantu, R., Wu, L., & Doolan, P., et al. (2002). *Constraint-based LSP Setup Using LDP, RFC 3212*.

Janssen, J., de Vleeschauwer, D., & Petit, G. H. (2000). Delay and distortion bounds for packetized voice calls of traditional pstn quality. In *IPtel 2000*. Berlin: Alcatel.

Jensen, T., Grgic, I., & Espvik, O. (1999). *Managing Quality of Service in Multi-Provider Environment*. Paper presented at the TELECOM 99.

Johannesson, N. O. (1997). *The etsi computation model: A tool for transmission planning of telephone networks. IEEE Communications* (pp. 1–10). Washington, DC: IEEE.

Jorge, L., & Gomes, T. (2006). Survey of Recovery Schemes in MPLS Networks. *International Conference on Dependability of Computer Systems (DepCos-RELCOMEX '06)*, (pp. 110-118).

Juran, J. M. (1999). *Juran's Quality Handbook*. New York: McGraw-Hill.

Kamel, T., Elzarki, M., Eissa, H. & Abd El-kader, S., (2002). Bandwidth and Capacity Study for Multimedia Applications over IP Backbone Networks. US-Egypt Science & Technology Joint Fund, ID Code: OTH3-009-001.

Kamien, M., & Schwartz, N. (1982). *Market structure and innovation*. Cambridge, UK: Cambridge University Press.

Kang, Y.-H., & Lee, J.-H. (2005). The implementation of the premium services for MPLS IP VPNs. In *The 7th International Conference on Advanced Communication Technology (ICACT 2005)*, (pp. 1107-1110).

Kano, N. (1984). Attractive quality and must-be quality. *The Journal of the Japanese Society for Quality Control*, *14*(2), 39–48.

Karl, H., & Willig, A. (2005). *Protocols and Architectures for Wireless Sensor Networks*. Chichester, UK: John Wiley & Sons. doi:10.1002/0470095121

Karn, P. (1990). MACA - A New Channel Access Protocol for Packet Radio. Proceedings of the ARRL/CRRL Amateur Radio Ninth Computer Networking Conference (pp. 134.140).

Karystinos, G., & Pados, D. (2000). On Overfitting, Generalization, and Randomly Expanded Training Sets. *IEEE Transactions on Neural Networks*, *11*(5), 1050–1057. doi:10.1109/72.870038

Katz, D., Kompella, K., & Yeung, D. (2003, September). *Traffic Engineering (TE) Extensions to OSPF Version 2*. RFC 3630. IETF.

Kazantzidis, M., & Gerla, M. (2002). End-to-end versus explicit feedback measurement in 802.11 networks. In *Proceedings of the 7th IEEE International Symposium on Computers and Communications (ISCC)* (pp.429–434).

Kelly, F. P. (1991). Effective bandwidths at multi-class queues. *Queueing Systems*, *9*(1-2), 5–16. doi:10.1007/BF01158789

Kelly, F. P. (1996). Notes on effective bandwidths. In Kelly, F. P., Zachary, S., & Ziedins, I. (Eds.), *Stochastic Networks: Theory and Applications* (pp. 141–168). Oxford, UK: Oxford University Press.

Kim, S., & Lee, M. (2001). Server based QoS routing with implicit network state updates. *IEEE GLOBECOM*, *4*, 2182–2187.

Knoll, T. (2009). *BGP Extended Community Attribute for QoS Marking*. draftknollidrqos-attribute02, work in progress, IETF.

Kobayashi, K., & Takahashi, Y. (1997). Tail probability of a Gaussian fluid queue under finite measurement of input processes. In *Proceedings of the IFIP TC6 / WG6.3 & WG7.3 International Conference on the Performance and Management of Complex Communication Networks*, (pp. 43-58).

Kodialam, M., & Lakshman, T. V. (2000). Minimum interference routing with applications to MPLS traffic engineering. In *IEEE INFOCOM* (*Vol. 2*, pp. 884–893). Piscataway, NJ: IEEE Computer Society.

Kondratief, N. D. (1935, November). The long waves in economic life. *The Review of Economics and Statistics*, *17*(6), 105–115. doi:10.2307/1928486

Koubâa, A., Alves, M., Tovar, E., & Cunha, A. (2008). An Implicit GTS Allocation Mechanism in IEEE 802.15.4 for Time-sensitive Wireless Sensor Networks: Theory and Practice. *ACM Real-Time Systems*, *39*(1-3), 169–204. doi:10.1007/s11241-007-9038-x

Krishna, P. M., Gadre, V. M. & Desai, U. B. (2003). Multifractal based network traffic modeling. Boston: Kluwer Academic Publishers.

Krishna, P. M., Gadre, V. M., & Desai, U. B. (2001). Global Scaling Exponent for Variable Variance Gaussian Multiplicative (VVGM) Multifractal Cascades. In *Proceedings of the Sixth Biennial Conference on Signal Processing and Communications (SPCOM'01)*, (pp. 19-25).

Kuipers, F., Korkmaz, T., Krunz, M., & Mieghem, P. V. (2004). Performance evaluation of constraint-based path selection algorithms. *IEEE Network*, *18*, 16–23. doi:10.1109/MNET.2004.1337731

Kuipers, F., Van Mieghem, P., Korkmaz, T., & Krunz, M. (2002). An overview of constraintbased path selection algorithms for QoS routing. *IEEE Communications Magazine*, *40*(12), 50–55. doi:10.1109/MCOM.2002.1106159

Kulik, J., Heinzelman, W. R., & Balakrishnan, H. (2002). Negotiation-based protocols for disseminating information in wireless sensor networks. *Wireless Networks*, *8*(2/3), 169–185. doi:10.1023/A:1013715909417

Kumar, N., & Saraph, G. (2006). EndtoEnd QoS in Interdomain Routing. In *ICNS '06: Proceedings of the international conference on networking and services* (pp. 82). Washington, DC: IEEE Computer Society.

Kummerle, K. (1974). Multiplexer Performance for Integrated Line- and Packet-Switched Traffic, *Proceedings of the ICCC*, Stockholm (pp. 508-515).

Lage, A. L., Martins, J. S. B., & Oliveira, J. C. (2004). A quality of service framework for tele-medicine applications. In *Conference on WebMedia and LA-Web*, (pp. 18 – 20).

Lai, W. (2005). *Bandwidth Constraints Models for Differentiated Services (Diffserv)-aware MPLS Traffic Engineering: Performance Evaluation, RFC 4128.*

Lancaster, K. J. (1966). A New Approach to Consumer Theory. *The Journal of Political Economy*, *74*(2), 132. doi:10.1086/259131

Le Faucheur, F. (2003). *Requirements for support of Differentiated Services-aware MPLS Traffic Engineering, RFC 3564.*

Le Faucheur, F., Wu, L., Davie, B., Davari, S., Vaananen, P., Krishnan, R., Cheval, P., & Heinanen, J., (2002). *Multi-Protocol Label Switching (MPLS) Support of Differentiated Services, RFC 3270.*

Lee, B., Ahn, G. S., Zhang, X., & Campbell, A. T. (2000). INSIGNIA: an IP-based quality of service framework for mobile ad hoc networks. *Journal of Parallel and Distributed Computing*, *60*(4), 374–406. doi:10.1006/jpdc.1999.1613

Lee, H. H., & Un, C. K. (1987). A Study of On-Off Characteristics of Conversational Speech. *IEEE Transactions on Communications*, 630–637.

Lee, S. C., Lee, Y. D., & Chung, W. Y. (2008). Design and Implementation of Reliable Query Process for Indoor Environmental and Healthcare Monitoring System. In *The Third International Conference on Convergence and Hybrid Information Technology*, (pp. 398 – 402). Busan, Republic of Korea: IEEE Computer Society.

Lee, S.-B., Ahn, G. S., Zhang, X., & Campbell, A. T. (2000). INSIGNIA: an IPbased quality of service framework for mobile ad hoc networks. *Journal of Parallel and*

Distributed Computing, *60*(4), 374–406. doi:10.1006/jpdc.1999.1613

Lee, W. C. Y. (1982). *Mobile Communications Engineering*. New York: McGraw-Hill.

Lee, W. C. Y. (1989). *Mobile Cellular Telecommunications Systems*. New York: McGraw-Hill.

Lee, W. C. Y. (1991). Overview of Cellular CDMA. In IEEE Transactions on Vehicular Technology, (pp. 291-302).

Lee, Y. D., Lee, D. S., Walia, G., Alasaarela, E., & Chung, W. Y. (2007). Design and Evaluation of Query Supported Healthcare Information System Using Wireless Sensor Ad-hoc Network. *The International Conference on Convergence Information Technology,* (pp. 997-1002). Bangladesh: United International University.

Lee, Y., et al. (2002, April). A Constrained Multipath traffic Engineering Scheme for MPLS Networks. In International conference on communications (ICC). New York: IEEE Communications Society.

Lehman, T. (2006). InterDomain Peering and Provisioning via GMPLS and Web Services. In 6th Global Lambda Workshop, Tokyo, Sep. 1-13, 2006.

Leinwand, A., & Fang, K. (1993). *Network management: a practical perspective*. Boston: AddisonWesley Longman Publishing Co., Inc.

Leland, W. E., Taqqu, M. S., Willinger, W., Wilson, D. V., & Bellcore, M. (1994). On the self-similar nature of Ethernet traffic (extended version). *Networking, IEEE/ACM Transactions on,* *2*(1), 1-15.

Leonard-Barton, K. (1992). Core capabilities and core rigidities: A paradox in managing new product development. *Strategic Management Journal*, *28*(2), 228–247.

Leung, F., Flidr, J., Tracy, C., Yang, X., Lehman, T., Jabbari, B., Riley, D. & Sobieski, J. (2006). The DRAGON Project and Application Specific Topologies. In *Broadnets 2006,* San Jose, CA.

Lévy Véhel, J., & Riedi, R. (1997). Fractional Brownian motion and data traffic modeling: The other end of the spectrum. In Lévy Véhel, J., Lutton, E., & Tricot, C. (Eds.), *Fractals in engineering: from theory to industrial applications* (pp. 185–202). Berlin: Springer.

Lévy Véhel, J., & Riedi, R. H. (1997). *TCP traffic is multifractal: a numerical study. INRIA research report No. 3129*. INRIA - Institut National de Recherche en Informatique et en Automatique.

Li, Q., & Mills, D. L. (1999). Investigating the scaling behavior, crossover and anti-persistence of Internet packet delay dynamics. In *Proceedings of the Global Telecommunications Conference, 1999 (GLOBECOM '99), 3,* (pp. 1843-1852).

Li, T. & Smit, H. (2008, October). *ISIS Extensions for traffic Engineering*. RFC 5305. IETF.

Li, T., Iraqi, Y., & Boutaba, R. (2003). Traffic-Based Pricing and Admission Control for DiffServ Networks. In *IFIP/IEEE 8th International Symposium on Integrated Network Management,* (pp. 73-86).

Li, T., Iraqi, Y., & Boutaba, R. (2004). Pricing and admission control for QoS-enabled Internet. In *Computer Networks*. New York: Elsevier.

Li, Y., Chen, C. S., Song, Y.-Q., & Wang, Z. (2007). Realtime QoS support in wireless sensor networks: a survey. In *7th IFAC International Conference on Fieldbuses & Networks in Industrial & Embedded Systems (FeT'2007),* Toulouse, France.

Lim, H., & Singh, V. K. (2005). Design of Healthcare System for Disabled Person Using Eye Blinking. In *The Fourth Annual ACIS International Conference on Computer and Information Science,* (pp. 551-555). Jeuu Island, South Korea: IEEE Computer Society.

Lima, S. R., Carvalho, P., & Freitas, V. (2004). Distributed Admission Control for QoS and SLS Management. *Journal of Network and Systems Management. Special Issue on Distributed Management*, *12*(3), 397–426.

Lin, Y. B. (1994). Determining the User Locations for Personal Communications Services Networks. *IEEE Transactions on Vehicular Technology*, *43*(3), 466–473. doi:10.1109/25.312799

Liu, C. L., & Layland, J. W. (1973). Scheduling algorithms for multiprogramming in hard real-time environment. *Journal of the ACM*, *20*(1), 40–61. doi:10.1145/321738.321743

Liu, G., & Ramakrishnan, K. (2001). A*prune: An algorithm for finding k shortest paths subject to multiple constraints. In *Twentieth Annual Joint Conference of the IEEE Computer and Communications Societies (INFOCOM)*, (vol. 2, pp. 743-749).

Liu, M., & Papantoni-Kazakos, P. (1992). A Random Access Algorithm for Data Networks Carrying High Priority Traffic. *IEEE Transactions on Communications*, *40*, 84–96. doi:10.1109/26.126710

Liu, M., & Papantoni-Kazakos, P. (1993). A Protocol for Cellular Radio Signaling Channels Carrying Data and High Priority Accessing Requests. *IEEE Transactions on Communications*, *41*, 570–582. doi:10.1109/26.223781

Loukola, M. V., & Skytta, J. (2003). *New possibilities offered by IPv6*. Retrieved from http://www.hut.fi/~mloukola/pub7/p1.pdf

Lu, B., & Pooch, U. W. (2005). Security in QoS signaling systems for mobile ad hoc networks. In *Proceedings of IEEE International Conference on Wireless And Mobile Computing, Networking. Communications*, *3*, 213–220.

Lubrin, E., Lawrence, E., & Navarro, K. F. (2005). Wireless Remote Healthcare Monitoring with Motes. In *The International Conference on Mobile Business (ICMB'05)*, (pp.235-241). Sydney, Australia: IEEE Computer Society.

Ma, Q., & Steenkiste, P. (1997). On path selection for traffic with bandwidth guarantees. In *Proceedings of IEEE International Conference on Network Protocols* (pp. 191-202). Washington, DC: IEEE Computer Society.

Ma, Q., & Steenkiste, P. (1997). Quality of service routing with performance guarantees. *4th International IFIP Workshop on QoS*, (pp. 1-12). Boca Raton, FL: Chapman & Hall.

Mackie-Masson, J. K., & Varian, H. R. (1994, March). Pricing the Internet. In *International Conference of Telecommunication Systems Modelling*, Nashville, TN, (pp.378-93). Retrieved from http://www.spp.umich.edu/papers/listing.html

Madhow, U., Honig, M. L., & Steiglitz, K. (1994). Optimization of Wireless Resources for Personal Communications Mobility Tracking. *Proceedings - IEEE INFOCOM*, *94*, 577–584.

Maes, P. (1997). *Agents That Reduce Work and Information Overload. Software Agents*. Cambridge, MA: MIT Press.

Mahajan, R., Wetherall, D., & Anderson, T. (2004). Towards coordinated interdomain traffic engineering. In SIGCOMM workshop on hot topics in networking (HotNets). New York: ACM.

Mahajan, R., Wetherall, D., & Anderson, T. (2005). Negotiation-based routing between neighboring ISPs. In *NSDI'05: Proceedings of the 2nd conference on symposium on networked systems design & implementation*, (pp. 29-42). Berkeley, CA: USENIX Association.

Mahapatra, A., Anand, K., & Agrawal, D. P. (2006). QoS and Energy Aware Routing for Real-time Traffic in Wireless Sensor Networks. *Computer Communications*, *29*(4), 437–445. doi:10.1016/j.comcom.2004.12.028

Mandelbrot, B. B., & Van Ness, J. W. (1968). Fractional Brownian motions, fractional noises and applications. *SIAM Review*, *10*(4), 422–437. doi:10.1137/1010093

Mandelbrot, B. B., & Wallis, J. R. (1969). Computer experiments with fractional Gaussian noises, parts 1, 2 and 3. *Water Resources Research*, *5*(1), 228–267. doi:10.1029/WR005i001p00228

Mandelbrot, B. B., Fisher, A. J., & Calvet, L. E. (1997). *A Multifractal Model of Asset Returns*. Cowles Foundation Discussion Paper No. 1164. Cowles Foundation for Research in Economics at Yale University, New Haven, CT.

Manjeshwar, A., & Agarwal, D. P. (2001). TEEN: a routing protocol for enhanced efficiency in wireless sensor networks. In *Proceeding of 15th International Parallel and Distributed Processing Symposium (IPDPS 2001)*, (pp. 2009-2015).

Manjeshwar, A., & Agarwal, D. P. (2002). APTEEN: A hybrid protocol for efficient routing and comprehensive information retrieval in wireless sensor networks. In *Proceeding of 16th Proceedings International Parallel and Distributed Processing Symposium (IPDPS 2002)*, (pp. 195-202).

Manjunath, R. & Gurumurthy, K.S. (2003), Bayesian decision on differentially fed hyperplanes. *ITSim2003.*

Manjunath, R. & Gurumurthy, K.S. (2003). System Design using differentially fed Artificial Neural Network. *ICAAI'03.*

Manjunath, R. & Gurumurthy, K.S. (2003). *Tensor domain analysis of differentially fed artificial neural networks, ITSim2003.*

Manjunath, R. & Gurumurthy, K.S. (2003a). Wavelet Representation of Differentially Fed ANN. *WSEAS Transactions On Circuits and systems*, Oct. 2003.

Manjunath, R. & Gurumurthy, K.S. (2004) Maintaining Long-range dependency of traffic in a network. *CODEC'04.*

Manjunath, R. & Shyam, V. (2008). *Improving Quality of Service through shifted prediction feedback*, CCNC'08.

Manjunath, R. (2006). *Compact architecture for the analysis and processing of subnet signals using differentiators as building blocks.* Unpublished doctoral dissertation, University of Bangalore, India

Manjunath, R., & Gurumurthy, K. S. (2002). *Information geometry of differentially fed artificial neural networks* (*Vol. 3*, pp. 1521–1525). TENCON.

Mao, G. (2005, February). A Real-Time Loss Performance Monitoring Scheme. *Computer Communications*, *28*(2), 150–161. doi:10.1016/j.comcom.2004.06.007

Marquardt, D. W. (1963). An Algorithm for Least-Squares Estimation of Nonlinear Parameters. *SIAM Journal on Applied Mathematics*, *11*(2), 431–441. doi:10.1137/0111030

Marsan, M. A., et.al. (2005). Using Partial Differential Equations to Model TCP Mice and Elephants in Large IP Networks. *IEEE/ACM Transactions on Networking*, *13*(6), 1289-1301.

Marsan, M., Casetti, A. C., Mardente, G., & Mellia, M. (2007). A framework for admission control and path allocation in DiffServ networks. *Computer Networks*, *51*(10), 2738–2752. doi:10.1016/j.comnet.2006.11.022

Martínez, J. F., García, A. B., Corredor, I., López, L., Hernández, V., & Dasilva, A. (2007). QoS in wireless sensor networks: survey and approach. In *Proceedings of the 2007 Euro American conference on Telematics and Information Systems (EATIS '07).*

Marwaha, S., Indulska, J., & Portmann, M. (2008). Challenges and Recent Advances in QoS Provisioning, Signaling, Routing and MAC protocols for MANETs. In. *Proceedings of Telecommunication Networks and Applications Conference*, *2008*, 97–102.

Marzo, J., Calle, E., Scoglio, C., & Anjah, T. (2003). QoS online routing and MPLS multilevel protection: a survey. *IEEE Communications Magazine*, *41*, 126–132. doi:10.1109/MCOM.2003.1235604

Mateo, R. M., Salvo, M. A., & Lee, J. (2008). Balanced Clustering using Mobile Agents for the Ubiquitous Healthcare Systems. In *The Third International Conference on Convergence and Hybrid Information Technology.* (pp.686-691). Busan, Korea: IEEE Computer Society.

McPherson, D. & Gill, V. (2006, March). *BGP MULTI_EXIT_DISC (MED) Considerations.* RFC 4451. IETF.

Medina, A., Lakhina, A., Matta, I., & Byers, J. (2001). BRITE: An Approach to Universal Topology Generation. In *Proc. of MASCOTS'01*, (pp. 346-354).

Medina, A., Matta, I., & Byers, J. (2000). *Brite: A flexible generator of internet topologies. Technical Report: 2000-005.* Boston: Boston University.

Meier-Hellstern, K. S., Pollini, G. P., & Goodman, D. J. (1991). A Wireless Service for the IEEE 802.6 Metropolitan Area Network. In *Proceedings. IEEE GLOBECOM '91*, (pp. 1964-1968).

Mermelstein, P., Jalali, A., & Leib, H. (1993). Integrated Services on Wireless Multiple Access Networks. In IEEE ICC '93, (pp. 863-867).

Miller, L. E. (2005). *Wireless Technologies and the SAFECOM SoR for Public Safety Communications, Leonard E. Miller, Wireless Communication Technologies Group. National Institute of Standards and Technology.* Report, Maryland, USA: NIST.

Minacom. (2003). *Extended e-model solution.* Retrieved January 22, 2005 from http://www.minacom.com/products/pp6000_files/Extended%20E-Model%20Solution%20Sheet%20001-000104-101_A.pdf

Mirhakkak, M., Schult, N., & Thomson, D. (2000). Dynamic quality-of-service for mobile ad hoc networks. In ACM International Symposium on Mobile ad hoc networking & computing (pp. 137 – 138).

Mirrokni, V. S., Thottan, M., Uzunalioglu, H., & Paul, S. (2004, March). A Simple Polynomial Time Framework For ReducedPath Decomposition in MultiPath Routing. In *IEEE INFOCOM* (*Vol. 1*, p. 739749). Washington, DC: IEEE Computer Society.

Mitra, D., & Ramakrishnan, K. (1999). A case study of multiservice, multipriority traffic engineering design for data networks. *IEEE Global Telecommunications Conference, 1999. GLOBECOM '99*, 1B, 10771083.

Mitra, D., & Wang, Q. (2003). Stochastic traffic engineering with applications to network revenue management. In *Twenty-Second Annual Joint Conference of the IEEE Computer and Communications Societies (INFOCOM)*, (vol. 1, pp. 396-405).

Mohan, S., & Jain, R. (1994). Two User Location Strategies for Personal Communications Services. *IEEE Personal Communications*, *1*(1), 42–50.

Molnár, S., Dang, T. D., & Maricza, I. (2002). On the queue tail asymptotics for general multifractal traffic. In *Proceedings of the Second International IFIP-TC6 Networking Conference on Networking Technologies, Services, and Protocols; Performance of Computer and Communication Networks; and Mobile and Wireless Communications, 2002 (IFIP Networking '02)* (Vol. LNCS 2345, pp. 105-116). Berlin: Springer-Verlag.

Nanda, S., Goodman, D. J., & Timor, U. (1991). Performance of PRMA: A Packet Voice Protocol for Cellular Systems. *IEEE Transactions on Vehicular Technology*, *40*, 584–598. doi:10.1109/25.97513

Nelakuditi, S., Zhang, Z., Tsang, R., and Du, D.H.C, (2002). Adaptive proportional routing: A localized QoS routing approach. *IEEE/ACM Transactions on Networking*, *10*(6), 790 - 804.

Nelson, R. R., & Wright, G. (1992). The rise and fall of american technological leadership: The postwar era in historical perspective. *Journal of Economic Literature*, *30*(4), 1931–1964.

Nicholas, K., Blake, S., Baker, F., & Black, D. (1998). (DS Field) in the IPv4 and IPv6 Headers. In *Internet Engineering Task Force Request for Comment – IETF RFC 2474.* Definition of the Differentiated Services Field.

Nichols, K. & Carpenter, B. (2001 April). *Definition of Differentiated Services Per Domain Behaviors and Rules for their Specification, RFC 3086.*

Nichols, K., Blake, S. Baker, F. & Black, D. (1998). Definition of the Differentiated Services Field (DS Field) in the IPv4 and IPv6 Headers. RFC 2474.

Nichols, K., Jacobson, V., & Zhang L. (1999). *A two-bit differentiated services architecture for the Internet, RFC 2638.*

Norros, I. (1994). A storage model with self-similar input. *Queueing Systems*, *16*(3), 387–396. doi:10.1007/BF01158964

Norros, I. (1995). On the use of fractional Brownian motion in the theory of connectionless networks. *IEEE Journal on Selected Areas in Communications*, *13*(6), 953–962. doi:10.1109/49.400651

NS-2 The Network Simulator ns-2. (n.d.). Retrieved Oct. 30, 2004 from http://www.isi.edu/nsnam/ns/

Nwana, H. (1996). Software agents: an overview. *The Knowledge Engineering Review*, *11*(3). doi:10.1017/S026988890000789X

Okumu, I. T., Mantar, H. A., Hwang, J., & Chapin, S. J. (2005). Inter-domain QoS routing on DiffServ networks: a region-based approach. *Computer Communications*, *28*(2), 174–188. doi:10.1016/j.comcom.2004.08.018

Oodan, A. P. Ward, K.E., Savolaine, C.G., Daneshmand, M. & Hoath, P. (2003). Telecommunications Quality of Service Management: from legacy to emerging services. Stevenage, UK: Institution of Engineering and Technology.

P906. E. P. I. P. (2000). Project P906: QUASIMODO - *Quality of Service MethODOlogies and solutions within the service framework: measuring, managing and charging QoS.*

Pados, D. A., & Papantoni-Kazakos, P. (1995). New Non-Least-Squares Neural Network Learning Algorithms for Hypothesis Testing. *IEEE Transactions on Neural Networks*, *6*(3), 596–609. doi:10.1109/72.377966

Pados, D. A., Papantoni-Kazakos, P., Kazakos, D., & Kogiantis, A. (1994). On-Line Threshold Learning for Neyman-Pearson Distributed Detection. *IEEE Transactions on Systems, Man, and Cybernetics*, *24*(10), 1519–1531. doi:10.1109/21.310534

Pan, J., Li, S., & Wu, Z. (2008). Towards a Novel In-community Healthcare Monitoring System over Wireless Sensor Networks. In *The International Conference on Internet Computing in Science and Engineering.* (pp.160-165). Harbin, China: IEEE Computer Society.

Pan, P., Hahne, E., & Schulzrinne, H. (2000). BGRP: A Tree-Based Aggregation Protocol for Inter-domain Reservations. *Journal of Communications and Networks*, *2*(2), 157–167.

Papantoni-Kazakos, P. (1979). Algorithms for Monitoring Changes in Quality of Communications Links. *IEEE Transactions on Communications*, *27*(4), 682–692. doi:10.1109/TCOM.1979.1094443

Papantoni-Kazakos, P. (1979). The Potential of End-to-End Observations in Trouble Localization and Quality Control of Network Links. *IEEE Transactions on Communications*, *27*(1), 16–30. doi:10.1109/TCOM.1979.1094254

Papantoni-Kazakos, P. (1992). Multiple Access Algorithms for a System with Mixed Traffic: High and Low Priority. *IEEE Transactions on Communications*, *40*, 541–555. doi:10.1109/26.135724

Papantoni-Kazakos, P. (1994). Accessing Protocols and Network Reconfiguration for Cellular-ISDN Systems. In. *Proceedings of IEEE ICC*, *94*, 1285–1296.

Papantoni-Kazakos, P., Delic, H., Paterakis, M., & Liu, M. (1993). Transmission Algorithms for a Multi-Channel Packet Radio System with Priority Users. *IJDACS*, *6*(4), 193–212.

Papantoni-Kazakos, P., Likhanov, N., & Tsybakov, B. S. (1995). A Protocol for Random Multiple Access of Packets with Mixed Priorities in Wireless Networks. *IEEE JSAC*, *13*(7), 1324–1331.

Parasuraman, A., Zeithaml, V. A., & Berry, L. L. (1996). The Behavioral Consequences of Service Quality. *Journal of Marketing*, *60*(2), 31–46. doi:10.2307/1251929

Park, K., & Tuan, T. (2000). Performance evaluation of multiple time scale TCP under self-similar traffic conditions. *ACM Transactions on Modeling and Computer Simulation*, *10*(2), 152–177. doi:10.1145/364996.365005

Park, K., & Willinger, W. (2000). *Self-Similar Network Traffic and Performance Evaluation.* New York: Wiley-Interscience. doi:10.1002/047120644X

Paterakis, M., & Papantoni-Kazakos, P. (1989). A Simple Window Random Access Algorithm with Advantageous Properties. *IEEE Transactions on Information Theory*, *35*, 1124–1130. doi:10.1109/18.42234

Paterakis, M., Georgiadis, L., & Papantoni-Kazakos, P. (1989). A Full Sensing Window Random-Access Algorithm for Messages with Strict Delay Constraints. *Algorithmica*, *4*(3), 313–329. doi:10.1007/BF01553894

Patrick, A. S., Singer, J., Corrie, B., Noel, S., El Khatib, K., Emond, B., et al. (2004). *A QoE sensitive architecture for advanced collaborative environments.* Paper presented at the Quality of Service in Heterogeneous Wired/Wireless Networks, Dallas, TX.

Pavlovski, C., Kim, H., & Wood, D. (2004).Ubiquitous Mobility in Clinical Healthcare. In *IDEAS Workshop on Medical Information Systems: The Digital Hospital.* (pp.147-153). Beijing, China: IEEE Computer Society.

Paxson, V. & Floyd, S. (1995). Wide area traffic: the failure of Poisson modeling. *Networking, IEEE/ACM Transactions on, 3*(3), 226-244.

Pelsser, C., & Bonaventure, O. (2006). Path Selection Techniques to Establish Constrained Interdomain MPLS LSPs. In *Proc. of IFIP Networking,* Coimbra, Portugal.

Peltier, R. F., & Lévy Véhel, J. (1995). *Multifractional Brownian motion: definition and preliminary results. INRIA research report No. 2645.* INRIA - Institut National de Recherche en Informatique et en Automatique.

Pereira, A., & Monteiro, E. (2006). Admission Control in IntServ to DiffServ mapping. *International conference on Networking and Services (ICNS '06),* (pp. 83).

Pereira, M., Amorim, C., & Castro, M. (2003). Tutorial sobre Redes de Sensores. Universidade do Estado do Rio de Janeiro, Cadernos do IME. *Série Informática, 14*, 39–53.

Perkins, C. E. (2001). *Ad hoc Networking.* Boston: Addison Wesley.

Perkins, C. E., & Belding-Royer, E. M. (2001). Quality of Service for Ad Hoc On-Demand Distance Vector Routing. *Internet Draft.* Retrieved August 9, 2009, from http://tools.ietf.org

Perkins, C. E., & Bhagwat, P. (1994). Highly Dynamic Destination-Sequenced Distance-Vector Routing (DSDV) for Mobile Computers. ACM Special Interest Group on Data Communications (SIGCOMM) Conference, 24(4), 234-244.

Perkins, C. E., & Royer, E. M. (1999). Ad hoc On-Demand Distance Vector Routing. IEEE Workshop on Mobile Computing Systems and Applications (pp. 90-100).

Perkins, C.E., Royer, E.M. & Das, S.R. (2000). Quality of Service for Ad hoc On-Demand Distance-vector Routing. IETF MANET WG Draft: draft-ietf-manet-aodvqos-00.txt

Perrig, A., Szewczyk, R., Wen, V., Culler, D., & Tygar, J. (2001). SPINS: Security protocols for sensor networks. In *Proc. of ACM MobiCom'01, Italy.*

Pfeffer, J., & Salancik, G. R. (1978). *The external control of organizations: A resource dependence perspective.* New York: Harper & Row.

Philip, N., & Istepanian, R. S. H. (2007). Medical Quality of Service for Wireless Ultrasound Streaming in Robotic Tele-Ultrasonography System. In *The IEEE International Conference on Networking, Sensing and Control,* (pp. 245 – 250). London: IEEE Computer Society.

Polastre, J., Hill, J., & Culler, D. (2004). Versatile low power media access for wireless sensor networks. In *Proceedings of the 2nd International Conference on Embedded Networked Sensor Systems (SenSys '04),* 95--107, New York.

Polastre, J., Szewczyk, R., Mainwaring, A., & Culler, D. (2004). Analysis of Wireless Sensor Networks for Habitat Monitoring. In Raghavendra, C. S., Sivalingam, K. M., & Znati, T. (Eds.), *The book Wireless Sensor Networks.* Amsterdam: Kluwer Academic Publishers.

Postigo-Boix, M., Garcia-Haro, J., & Melus-Moreno, J. L. (2007). A cost-efficient method for streaming stored content in a guaranteed QoS Internet. *Computer Networks, 51*(1), 309–335. doi:10.1016/j.comnet.2006.05.002

Postigo-Boix, M., Melu's-Moreno, J. (2007). Performance evaluation of RSVP extensions for a guaranteed delivery scenario. Computer Communications. ScienceDirect., 30, 2113–2121.

Pracht, S., Newman, D., & Douskalis, B. (2000). Now hear this. *Telephony, 239*(6), 58–65.

Prakash, R., Shivaratrai, N. G., & Singhal, M. (1995). Distributed Dynamic Channel Allocation For Mobile Computing. In *Proceedings of the Fourth Annual ACM Symposium on Principles on Distributed Computing,* (pp. 47-56).

Proakis, J. G. (1995). *Digital Communications* (3rd ed.). New York: McGraw-Hill.

Quoitin, B., Pelsser, C., Bonaventure, O., & Uhlig, S. (2005). A performance evaluation of BGP based traffic engineering. *International Journal of Network Management, 15*, 177–191. doi:10.1002/nem.559

Quoitin, B., Pelsser, C., Swinnen, L., Bonaventure, O., & Uhlig, S. (2003, May). Interdomain traffic engineering with BGP. *IEEE Communications Magazine, 41*(5), 122–128. doi:10.1109/MCOM.2003.1200112

Raghavachari, B., & Veerasamy, J. (1999). Approximation algorithms for mixed postman problem. *SIAM Journal on Discrete Mathematics, 12*(4), 425–433. doi:10.1137/S0895480197331454

Raj, A., & Oliver, C. I. (2007). A survey of IP and multiprotocol label switching fast reroute schemes. *Computer Networks, 51*(8), 1882–1907. doi:10.1016/j.comnet.2006.09.010

Rajahalme, J., Couta, A., Carpenter, A. & Deering, S. (2003). *IPv6 Flow label specification.* Retrieved March from draft-ietf-ipv6flow-label-0.1.txt

Rajendran, V., Obraczka, K., & Garcia-Luna-Aceves, J. J. (2003). Energy-Efficient, Collision-Free Medium Access Control for Wireless Sensor Networks. In *Proc. ACM SenSys'03, Los Angeles, CA,* (pp. 181-92).

Ramakrishnan K., Floyd S. & Black D. (2001). The Addition of Explicit Congestion Notification (ECN) to IP. IETF RFC: 3168.

Raman, R. S., Jagannathan, V., & Reddy, R. (1997). Security Collaboration Technology for Healthcare Enterprises. In Sixth IEEE Workshops on Enabling Technologies: Infrastructure for Collaborative Enterprises. (pp. 263-268). Cambridge, UK: IEEE Computer Society.

Ramanathan, N., Chang, K., Kapur, R., Girod, L., Kohler, E., & Estrin, D. (2005). Sympathy for the Sensor Network Debugger. In *Proc. of 3rd Embedded networked sensor systems.*

Rangwala, S., Gummadi, R., Govindan, R., & Psounis, K. (2006). Interference-aware fair rate control in wireless sensor networks. *ACM SIGCOMM. Computer Communication Review, 36*(4), 63–74. doi:10.1145/1151659.1159922

Ray, P., & Weerakkody, G. (1999). Quality of Service Management in Healthcare Organizations: A Case Study. In *The 12th IEEE Symposium on Computer-Based Medical Systems,* (pp. 80 – 85). Stamford, CT: IEEE Computer Society.

Raychaudhuri, D. (1994). ATM Based Transport Architecture for Multi-services Wireless Personal Communications Networks. *Proceedings of the IEEE, 94*, 559–565.

Raychaudhuri, D., & Wilson, N. (1993). Multimedia Transport in Next-Generation Personal Communications Networks. *Proceedings of the IEEE, 93*, 858–862.

Raz, D., & Shavitt, Y. (1999). An Active Network Approach to Efficient Network Management. In *IWAN'99: Proceedings of the first international working conference on active networks* (pp. 220-231). London: SpringerVerlag.

Reddy, T. B., John, J. P., & Murthy, C. S. R. (2007). Providing MAC QoS for multimedia traffic in 802.11e based multi-hop ad hoc wireless networks. Computer Networks. *The International Journal of Computer and Telecommunications Networking, 51*(1), 153–176.

Reid, D. & Katchabaw, M. (2006). Achieving Quality of Service through SCalable Aggregate Reservations. *INFOCOMP - Journal of Computer Science, 5*(4), 9-18.

Reinganum, J. (1983). Uncertain innovation and the persistence of monopoly. *The American Economic Review, 73*(4), 741–748.

Reinisch, C., Kastner, W., Neugschwandtner, G., & Granzer, W. (2007). Wireless Technologies in Home and Building Automation. In *Proceedings of the 5th IEEE International Conference on Industrial Informatics, 1,* 93-98.

Reinisch, C., Kastner, W., Neugschwandtner, G., & Granzer, W. (2007). Wireless Technologies in Home and Building Automation. In Fifth IEEE Industrial Informatics International Conference, (Vol. 1, pp. 93-98).

Rekhter, Y., Li, T. & Hares, S. (2006, January). *A Border Gateway Protocol 4 (BGP4).* RFC 4271. IETF.

Rentala, P., Musunuri, R., Gandham, S., & Saxena, U. (2002). *Survey on Sensor Networks.* Technical Report No.UTDCS-33-02, University of Texas, Dallas, TX.

RFC3031 & Rosen, E., et al (2001, January). *IETF RFC 3031, Multiprotocol Label Switching Architecture.*

RFC3945 & Mannie, E., (2004 October). IETF RFC 3945. *Generalised Multi-Protocol Label Switching (GMPLS) Architecture.*

RFC4655, Farrel, A., & Vasseur, J.-P. (2006 August). A Path Computation Element (PCE)-Based Architecture. *IETF RFC 4655.*

Rhee, I., Warrier, A., Aia, M., & Min, J. (2005). Z-MAC: a Hybrid MAC for Wireless Sensor Networks. In *Proceedings of the 3rd International Conference on Embedded Networked Sensor Systems (SenSys'05)*, (pp. 90 – 101), San Diego, CA.

Ribeiro, V. J., Riedi, R. H., Crouse, M. S., & Baraniuk, R. G. (2000). Multiscale Queuing Analysis of Long-Range-Dependent Network Traffic. In *Proceedings of the Nineteenth Annual Joint Conference of the IEEE Computer and Communications Societies (INFOCOM 2000). 2,* (pp. 1026-1035).

Richters, J. S., & Dvorak, C. A. (1988). A framework for defining the quality of communications services. *IEEE Communications Magazine, 26*(10), 17–23. doi:10.1109/35.7663

Riedi, R. H., Crouse, M. S., Ribeiro, V. J., & Baraniuk, R. G. (1999). A multifractal wavelet model with application to network traffic. *IEEE Transactions on Information Theory, 45*(3), 992–1018. doi:10.1109/18.761337

Rix, A. W., & Hollier, M. P. (2000). The perceptual analysis measurement system for robust end-to-end speech quality assessment. In *IEEE ICASSP.* BT Advanced Communications Research.

Rolls, D. A., Michailidis, G., & Hernández-Campos, F. (2005). Queueing analysis of network traffic: methodology and visualization tools. *Computer Networks, 48*(3), 447–473. doi:10.1016/j.comnet.2004.11.016

Rosen, E., Viswanathan, A. & Callon, R. (2001, January). *Multiprotocol Label Switching Architecture.* RFC 3031. IETF.

Ross, M. J., Gottschalck, J. H., & Harrington, E. A. (1980). An Architecture for a Flexible Integrated Voice/Data Switch. In *Conference. Rec. 1980 International Conference on Communications* (pp. 21.6-1-- 21.6-5).

Rozenbaum, Y., Papantoni-Kazakos, P., & Kazakos, D. (1995). Semidynamic and Dynamic Transmission Algorithms for Multiplexing Voice with Data. *Telecommunication Systems, 3,* 341–378. doi:10.1007/BF02110311

Russell, S. & Norvig, (1995). *Artificial Intelligence: A Modern Approach.* New York: Prentice Hall.

Ryu, B. K., & Elwalid, A. (1996). The importance of long-range dependence of VBR video traffic in ATM traffic engineering: Myths and realities. *ACM SIGCOMM Computer Communication Review, 26*(4), 3–14. doi:10.1145/248157.248158

Sahal, D. (1981). *Patterns of technological innovation.* London: Addison-Wesley.

Sánchez-Macián, A., López de Vergara, J. E., Pastor, E., & Bellido, L. (2008). A system for monitoring, assessing and certifying Quality of Service in telematic services. *Knowledge-Based Systems, 21*(2), 101–109. doi:10.1016/j.knosys.2007.02.003

Sanjay, S., & Hassan, M. (2002). *Engineering Internet QoS.* Norwood, MA: Artech House.

Saxena, N., Roy, A., & Shin, J. (2008). A QoS-Based Energy-Aware MAC Protocol for Wireless Multimedia Sensor Networks. In *Proc. of IEEE VTC'08*, (pp. 183-187).

Scherer, F. M. (1992). Schumpeter and plausible capitalism. *Journal of Economic Literature, 30*(3), 1416–1433.

Schmutzler, J., Foley, C., Michaelis, S., van der Meer, S., & Wietfeld, C. (2008). Dynamic group management as an enhancement to emergency healthcare using policies. In e-health Networking, Applications and Services (HealthCom 2008). Biopolis, Singapore: IEEE computer Society.

Schumpeter, J. A. (1942). *Capitalism, socialism and democracy.* New York: Harper & Row.

Schwartz, M. (1987). *Telecommunication Networks: Protocols, Modeling and Analysis.* Reading, MA: Addison-Wesley.

Seitz, N. B., Wolf, S., Voran, S., & Bloomfield, R. (1994). User-oriented measures of telecommunication quality. *IEEE Communications Magazine*, *32*(1), 56–66. doi:10.1109/35.249792

Sekhar, A., Manoj, B. S., & Murthy, C. S. R. (2004). MARVIN: movement-aware routing over interplanetary networks. IEEE Sensor and Ad Hoc Communications and Networks conference (pp. 245- 254).

SEQUIN. (2002). *SEQUIN (IST-1999-20841)*

Seshadri, K., Liotta, L., Gopal, R., & Liotta, T. (2001). A Wireless Internet Application for Healthcare. In *The 14th IEEE Symposium on Computer-Based Medical Systems,* (pp.109-114). Bethesda, MD: IEEE Computer Society.

Shah, G. A., Akan, O. B., & Bozyigit, M. (2006). (MEAC) Protocol for Heterogeneous Wireless Sensor Networks. In *Proc. of Mediterranean Ad Hoc Networking Workshop (MedHoc-Net'06).* Multi-Event Adaptive Clustering.

Shaikh, F. A., McClellan, S., Singh, M., & Chakravarthy, S. (2002). End-to-End Testing of IP QoS Mechanisms. *IEEE Computer Magazine*, *35*(5), 80–87.

Shanshan, L., Xiangke, L., Shaoliang, P., Peidong, P., & Jie, J. (2007). Credit based fairness control in wireless sensor network. In *Proc. of 8th ACIS, International Conference on SNPD, Qingdao, China, (*pp. 817-822).

Shen, C. C., Rajagopalan, S., Borkar, G., & Jaikaeo, C. (2004). A flexible routing architecture for ad hoc space networks. *International Journal of Computer and Telecommunications Networking*, *46*(3), 389–410.

Shenker, S., Clark, D., Estrin, D., & Herzog, S. (1996). Pricing in Computer Networks: Reshaping the Research Agenda. *ACM Computer Communication Review*, *26*(2), 19–43. doi:10.1145/231699.231703

Shenker, S., Partridge, C., & Guerin, R. (1997). Specification of Guaranteed Quality of Service. In Internet Engineering Task Force Request for Comment – RFC 2212.

Shier, D. (1979). On algorithms for finding the k shortest paths in a network. *Networks*, *9*(3), 195–214. doi:10.1002/net.3230090303

Shigang, C., & Na, Y. (2006). Congestion avoidance based on light-weight buffer management in sensor networks. *IEEE Transactions on Parallel and Distributed Systems*, *17*(9), 934–946. doi:10.1109/TPDS.2006.115

Shioda, S. & Mase, K. (2005). Performance comparison between IntServ-based and DiffServ-based networks. *GLOBECOM*, 2005

Shrimali, G., Akella, A., & Mutapcic, A. (2007, May). Cooperative InterDomain traffic Engineering Using Nash Bargaining and Decomposition. In *IEEE INFOCOM* (p. 330338). Piscataway, NJ: IEEE Computer Society.

Sichitiu, M. L. (2004). Cross-layer scheduling for power efficiency in wireless sensor networks. In *Proc. of IEEE INFOCOM'04.*

Siller, M. (2003). *Improving Quality of Experience for Multimedia Services by QoS Arbitration on a QoE Framework.* Paper presented at the 13th Packed Video Workshop Nantes.

Siller, M., & Woods, J. C. (2003). *QoS arbitration for improving the QoE in multimedia transmission.* Paper presented at the Visual Information Engineering.

Soldatos, J., Vayias, E., & Kormentzas, G. (2005). First Quarter). On the building blocks of quality of service in heterogeneous IP networks. *IEEE Communications Surveys and Tutorials*, *7*(1), 69–88. doi:10.1109/COMST.2005.1423335

Srivastava, S., Thirumalasetty, S. R., & Medhi, D. (2005). Network traffic Engineering with varied levels of Protection in Next Generation Internet. In A. Girard, B. Sanso, & F. VazquezAbad (Eds.), Performance evaluations and planning methods for the next generation internet (pp. 99-124). New York: Springer US.

Staddon, J. Balfanz, D. & Durfee, G. (2002). Efficient Tracing of Failed Nodes in Sensor Networks. In *Proc. of 1st ACM International Workshop on Wireless Sensor Networks and Applications, USA*.

Stader, R. (2001). *QoS Provisioning for IP Telephony Networks by Advanced bandwidth management.* Masters of Science Thesis, Hochschule Konstanz Technik, Wirtschaft und Gestaltung.

Stallings, W. (1996). IPv6: The New Internet Protocol. *IEEE Communications Magazine*, (July): 96–108. doi:10.1109/35.526895

Steele, R. (1994). The Evolution of Personal Communications. *IEEE Personal Communications, 2*, 6–11. doi:10.1109/MPC.1994.298461

Stern, H. P., Mahmoud, S. A., & Wong, K. K. (1994). A Model for Generating On-Off Patterns in Conversational Speech, Including Short Silence Gaps and the Effects of Interaction between Parties. *IEEE Transactions on Vehicular Technology*, 1094–1100. doi:10.1109/25.330173

Stiliadis, D. & Varma, A. (1998, April). Rate-Proportional Servers: A Design Methodology Fair Queuing Algorithms. *IEEE/ ACM Trans. on Networking.*

Strassner, J. C. (2003). *Policybased network management.* San Francisco, CA: Morgan Kaufmann Publisher.

Subramanian, L., Agarwal, S., Rexford, J., & Katz, R. H. (2002). Characterizing the Internet Hierarchy from Multiple Vantage Points. In *Proc. of INFOCOM'02, 2*, (pp. 618-627), New York.

Subramanian, L., Caesar, M., Tien, C., Handley, M., Mao, M., Shenker, S., et al. (2005). HLP: a next generation inter-domain routing protocol. In *Proc. of SIGCOMM '05* (pp. 13-24). Philadelphia, PA: ACM Press.

Suri, S., Waldvogel, M., & Warkhede, P. R. (2001, September). ProfileBased Routing: A New Framework for MPLS traffic Engineering. In F. Boavida (Ed.), Quality of future internet services (Vol. 2156, pp. 138–157). Berlin: Springer Verlag.

Sycara, K., Dekker, K., Pannu, A., Williamson, M., & Zeng, D. (1996). Distributed Intelligent Agents. In IEEE Expert systems.

Szewczyk, R., Mainwaring, A., Polastre, J., & Culler, D. (2004). An Analysis of a Large Scale Habitat Monitoring Application. *ACM Conference on Embedded Networked Sensor Systems.*

Talwar, V., Nath, S. K., & Nahrstedt, K. (2001). RSVP-SQoS: A Secure RSVP Protocol. In *Proceedings of International Conference on Multimedia and Exposition* (pp.579-582).

Tanchotsrinon, W., & Bhattarakosol, P. (2008). Enhancing Services in Healthcare System using Overlapping Network Models. In *The 7th International Conference on e-Business*, (pp.128 – 134). Bangkok: Rangsit University Press.

Tang, P., & Charles, T. (1999). Network Traffic Characterization Using Token Bucket Model. In Proceedings of the Conference on Computer Communications (IEEE Infocom).

Tartarelli, S., Falkner, M., Devetsikiotis, M., Lambadaris, I., & Giordano, S. (2000). Empirical effective bandwidths. In *Proceedings of the IEEE Global Telecommunications Conference, 2000 (GLOBECOM '00), 1*, (pp. 672-678).

Teitelbaum, B. (1999). QBone Architecture (v1.0).

Teitelbaum, B., & Shalunov, S. (2002). *Why Premium IP Service Has Not Deployed.* Retrieved 01/12/2009 from http://qbone.internet2.edu/papers/non-architectural-problems.txt

Teixeira, R., Shaikh, A., Griffin, T. G., & Rexford, J. (2008, Dec.). Impact of HotPotato Routing Changes in IP Networks. *IEEE/ACM Transactions on Networking, 16*(6), 12951307.

Tentori, M., & Favela, J. (2008). Activity-Aware Computing for Healthcare. *IEEE Pervasive Computing / IEEE Computer Society [and] IEEE Communications Society, 7*(2), 51–57. doi:10.1109/MPRV.2008.24

TEQUILA. (2002). *TEQUILA: Traffic Engineering for Quality of Service in the Internet at Large Scale* (IST-1999-11253).

Thai, M. T., Wang, F., Du, H., & Jia, X. (2008). Coverage Problems in Wireless Sensor Networks: Designs and Analysis. *International Journal of Sensor Networks*, *3*(3), 191–200. doi:10.1504/IJSNET.2008.018482

The Internet Singularity, Delayed: Why Limits in Internet Capacity Will Stifle Innovation on the Web. (2007, November). Mokena, IL: Nemertes Research.

The Working Group for WLAN Standards. (1997). *Ieee 802.11tm Wireless Local Area Networks*. Retrieved from http://www.ieee802.org/11/

Tien, C., & Bajcsy, R. (2004). Congestion control and fairness for many-to-one routing in sensor networks. In *Proc. of 2nd International Conference on Embedded Networked Sensor Systems (SenSys), Baltimore, MD,* (pp. 148-161).

Tilak, S., Abu-Ghazaleh, N., & Heinzelman, W. (2002). A taxonomy of wireless micro-sensor network communication models. In ACM Mobile Computing and Communication Review(MC2R).

TISPAN. (2008, May). *Resource and Admission Control SubSystem (RACS): Functional Architecture*. ETSI ES 282 003 v2.0.0.

TMF, Telemanagement Forum (2005). SLA Management Book - Volume 2- Concepts and Principles (Vol. 2).

TMF. (2005). *Telemanagement Forum* (*Vol. 2*, p. 0). SLA Handbook Solution Suite.

TMF, Telemanagement Forum. (1999). *enhanced Telecom Operations Map (eTOM)*. Retrieved February 1st, 2009 from http://www.tmforum.org/BusinessProcessFramework/1647/home.html

Toh, C.-K. (2007). Future Application Scenarios for MANET-Based Intelligent Transportation Systems. In Future Generation Communications and Networking International Conference: (Vol. 2, pp. 414-417). Washington, DC: IEEE Computer Society Press.

Toh, C.-K. (2007). Future Application Scenarios for MANET-Based Intelligent Transportation Systems. In *Proceedings of Future Generation Communication and Networking (FGCN 2007),* (Vol.2, pp. 414-417).

Torab, P., Jabbari, B., Xu, Q., Gong, S., Yang, X., Lehman, T., et al. (2006). On Cooperative InterDomain Path Computation. In *ISCC '06: Proceedings of the 11th IEEE symposium on computers and communications* (pp. 511-518). Washington, DC: IEEE Computer Society.

Tripsas, M. (1997). Unraveling the process of creative destruction: Complementary assets and incumbent survival in teh typesetter industry. *Strategic Management Journal*, *18*(6), 119–142. doi:10.1002/(SICI)1097-0266(199707)18:1+<119::AID-SMJ921>3.3.CO;2-S

Troubleyn, E., Poorter, E., Moerman, I., & Demeester, P. (2008). AMoQoSA: Adaptive Modular QoS Architecture for Wireless Sensor Networks. In *2nd IEEE International Conference on Sensor Technologies and Applications (SENSORCOMM 2008)*, (pp. 172 – 178), Cap Esterel, France.

Tsybakov, B. S., & Mikhailov, V. A. (1979). Ergodicity of Slotted ALOHA System. *Probability. Peredachi Information*, *15*, 73–87.

Tushman, M. L., & Anderson, P. (1986). Technological discontinuities and organizational environments. *Administrative Science Quarterly*, *31*, 439–465. doi:10.2307/2392832

Tzamaloukas, A., & Garcia-Luna-Aceves, J. J. (2001). A Receiver-Initiated Collision-Avoidance Protocol for Multi-Channel Networks. IEEE INFOCOM, Twentieth Annual Joint Conference of the IEEE Computer and Communications Societies, (Vol.1, pp. 189-198).

Ulrich, D., & Barney, J. (1984). Perspectives in organizations: Resource dependence, eficiency, and population. *The Academy of Management Review*, *9*(3), 471–481. doi:10.2307/258287

Van Mieghem, P., De Neve, H., & Kuipers, F. A. (2001). Hop-by-hop Quality of Service Routing. *Computer Networks*, *37*(3-4), 407–423. doi:10.1016/S1389-1286(01)00222-5

Varga, P., Kún, G., Sey, G., Moldován, I., & Gelencsér, P. (2006). Experimenting with QoE. In *Autonomic Principles of IP Operations and Management* (pp. 218–221). Correlating User Perception and Measurable Network Properties. doi:10.1007/11908852_19

Varshney, U. (2006).Transmission of Emergency Messages in Wireless Patient Monitoring: Routing and Performance Evaluation. In *The 39th Annual Hawaii International Conference on System Sciences,* (pp.91a). Manoa, HI: University of Hawaii.

Vasseur, J. P. & Le Roux, J. L. (2009, March). *Path Computation Element (PCE) Communication Protocol (PCEP).* RFC 5440, IETF.

Vasseur, J. P., Zhang, R., Bitar, N., & Le Roux, J. L. (2009, April). *A Backward Recursive PCE-based Computation (BRPC) Procedure to Compute Shortest Constrained Interdomain traffic Engineering Label Switched Paths.* RFC 5441, IETF.

Vasseur, J., Ayyangar, A., & Zhang, R. (2008, February). *A PerDomain Path Computation Method for Establishing InterDomain traffic Engineering (TE) Label Switched Paths (LSPs).* RFC 5152. IETF.

Vázquez, E., Álvarez-Campana, M., & García, A. B. (2004). Network Convergence over MPLS. In *High Speed Networks and Multimedia Communications* (*Vol. 3079*, pp. 290–300). Berlin: Springer Verlag.

Veciana, G., Courcoubetis, C., & Walrand, J. (1994). Decoupling bandwidths for networks: a decomposition approach to resource management. In *Proceedings of the Thirteenth Annual Joint Conference of the IEEE Computer and Communications Societies (INFOCOM '94), 2,* (pp. 466-473).

Veciana, G., Kesidis, G., & Walrand, J. (1995). Resource management in wide-area ATM networks using effective bandwidths. *IEEE Journal on Selected Areas in Communications, 13*(6), 1081–1090. doi:10.1109/49.400663

Vidhyapriya R. & Vanathi, P. T. (2007). Energy Efficient Adaptive Multipath Routing for Wireless Sensor Networks. *International Journal of Computer Science.*

Vieira, F. H. T., & Lee, L. L. (2006). Queueing analysis for multifractal traffic through network calculus and global scaling parameter. In *Proceedings of the IEEE International Telecommunications Symposium, 2006 (ITS 2006),* (pp. 181-186).

Vieira, F. H. T., & Ling, L. L. (2006). Performance bounds for a cascade based multifractal traffic model with generalized multiplier distributions. *Journal of Communication and Information Systems, 21,* 1.

Vieira, F. H. T., & Ling, L. L. (2007). Limitantes de Desempenho de Fila para Tráfego Multifractal de Redes. *INFOCOMP - Journal of Computer Science, 6*(4), 100-110.

Vieira, F. H. T., & Ling, L. L. (2009). Adaptive Wavelet Based Multifractal Model Applied to the Effective Bandwidth Estimation of Network Traffic Flows. *IET Communications, 3*(6), 906–919. doi:10.1049/iet-com.2008.0078

Vieira, F. H. T., Bianchi, G. R., & Ling, L. L. (2008). A Network Traffic Prediction Approach Based on Multifractal Modeling. *Journal of High Speed Networks.*

Vieira, F. H. T., Garcez, S. G., & Miranda, W. F. (2008). Uma Abordagem para Estimação de Probabilidade de Perda em Redes Através da Teoria de Muitas Fontes e Modelagem Multifractal de Tráfego. In *7th International Information and Telecommunication Technologies Symposium (I2TS 2008).*

Vieira, F. H. T., Lee, L. L., & Jorge, C. (2008). An improved GPS scheduling discipline based on multifractal traffic characteristics. In *Proceedings of the IEEE/IFIP Network Operations and Management Symposium, 2008 (NOMS 2008),* (pp. 987-990).

VIOLA project - Vertically Integrated Optical Testbed for Large Applications in DFN. (n.d.). Retrieved from http://www.viola-testbed.de/

Vladimirova, T., Wu, X., & Bridges, C. P. (2008). Development of a Satellite Sensor Network for Future Space Missions. IEEE Aerospace Conference (pp.1 – 10).

Vuran, M. C. & Akyildiz, I. F. (2006). Spatial Correlation-based Collaborative Medium Access Control in Wireless Sensor Networks. *IEEE/ACM Transactions on Networking, 14*(2), 316-329.

Vuran, M. C., Gungor, V. B., & Akan, O. B. (2005). On the interdependency of congestion and contention in wireless sensor networks. In *Proc. of SENMETRICS'05.*

Wang, C., Daneshmand, M., Li, B. & Sohraby, K., (2006). A survey of transport protocols for wireless sensor networks. *IEEE Journal of Network.*

Wang, C., Li, B., Sohraby, K., Daneshmand, M., & Hu, Y. (2007). Upstream congestion control in wireless sensor networks through cross-layer optimization. *IEEE Journal on Selected Areas in Communications, 25*(4), 786–795. doi:10.1109/JSAC.2007.070514

Wang, J. Z. (1993). A Fully Distributed Location Registration Strategy for Universal Personal Communication Systems. *IEEE Journal on Selected Areas in Communications, 11*(6), 850–860. doi:10.1109/49.232294

Wang, N., Ho, K., Pavlou, G., & Howarth, M. (2008). First Quarter). An overview of routing optimization for Internet traffic engineering. *IEEE Communications Surveys and Tutorials, 10*(1), 3656. doi:10.1109/COMST.2008.4483669

Wang, Y., Liu, X., & Yin, J. (2006). Requirements of Quality of Service in Wireless Sensor Networks. In *Proceedings of the International Conference on Networking, International Conference on Systems an International Conference on Mobile Communications and Learning Technologies (ICNICONSMCL'06).*

Wang, Y., Tsai, C., & Mao, H. (2006). HMRP: Hierarchy-Based Multipath Routing Protocol for Wireless Sensor Networks. *Journal of Science and Engineering, 9*(3), 255–264.

Wang, Z. (2001). *Internet QoS: Architectures and Mechanisms for Quality of Service.* San Mateo, CA: Morgan Kaufmann Publishers.

Waxman, B. (1988). Routing of multipoint connections. *IEEE Journal on Selected Areas in Communications, 6*(9), 1617–1622. doi:10.1109/49.12889

Weisser, M.-A., & Tomasik, J. (2006). A distributed algorithm for inter-domain resources provisioning. In *Proc. of Second EuroNGI Conference*, (pp. 9-16), Valencia, Spain.

Weisser, M.-A., & Tomasik, J. (2007). Automatic induction of inter-domain hierarchy in randomly generated network topologies. In *Proc. of CNS'07* (pp. 77-84), Norfolk, VA. Retrieved from http://wwwsi.supelec.fr/~weisser/

Weisser, M.-A., & Tomasik, J. (2007). *Innapproximation proofs for directed Steiner tree and network problems. PRiSM Laboratory, University of Versailles Saint Quentin.* UVSQ.

Weisser, M.-A., Tomasik, J., & Barth, D. (2008). Congestion avoiding mechanism based on inter-domain hierarchy. IFIP Networking. (LNCS 4982, pp. 470-481). Singapore: Springer.

White, H. (1989). Some Asymptotic Results for Learning in Single Hidden-Layer Feedforward Network Models. *Journal of the American Statistical Association, 84*, 1003–1013. doi:10.2307/2290076

White, P. P. (1997). RSVP and Integrated Services in the Internet: A Tutorial. *IEEE Communications Magazine*, 100–106. doi:10.1109/35.592102

Willinger, W., Taqqu, M. S., & Erramilli, A. (1996). A bibliographical guide to self-similar traffic and performance modeling for modern high-speed networks. In Kelly, F. P., Zachary, S., & Ziedins, I. (Eds.), *Stochastic Networks: Theory and Applications* (*Vol. 4*, pp. 339–366). Oxford, UK: Oxford University Press.

Willinger, W., Taqqu, M.S., Sherman, R. & Wilson, D.V. (1997). Self-similarity through high Variability: Statistical analysis of Ethernet LAN traffic at the source level. *IEEE/ACM transaction on networking, 5*, 71-86.

Winters, J. H. (1993). Signal Acquisition and Tracking with Adaptive Arrays in the Digital Mobile Radio System IS-54 with Flat Fading. *IEEE Transactions on Vehicular Technology, 42*(4), 377–380. doi:10.1109/25.260776

Wischik, D. J. (1999). The output of a switch, or, effective bandwidths for networks. *Queueing Systems, 32*(4), 383–396. doi:10.1023/A:1019107708752

Wolff, R. S., Dunkle, D., Nugent, P., & Overcast, M. (2005, July). Ad-hoc Networking in Rugged and Remote Areas: Intermittently Connected Networking. Paper presented at the 17th International Conference on Wireless Communications, Calgary, Canada.

Woodruff, G., & Kositpaiboon, R. (1990). *Multimedia Traffic Management Principles for Guaranteed ATM Network Performance*. IEEE Journal on Selected Areas in Communications.

Wroclawski, J. (1997). Specification of the Controlled-load Network Element Service. In Internet Engineering Task Force Request for Comment – IETF RFC 2211.

Wu, J., Campbell, S., Savoie, J. M., Zhang, H., Bochmann, G. v., & St.Arnaud, B. (2003, Sept. 7-11). User-managed end-to-end lightpath provisioning over CA*net 4. In *Proceedings of the National Fiber Optic Engineers Conference (NFOEC)*, Orlando, FL, (pp. 275-282).

Wu, T., Wu, S. F., Fu, Z., Huang, H., & Gong, F. (1999). Securing QoS: Threats to RSVP Messages and Their Countermeasures. In *Proceedings of the Seventh International Workshop on Quality of Service* (pp. 62-64).

Xia, F. (2008). QoS Challenges and Opportunities in Wireless Sensor/Actuator Networks. *Sensors, 8*(2), 1099–1110. doi:10.3390/s8021099

Xiao, J., & Boutaba, R. (2007). Assessing Network Service Profitability: Modeling From Market Science Perspective. *IEEE/ACM Transactions on Networking, 15*(6), 1307-1320.

Xiao, J., Boutaba, R., & Aib, I. (2008). *CyberPlanner: A comprehensive toolkit for network service providers.* Paper presented at the Network Operations and Management Symposium, 2008. NOMS 2008 Salvador, Bahia.

Xiao, L., Lui, K. S., Wang, J., & Nahrstedt, K. (2002). QoS extension to BGP. In *Proc. of ICNP '02*, (pp. 100-109), Paris, France.

Xiao, X., & Ni, L. M. (1999). Internet QoS: a big picture. *IEEE Network, 13*(2), 8–18. doi:10.1109/65.768484

Xiao,V., Ni, L.M., (1999). Internet QoS: The Big Picture. *IEEE Network Magazine (*March/April), 8-18.

Yaghmaee, M. H., Menhaj, M. B., & Amintoosi, H. (2005). Design and performance evaluation of a fuzzy based traffic conditioner for differentiated services. *Journal on Computer Networks, Elsevier, 47*(6), 847–869. doi:10.1016/j.comnet.2004.09.003

Yang, G., Cao, Y., Chen, J., Tenhunen, H., & Zheng, L. R. (2008). An Active-Cable Connected ECG Monitoring System for Ubiquitous Healthcare. In *The Third International Conference on Convergence and Hybrid Information Technology*, (pp. 392-397). Busan, Korea: IEEE Computer Society.

Yang, X., Clark, D. & Berger, A. W. (2007). NIRA: a new interdomain routing architecture. *IEEE/ACM Transactions on Networking, 15*(4), 775-788.

Yangfan, Z., Micheal, R. L., Jiangchuan, L., & Hui, W. (2005). PORT: A price-oriented reliable transport protocol for wireless sensor networks. In *Proc. of 16th IEEE International Symposium on Software Reliability Engineering (ISSRE),* (pp. 117-126).

Yates, D. J., Nahum, E. M., Kurose, J. F., & Shenoy, P. (2008). Data quality and query cost in pervasive sensing systems. *Pervasive and Mobile Computing, 4*(6), 851–870. doi:10.1016/j.pmcj.2008.09.003

Yau, C. L., & Chung, W. Y. (2007). IEEE 802.15.4 Wireless Mobile Application for Healthcare System. In *The 2007 International Conference on Convergence Information Technology*, (pp.1433-1438). Gyeongju, Korea: IEEE Computer Society.

Ye W., Heidemann, J. & Estrin, D. (2004). Medium Access Control with Coordinated Adaptive Sleeping for Wireless Sensor Networks. *IEEE/ACM Transaction on Network, 12*(3), 493-506.

Yessad, S., Abdesselam, F. N., Taleb, T., & Bensaou, B. (2007). R-MAC: Reservation Medium Access Control Protocol for Wireless Sensor Networks. In *Proc. of*

32nd IEEE Conference on Local Computer Networks, (pp. 719-724.)

Yoon, S., & Shahabi, C. (2005). Exploiting Spatial Correlation Towards an Energy Efficient Clustered AGgregation Technique (CAG). In *Proc. of ICC'05.*

Younis, O., & Fahmy, S. (2003). ConstraintBased Routing in the Internet: Basic Principles and Recent Research. *IEEE Communications Surveys and Tutorials, 5,* 2–13. doi:10.1109/COMST.2003.5342226

Younis, S., & Fahmy, O. (2004). HEED: A Hybrid, Energy-Efficient, Distributed Clustering Approach for Ad Hoc Sensor Networks. *IEEE Transactions on Mobile Computing, 3*(4). doi:10.1109/TMC.2004.41

Yu, M., Mokhtar, H., & Merabti, M. (2007). A Survey on Fault Management in Wireless Sensor Networks. In *Proc. of 8th Annual Postgraduate Symposium.*

Zhang, C. G., Hafez, H. M., & Falconer, D. (1994). Traffic Handling Capacity of Broadband Indoor Network Using CDMA Multiple Access. *IEEE JSAC, 12*(12), 645–652.

Zhang, G., & Mouftah, H. T. (2001). End-to-end QoS guarantees over Diffserv networks. In *Proceedings of the Sixth IEEE Symposium on Computers and Communications,* (pp. 302-309).

Zhang, R. & Vasseur, J.P. (2005, November). *MPLS InterAutonomous System (AS) traffic Engineering (TE) Requirements.* RFC 4216. IETF.

Zhao, L., Xu, C., Xu, Y., & Li, X. (2006). Energy-Aware QoS Control for Wireless Sensor Network. In *1st IEEE Conference on Industrial Electronics and Applications (ICIEA 2006),* 1–6.

Zhu, H., Li, M., Chlamtac, I., & Prabhakaran, B. (2004). A Survey of Quality of Service in IEEE 802.11 Networks. *IEEE Wireless Communications, 11*(4), 6–14. doi:10.1109/MWC.2004.1325887

Zhu, Y., Keoh, S. L., Sloman, M., Lupu, E., Dulay, N., & Pryce, N. (2008). An Efficient Policy System for Body Sensor Networks. In *14th IEEE International Conference on Parallel and Distributed Systems.* (pp. 383, 390). Melbourne, Australia: IEEE Computer Society.

Zook, C., & Allen, J. (2001). *Profit from the core.* Boston: Harvard Business School.

Zorzi, M., & Rao, R. (2003). Geographic random forwarding (GeRaF) for ad hoc and sensor networks: multihop performance. *IEEE Transactions on Mobile Computing, 2*(4), 337–348. doi:10.1109/TMC.2003.1255648

Zouridaki, C., Hejmo, M., Mark, B. L., Thomas, R. K., & Gaj, K. (2005). Analysis of Attacks and Defense Mechanisms for QoS Signaling Protocols in MANETs. In Proceedings of Wireless Information Systems (WIS) Workshop, 2005, (pp.61–70).

About the Contributors

Pattarasinee Bhattarakosol is an Assistant Professor in the Computer Science Program, Department of Mathematics, Faculty of Science, Chulalongkorn University, Thailand. She graduated from Wollongong University since 1996. Her interested area is in the computer network and software engineering. Her main research is focusing on the quality of services over networks. Currently, she has many international publications both journal and proceedings.

* * *

Rehab Alnemr is a PhD student at Hasso-Plattner Institute. She is a graduate of faculty of Computers & Information, Information Technology department,Cairo University in Egypt. On 2006, she has her master degree in the field of security for mobile networks. Since 2007, she is a member of the associated Service-oriented Research School in Hasso-Plattner Institute. Her research interests are in the area of security, mobile networks, Internet technologies and trust management. Her PhD topic is focusing on reputation management systems and the use of service oriented architecture and quality processes to enhance them.

Dominique Barth defended a PhD thesis in Computer Science (1994) at the University of Bordeaux and defended a HDR (Habilitation à Diriger des Recherches) (1999) at the University Paris-Sud. He was an assistant professor at the University Paris-Sud in Orsay between 1994 and 1999, and starting from 1999 has been a professor in the PRiSM laboratory at the University of Versailles St Quentin. He created and led the Algorithmic, Combinatoric and Application team of PRiSM. His main research interests concern graph theory and graph algorithms applied to many research domains, notably telecommunication network and computational biology. In the field of telecommunication networks, his work focuses on QoS routing and multicast. He is and has been a leader of his team in many European and national research projects.

Gilles Bertrand received his M.Sc. degree in telecommunications engineering from Telecom SudParis, Evry, France and a Dipl-Ing. degree in electrical engineering from the University of Stuttgart, Germany in 2006. Since 2006, he has been working toward the Ph.D. degree in computer science at the Network, Multimedia, and Security department of Telecom Bretagne, Rennes, France. In the scope of his research, he is involved in the French project NextTV4all, which designs new audiovisual interactive services (IPTV) for fixed and mobile networks based on the IP Multimedia Sub-system (IMS). In the past, he has been involved, to various degrees, in the project VoD@IMS and the European networks of excellence (NoE) EuroNGI, EuroFGI, and EuroNF. His current research interests include convergent networks, methods for end-to-end quality of service, inter-domain traffic engineering in the Path Computation Element (PCE) framework, and various optimization problems.

Christos Bouras obtained his Diploma and PhD from the Computer Science and Engineering Department of Patras University (Greece). He is currently a Professor in the above department. He is also a scientific advisor of Research Unit 6 in Research Academic Computer Technology Institute (CTI), Patras, Greece. His research interests include Analysis of Performance of Networking and Computer Systems, Computer Networks and Protocols, Telematics and New Services, QoS and Pricing for Networks and Services, e – learning, Networked Virtual Environments and WWW Issues. He has extended professional experience in Design and Analysis of Networks, Protocols, Telematics and New Services. He has published 300 papers in various well-known refereed conferences and journals. He is a co-author of 8 books in Greek. He has been a PC member and referee in various international journals and conferences.

George Emmanuel Bozinis recieved his B.Sc., M.Sc. and Ph.D degrees in Electrical Engineering from the State University of Campinas (UNICAMP) in 1994, 1998 and 2007, respectively. Participated as the project coordinator from 2004 to 2008 at Innovatech Telecom in the research and development of a 2nd generation GSM femto-cell, funded by grants from the State of Sao Paulo Research Foundation (FAPESP). Currently holds a post-doctoral Scientific Regional Development (DCR) position at the Federal University of Goias (UFG) funded by grants from the National Council for Research (CNPq) and the State of Goias Research Support Foundation (FAPEG). E-mail: bozinis@gmail.com

Justus Bross, M.Sc. & MBE, 1979, is a doctoral candidate of the chair "Internet Technologies and Systems" at the Hasso-Plattner Institute in Potsdam. His area of research lies within the field of collaborative working and discussion platforms (weblogs). He graduated in International Business studies at the University of Maastricht in the Netherlands, earned the master's degree of Business and Engineering at the German Steinbeis Association and the D.E.L.E degree at the University of Salamanca in Spain. He has several publications in the research area of the collaborative and social web with a focus on the global blogosphere.

Anthony T. Burrell received the B.A. degree in Computer Science from the University of California at Santa Barbara, California, in 1982, the M.S. degree in Computer Science from West Coast University, Los Angeles, California, in 1986, and the Ph.D. degree in Computer Science in August 1994, from the University of Virginia, Charlottesville, Virginia. From 1982 to 1988, he worked as systems analyst and programmer at various companies including Unisys Corporation and William O'Neil & Company. Concurrently, he joined the faculty at West Coast University as an instructor, teaching graduate level computer science courses. In January 1994, he was employed as a research associate at the University of Ottawa, Canada, performing research in high-speed networks. From September 1994 to August 1999 he was faculty at the department of electrical & computer engineering at the University of Alabama in Tuscaloosa. In August of 1999, he joined the Computer Science department at Oklahoma State University in Stillwater, Oklahoma. Dr. Burrell's research interests include operating systems, artificial intelligence, and high-speed computer-communication networks, with special emphasis on ATM in the Broadband Integrated Services Digital Network environment.

Abd El-Kader has her M.Sc., & Ph.D. degrees from the Electronics & Communications Dept. & Computers Dept., Faculty of Engineering, Cairo University, at 1998, & 2003. Dr. Abd El-kader is an Associate Prof., Computers & Systems Dept., at the Electronics Research Institute (ERI). She is currently supervising 3 Ph.D. student, and 8 M.Sc. students. Dr. Abd El-kader has published more than 15 papers in computer networking area. She is working in many computer networking hot topics such as; Wi-MAX, Wi-Fi, IP Mobility, QoS, Wireless sensors Networks, Ad-Hoc Networking, real-time traffics, Bluetooth, and IPv6. She is an Associate Prof., at Faculty of Engineering, Akhbar El Yom Academy from 2007 till now. Also she is a technical reviewer for many international Journals. She is heading the Internet and Networking unit at ERI from 2003 till now. She is supervising many automation and web projects for ERI. She is supervising many Graduation Projects from 2006 till now. She is also a technical member at both the ERI projects committee and at the telecommunication networks committee, Egyptian Organization for Standardization & Quality since February 2007 till now. Finally, Dr. Abd El-kader is the main researcher at two US-EG joint funded projects with University of California at Irvine, CA, USA since 2001.

El-Bahlul Fgee is a Lecturer at the Academy of Graduate Studies, School of Applied Science and Engineering, Department of Computer Engineering and Information Technology, Tripoli-Libya. He earned his BSc in 1986 from the Department of Electrical and Computer Engineering at AlFateh University, Tripoli, Libya. He earned his Master's degree in 1999 from the Department of Electrical and Computer Engineering, and PhD in 2005 from the Department Internetworking and Engineering Mathematics at Dalhousie University, Halifax, Canada. His research interests are Internet Quality of Service, Sensor Networks, Networks security and management.

Apostolos Gkamas obtained his Diploma, Master Degree and Ph.D from the Computer Engineering and Informatics Department of Patras University (Greece). He is currently an R&D Computer Engineer at the Research Unit 6 of the Research Academic Computer Technology Institute, Patras, Greece. He is also teaching at the Hellenic Open University in the Informatics Curriculum. His research interests include Computer Networks, Telematics, Distributed Systems, Multimedia and Hypermedia. More particular he is engaged in transmission of multimedia data over networks and multicast congestion control. He has published more than 60 papers in international Journals and well-known refereed conferences. He is also co-author of three books (one with subject Multimedia and Computer Networks one with subject Special Network Issues and one with subject IPv6). He has participated in R&D projects such as IST, eLearning, PENED, EPEAEK, Information Society.

Wayne Goodridge earned his Bachelors and Master degrees at the University of the West Indies, Cave Hill, Barbados. He graduated from Dalhousie University in 2005 with a PhD in Internetworking and Engineering Mathematics. He is currently a Lecturer at the University of the West Indies St. Augustine, Trinidad. His main goal is to convert concepts into useful products for use in business. His research and business interests are student management systems, decision support systems, case based reasoning, medical applications, IP traffic engineering, song finger printing algorithms and the time tabling problem.

Sunyoung Han is the Dean and Professor at College of Information & Telecommunications, Konkuk University, Hwayangdong Kwangjinku, Seoul, Korea. He is a specialist in the area of computer network and has many publications related to Internet, Mobile IP, Multicasting, Wireless/Mobile Networks, Future Internet, Distributed Systems, including Web Services.

Faisal Bashir Hussain received his MS in computer science degree from department of computer science, International Islamic University Pakistan and PhD from department of computer engineering, Dokuz Eylul University, Izmir Turkey in 2008 as a cultural exchange scholar. He is currently working as Assistant Professor at department of Computer Science, Military College of Signals, a constituent college of National University of Sciences & Technology (NUST). His research interests mainly include wireless sensor networks, next generation networks.

Eva Ibarrola received the B.S. and M.S. degrees in Telecommunications Engineering from the University of the Basque Country, Spain, in 1991. She is currently a lecturer at the Faculty of Engineering in Bilbao. She was previously working in the CNSO (National Centre for Supervision and Operations) of Telefónica from 1991-2000. Her research interests focus mainly on user's oriented Quality of Service (QoS) management models and frameworks. She has been cooperating in different R&D projects related with telecommunications QoS evaluation and measurement. Currently, she is working on her PhD thesis in the area of QoS deployment methodologies.

Jadwiga Indulska is a Professor in the School of Information Technology and Electrical Engineering at The University of Queensland. Her research interests include pervasive/ubiquitous computing, wireless networks, autonomic networks and mobile computing. In the past she led projects on mobile and pervasive computing in the Collaborative Research Centre on Distributed Systems Technology and currently she is a Research Leader in National ICT Australia (NICTA). She is a member of the IEEE Computer Society and the ACM.

Vikas Jain is currently working at Philips, Bangalore. He has about 14 years of software development experience in the area of UI/Application, User Experience, DLNA/UPnP, DRM development, know-how generation and architecting solutions for resource constrained embedded platforms. His areas of interests include User Experience, content management, connectivity etc.

Samer Lahoud was graduated at the Faculty of Engineering, Saint Joseph University, Beirut, in 2002. In 2006, he received the Ph.D degree in computer science from Telecom Bretagne, Rennes. After his Ph.D. he spent one year with Alcatel-Lucent Bell Labs Europe working as a research engineer. Since 2007, he has been with the University of Rennes I, where he is working as assistant professor, and with IRISA of Rennes, where he is taking part in the research activities. His main research activity is in network design, combinatorial optimization and engineering algorithms for communication networks. His research results are mainly from the following domains: fast polynomial approximation for combinatorial problems, routing algorithms for traffic engineering and survivability design. He has been involved in many research programs at the national and the European level.

Lina Maria Pestana Leão de Brito holds a degree in Systems and Computing Engineering from the University of Madeira (1999), Portugal, and an MSc. degree in Electronic and Telecommunications Engineering from the University of Aveiro (2004), Portugal. Since 2006, she is a PhD candidate in the Mathematics and Engineering Department at University of Madeira, in Distributed Systems and Networks. She is a teaching assistant at the University of Madeira since 1999. Her research interests cover the areas of wireless sensor networks, wireless networks, CSCW and Quality of Service.

Fidel Liberal received the B.S. and M.S. degrees in Telecommunications Engineering from the University of the Basque Country, Spain, in 2001. In 2005 he received the Ph.D. in Telecommunications Engineering from the same University for his work in the area of holistic management of quality (both NQoS and PQoS-QoE) in telecommunications services. He currently works as a lecturer in the Faculty of Engineering in Bilbao and cooperates in different National and International R&D projects. He has large experience in the management of national R&D projects and his research interests include objective/subjective evaluation of the perceived quality of multimedia.

Shivanajay Marwaha is pursuing his PhD at The University of Queensland, School of Information Technology and Electrical Engineering and National ICT Australia, Queensland Research Laboratory. His research interests are in Wireless Mesh Networks, Multimedia Networking and Computational Intelligence. He has numerous publications in the field of Computer Networks. He has previously worked with Panasonic and Motorola. He is a student member of IEEE, IEEE Communications Society and the Australian Computer Society.

Eduardo Miguel Dias Marques obtained his MSc. degree in Multimedia Technologies from University of Oporto, Portugal, in March 2005. He is currently a Ph.D. candidate in Informatics Engineering at University of Madeira, in Portugal. He is a teaching assistant at the University of Madeira since 2001. His research interests include Quality of Service and network simulation with emphasis in network simulation description languages and simulation interfaces.

Miklos Molnar was graduated at the Faculty of Electrical Engineering, Technical University of Budapest (Hungary) in 1976. He received the Ph.D. degree in computer science from the University of Rennes 1 (France) in 1992 and the "Habilitation à Diriger des Recherches" (HDR) scientific degree in France in 2008, respectively. Since 1989, he has been with the INSA of Rennes, where he is working as an associate professor in the Computer Science Department and also with the research laboratory IRISA of Rennes. His main results are from the stochastic control, combinatorial optimization and management algorithms for communication networks. His current research activity deals with efficient heuristics for NP-hard optimization problems, routing algorithms for unicast, in-cast and multicast communications in WDM and WLAN networks, dependable communications, energy aware protocols and optimizations. Miklos Molnar is coauthor of several papers about heuristic and exact solutions of hard optimization problems. He has been a session organizer and a member of the Program Committee of several international symposiums.

P. Papantoni-Kazakos received the Diploma in Electrical, Mechanical and Industrial Engineering from the National Technical University of Athens, Greece, in 1968; the M.S, degree from Princeton University, Princeton, NJ, in 1970; and the Ph.D. from the University of Southern California, Los Angeles, CA, in 1973, both in Electrical Engineering with specialization in Statistical Communications and with minor in Mathematics. Since 1973, she has been professor of Electrical Engineering at Rice University, Houston, Texas, at the University of Connecticut, Storrs, Connecticut, at the University of Virginia, Charlottesville, Virginia, at the University of Ottawa, Ottawa, Canada and at the University of Alabama, Tuscaloosa, Alabama. She is presently professor of Electrical Engineering at the University of Colorado Denver, Colorado. Her research interests include Statistical Decision Theory, Distributed Processing and Neural Network Structures, Statistical-Communications, Information Theory, Robust Statistical and Encoding Methods, Stochastic Processes, Computer-Communication Networks, Sensor Networks and organizational networks. She is coeditor and contributor to the book: Nonparametric Methods in Communications (New York, Marcel Dekker, 1977). She is also coauthor of the book: Detection and Estimation (Computer Science Press, 1989). In addition to these books, she has published over 225 refereed technical papers. Dr. Papantoni is a Fellow of IEEE; for "Contributions to Communication Networks and to Detection and Estimation Theory".

Laura Margarita Rodríguez Peralta is Assistant Professor at University of Madeira (Portugal) since 2004. She obtained her PhD degree on Informatics and Telecommunications from the Institut National Polytechnique de Toulouse (ENSEEIHT/INPT), France. Her PhD work was carried out at Laboratory of Analysis and Architecture of Systems from the CNRS (LAAS-CNRS) in Toulouse (France). She worked as a research fellow (post-doc) at the Institute of Mechanical Engineering of the State University of Campinas, with the collaboration of the research laboratory Centro de Pesquisas Renato Archer (CenPRA) in 2003-2004. She is a researcher in the Centro de Ciências Matemáticas (CCM) of the University of Madeira since 2004, and she is a faculty member of the M.Sc. Program in Human-Computer Interaction under the Carnegie Mellon University - Portugal Program since 2007. Among her research interests are the collaborative engineering (CSCW), groupware, web technologies, database, distributed systems, parallel systems, computer networks, collaborative wireless sensor networks and multimedia applications.

William Phillips is Professor and Head of the Department of Engineering Mathematics and Internetworking in the Faculty of Engineering at Dalhousie University. He holds a B.Sc. in Mathematics and Engineering from Queen's University, an M.Sc. in Mathematics, also from Queen's University, and a Ph.D. in Mathematics from the University of British Columbia. Dr. Phillips' research program is aimed at the development of algorithms and implementations for communication networks.

Marius Portmann is a Senior Lecturer at School of Information Technology and Electrical Engineering at The University of Queensland, and a Project Leader at National ICT Australia's Queensland Research Lab. His research interests include Pervasive Computing, Wireless Mesh Networks, P2P Computing and Network Security. He has a PhD in Electrical Engineering from the Swiss Federal Institute of Technology (ETH), Zurich. The main focus of his research currently is Wireless Mesh Networks technology for Public Safety, Emergency Response and Disaster Recovery situations. He is a member of IEEE.

Manjunath Ramachandra is currently working at Philips, Bangalore. He has about 14 years of industrial and academic experience in the overlapping verticals of Signal processing, including Wireless, mobile and data networking, Multimedia, information and supply chain management. Research in the same field led to PhD thesis, about 75 international publications, patent disclosures etc. He has chaired about 10 international conferences and Figures in Marquis Who's Who 2008. His areas of interests include Signal processing, database architecture, networking etc.

William Robertson earned his B.Sc (Hons., Eng) and his M.Sc. from Aberdeen University and his Ph.D. from the Technical University of Nova Scotia. Since 1985 he has held various professorial positions at the Technical University of Nova Scotia which was amalgamated in 1997 with Dalhousie University. His research has covered computer architecture, digital signal processing, neural networks, and network protocols. He has been the principal investigator in strategic and Canada Foundation for Innovation research projects. He was the Head of Electrical and Computer Engineering from 1994 to 1998 and has been the Director of the Internetworking Program at Dalhousie University since 1997. Current research interests are in the internetworking area include wireless sensor networks, and routing in optical based systems.

Paulo Nazareno Maia Sampaio is Assistant Professor at University of Madeira (Portugal), and he holds a PhD degree in Informatics and Telecommunications from University Paul Sabatier - Toulouse II. His PhD work was carried out at Laboratory of Analysis and Architecture of Systems (LAAS-CNRS) in Toulouse (France). He is a researcher in the Centro de Ciências Matemáticas (CCM) of the University of Madeira, and he is a faculty member of the M.Sc. Program in Human-Computer Interaction under the Carnegie Mellon University - Portugal Program. His research interests are: the project and development of distributed multimedia systems, web engineering, integration of multimedia content inside virtual and augmented reality environments and multimodal systems.

Ghalib Asadullah Shah is an Assistant Professor at Department of Computer Engineering, College of Electrical & Mechanical Engineering campus of National University of Sciences & Technology (NUST). He earned his MSc and PhD degrees from Department of Computer Science, Bahauddin Zakariya University Multan and Middle East Technical University Ankara Turkey respectively. He was awarded cultural exchange scholarship, a joint program by the ministries of education Pakistan and Turkey during 2002-2007. Recently, he is awarded a Post-Doc fellowship under French Embassy Sandwich PhD and Post-Doc Fellowship program in Science & technology to be carried at Universite BORDEAUX 1, France. His research mainly focus on mobile ad hoc networks, wireless sensor networks, wireless mesh networks.

Shyamala C. Sivakumar obtained her B.Eng (Electrical) from Bangalore University, India in 1984. She worked as a Design Engineer in the Avionics Design Bureau at Hindustan Aeronautics Limited, Bangalore, India until 1989. She obtained her M.A. Sc (Eng) and Ph.D from the Department of Electrical Engineering at the Technical University of Nova Scotia (now Dalhousie University), Canada in 1992 and 1997 respectively. She is currently an Associate Professor of Computing and Information Systems at the Sobey School of Business, Saint Mary's University, Halifax, NS. Her research interests include Quality of Service and pricing issues in wired and wireless networks, algorithms & energy efficient architectures for wireless sensor networks, applying internetworking technology for innovative applications in e-education, telemedicine and e-commerce.

Shaleeza Sohail received the BE degree in civil engineering from the University of Engineering, Taxila, Pakistan, in 1998 and the MS degree in computer engineering from the University of New South Wales, Sydney, Australia, in 2000. She completed her doctorate in computer science at the University of New South Wales, Sydney, Australia in 2005. She is currently with department of Computer Engineering, College of E & ME, National University of Sciences & Technology (NUST). Her current research interests include quality-of-service in computer networks and grid computing.

Ohm Sornil is an Assistant Professor at the Department of Computer Science, National Institute of Development Administration, Thailand. He holds a Ph.D. in Computer Science from Virginia Polytechnic Institute and State University (Virginia Tech), an M.S. in Computer Science from Syracuse University, an M.B.A. in Finance from Mahidol University, and a B.Eng. in Electrical Engineering from Kasetsart University. His main research interests include computer and network security, artificial intelligence, information retrieval, data mining, and related areas.

Kostas Stamos obtained his Diploma, Master Degree and Ph.D from the Computer Engineering and Informatics Department of Patras University (Greece). He has worked for the Networking Technologies Sector of CTI, Research Unit 6 of CTI and the Greek Research and Education Network (Grnet). He is also teaching at the Computer Engineering and Informatics Department at the University of Patras, and at the Technological Educational Institute of Patras. He has published 7 articles in Journals and 28 papers in well-known refereed conferences. He is also co-author of 2 technical books, several encyclopaedia articles and of a Global Grid Forum (GGF) standard document.

Watcharaporn Tanchotsrinon graduated from the Master Program in Computer Science and Information Technology in the year 2009. Her major area is the performance management in the computer network.

Géraldine Texier is an assistant professor of the Network, Multimedia and Security department at Telecom Bretagne, Rennes, France. She. received her PhD degree on the management of the cooperation and the awareness in computer supported collaborative work in 2000 from the University of Rennes 1 (France). She is involved in EuroNF and was previously contributing to EuroNGI and EuroFGI Networks of Excellence (NoE). Her current research fields are routing protocols in both Networks and Network on Chips with a focus on QoS management and routing optimization and especially in inter-domain context. She is participating to the national projects Afana on NoCs and NextTV4all on the study of IPTV on the IMS architecture.

Joanna Tomasik received her magisterium diplomas in applied mathematics and in computer science at the University of Technology in Gliwice, Poland, in 1988 and 1989, respectively. She obtained her PhD in 1989 from the same university. In 1988 she started to work at the Institute of Theoretical and Applied Computer Science of the Polish Academy of Sciences in Gliwice. She spent an academic year as a research fellow at the University of Edinburgh, the UK. She also worked in France at the University of Versailles and the National Institute of Telecommunications. Since 2002 Joanna Tomasik has worked permanently in France and she is a professor in the Computer Science Department of SUPELEC, one of the leading French engineering schools. Her main research domains concern performance of computer systems, and in particular of telecommunication networks, i.e. analytical methods, simulation, formalisms of compositional methods for generation of Markov chain matrices and algorithms for the QoS in the Internet.

Armando Ferro Vázquez graduated in 1987 from the Faculty of Engineering in Bilbao. He counts with 20 years of communications engineering experience. The first 10 years working in industrial companies. At first he participated in the national development of SPRITEL program that received an ESA-IRS European Information Technology Trophy awarded by European Information Industry Association in 1991. He also has participated in several European projects. Since 1997 he has been making researches in security systems and Quality of Service. He received Ph.D. degree in Communications Engineering (University of the Basque Country) in 2002. He was habilitated in 2004 and is an assistance professor since 2005. He has large experience in the management of national R&D projects and actually is a research responsible within a contract with European Commission monitoring CORDIS′ services. Currently he is involved in 7FP STREP project ADAMANTIUM (2008-2011).

Flavio Henrique Teles Vieira received his B.Sc. degree in Electrical Engineering from the Federal University of Goias (UFG) in 2000, the M.Sc. degree in Electrical and Computer Engineering from UFG in 2002 and the doctorate degree in Electrical and Computer Engineering at State University of Campinas (FEEC-UNICAMP) in 2006. Since 2008, he has been a Professor at the Federal University of Goias in Brazil. He acts in the following research areas: Network Traffic Modeling and Control and Communication Networks and Protocols. E-mail: flavio@eeec.ufg.br

Long Wang is currently a PhD student at the chair "Internet Technologies and Systems" of the Hasso-Plattner Institute in Potsdam since 2005. Before that, he got his master degree in computer science in 2002 from Beijing University of Technology. His research interest lies in data mining, information retrieval, e-learning and social media analysis. In recent years, he has published several papers on discovering and monitoring usage interest on information portal sites, e-learning environments and online social communities.

Marc-Antoine Weisser defended a PhD thesis in Computer Science (2007) at SUPELEC, one of the leading French engineering schools. He was a post-doctoral fellow in 2008 at the University of Versailles Saint Quentin and a member of Alcaap team (Algorithmic, Combinatoric and Application team of PRiSM laboratory). Since September 2008 he has been an assistant professor in Computer Science Department of SUPELEC. His main research interests concern the graph theory and graph algorithms applied to telecommunication networks. He mainly focuses on QoS routing and multicast in inter-domain networks as well as mobile networks in which related graph problems are variants of Steiner tree problems.

Index

U

V

W